13.14

DM 1/01

THE BRITISH
MEDICAL ASSOCIATION

NEW GUIDE TO

Medicines
& Drugs

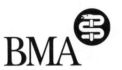

BMA
THE BRITISH
MEDICAL ASSOCIATION

NEW GUIDE TO

Medicines
& Drugs

Chief Medical Editor
Professor John A. Henry MB FRCP

St Mary's Hospital,
London

A DORLING KINDERSLEY BOOK

Dorling **DK** Kindersley

LONDON, NEW YORK, SYDNEY, DELHI, PARIS,
MUNICH AND JOHANNESBURG

BRITISH MEDICAL ASSOCIATION

Chairman of the Council Dr. Ian Bogle
Treasurer Dr. W.J. Appleyard
Chairman of the BMA Journal Committee Sir Anthony Grabham
Associate Editor, British Medical Journal Dr. Tony Smith

Chief Medical Editor Professor John A. Henry MB FRCP
Drug Information Reviewer Michael Rogers BPharm, MRPharmS, DipInfSc, MIInfSc
Contributors Stephanie Barnes, Principal Formulary Pharmacist; Margaret-Anne Faulds
Dip. Pharm (NZ), MRPharmS; Meera Gill BPharmS, MRPharmS, Dip. Clin (Lon) DMS (OU);
Susanna Gilmour-White BPharm, MRPharmS; David Hands BPharm; Sarah King BPharm
MRPharmS, DipClinPharm; Dr. Jeevan Kumaradeevan MRCP; Frank Leach PhD, MSc,
BPharm, MRPharmS; Caroline Nathan BPharm MRPharmS; Kathy Reed BPharm,
MRPharmS; Dr. K.S. Sandhu MA MRCP (UK); Dr. Brian Saunders MD MRCP; Karen J.
Sorensen SRD; Dr. Maxwell Summerhayes BPharm, PhD, MRPharmS; Dr. Frances Williams
MB BChir MRCP DTM&H

Dorling Kindersley would like to thank John Ramsey of St George's Hospital Toxicology
Unit, London, for supplying drugs for photography in the Colour Identification Guide; Dr. Susan
Davidson MB MRCP MRCGP; The Malaria Reference Laboratory; Sir Peter Beale KBE FRCP
FFCM FFOM DTM&H, Chief Medical Adviser, British Red Cross; Kay Wright, indexer.

DORLING KINDERSLEY LIMITED

FIFTH EDITION
Senior Editor Heather Jones
Project Editor Teresa Pritlove
Senior Managing Editor Martyn Page
Photography Steve Gorton
Illustrators Karen Cochrane, Richard Tibbitts

Senior Designer Louise Dick
Designer Corinne Manches
DTP Design Jason Little
Deputy Art Director Bryn Walls
Production Elizabeth Cherry

PREVIOUS EDITIONS
Senior Project Editor: Cathy Meeus; Editors: Jill Hamilton, Marian Broderick, Louise Clairmonte,
Deirdre Clark, Christiane Gunzi, Stephanie Jackson, Mary Lindsay, Teresa Pritlove, Terence
Monaighan, Penny Gray, David Bennett; Art Editors: Philip Ormerod, Chez Picthall, Clare Shedden,
Anne Renel; Designers: Nicola Hampel, Debra Lee, Gail Jones, Sandra Schneider, Christina Betts;
Illustrators: Karen Cochrane, Tony Graham, Kevin Marks, Coral Mula, Lynda Payne; Photography:
Steve Gorton. Dorling Kindersley would like to thank Dr. Sheila Bingham, Stephen and Nikki Carroll,
Peter Cooling, and Guy's Hospital Pharmacy.

First published in Great Britain in 1988
by Dorling Kindersley Limited,
9 Henrietta Street, London WC2E 8PS
First published in paperback 1989, reprinted 1990
Second edition 1991, reprinted 1992, 1993
Third edition 1994, reprinted 1995
Fourth edition 1997, reprinted 1998, 1999
Fifth edition 2001

A CIP catalogue record for this book is available from the British Library.

ISBN 0-751-327-379

Colour reproduction by IGS, Bath, England

Printed and bound in China by Sun Fung Offset Binding Company Limited.

See our complete catalogue at
www.dk.com

PREFACE

Doctors no longer hand out prescriptions without any explanation, and the days are long gone when pharmacists solemnly handed bottles labelled "the mixture" or "the tablets" to the patients and expected no questions. Most patients today are critical consumers; they want to know what drugs they are taking, the actions of these drugs, their side effects, and their possible risks.

However, information given by word of mouth at the end of a consultation may be difficult to remember. Researchers have shown that the most effective way of providing information about drugs is in the form of printed notes or data sheets. Although leaflets of this kind are generally available in Britain, many people want a deeper understanding about the drugs and medicines they take.

The main section of this book consists of structured information on 249 of the most widely used drugs, presented in a clear, easy-to-understand format. These drug profiles provide the essential information for the patient, including the effects of the drug, potential problem areas, and what to do if a dose is forgotten. But these basic facts are not enough for an understanding of how the drug works. The first and third sections of this book give a fuller account of the way drugs affect body systems and outline the actions of the main classes of drugs. The second section provides a comprehensive directory of drugs and brand names, and a colour identification guide to tablets, capsules, patches, and pens. Other sections include profiles of vitamins, minerals, drugs of abuse, and alternative medicine, as well as important considerations pertaining to sport and travel.

The British Medical Association NEW GUIDE TO MEDICINES AND DRUGS has been compiled by doctors and pharmacists familiar with the sorts of questions patients ask. The detailed, factual content has been checked and verified by specialists. The book is not intended to supersede the information given to the individual patient by his or her doctor. Choosing the most suitable drug and advising on use depends on the doctor's knowledge of your previous health and medical background.

This guide should, however, help patients and their families to understand more about the treatment they have been prescribed, it should alert them to early warning signs of adverse effects, and it should act as a ready reference source for information that might otherwise have been forgotten. We believe the book will improve relationships between patients and their doctors, and contribute to the effectiveness and safety of the drugs people take.

Dr. Tony Smith
Associate Editor
British Medical Journal

CONTENTS

4 A–Z OF DRUGS

5 GLOSSARY AND INDEX

INTRODUCTION

The British Medical Association New Guide to Medicines and Drugs has been planned and written to provide clear information and practical advice on drugs and medicines in a way that can be readily understood by a non-medical reader. The text reflects current medical knowledge and standard medical practice in this country. It is intended to complement and reinforce the advice of your doctor.

How the book is structured
The book is divided into five parts. The first part, Understanding and Using Drugs, provides a general introduction to the effects of drugs and gives general advice on practical questions, such as the administration and storage of drugs. The second part, the Drug Finder Index, provides the means of locating information on specific drugs through a colour identification guide and an index to over 2,500 generic and brand-name drugs. Part 3, Major Drug Groups, will help you understand the uses and mechanisms of action of the principal classes of drugs. Part 4, the A–Z of Drugs, consists of 249 detailed profiles of commonly prescribed generic drugs, profiles of vitamins, minerals, and drugs of abuse, and information on drugs in sport and travel. Part 5 contains a glossary of drug-related terms (italicized in the text) and a general index.

Finding your way into the book
The information you require, whether on the specific characteristics of an individual drug or on the general effects and uses of a group of drugs, can be easily obtained without prior knowledge of the medical names of drugs or drug classification through one of the two indexes: the Drug Finder or the General Index. The diagram on the facing page shows how you can obtain information throughout the book on the subject concerning you from each of these starting points.

1 UNDERSTANDING AND USING DRUGS

The introductory part of the book, Understanding and Using Drugs, gives a grounding in the fundamental principles underlying the medical use of drugs. Covering such topics as classifications of drugs, mechanisms of action, and the proper use of medicines, it provides valuable background information that backs up the more detailed descriptions and advice given in Parts 3 and 4. You should read this section before seeking further specific information.

2 DRUG FINDER INDEX

This is composed of two elements. The Colour Identification Guide contains photographs of over 240 brand-name drug products to help you identify medications. The Drug Finder helps you to find information on specific brand-name drugs and generic substances.

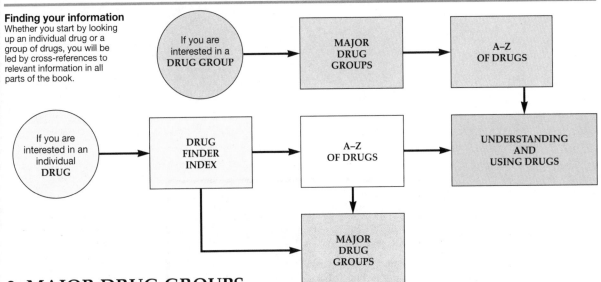

Finding your information
Whether you start by looking up an individual drug or a group of drugs, you will be led by cross-references to relevant information in all parts of the book.

If you are interested in a **DRUG GROUP**

MAJOR DRUG GROUPS

A–Z OF DRUGS

If you are interested in an individual **DRUG**

DRUG FINDER INDEX

A–Z OF DRUGS

UNDERSTANDING AND USING DRUGS

MAJOR DRUG GROUPS

3 MAJOR DRUG GROUPS

Subdivided into sections dealing with each body system (for example, heart and circulation) or major disease grouping (for example, malignant and immune disease), this part of the book contains descriptions of the principal classes of drugs. Information is given on the uses, actions, effects, and risks associated with each group of drugs and is backed up by helpful illustrations and diagrams. Individual drugs in each group are listed to allow cross-reference to Part 4.

4 A–Z OF DRUGS

This part contains profiles of 249 generic drugs, written to a standard format to help you find specific information quickly and easily; cross-references to the relevant major drug groups are provided. Supplementary sections profile vitamins and minerals, drugs of abuse, alternative medicine, and drugs in sport and travel.

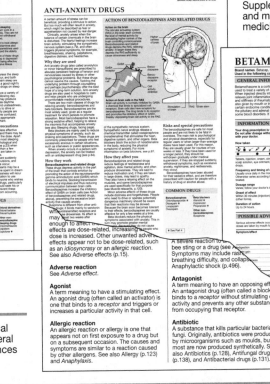

5 GLOSSARY AND INDEX

A glossary of terms explains technical words italicized in the text. The general index enables you to look up references throughout the book.

Adverse reaction
See *Adverse effect*.

Agonist
A term meaning to have a stimulating effect. An agonist drug (often called an activator) is one that binds to a *receptor* and triggers or increases a particular activity at that cell.

Allergic reaction
An allergic reaction or allergy is one that appears not on first exposure to a drug but on a subsequent occasion. The causes and symptoms are similar to a reaction caused by other allergens. See also *Allergy* (p.123) and *Anaphylaxis*.

Antagonist
A term meaning to have an opposing effect. An antagonist drug (often called a blocker) binds to a *receptor* without stimulating cell activity and prevents any other substance from occupying that receptor.

Antibiotic
A substance that kills particular bacteria or fungi. Originally, antibiotics were produced by microorganisms such as moulds, but most are now produced synthetically. See also *Antibiotics* (p.128), *Antifungal drugs* (p.138), and *Antibacterial drugs* (p.131).

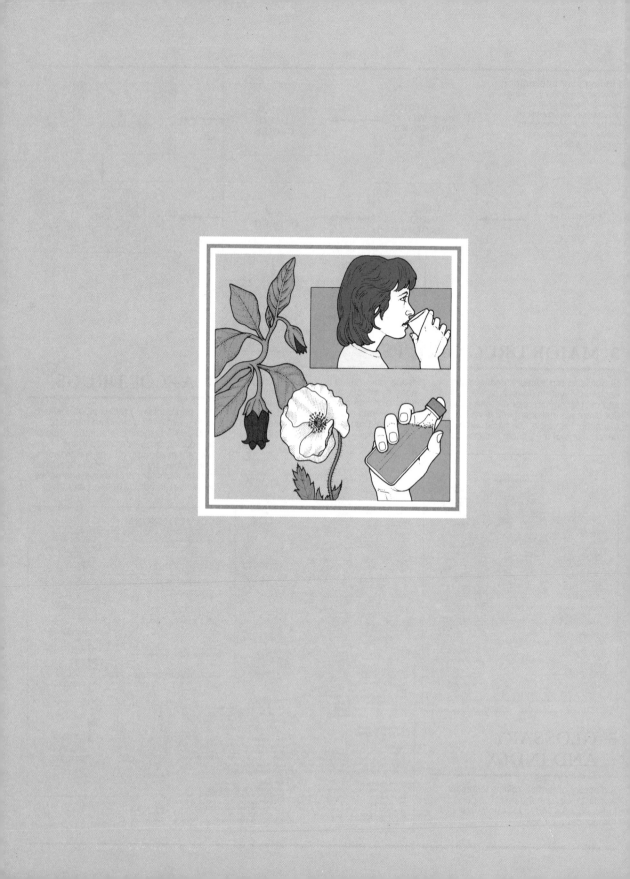

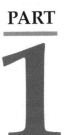

PART 1

UNDERSTANDING AND USING DRUGS

WHAT ARE DRUGS?

The medical and nursing professions use the word "drugs" to refer to medicines – substances that can cure or arrest disease, relieve symptoms, ease pain, and provide other benefits. This definition includes essential vitamins and minerals that may be given to correct deficiency diseases.

Powerful drugs often have marked *adverse effects*. Commonly used drugs with less potential to cause harm are sold over the counter in pharmacies and supermarkets. More powerful drugs (those that the Medicines Commission has ruled cannot be used safely without medical supervision) require a doctor's prescription.

A different use of the word "drugs" refers to those substances on which a person may become dependent. These range from mild stimulants such as caffeine (found in tea and coffee) to powerful agents that alter mood and behaviour. Some addictive drugs have no medical use and cannot be obtained legally.

Where drugs come from

At one time, the only available drugs were substances extracted from plants, or, in some cases, animals. Herbalism, the study and medicinal use of plants, was practised by the Chinese more than 5,000 years ago and is becoming popular in many parts of the world today.

Virtually all the drugs in current use have been developed in the laboratory and are manufactured through various chemical processes. About a quarter of these are derived from plants or other organisms. Most drugs are synthetic chemical copies, but some are still extracted from natural sources. For example, the opioid drugs, including morphine, are made from a species of poppy. Many antibiotics and some anticancer drugs are still of natural origin. The main difference between drugs of plant origin and "herbal medicines" is that drugs have been thoroughly tested to prove that they work and are safe.

Some drugs can now be made through genetic engineering, in which the genes (which control a cell's function) of certain microorganisms are altered, changing the products of cell activity to the desired drug. For example, the hormone insulin can now be manufactured by genetically engineered bacteria. This could eliminate the need to extract insulin from animal pancreas glands, the source until recently, benefiting those people who experience adverse reactions to material derived from animal sources.

Purely synthetic drugs are either modifications of naturally occurring ones, with the aim of increasing effectiveness or safety, or drugs developed after scientific investigation of a disease process with the intention of changing it biochemically.

Developing and marketing new drugs

Pharmaceutical manufacturers find new products in a variety of ways. New drugs are usually developed for one purpose but quite commonly a variant will be found that will be useful for something entirely different.

When a new drug is discovered, the manufacturer often undertakes a programme of molecular tinkering, or elaboration. This refers to investigations into variants of the drug to see if the substance can be made more effective or more free of adverse effects. In some cases that experimental process has unexpected results. The elaboration process, for example, transformed some sulpha drugs, which were originally valued for their antibacterial properties, into widely used oral antidiabetics, diuretics, and anticonvulsants.

All new drugs undergo a long, careful test period before they are approved for marketing by the Committee on Safety of Medicines (CSM) (see Testing and approving new drugs). Once approval has been given, the manufacturer can then market the drug under a brand or trade name. Technically, patent protection gives the manufacturer exclusive rights for 20 years, but this protection starts from when the drug is first identified. The time remaining after CSM approval can be much less than 20 years.

When patent protection ends, other manufacturers may produce the drug, although they must use a different brand name or the generic name (see How drugs are classified, facing page).

Testing and approving new drugs

Before a drug is cleared by the CSM, it undergoes a cautious, step-by-step period of testing, often lasting six to ten years. By law, a drug must be both safe and medically effective. Safety is established through various means, including tests on animals and human volunteers. Efficacy is proven through complex tests (including *double-blind* trials) on groups of healthy and ill patients. The testing is done in various research institutions under government-approved procedures.

The approval process also involves weighing a new drug's risks against its benefits. A dangerous drug whose only potential might be the relief of an ordinary headache undoubtedly would not win approval. Yet an equally *toxic* drug, effective against cancer, might. Medical judgment is an important part of the approval process.

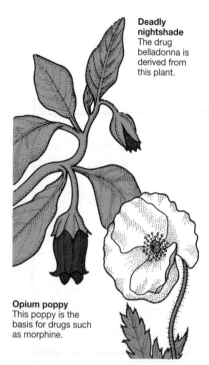

Deadly nightshade
The drug belladonna is derived from this plant.

Opium poppy
This poppy is the basis for drugs such as morphine.

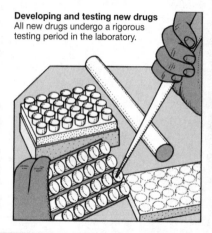

Developing and testing new drugs
All new drugs undergo a rigorous testing period in the laboratory.

HOW DRUGS ARE CLASSIFIED

The 5,000 or so substances loosely called drugs are described in many ways. Scientists and pharmacologists, interested in chemical structure, use one system. Doctors, concerned with use, employ another. Manufacturers and advertisers, promoting the benefits of their products, use simpler, more appealing names. Government regulators, wary of the harm some drugs may do, classify them in a different manner altogether, according to their legal status.

Specific names

All drugs in general use rely on three terms: the generic, brand, and chemical names. The generic name, which is the official medical name for the basic active substance, is chosen by the Nomenclature Committee of the British Pharmacopoeia Commission.

The brand name is chosen by the manufacturer, usually on the basis that it can be easily pronounced, recognized, or remembered. There may be several brands (each by a different manufacturer) containing the same generic substance. Differences between the brands may be slight but may relate to absorption rate (bioavailability), convenience, and digestibility. A drug may be available in generic form, as a brand-name product, or both. Some brand-name products contain several generic drugs. The chemical name is a technical description of the drug, and is not used in this book.

For example, the three names for a drug used to help those with AIDS are as follows. The generic name is zidovudine; the brand name is Retrovir (generic names are not capitalized, brand names are); and the chemical name is 3-azido-3-deoxythymidine.

General terms

Drugs may be grouped according to chemical similarity, for example, the benzodiazepines. More often, though, drugs are classified according to use (antihypertensive) or biological effect (diuretic). Most drugs fit into one group, although many have multiple uses and are listed in several categories.

Because this book is aimed at the lay person, we have grouped drugs according to use, although a chemical description may be added to distinguish one group of drugs from others used to treat the same disorder (for example, benzodiazepine sleeping drugs).

Legal classification

Besides specifying which drugs can be sold over the counter and which require a doctor's prescription, government regulations determine the degree of availability of many substances that have an abuse potential. Regulated drugs are also classified by how harmful they are when abused (see the box below).

CONTROLLED DRUGS

The Misuse of Drugs Act 1971 prohibits activities relating to the manufacture, sale, and possession of particular drugs. The drugs are graded in three classes according to their harmfulness if misused. Offences that involve Class A drugs, potentially the most harmful when abused, carry the highest penalties, while those involving Class C drugs carry the lowest penalties.

Class A	These include: cocaine, dextromoramide, diamorphine (heroin), lysergic acid (LSD), methadone, morphine, opium, pethidine, phencyclidine, and injectable preparations of class B drugs.
Class B	These include: amphetamines (oral), barbiturates, codeine, glutethimide, marijuana (cannabis), pentazocine, and pholcodine.
Class C	These include: drugs related to the amphetamines (for example, chlorphentermine), anabolic and androgenic steroids, most benzodiazepines, buprenorphine, human chorionic gonadotrophin (HCG), mazindol, meprobamate, pemoline, phenbuterol, and somatropin.

The Misuse of Drugs Regulations 1985 define those people who are authorized in their professional capacity to supply and possess controlled drugs. The Regulations also describe the requirements for legally undertaking these activities, such as storage of the drugs and limits on their prescription. Drugs are divided into five schedules based on their potential for abuse if misused.

Schedule I	Virtually all the drugs in this group are prohibited, except in accordance with Home Office authority. All of them have a high potential for abuse and are not used medicinally. **Examples** Marijuana (cannabis), LSD.
Schedule II	Like Schedule I drugs, these have a high potential for abuse and can lead to physical and psychological dependence. They have an accepted medical use, but are subject to full controlled drug requirements. Most of them are stimulants, opioids, or depressants. Prescriptions cannot be renewed. **Examples** Amphetamines, cocaine, diamorphine (heroin), glutethimide, morphine, pethidine, secobarbital.
Schedule III	Drugs in this group have a lower potential for abuse than those in Schedules I and II, but they are nevertheless subject to special prescription requirements. Prescriptions for Schedule III drugs may be repeated if authorized. **Examples** Barbiturates, flunitrazepam, mazindol, meprobamate, methyprylone, pentazocine, phentermine, temazepam.
Schedule IV	The drugs in this group have a lower potential for abuse than Schedule I–III drugs and are subject to minimal control. Special prescription requirements do not apply. **Examples** Benzodiazepines, other than those in Schedule III.
Schedule V	These drugs have a low potential for abuse because of their low strength. For the most part, they are preparations that contain small amounts of opioid drugs, but are exempt from controlled drug requirements. **Examples** Kaolin and morphine (an antidiarrhoeal), codeine linctus (a cough suppressant), DF118 tablets (an opioid analgesic containing dihydrocodeine).

HOW DRUGS WORK

Before the discovery of the sulpha drugs in 1935, medical knowledge of drugs was limited to possibly only a dozen or so drugs that had a clear medical value. Most of these were the extracts of plants (such as digitalis, from foxgloves), while others, such as aspirin, were chemically closely related to plant extracts (in this case, salicylic acid, from the willow tree). It was soon realised, however, that crude plant extracts had two disadvantages: they were of variable potency, and the same plant could contain a number of different substances with different actions. These might even oppose each other, or cause serious *adverse effects*. Now, thousands of effective drugs are available and scientific knowledge regarding drugs and their actions has virtually exploded.

Today's doctor understands the complexity of drug actions in the body, both beneficial and adverse. As a result of extensive research and clinical experience, the doctor can now also recognize that some drugs interact harmfully with others, or with certain foods and alcohol.

DRUG ACTIONS

While the exact workings of some drugs are not fully understood, medical science provides clear knowledge as to what most of them do once they enter or are applied to the human body. Drugs serve different purposes: sometimes they cure a disease, sometimes they only alleviate symptoms. Their impact occurs in various parts of the anatomy. Although different drugs act in different ways, their actions generally fall into one of three categories.

Replacing chemicals that are deficient

To function normally, the body requires sufficient levels of certain chemical substances. These include vitamins and minerals, which the body obtains from food. A balanced diet usually supplies what is needed. But when deficiencies occur, various deficiency diseases result. Lack of vitamin C causes scurvy, iron deficiency causes anaemia, and lack of vitamin D leads to rickets in children and osteomalacia in adults.

Other deficiency diseases arise from a lack of various *hormones* which are the chemical substances produced by glands. Hormones act as internal "messengers". Diabetes mellitus, hypothyroidism, and Addison's disease all result from deficiencies of different hormones.

Deficiency diseases are treated with drugs that replace the substances that are missing or, in the case of some hormone deficiencies, with animal or synthetic replacements.

Interfering with cell function

Many drugs can change the way cells work by increasing or reducing the normal level of activity. Inflammation, for example, is due to the action of certain natural hormones and other chemicals on blood vessels and blood cells . Anti-inflammatory drugs block the action of the hormones or slow their production. Drugs that act in a similar way are used in the treatment of a variety of conditions: hormone disorders, blood clotting problems, and heart and kidney diseases.

Many such drugs do their work by altering the transmission system by which messages are sent from one part of the body to another.

A message – to contract a muscle, say – originates in the brain and enters a nerve cell through its receiving end. The message, in the form of an electrical impulse, travels the nerve cell to the sending end. Here a chemical substance called a *neurotransmitter* is released, conducting the message across the tiny gap (synapse) separating it from an adjacent nerve cell. That process is repeated until the message reaches the appropriate muscle.

Many drugs can alter this process, often by their effect on receptor sites on cells (see left). Some drugs (*agonists*) intensify cell activity, while other drugs (*antagonists*) reduce activity in the cells.

Acting against invading organisms or abnormal cells

Infectious diseases are caused by viruses, bacteria, protozoa, and fungi invading the body. We now have a wide choice of drugs that destroy these microorganisms, either by halting their multiplication or by killing them directly. Other drugs treat disease by killing abnormal cells produced by the human body – cancer cells, for example.

RECEPTOR SITES

Many drugs produce their effects through their action on special sites called *receptors* on the surface of body cells. Natural body chemicals such as *neurotransmitters* bind to these sites, initiating a response in the cell. A cell may have many types of receptors, each of which has an affinity for a different chemical in the body. Drugs may also bind to receptors, either adding to the effect of the body's natural chemicals and enhancing cell response (agonists) or preventing such a chemical from binding to its receptor, and thereby blocking a particular cell response (antagonists).

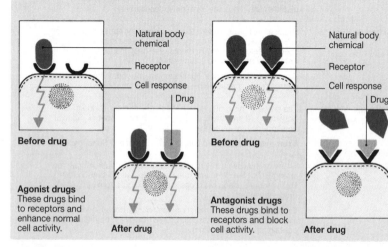

Natural body chemical
Receptor
Cell response
Drug

Before drug

Agonist drugs
These drugs bind to receptors and enhance normal cell activity.

After drug

Natural body chemical
Receptor
Cell response
Drug

Before drug

Antagonist drugs
These drugs bind to receptors and block cell activity.

After drug

THE EFFECTS OF DRUGS

Before a doctor selects a drug to be used in the treatment of a sick person, he or she carefully weighs the benefits and the risks. Obviously, the doctor expects a positive result from the drug – a cure of the condition or at least the relief of symptoms. At the same time, the doctor has to consider the risks, since all drugs are potentially harmful, some of them considerably more so than others.

Reaction time

Some drugs can produce rapid and spectacular relief from the symptoms of disease. Glyceryl trinitrate frequently provides almost immediate relief from the pain of angina; other drugs can quickly alleviate the symptoms of an asthmatic attack. Conversely, some drugs take much longer to produce a response. It may, for example, require several weeks of treatment with an antidepressant drug before a person experiences maximum benefit. This can add to anxiety unless the doctor has warned of the possibility of a delay in the onset of beneficial effects.

Adverse effects

The *adverse effects* of a drug (also known as side effects or adverse reactions) are its undesired effects. When drugs are taken, they are distributed throughout the body and their effects are unlikely to be restricted just to the organ or tissue we want them to affect. Other parts of the body contain receptor sites like those the drug is targeting. In addition, the drug molecule may fit other, different receptors well enough to activate or block them too.

For example, *anticholinergic* drugs, given to relieve spasm of the intestinal wall, may also cause blurred vision, dry mouth, and retention of urine. Such effects may gradually disappear as the body becomes used to the drug. If they persist, the dose may have to be reduced, or the time between doses may need to be increased. Reducing the dose will often reduce the severity of the adverse effect for those effects that are called "dose-related".

DOSE AND RESPONSE

People respond in different ways to a drug, and often the dose has to be adjusted to allow for a person's age, weight, or general health.

The dose of any drug should be sufficient to produce a beneficial response but not so great that it will cause excessive adverse effects. If the dose is too low, the drug may not have any effect, either beneficial or adverse; if it is too high, it will not produce any additional benefits and may produce adverse effects.

The aim of drug treatment is to achieve a concentration of drug in the blood or tissue that lies between the minimum effective level and the maximum safe concentration. This is known as the therapeutic range.

For certain drugs, such as digitalis drugs, the therapeutic range is quite narrow, so the margin of safety/effectiveness is small. Other drugs, such as penicillin antibiotics, have a much wider therapeutic range.

Wide therapeutic range

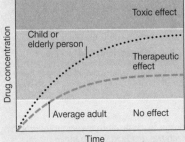

Dosage of drugs with a wide therapeutic range can vary considerably without altering the drug's effect. The effect is greater in children and the elderly.

Narrow therapeutic range

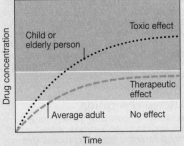

Dosage of drugs with a narrow therapeutic range must be carefully calculated to achieve the desired effect without toxicity. Children or the elderly experience toxic levels earlier.

Adverse effects of some drugs can be quite serious. Such drugs are given because they may be the only treatment for an otherwise fatal disease. But all drugs are chemicals, with a potential for producing serious, *toxic* reactions.

Some adverse effects seem not to be dose-related, and where the effect appears on first use and is unexpected, the phenomenon is called *idiosyncrasy*. People are genetically different and, as a result, their response to drugs differs, perhaps because they lack a particular enzyme or because it is less active than usual. For this reason, not everybody suffers even the "common" adverse effects; but, occasionally, a new adverse

effect, due to a rare and unsuspected genetic variation, will be discovered only after the drug has been taken by a large number of people.

Other adverse effects that are not dose-related are *allergic reactions*. These reactions do not usually appear on the first exposure to the drug but on a subsequent occasion. The symptoms are similar to those caused by other allergens and, in extreme cases, may cause anaphylactic shock (see p.496).

Beneficial vs. adverse effects

In evaluating the risk/benefit ratio of a prescribed drug, the doctor has to weigh the drug's therapeutic benefit to the sick person against the possible adverse effects. For example, such side effects as nausea, headache, and diarrhoea may result from taking an antibiotic. But the possible risks of the drug's side effects will certainly be considered acceptable if the problem is a life-threatening infection requiring immediate medical treatment. On the other hand, such side effects would be considered unacceptable for an over-the-counter drug for the relief of headaches.

Because some people are more at risk from adverse drug reactions than others (particularly those who have a history of drug allergy), the doctor normally checks whether there is any reason why a certain drug should not be prescribed (see Drug treatment in special risk groups, p.20).

PLACEBO RESPONSE

The word placebo – Latin for "I will please" – is used to describe any chemically inert substance given as a substitute for a drug. Any benefit gained from taking a placebo occurs because the person taking it believes that it will produce good results.

New drugs are almost always tested against a placebo preparation in clinical trials as a way of assessing the efficacy of a drug before it is marketed. The placebo is made to look identical to the active preparation, and the volunteers are not told whether they have been given the active drug or the placebo. Sometimes the doctor is also unaware of which preparation an individual has been

given. This is known as a *double-blind* trial. In this way, the purely placebo effect can be eliminated and the effectiveness of the drug determined more realistically.

Sometimes the mere taking of a medicine has a psychological effect that produces a beneficial physical response. This type of placebo response can make an important contribution to the overall effectiveness of a chemically active drug. It is most commonly seen with analgesics, antidepressants, and anti-anxiety drugs. Some people, known as placebo responders, are more likely to experience this sort of reaction than the rest of the population.

DRUG INTERACTIONS

When two different drugs are taken together, or when a drug is taken in combination with certain foods or with alcohol, this may produce effects different from those produced when the drug is taken alone. Often, this is beneficial and doctors frequently make use of interactions to increase the effectiveness of a treatment. Very often, more than one drug may be prescribed to treat cancer or high blood pressure (hypertension).

Other interactions, however, are unwanted and may be harmful. They may occur not only between prescription drugs, but also between prescription and over-the-counter drugs. It is important to read warnings on drug labels and tell your doctor if you are taking any preparations – both prescription and over-the-counter, and even herbal or homeopathic remedies.

A drug may interact with another drug or with food or alcohol for a number of reasons (see below).

Altered absorption

Alcohol and some drugs (particularly *opioids* and drugs with an *anticholinergic* effect) slow the digestive process that empties the stomach contents into the intestine. This may delay the absorption, and therefore the effect, of another drug. Other drugs (for example, metoclopramide, an anti-emetic drug) may speed the rate at which the stomach empties and may, therefore, increase the rate at which another drug is absorbed and takes effect.

Some drugs also combine with another drug or food in the intestine to form a compound that is not absorbed as readily. This occurs when tetracycline and iron tablets or antacids are taken together. Milk and dairy products also reduce the absorption of tetracycline and some other

Drug absorption in the intestine

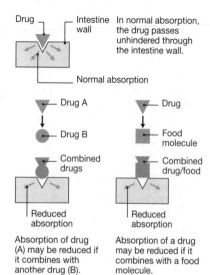

In normal absorption, the drug passes unhindered through the intestine wall.

Normal absorption

Absorption of drug (A) may be reduced if it combines with another drug (B).

Absorption of a drug may be reduced if it combines with a food molecule.

EXAMPLES OF IMPORTANT INTERACTIONS

Adverse interactions between drugs may vary from a simple blocking of a drug's beneficial effect to a serious reaction between two drugs that may be life-threatening. Some of the more serious adverse interactions occur between the following:

Drugs that depress the central nervous system (opioids, most antihistamines, sleeping drugs, and alcohol). The effects of two or more of these drugs together may be additive, causing dangerous oversedation.

Drugs that lower blood sugar levels and such drugs as sulphonamides and alcohol. The drug interaction increases the effect of blood sugar-lowering drugs, thus further depressing blood sugar levels.

Oral anticoagulants and other drugs, particularly aspirin and antibiotics. As these drugs may increase the tendency to bleed, it is essential to check the effects in every case.

Monoamine oxidase inhibitors (MAOIs). Many drugs and foods can produce a severe increase in blood pressure when taken with MAOIs. Such drugs include amphetamines and decongestants; foods include cheese, herring, chocolate, red wine, and beer. Some of the newer MAOIs, however, are much less likely to interact with food and drugs.

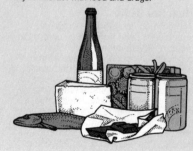

drugs, such as ciprofloxacin, by combining with the drugs in this manner.

Enzyme effects

Some drugs increase the production of *enzymes* in the liver that break down drugs, while others inhibit or reduce enzyme production. Thus they affect the rate at which other drugs are activated or inactivated.

Excretion in the urine

A drug may reduce the kidneys' ability to excrete another drug, raising the drug level in the blood and increasing its effect.

Receptor effects

Drugs that act on the same *receptor sites* (p.14) sometimes add to each other's effect on the body, or compete with each other in occupying certain receptor sites. For example, naloxone blocks receptors used by opioid drugs, thereby helping to reverse the effects of opioid poisoning.

Similar or opposite effects

Drugs that produce similar effects (but act on different receptors) add to each others' actions. Often, lower doses are possible as a result, with fewer *adverse effects*. This is common practice in the treatment of high blood pressure and cancer. Antibiotics are given together as the infecting organisms are less likely to develop resistance to the drugs. Drugs with *antagonistic* effects reduce the useful activity of one or both drugs. For example, some antidepressants oppose the effects of anticonvulsants.

Reduced protein binding

Some drugs circulate around the body in the bloodstream with a proportion of the drug attached to the proteins of the blood

plasma. The amount of drug attached to the plasma proteins is inactive. If another drug is taken, some of the second drug may also bind to the plasma proteins and displace the first drug; more of the first drug is then active in the body.

Interaction between protein-bound drugs

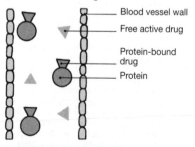

Blood vessel wall

Free active drug

Protein-bound drug

Protein

Protein-bound drug taken alone
Drug molecules that are bound to proteins in the blood are unable to pass into body tissues. Only free drug molecules are active.

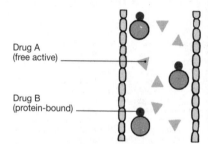

Drug A (free active)

Drug B (protein-bound)

Taken with another protein-bound drug
If a drug (B) with a greater ability to bind with proteins is also taken, drug (A) is displaced, increasing the amount of active drug.

METHODS OF ADMINISTRATION

The majority of drugs must be absorbed into the bloodstream in order for them to reach the site where their effects are needed. The method of administering a drug determines the route it takes to get into the bloodstream and the speed at which it is absorbed into the blood.

When a drug is meant to enter the bloodstream it is usually administered in one of the following ways: through the mouth or rectum, by injection, or by inhalation. Drugs that are implanted under the skin or enclosed in a skin patch also enter the bloodstream. These types are discussed under Slow-release preparations (p.18).

When it is unnecessary or undesirable for a drug to enter the bloodstream in large amounts, it may be applied *topically* so that its effect is limited mainly to the site of the disorder, such as the surface of the skin or mucous membranes (the membranes of the nose, eyes, ears, vagina, or rectum). Drugs are administered topically in a variety of preparations, including creams, sprays, drops, and suppositories. Most inhaled drugs also have a local effect on the respiratory tract.

Very often, a particular drug may be available in different forms. Many drugs are available both as tablets and injectable fluid. The choice between a tablet and an injection depends on a number of factors, including the severity of the illness, the urgency with which the drug effect is needed, the part of the body requiring treatment, and the patient's general state of health, in particular his or her ability to swallow.

The various administration routes are discussed in greater detail below. For a description of the different forms in which drugs are given, see Drug forms (p.19).

ADMINISTRATION BY MOUTH

Giving drugs by mouth is the most common method of administration. Most of the drugs that are given by mouth are absorbed into the bloodstream through the walls of the intestine. The speed at which the drug is absorbed and the amount of active drug that is available for use depend on several factors, including the form in which the drug is given (for example, as a tablet or a liquid) and whether it is taken with food or on an empty stomach. If a drug is taken when the stomach is empty (before meals, for example) it may act more quickly than a drug that is taken after a meal when the stomach is full.

Some drugs (like antacids, which neutralize stomach acidity) are taken by mouth to produce a direct effect on the stomach or digestive tract.

In-mouth administration
Products are available that are placed in the mouth but not swallowed. They are absorbed quickly into the bloodstream through the lining of the mouth, which has a rich supply of blood vessels. Sublingual tablets are placed under the tongue, wafers are placed on the tongue, and buccal tablets are placed in the pouch between the cheek and teeth.

HOW DRUGS PASS THROUGH THE BODY

Most drugs taken by mouth reach the bloodstream by absorption through the wall of the small intestine. Blood vessels supplying the intestine then carry the drug to the liver, where it may be broken down into a form that can be used by the body. The drug (or its breakdown product) then enters the general circulation, which carries it around the body. It may pass back into the intestine before being reabsorbed into the bloodstream. Some drugs are rapidly excreted via the kidneys; others may build up in fatty tissues in the body.

Certain insoluble drugs cannot be absorbed through the intestinal wall and pass through the digestive tract unchanged. These drugs are useful for treating bowel disorders, but if they are intended to have *systemic* effects elsewhere they must be given by intravenous injection.

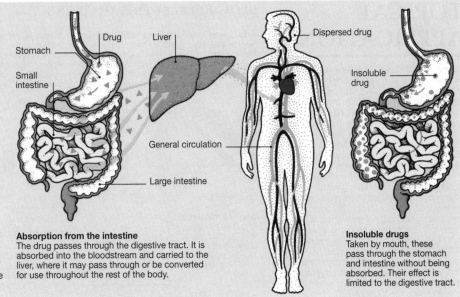

Stomach
Small intestine
Drug
Liver
Large intestine
General circulation
Dispersed drug
Insoluble drug

Absorption from the intestine
The drug passes through the digestive tract. It is absorbed into the bloodstream and carried to the liver, where it may pass through or be converted for use throughout the rest of the body.

Insoluble drugs
Taken by mouth, these pass through the stomach and intestine without being absorbed. Their effect is limited to the digestive tract.

RECTAL ADMINISTRATION

Drugs intended to have a *systemic* effect may be given in the form of suppositories inserted into the rectum, from where they are absorbed into the bloodstream. This method may be used to give drugs that might be destroyed by the stomach's digestive juices. It is also sometimes used to administer drugs to people who cannot take medication by mouth, such as those who are suffering from nausea and vomiting.

Drugs may also be given rectally for local effect, either as suppositories (to relieve haemorrhoids) or as enemas (for ulcerative colitis).

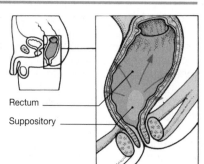

Rectum

Suppository

INHALATION

Drugs may be inhaled to produce a *systemic* effect or a direct local effect on the respiratory tract.

Gases to produce *general anaesthesia* are administered by inhalation and are absorbed into the bloodstream through the lungs, producing a general effect on the body, particularly the brain.

Bronchodilators, used to treat certain types of asthma, emphysema, and bronchitis, are a common example of drugs administered by inhalation for their direct effect on the respiratory tract, although some of the active drug also reaches the bloodstream. (See also p.92.)

ADMINISTRATION BY INJECTION

Drugs may be injected into the body to produce a *systemic* effect. One reason for injecting drugs is the rapid response that follows. Other circumstances that call for injection are when: a person is intolerant to the drug when taken by mouth; the drug would be destroyed by the stomach's digestive juices (insulin, for example); or the drug cannot pass through the intestinal walls into the bloodstream. Drug injections may also be given to produce a local effect, as is often done to relieve the pain of arthritis.

The three most common methods of injection – intramuscular, intravenous, and subcutaneous – are described in the illustration (see right). The type of injection depends both on the nature of the drug and the condition being treated.

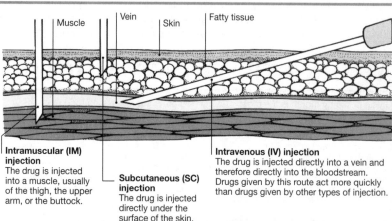

Muscle — Vein — Skin — Fatty tissue

Intramuscular (IM) injection
The drug is injected into a muscle, usually of the thigh, the upper arm, or the buttock.

Subcutaneous (SC) injection
The drug is injected directly under the surface of the skin.

Intravenous (IV) injection
The drug is injected directly into a vein and therefore directly into the bloodstream. Drugs given by this route act more quickly than drugs given by other types of injection.

TOPICAL APPLICATION

In treating localized disorders such as skin infections and nasal congestion, it is often preferable when a choice is available to prescribe drugs in a form that has a *topical*, or localized, rather than a *systemic* effect. The reason is that it is much easier to control the effects of drugs administered locally and to ensure that they produce the maximum benefit with minimum *adverse effects*.

Topical preparations are available in a variety of forms, from skin creams, ointments, and lotions to inhalers, nasal sprays, ear and eye drops, bladder irrigations, and vaginal pessaries. It is important when using topical preparations to follow instructions carefully, avoiding a higher dose than recommended or application for longer than necessary. This will help to avoid adverse systemic effects caused by the absorption of larger amounts into the bloodstream.

SLOW-RELEASE PREPARATIONS

A number of disorders can be treated with drug preparations that have been specially formulated to release their active drug slowly over a given period of time. Such preparations may be beneficial when it is inconvenient for a person to visit the doctor on a regular basis to receive treatment by injection, or when it is necessary to control accurately the release of small amounts of the drug into the body. Slow release of drugs can be achieved by *depot injections*, *transdermal patches*, slow-release capsules and tablets, and implants.

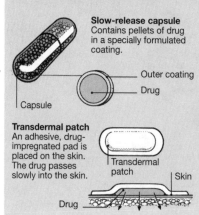

Slow-release capsule
Contains pellets of drug in a specially formulated coating.

Outer coating

Drug

Capsule

Transdermal patch
An adhesive, drug-impregnated pad is placed on the skin. The drug passes slowly into the skin.

Transdermal patch

Skin

Drug

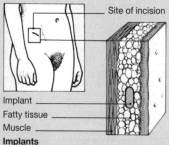

Site of incision

Implant

Fatty tissue

Muscle

Implants
A pellet containing the drug is implanted under the skin. By this rarely used method, a drug (usually a hormone) is slowly released into the bloodstream over a period of months.

DRUG FORMS

Most drugs are specially prepared in a form designed for convenience of administration. This helps to ensure that dosages are accurate and that taking the medication is as easy as possible. Inactive ingredients (those with no therapeutic effect) are sometimes added to flavour or colour the medicine, or to improve its chemical stability, extending the period during which it is effective.

The more common drug forms are described in detail below.

Tablets

This contains the drug compressed with other ingredients (see right) into a solid plug. Some are coated with a membrane that allows the drug to be slowly released, to produce a sustained effect; others are composed of granules that are individually layered to give the slow release.

Capsules

The drug is contained in a cylindrically shaped gelatin shell that breaks open after the capsule has been swallowed, releasing the drug. Slow-release capsules contain pellets that dissolve in the gastrointestinal tract, releasing the drug slowly (facing page).

Wafers

The drug is contained in a small wafer, which is placed on the tongue and allowed to dissolve.

Liquids

Some drugs are available in liquid form, the active substance being combined in a solution, suspension, or emulsion with other ingredients – preservatives, solvents, and flavouring or colouring agents. Many liquid preparations should be shaken before use to ensure that the active drug is evenly distributed. If it is not, inaccurate dosages may result.

Mixture

A mixture is one or more drugs, either dissolved to form a solution or suspended in a liquid (often water).

Elixir

An elixir is a solution of a drug in a sweetened mixture of alcohol and water. It is often highly flavoured.

Emulsion

An emulsion is a drug dispersed in oil and water. An emulsifying agent is often included to stabilize the product.

Syrup

A syrup is a concentrated solution of sugar containing the active drug, with flavouring and stabilizing agents added.

Topical skin preparations

These are preparations designed for application to the skin and other surface

WHAT A TABLET CONTAINS

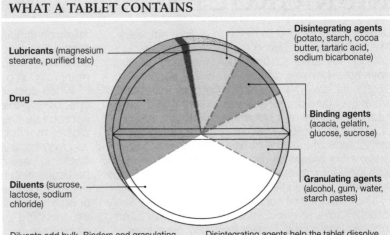

Lubricants (magnesium stearate, purified talc)

Drug

Diluents (sucrose, lactose, sodium chloride)

Disintegrating agents (potato, starch, cocoa butter, tartaric acid, sodium bicarbonate)

Binding agents (acacia, gelatin, glucose, sucrose)

Granulating agents (alcohol, gum, water, starch pastes)

Diluents add bulk. Binders and granulating agents bind the ingredients. Lubricants ensure a smooth surface by allowing the ingredients to flow during the manufacturing process.

Disintegrating agents help the tablet dissolve. A sugar coating or a transparent film protects the surface or modifies the drug's release rate. Dyes and imprints make it recognizable.

tissues of the body. Preservatives are usually included to reduce the growth of bacteria. The most commonly used types of skin preparations are described below. For a more detailed discussion, see Bases for skin preparations, p.175.

Cream

A cream is a non-greasy preparation that is used to apply drugs to an area of the body or to cool or moisten the skin. It is less noticeable than an ointment.

Ointment

An ointment is a greasy preparation used to apply drugs to an area of the body, or as a protective or lubricant layer for the relief of dry skin conditions.

Lotion

A lotion is a solution or suspension applied to unbroken skin to cool and dry the affected area. Some are more suitable for use in hairy areas because they are not as sticky as creams or ointments.

Injection solutions

Solutions used for injections are sterile (germ-free) preparations of a drug that are dissolved or suspended in a liquid. Other chemicals (such as anti-oxidants and buffers) are often added to preserve the stability of the drug or to regulate the acidity or alkalinity of the solution. Most injectable drugs used today are packaged in sterile, disposable syringes. This reduces the chance of contamination. Certain drugs are still available in multiple- dose vials, and a chemical bactericide is added to prevent the growth of bacteria when the needle is reinserted through the rubber

seal. For details on different types, see Administration by injection, facing page.

Suppositories and pessaries

These are solid, bullet-shaped dosage forms designed for easy insertion into the rectum (rectal suppository) or vagina (pessary). They contain a drug and an inert (pharmacologically and chemically inactive) substance often derived from cocoa butter or vegetable oil. The drug is gradually released in the rectum or vagina as the suppository or pessary dissolves at body temperature.

Eye drops

A sterile drug solution (or suspension) dropped behind the eyelid.

Ear drops

A solution (or suspension) containing a drug introduced into the ear by dropper. Ear drops are usually given to produce an effect on the outer ear canal.

Nasal drops/spray

A solution of a drug for introduction into the nose to produce a local effect.

Inhalers

Aerosol inhalers contain a solution or suspension of a drug under pressure. A valve ensures delivery of a recommended dosage when the inhaler is activated. A mouthpiece facilitates inhalation as the drug is released from the canister. The correct technique is important; the printed instructions should be followed carefully or your doctor, pharmacist, or nurse will show you. Aerosol inhalers are used for respiratory conditions such as asthma (see also p.92).

DRUG TREATMENT IN SPECIAL RISK GROUPS

Different people tend to respond in different ways to drug treatment. Taking the same drug, one person may suffer *adverse effects* while another does not. However, doctors know that certain people are always more at risk from adverse effects when they take drugs; the reason is that in those people the body handles drugs differently, or the drug has an atypical effect. Those people at special risk include infants and children, women who are pregnant or breast-feeding, the elderly, and people with long-term medical conditions, especially those who have impaired liver or kidney function.

The reasons that such people may be more likely to suffer adverse effects are discussed in detail on the following pages. Others who may need special attention include those already taking regular medication who may risk complications when they take another drug. Drug interactions are discussed more fully on p.16.

When doctors prescribe drugs for people at special risk, they take extra care to select appropriate medication, adjust dosages, and closely monitor the effects of treatment. If you think you may be at special risk, be sure to tell your doctor in case he or she is not fully aware of your particular circumstances. Similarly, if you are buying over-the-counter drugs, you should ask your doctor or pharmacist if you think you may be at risk of experiencing any possible adverse effects or hazardous drug interactions.

INFANTS AND CHILDREN

Infants and children need a lower dosage of drugs than adults because children have a relatively low body weight. In addition, because of differences in body composition and the distribution and amount of body fat, as well as differences in the state of development and function of organs such as the liver and kidneys at different ages, children cannot simply be given a proportion of an adult dose as if they were small adults. Dosages need to be calculated in a more complex way, taking into account the child's age and weight. While newborn babies often have to be given very small doses of drugs, older children may need relatively large doses of some drugs compared to the adult dosage.

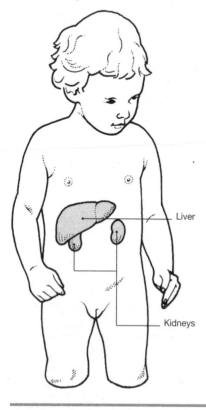

Liver

Kidneys

The liver
The liver's enzyme systems are not fully developed when a baby is born. This means that drugs are not broken down as rapidly as in an adult, and may reach dangerously high concentrations in the baby's body. For this reason, many drugs are not prescribed for babies or are given in very reduced doses. In older children, because the liver is relatively large compared to the rest of the body, some drugs may need to be given in proportionately higher doses.

The kidneys
During the first six months, a baby's kidneys are unable to excrete drugs as efficiently as an adult's kidneys. This may lead to a dangerously high concentration of a drug in the blood. The dose of certain drugs may therefore need to be reduced. Between one and two years of age, kidney function improves, and higher doses of some drugs may then be needed.

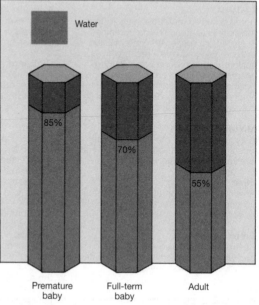

Water

85%

70%

55%

Premature baby

Full-term baby

Adult

Body composition
The proportion of water in the body of a premature baby is about 85 per cent of its body weight, that of a full-term baby is 70 per cent, and that of an adult is only 55 per cent. This means that drugs that stay in the body water will not be as concentrated in an infant's body as in an adult's, unless a higher dose relative to body weight is given.

PREGNANT WOMEN

Great care is needed during pregnancy to protect the fetus so that it develops into a healthy baby. Drugs taken by the mother can cross the placenta and enter the baby's bloodstream. With certain drugs, and at certain stages of pregnancy, there is a risk of developmental abnormalities, retarded growth, or post-delivery problems affecting the newborn baby. In addition, some drugs may affect the health of the mother during pregnancy.

Many drugs are known to have *adverse effects* during pregnancy; others are known to be safe, but in a large number of cases there is no firm evidence to decide on risk or safety. Therefore, the most important rule if you are pregnant or trying to conceive is to consult your doctor before taking any prescribed or over-the-counter medication.

Drugs such as marijuana, nicotine, and alcohol should also be avoided during pregnancy. A high daily intake of caffeine should be reduced if possible. Your doctor will assess the potential benefits of drug treatment against any possible risks to decide whether or not a drug should be taken. This is particularly important if you need to take medication regularly for a chronic condition such as epilepsy, high blood pressure, or diabetes.

Drugs and the stages of pregnancy

Pregnancy is divided into three three-month stages called trimesters. Depending on the trimester in which they are taken, drugs can have different effects on the mother, the fetus, or both. Some drugs may be considered safe during one trimester, but not during another. Doctors, therefore, often need to substitute one medication for another given during the course of pregnancy and/or labour.

The trimesters of pregnancy

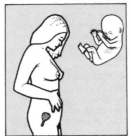
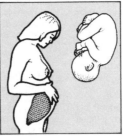
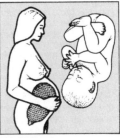

First trimester
During the first three months of pregnancy – the most critical period – drugs may affect the development of fetal organs, leading to congenital malformations. Very severe defects may result in miscarriage.

Second trimester
From the fourth to the sixth month some drugs may retard the growth of the fetus. This may also result in a low birth weight. Other drugs may affect the development of the nervous system.

Third trimester
During the last three months of pregnancy, major risks include breathing difficulties in the newborn baby. Some drugs may also affect labour, causing it to be premature, delayed, or prolonged.

How drugs cross the placenta
The placenta acts as a filter between the mother's bloodstream and that of the baby. It allows small molecules of nutrients to pass into the baby's blood, while preventing larger particles such as blood cells from doing so. Drug molecules are comparatively small and pass easily through the placental barrier.

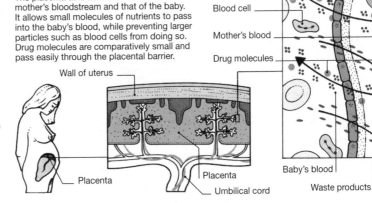

Wall of uterus
Placenta
Placenta
Umbilical cord
Nutrients
Blood cell
Mother's blood
Drug molecules
Baby's blood
Waste products

BREAST-FEEDING

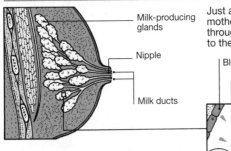

How drugs pass into breast milk
The milk-producing glands in the breast are surrounded by a network of fine blood vessels. Small molecules of substances such as drugs pass from the blood into the milk. Drugs that dissolve easily in fat may pass across in greater concentrations than other drugs.

Milk-producing glands
Nipple
Milk ducts

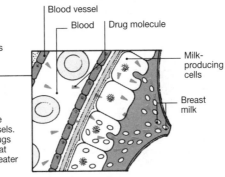

Blood vessel
Blood
Drug molecule
Milk-producing cells
Breast milk

Just as drugs may cross from the mother's bloodstream into the baby's through the placenta, they may also pass to the baby from the mother's milk. This means that a breast-fed baby will receive small doses of whatever drugs the mother is taking. In many cases this is not a problem, because the amount of drug that passes into the milk is too small to have any significant effect on the baby. However, some drugs can produce unwanted effects on the baby. Antibiotics may sensitize the infant and consequently prevent their use later in life. Sedative drugs may make the baby drowsy and cause feeding problems. Moreover, some drugs may reduce the amount of milk produced by the mother.

Doctors usually advise breast-feeding women to take only essential drugs. When a mother needs to take regular medication while breast-feeding, her baby may also need to be closely monitored for possible adverse effects.

THE ELDERLY

Older people are particularly at risk when taking drugs. This is partly due to the physical changes associated with ageing, and partly because many elderly people need to take several different drugs at the same time. They may also be at risk because they may be unable to manage their treatment properly, or they may lack the information to do so.

Physical changes

Elderly people have a greater risk of accumulating drugs in their body tissues because the liver is less efficient at breaking drugs down and the kidneys are less efficient at excreting them. Because of this, in some cases the normal adult dose will produce side effects, and a smaller dose may be needed to produce a therapeutic effect without the side effects. (See also Liver and kidney disease, below.)

Older people tend to take more drugs than younger people – many take three or more drugs at the same time. Apart from increasing the number of drugs in their systems, adverse drug interactions (see p.16) are more likely.

As people grow older, some parts of the body, such as the brain and nervous system, become more sensitive to drugs, thus increasing the likelihood of adverse reactions from drugs acting on those sites (see right). A similar problem may occur due to changes in the body's ratio of body fat. Although allergic reactions (see Allergy, p.123) do not become commoner due to increasing age, they are more likely because more drugs are prescribed. Accordingly, doctors prescribe more carefully for older people, especially those with disorders that are likely to correct themselves in time.

Incorrect use of drugs

Elderly people often suffer harmful effects from their drug treatment because they fail to take their medication regularly or correctly. This may happen because they have been misinformed about how to take it or receive vague instructions. Problems arise sometimes because the elderly person cannot remember whether he or she has taken the drug and takes a double dose (see Exceeding the dose, p.30). Problems may also occur because the person is confused; this is not necessarily due to age or illness, but can arise as a result of drug treatment, especially if an elderly person is taking a number of different drugs or a sedative.

Prescriptions for the elderly should be clearly and fully labelled, and/or information about the drug and its use should be provided either for the individual or for the person taking care of him or her. When appropriate, containers with memory aids should be used to dispense the medication in single doses.

Elderly people often find it difficult to swallow medicine in capsule or tablet

Effect of drugs that act on the brain

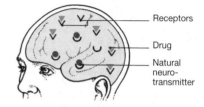

In young people
There are plenty of receptors to take up the drug as well as natural *neurotransmitters*.

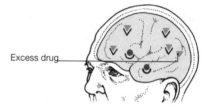

In older people
There are fewer receptors so that even a reduced drug dose may be excessive.

form; they should always take capsules or tablets with a full glass or cup of liquid. A liquid medicine may be prescribed instead.

LIVER AND KIDNEY DISEASE

Long-term illness affects the way in which people respond to drugs. This is especially true of liver and kidney problems. The liver alters the chemical structure of many drugs that enter the body (see How drugs pass through the body, p.17) by breaking them down into simpler substances, while the kidneys excrete drugs in the urine. If the effectiveness of the liver or kidneys is reduced by illness, the action of drugs on the individual can be significantly altered. In most cases, people with liver or kidney disease will be prescribed a smaller number of drugs and lower doses. In addition, certain drugs may, in rare cases, damage the liver or kidneys. For example, tetracycline can cause kidney failure in those with poor kidney function. A doctor may be reluctant to prescribe such a drug to someone with already reduced liver or kidney function in order to avoid the risk of further damage.

Drugs and liver disease

Severe liver diseases, such as cirrhosis and hepatitis, affect the way the body breaks down drugs. This can lead to a dangerous accumulation of certain drugs in the body. People suffering from these diseases should consult their doctor before taking any medication (including over-the-counter drugs) or alcohol. Many drugs must be avoided completely, since they could cause coma in someone with liver damage.

Drugs and kidney disease

People with poor kidney function are at risk from drug side effects. There are two reasons for this. First, drugs build up in the system because smaller amounts are excreted in urine. Second, kidney disease can cause protein loss through the urine, which lowers the level of protein in the blood. Some drugs bind to blood proteins, and if there are fewer protein molecules, a greater proportion of drug becomes free and active in the body.

Drug passing through body

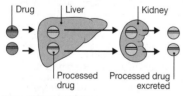

Normal liver and kidneys
Drugs are processed in the liver before being excreted by the kidneys.

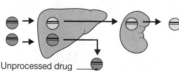

In liver damage
The liver cannot process sufficient drug and this builds up in the body tissues.

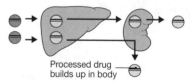

In kidney damage
The kidneys cannot excrete the processed drug in the urine and drug levels in the body rise.

DRUG TOLERANCE AND DEPENDENCE

In the course of treatment with many common drugs, the body acquires the ability to adapt to the drug's effect. This response is known as tolerance. As a result, the drug dose has to be increased to achieve the same effect as before. Tolerance is not always associated with dependence (often called addiction), which is the compulsion to continue taking a drug in order to experience a desired effect, or in order to avoid the unpleasant effects that occur when it is not taken. Dependence is almost always confined to drugs which act on the brain and nervous system, such as opiates, tobacco, and alcohol.

TOLERANCE

Drug tolerance occurs as the body adapts to a drug's actions. A person taking the drug needs larger and larger doses to achieve the original effect and as the dose increases, so too do the risks of toxic effects and dependence. Although people can develop a tolerance to many drugs, it is a dangerous characteristic of virtually all the drugs of dependence.

How tolerance develops

Drug tolerance can develop through a variety of different mechanisms, many of which are not fully understood. In some cases, the liver becomes more efficient at breaking the drug down to an inactive form. In other cases, the drug receptors adapt to the presence of the drug, In yet other cases, the drug exhausts the body's supply of chemicals necessary to produce a response.

Tolerance to one particular drug may result in the reduced effect of a drug that has similar properties or is processed in the body in the same way. This is known as cross tolerance. For example, a regular drinker, who can tolerate high levels of alcohol (a depressant), can have a dangerous tolerance to other depressants such as sleeping drugs and anti-anxiety drugs. While cross-tolerance can often cause problems, it sometimes has a beneficial effect in allowing a substance with a less addictive potential to replace the original drug. For example, the symptoms of alcohol withdrawal can be controlled by the anti-anxiety drug diazepam, which is also a depressant.

Tolerance to some drugs has its benefits. A person can develop tolerance to the side effects of a drug while still benefiting from its useful effects. For example, many people taking antidepressants find that side effects such as dry mouth slowly disappear, with the primary action of the drug continuing (see below).

Increasing drug tolerance has dangers. A person who has developed tolerance to a drug may keep raising the dose to sometimes toxic levels in order to achieve the desired effect.

Effects of tolerance

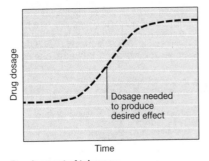

Development of tolerance
An gradually increasing dose of the drug is needed to produce the desired effect as tolerance develops over time.

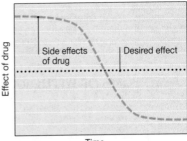

Beneficial effect of tolerance
During treatment with many drugs, the unwanted side effects decrease with time, while the desired effect of the drug is maintained.

DEPENDENCE

Drug dependence is defined as the compulsive use of a substance resulting in physical, psychological, or social harm to the user, with continued use despite the harm.

Drug dependence (now widely preferred as a term to the word addiction) applies far more widely than most people realize. It is usually thought of in association with the use of illegal drugs, such as heroin, or with excessive intake of alcohol. But millions of people are dependent on other drugs, including stimulants – such as caffeine found in coffee and tea, and nicotine in tobacco – and certain prescription medicines, such as analgesics, sleeping drugs, amphetamines, and tranquillizers.

Psychological and physical dependence

Drug dependence, implying that a person is reliant on the continued use of a substance with potential for abuse, is of two types. Psychological dependence is an emotional state of craving for a drug whose presence has a desired effect on the mind, or whose absence has an undesired effect. Physical dependence, which often accompanies psychological dependence, involves physiological adaptation to a medicine or alcohol that is characterized by severe physical disturbances – withdrawal symptoms – during a period of abstinence. Some drugs, such as laxatives, can produce physical dependence.

Drugs that cause dependence

Many people who need to take regular medication worry that they may become dependent on their drugs. In fact, only a few groups of drugs produce physical or psychological dependence, and most of them are substances that alter mood or behaviour. Such drugs include heroin and the *opioid* analgesics such as morphine and pethidine, sleeping and anti-anxiety drugs (benzodiazepines and barbiturates), depressants (alcohol), and nervous system stimulants (cocaine, caffeine, amphetamines, and nicotine).

Antidepressant drugs do not cause psychological dependence. When a depressive illness has been treated effectively, drugs can usually be stopped

DEPENDENCE continued

without any problems, although some people may experience physical withdrawal symptoms if drugs are stopped suddenly. Consult the drug profile in Part 4 of this book to discover the dependence rating of any drug you are taking.

The use of nicotine, in the form of tobacco, and of opioid analgesics, whether controlled or uncontrolled, invariably produces physical dependence if occurring regularly over a period of time. However, it is also true that not all regular users of alcohol become alcoholics. There is much argument over the definition of an alcoholic. A widely used definition is: a person who has experienced physical, psychological, social, or occupational impairment as a consequence of habitual, excessive consumption of alcohol.

Recognizing the dangers of drug dependence

Factors that determine a person's risk of developing physical dependence include the characteristics of the drug itself, the strength and frequency of doses, and the duration of use. However, the presence of these factors does not always result in dependence. Psychological and physiological factors that are unique to each individual also enter into the equation, and there may be other, as yet unknown, factors involved. For example, when the use of opioid analgesics is

DRUG MISUSE

The term is defined as any use of drugs that causes physical, psychological, economic, legal, or social harm to the user, or to persons who may be affected by the user's behaviour. Drug abuse commonly refers to taking drugs obtained illegally (such as heroin), but may also be used to describe the misuse of drugs generally obtainable legally (nicotine, alcohol), and to drugs obtainable through a doctor's prescription only (everything from sleeping drugs and tranquillizers to analgesics and stimulants).

The misuse of prescription drugs deserves more attention than it usually receives. The practice can include the personal use of drugs left over from a previous course of treatment, the sharing with others of drugs that have been prescribed for yourself, the deliberate deception of doctors, the forgery of prescriptions, and the theft of drugs from pharmacies. All of these practices can have dangerous consequences. Careful attention

to the advice in the section on Managing your drug treatment (p.25) will help to avoid inadvertent misuse of drugs. The dangers associated with abuse of individual drugs are discussed under Drugs of abuse (pp.450–459).

Commonly misused drugs	
Alcohol	Mescaline
Amphetamines	Nicotine
Barbiturates	Nitrates
Benzodiazepines	Opioids (including
Cocaine (including	heroin and
crack)	methadone
Ecstasy	Phencyclidine
GHB	Solvents
Ketamine	
Khat	
LSD	
Marijuana (cannabis)	

restricted to the short-term relief of pain in a medical setting, dependence is rare. Yet there is a high risk of physical dependence when opioid analgesics, or other drugs of abuse, are taken for non-medical reasons. There is also a risk in some cases of low-dose use when the drug is continued over a long period (e.g. with benzodiazepines, p.83). No one can

say for sure exactly what leads a person to drug-dependent behaviour. A person's psychological and physical make-up are thought to be factors, as well as his or her social environment, occupational pressures, and outlook on life.

The indiscriminate use of certain prescription drugs can also cause drug dependence. Benzodiazepine drugs can produce dependence, and this is one reason why doctors today discourage the use of any drug to induce sleep or calm anxiety for more than a few weeks. Appetite suppressants (see p.88) require close medical supervision. Amphetamines are no longer prescribed as appetite suppressants because of the frequency with which they are abused.

Treating drug dependence

Treatment for drug dependence can only be effective if the person is sufficiently motivated. There are two parts to treatment. The first part, detoxification, can take different forms. In some cases, if it is possible to do so, abstinence may be abruptly imposed. Sometimes, the drug may be gradually withdrawn or other safer substances substituted. For example, methadone (p.340) is substituted for heroin. Physical or mental withdrawal symptoms may need close monitoring, for instance, withdrawal from depressants such as barbiturates or alcohol may result in convulsions. Once the drug has been cleared from the body, the second part of treatment is directed at preventing a recurrence. This can involve psychological therapies to tackle the initial cause of the dependence, such as social problems or depression. Psychotherapy, personal counselling, and the work of support organizations, such as Alcoholics Anonymous, may all play a role in the rehabilitation of the alcoholic or addict.

SYMPTOMS OF WITHDRAWAL

These can range from the mild (sneezing, sweating) to the serious (vomiting, confusion) to the extremely serious (fits, coma). Alcohol withdrawal may be associated with delirium tremens, very occasionally fatal. Withdrawal from benzodiazepines can sometimes involve hallucinations and fits. But under medical guidance, withdrawal symptoms can be

relieved with doses of the original drug, or with less addictive substitutes.

Withdrawal symptoms occur because the body has adapted to the action of the drug (see Drug tolerance, p.23). When a drug is continuously present, the body may stop the release of a natural chemical necessary to normal function, like endorphins (below).

Pain and heroin withdrawal

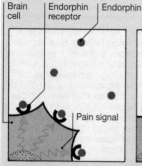

Normal brain
When no drug is present, natural substances called endorphins inhibit the transmission of pain signals.

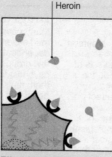

Effect of heroin
Heroin occupies the same receptors in the brain as endorphins, suppressing production of endorphins.

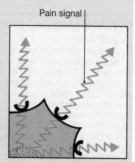

Heroin withdrawal
Abrupt withdrawal of heroin leaves the brain without a buffer to pain signals, even from minor stimuli.

MANAGING YOUR DRUG TREATMENT

A prescribed drug does not automatically produce a beneficial response. For a drug to have maximum benefit, it must be taken as directed by the doctor or manufacturer. It is estimated that two out of every five people for whom a drug is prescribed do not take it properly, if at all. The reasons include failure to understand or remember instructions, fear of adverse reactions, and lack of motivation, often arising from the disappearance of symptoms.

It is your responsibility to take a prescribed drug at the correct time, and in the manner stipulated. To do this, you need to know where to obtain information about the drug (see Questioning your doctor, p.26) and to make certain that you fully understand the instructions.

The following pages describe the practical aspects of drug treatment, from obtaining a prescription and buying over-the-counter drugs to storing drugs and disposing of old medications safely. Problems caused by mismanaging drug treatment – overdosing, underdosing, or stopping the drug altogether – and long-term drug treatment are dealt with on pp.28–31. Information regarding specific drugs is given in Part 4.

OVER-THE-COUNTER DRUGS

Over-the-counter drugs are those for which a prescription is not required. All are available from pharmacies (many only from pharmacies) but some, called General Sales List (GSL) medicines, are very widely sold, even by supermarkets.

It is generally accepted that over-the-counter drugs are suitable for self-treatment and are unlikely to produce serious adverse reactions if taken as directed. But, as with all medicines, they can be harmful if they are misused. The ease with which they can be purchased is no guarantee of their absolute safety. For this reason, the same precautions should be taken when using any over-the-counter medicine as when using a prescription drug.

Using over-the-counter drugs

A number of minor ailments and problems, ranging from coughs and colds to minor cuts and bruises, can be adequately dealt with by taking or using over-the-counter medicines. However, you must be sure to read the directions on the label and follow them carefully, particularly those advising on dosage and under what circumstances a doctor should be consulted. Most over-the-counter drugs are clearly labelled. They may warn of conditions under which the drug should not be taken, or advise you to consult a doctor if symptoms persist.

The pharmacist is a good source of information about over-the-counter drugs and can usually tell you what is suitable for your complaint. He or she can also determine when an over-the-counter drug may not be effective and can warn you if self-treatment or prolonged treatment is not advisable. When consulting the pharmacist regarding over-the-counter drugs, you should inform him or her if you are taking prescription drugs for any other illnesses.

It is important to speak to your doctor before buying over-the-counter drugs for children. Some symptoms, such as diarrhoea in young children, should be treated only by a doctor since they may be caused by a serious condition.

Buying over-the-counter medications
Various drugs are available over the counter, ranging from cough medicines to eye drops. Your pharmacist can often help you to select the appropriate medication.

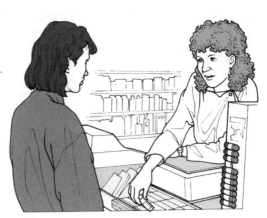

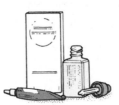
Eye preparations

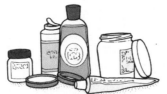
Medicated creams, lotions, and powders

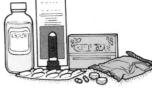
Cough and cold treatments

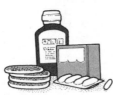
Laxatives

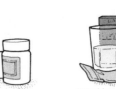
Analgesics

Antacids

PRESCRIPTION DRUGS

Drugs prescribed by your doctor are not necessarily "stronger" or more likely to have side effects than those you can buy without prescription. Indeed, doctors often prescribe drugs that are also available over the counter. Drugs that are available only on prescription are drugs whose safe use is difficult to ensure without medical supervision.

When a doctor prescribes a drug, he or she usually starts treatment at the normal dosage for the disorder being treated. The dosage may later be adjusted (lowered or increased) if the drug is not producing the desired effect or if there are adverse effects, and the doctor may also switch to an alternative drug that may be more effective.

Prescribing generic and brand-name drugs

When writing a prescription for a drug, the doctor often has a choice between a generic and a brand-name product. Although the active ingredient is the same, two versions of the same drug may act in slightly different ways, as each manufacturer may formulate their product differently. They may also look different. Generic drugs are sometimes cheaper than brand-name products. For this reason, certain brand-name products are not available on the National Health Service. For example, Valium, a well-known brand-name tranquillizer, is not prescribable on the NHS and a generic version of diazepam, the active drug, is always substituted. These are factors that a doctor must consider when writing a prescription.

Community pharmacists are obliged to dispense precisely what the doctor has written on the prescription form and are not allowed to substitute a generic drug when a brand-name has been specified.

However, if you are prescribed a generic drug, the pharmacist is free to dispense whatever version of this drug is available. This means that your regular medication may vary in appearance each time you renew your prescription.

Hospital pharmacies often dispense only generic versions of certain drugs. Therefore, if you are in hospital, the regular medication you receive may look different from that which you are used to at home.

Your prescription

It is advisable for you to obtain all of your prescription drugs from the same pharmacist or at least from the same pharmacy, so that your pharmacist can advise you about any particular problems you may have, and keep supplies of any unusual drugs you may be taking.

If you need to take drugs that are prescribed by more than one doctor, or by your dentist in addition to your doctor, the pharmacist is able to call attention to possible harmful interactions. Doctors do ask if you are taking other medicines, but your regular pharmacist provides valuable additional advice.

Questioning your doctor

Countless surveys unmistakably point to lack of information as the most common reason for drug failure. Responses like "The doctor is too busy to be bothered with a lot of questions" or "The doctor will think I'm stupid if I ask that" recur over and over. Be certain you understand the instructions for a drug before leaving the doctor, and don't leave with any questions unanswered.

It is a good idea to make a list of the questions you may want to ask before your visit, and to make a few notes while you are there about what you are told. It

is not uncommon to forget some of the instructions your doctor gives you during a consultation.

Know what you are taking

Your doctor should tell you the generic or brand name of the drug he or she is prescribing, and exactly what condition or symptom it has been prescribed to treat.

As well as telling you the name of the drug prescribed, your doctor should explain what dose you should take, how often to take it, and whether the prescription should be repeated. Be certain you understand the instructions about how and when to take the drug (see also Taking your medication, facing page). For example, does four times a day mean four times during the time you are awake, or four times in 24 hours? Ask your doctor how long the treatment should last; some medications cause harmful effects if you stop taking them abruptly, or do not have beneficial effects unless the course of drug treatment is completed.

To help you remember, the label on your dispensed medicine may repeat the instructions, and the pharmacist will give you a patient information leaflet that will give you detailed information about the drug. The pharmacist can also help by answering your questions, if you have forgotten to ask the doctor.

Risks and special precautions

All drugs have *adverse effects* (see The effects of drugs, p.15), and you should know what these are. Ask your doctor what the possible adverse effects of the drug are and what you should do if they occur. Also ask if there are any foods, activities, or other drugs you should avoid during treatment, and if you can drink alcohol while taking the drug.

Your prescription

Your prescription tells the pharmacist what to supply and what to put on the label. If the prescription and label differ, ask the pharmacist about it. The label will usually have a "do not use after" date. If it does not, ask the pharmacist to advise you. Usually, you will receive a Patient Information Leaflet, which gives details about the drug, its adverse effects, whether it is safe for you, when not to use it, and so on. Compare this with your doctor's instructions, and ask the pharmacist about any differences.

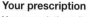

Patient's name and address

Drug name and strength

When to take

Quantity to be dispensed

Doctor's signature

Doctor's name and address

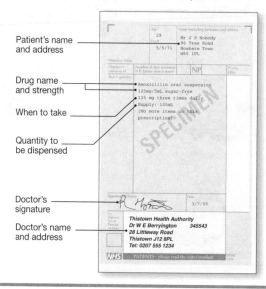

PRESCRIPTION TERMS

ac before meals	**pc** after meals
ad lib freely	**PM** evening
AM morning	**po** by mouth
bd twice a day	**prn** as needed
c with	**qds** four times
cap capsule	a day
cc cubic centimetre	**s** without
ext for external use	**sr** slow release
gtt drops	**stat** at once
mg milligrams	**tab** tablet
ml millilitres	**tds** three times
nocte at night	a day
od each day	**top** apply topically
om each morning	**ud** use as directed
on each night	**x** times

TAKING YOUR MEDICATION

Among the most important aspects of managing your drug treatment is knowing how often the drug is to be taken. Should it be taken on an empty stomach? With food? Mixed with something? Specific instructions on such points are given in the individual drug profiles in Part 4.

When to take your drugs

Certain drugs, such as analgesics and drugs for migraine, are taken only as necessary, when warning symptoms occur. Others are meant to be taken regularly at specified intervals. The prescription or label instructions can be confusing, however. For instance, does four times a day mean once every six hours out of 24 – at 8 am, 2 pm, 8 pm, and 2 am? Or does it mean take at four equal intervals during waking hours – morning, lunchtime, late afternoon, and bedtime? The latter is usually the case but you need to ask your doctor for precise directions.

The actual time of day that you take a drug is generally flexible, so you can normally schedule your doses to fit your daily routine. This has the additional advantage of making it easier for you to remember to take your drugs. For example, if you are to take the drug three times during the day, it may be most convenient to take the first dose at 7 am, the second at 3 pm, and the third at 11 pm, while it may be more suitable for another person on the same regimen to take the first dose at 8 am, and so on. You must, however, establish with your pharmacist or your doctor whether the drug should be taken with food, in which case you would probably need to take it with your breakfast, lunch, and dinner. Try to take your dose at the recommended intervals; if you take them too close

Four times a day?

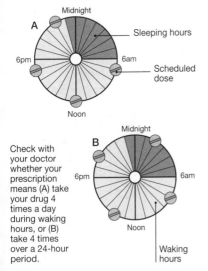

Check with your doctor whether your prescription means (A) take your drug 4 times a day during waking hours, or (B) take 4 times over a 24-hour period.

TIPS ON TAKING MEDICINES

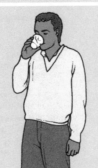

● Whenever possible, take capsules and tablets while standing up or in an upright sitting position, and take them with water. If you take them when you are lying down, or without enough water, it is possible for the capsules or tablets to become stuck in the oesophagus. This can delay the action of the drug and may damage the oesophagus.

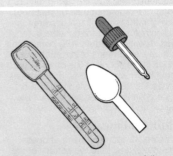

● Always measure your dose carefully, using a 5ml spoon or an accurate measure such as a dropper, children's medicine spoon, or oral syringe.

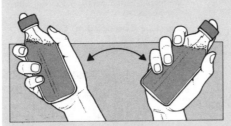

● When taking liquid medicines, shake the bottle before measuring each dose, or you may take improper dosages if the active substance has risen to the top or settled at the bottom of the bottle.

● A drink of cold water taken immediately after an unpleasantly flavoured medicine will often hide the taste.

together, the risk of side effects occurring is increased.

If you are taking several different drugs, ask your doctor if they can be taken together, or if they must be taken at different times in order to avoid any adverse effects or reduced effectiveness caused by an interaction between them.

How to take your drugs

If your prescription specifies taking your drug with food – or without food – it is very important to follow this instruction if you are to get the maximum benefit from your treatment.

Certain drugs, such as ampicillin and captopril, should be taken on an empty stomach (usually one to two hours before eating) so they will be absorbed more quickly into the bloodstream; others, such as ibuprofen, metronidazole, and allopurinol, should be taken with food to avoid stomach irritation. Similarly, you should comply with any instructions to avoid particular foods. Milk and dairy products may inhibit the absorption of some drugs, such as tetracycline; fruit juices can break down certain antibacterial drugs in the stomach and thereby decrease their effectiveness; alcohol is best avoided with many drugs. (See also Drug interactions, p.16.)

In some cases, when taking diuretics, for example, you may be advised to eat foods rich in potassium. But do not take potassium supplements unless you are advised to do so by your doctor (see Potassium, p.443). If you use any of the salt substitutes (all of which contain potassium), remember to tell your doctor.

GIVING MEDICINES TO CHILDREN

A number of over-the-counter medicines are specifically prepared for children. Many other medicines have labels that give both adult's and children's dosages. For the purposes of drug labelling, anyone 12 years of age or under is considered a child.

When giving over-the-counter medicines to children, you should always follow the instructions on the label exactly and under no circumstances exceed the dosage recommended for a child. Never give a child even a small amount of a medicine intended for adult use without the advice of your doctor.

Do not deceive your child about the medicine, such as pretending that tablets are sweets or that liquid medicines are soft drinks. Never leave a child's medicine within reach; he or she may be tempted to take an extra dose in order to hasten recovery.

MISSED DOSES

Missing a dose of your medication can be a problem only if you are taking the drug as part of a regular course of treatment. Missing a drug dose is not uncommon and it is not a cause for concern in most cases. The missed dose may sometimes produce a recurrence of symptoms or a change in the action of the drug, so you should know what to do when you have forgotten to take your medication. For advice on individual drugs, consult the drug profile in Part 4.

Additional measures

With some drugs, the timing of doses depends on how long the actions of the drugs last. When you miss a drug dose, the amount of drug in your body is lowered, and the effect of the drug may be diminished. You may therefore have to take other steps to avoid unwanted consequences. For example, if you are taking an oral contraceptive that contains progesterone only and you forget to take one pill at your usual time, you should take the pill as soon as you remember and for the next 48 hours use another form of contraception.

If you miss more than one dose of any drug you are taking regularly, you should tell your doctor. Missed doses are especially important with insulin and drugs for epilepsy.

If you frequently forget to take your medication, you should tell your doctor. He or she may be able to simplify your treatment schedule by prescribing a multi-ingredient preparation that contains several drugs, or a preparation that releases the drug slowly into the body over a period of time, and only needs to be taken once or twice daily.

REMEMBERING YOUR MEDICATION

If you take several different drugs, it is useful to draw up a chart to remind yourself of when each drug should be taken. This will also help anyone who looks after you, or a doctor who is unfamiliar with your treatment.

The example given here is of a dosage chart for an elderly woman suffering from arthritis and a heart condition who has trouble sleeping. Her doctor has prescribed the following treatment:

Bumetanide (a diuretic to counter fluid retention), one 1mg tablet in the morning.

Amiloride (another diuretic to counter the potassium loss caused by bumetanide), two 5mg tablets in the morning.

Ibuprofen (for arthritis), three 400mg tablets daily with meals.

Verapamil (to treat her heart condition), three 40mg capsules a day.

Zopiclone (a sleeping drug), one 3.75mg capsule at bedtime.

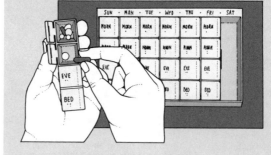

Dosage Chart

8am	1pm
1 x Bumetanide	1 x Ibuprofen
2 x Amiloride	1 x Verapamil
1 x Ibuprofen	
1 x Verapamil	
7pm	11pm
1 x Ibuprofen	1 x Verapamil
	1 x Zopiclone

Pill box
Using a pill box is a handy way of making sure you take your tablets in the right order. There is a strip for each day of the week, and compartments for morning, afternoon, evening, and bedtime.

ENDING DRUG TREATMENT

As with missed doses, ending drug treatment too soon can be a problem when you are taking a regular course of drugs. With medication that you take as required, you can stop treatment as soon as you feel better.

Advice on stopping individual drugs is given in the drug profiles in Part 4. Some general guidelines for ending drug treatment are given below.

Risks of stopping too soon

Suddenly stopping drug treatment before completing your course of medication may cause the original condition to recur or lead to other complications, including withdrawal symptoms. The disappearance of the symptoms does not necessarily mean that a disorder is cured. Even if you feel better, do not stop taking the drug unless your doctor advises you to do so. People taking antibiotics often stop too

soon, but the full course of treatment prescribed should always be followed.

Adverse effects

Do not stop taking a medication simply because it produces unpleasant side effects. Many adverse effects disappear or become bearable after a while. But if they do not, check with your doctor, who may want to reduce the dosage of the drug gradually or, alternatively, substitute another drug that does not produce the same side effects.

Gradual reduction

While many medications can be stopped abruptly, others need to be reduced gradually to prevent a reaction when treatment ends. This is the case with long-term corticosteroid therapy (see right) as well as with *dependence*-inducing drugs.

Phased reduction of corticosteroids

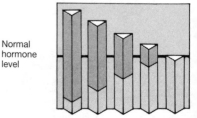

Corticosteroid drug

Natural adrenal hormone

Normal hormone level

Corticosteroid drugs suppress production in the body of natural adrenal hormones. A phased reduction of the dosage allows levels of the natural hormones to revert to normal. The last stages of withdrawal are made very slowly.

STORING DRUGS

Once you have completed a medically directed course of treatment, you should not keep any unused drugs. But most families will want to keep a supply of remedies for indigestion, headaches, colds, and so forth. Such medicines should not be used if they show any signs of deterioration, or if their period of effectiveness has expired (see When to dispose of drugs, right).

How to store drugs

All drugs, including cough medicines, iron tablets, and oral contraceptives, should be kept out of the reach of children. If you are in the habit of keeping your medicines where you will see them as a reminder to take them, leave an empty medicine container out instead, and put the drug itself safely out of reach.

Over-the-counter and prescription drugs should normally be stored in the container in which you purchased them. If it is necessary to put them into other containers, such as special containers designed for the elderly, make sure you keep the original container with the label, as well as any separate instructions, for future reference.

Make certain that caps and lids are replaced and tightly closed after use; loose caps may leak and spill, or hasten deterioration of the drug.

Where to store drugs

The majority of drugs should be stored in a cool, dry place out of direct sunlight, even those in plastic containers or tinted glass. Room temperature, away from sources of direct heat, is suitable for most medicines. A few drugs should be stored in the refrigerator. Storage information for individual drugs is given in the drug profiles in Part 4.

Wall cabinets that can be locked are ideal for storing drugs, as long as the cabinet itself is located in a cool, dry place and not, as often happens, in the bathroom, which is frequently warm and humid.

WHEN TO DISPOSE OF DRUGS

Old drugs should be flushed down the toilet or returned to the pharmacist, but not put in the dustbin. Always dispose of:

● Any drug that is past its expiry date.

● Aspirin and paracetamol tablets that smell of vinegar.

● Tablets that are chipped, cracked, or discoloured, and capsules that have softened, cracked, or stuck together.

● Liquids that have thickened or discoloured, or that taste or smell different in any way from the original product.

● Tubes that are cracked, leaky, or hard.

● Ointments and creams that have changed odour, or changed appearance by discolouring, hardening, or separating.

● Any liquid needing refrigeration that has been kept for over two weeks.

LONG-TERM DRUG TREATMENT

Many people require regular, prolonged treatment with one or more drugs. People who suffer from chronic or recurrent disorders often need lifelong treatment with drugs to control symptoms or prevent complications. Antihypertensive drugs for high blood pressure and insulin or oral antidiabetic drugs for diabetes mellitus are familiar examples. Many other disorders take a long time to cure; for example, people with tuberculosis usually need at least six months' treatment with antituberculous drugs. Long-term drug treatment may also be necessary to prevent a condition from occurring, and will have to be taken for as long as the individual is at risk. Antimalarial drugs are a good example.

Possible adverse effects

You may worry that taking a drug for a long period will reduce its effectiveness or that you will become dependent on it. However, *tolerance* develops only with a few drugs; most medicines continue to have the same effect indefinitely without necessitating an increase in dosage or change in drug. Similarly, taking a drug for more than a few weeks does not normally create dependence.

Changing drug treatment

If you are taking a drug regularly, you will need to know what to do if something else occurs to affect your health. If you wish to become pregnant, for example, you should ask your doctor right away if it is preferable to continue on your regular medicine or switch to another less likely to affect your pregnancy. If you contract a new illness, for which an additional drug is prescribed, your regular treatment may be altered.

There are a number of other reasons for changing a drug. You may have had an adverse reaction, or an improved preparation may have become available.

Adjusting to long-term treatment

You should establish a daily routine for taking your medication in order to reduce the risk of a missed dose. Usually you should not stop taking your medication, even if there are side effects, without consulting your doctor (see Ending drug treatment, facing page). If you fear possible side effects from the drug, discuss this with your doctor.

Many people deliberately stop their drugs because they feel well or their symptoms disappear. This can be dangerous, especially with a disease like high blood pressure, which has no noticeable symptoms. Stopping treatment may lead to a recurrence or worsening of a disease. If you are uncertain about why you have to keep taking a drug, ask your doctor.

Only a few drugs require an alteration in habits. Some drugs should not be taken with alcohol; with a few drugs you should avoid certain foods. If you require a drug that makes you drowsy, you should not drive a car or operate dangerous equipment.

If you are taking a drug that should not be stopped suddenly or that may interact with other drugs, it is a good idea to carry a warning card or bracelet, a Medic Alert for example. Such information might be essential for emergency medical treatment in an accident.

Monitoring treatment

If you are on long-term treatment, you need to visit your doctor for periodic check-ups. He or she will check your underlying condition and monitor any adverse effects of treatment. Levels of the drug in the blood may be measured. With insulin, in addition to checks with the doctor, you need to monitor blood or urine levels each day.

If a drug is known to cause damage to an organ, tests may be done to check the function of the organ. For example, blood and urine tests to check kidney function, or a blood count to check the bone marrow, may be indicated.

Medical check-ups
Blood pressure is commonly checked in people on long-term drug treatment.

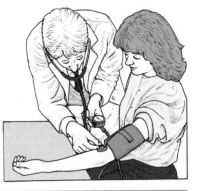

EXCEEDING THE DOSE

Most people associate drug overdoses with attempts at suicide or the fatalities and near fatalities brought on by abuse of street drugs. However, drug overdoses can also occur among people who deliberately or inadvertently exceed the stated dose of a drug that has been prescribed for them by their doctor.

A single extra dose of most drugs is unlikely to be a cause for concern, although accidental overdoses can create anxiety in the individual and his or her family, and may cause overdose symptoms, which can appear in a variety of different forms.

Overdose of some drugs, however, is potentially dangerous even when the dose has been exceeded by only a small amount. Each of the drug profiles in Part 4 gives detailed information on the consequences of exceeding the dose, symptoms to look out for, and what to do. Each drug has an overdose danger rating of low, medium, or high, which are described fully on p.186.

Taking an extra dose

People sometimes exceed the stated dose in the mistaken belief that by increasing dosage they will obtain more

Effects of repeated overdose
Repeated overdose of a drug over an extended period may lead to a build-up of high levels of the drug in the body, especially if liver or kidney function is reduced.

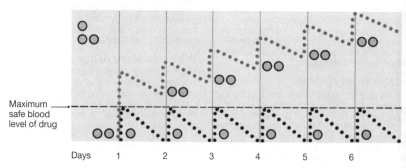

Maximum safe blood level of drug

Days   1   2   3   4   5   6

immediate action or a more effective cure. This action is a particular risk with *tolerance*-inducing drugs (see Drug tolerance and dependence, p.23). Others exceed their dose accidentally, by miscalculating the amount or forgetting that the dose has already been taken.

Taking extra doses is often a problem in the elderly, who may repeat their dose through forgetfulness or confusion. This is

a special risk with medicines that cause drowsiness (see also p.22).

In some cases, especially when liver or kidney function is impaired, the drug builds up in the blood because the body cannot break down and excrete the extra dose quickly enough, so that symptoms of poisoning may result. Symptoms of excessive intake may not be apparent for many days.

When and how to get help

If you are not sure whether or not you have taken your medicine, think back and check again. If you honestly cannot remember, assume that you have missed the dose and follow the advice given in the individual drug profiles in Part 4 of this book. If you cannot find your drug, consult your doctor. Make a note to use some system in the future which will help you remember to take your medicine.

If you are looking after an elderly person on regular drug treatment who suddenly develops unusual symptoms such as confusion, drowsiness, or unsteadiness, consider the possibility of an inadvertent drug overdose and consult the doctor as soon as possible.

Deliberate overdose

While many cases of drug overdose are accidental or the result of a mistaken belief that increasing the dose will enhance the benefits of drug treatment, sometimes an excessive amount of a drug is taken with the intention of causing harm or even as a suicide attempt. Whether or not you think a dangerous amount of a drug has been taken, deliberate overdoses of this kind should always be brought to the attention of your doctor. Not only is it necessary to ensure that no physical harm has occurred as a result of the overdose, but the psychological condition of a person who takes such action may indicate the need for additional medical help, especially when the person is elderly, has a physical illness, or is known to suffer from depression.

THE EFFECT OF DRUG OVERDOSE ON THE BODY

The effect of drug overdose on the body depends on the type of drug involved. Some drugs produce an exaggeration of the desired effect, for instance overdose of tranquillizers leads to unconsciousness. With many drugs, the toxic overdose effects are unrelated to the action or side effects of the drug when it is taken in normal doses.

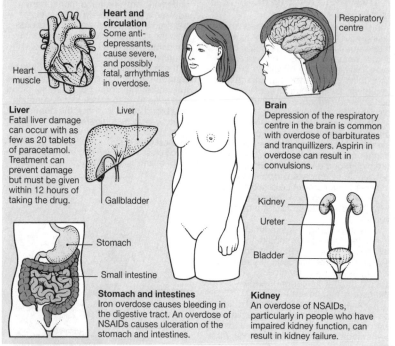

Heart and circulation
Some antidepressants, cause severe, and possibly fatal, arrhythmias in overdose.

Heart muscle

Liver
Fatal liver damage can occur with as few as 20 tablets of paracetamol. Treatment can prevent damage but must be given within 12 hours of taking the drug.

Liver

Gallbladder

Stomach

Small intestine

Brain
Depression of the respiratory centre in the brain is common with overdose of barbiturates and tranquillizers. Aspirin in overdose can result in convulsions.

Respiratory centre

Kidney

Ureter

Bladder

Stomach and intestines
Iron overdose causes bleeding in the digestive tract. An overdose of NSAIDs causes ulceration of the stomach and intestines.

Kidney
An overdose of NSAIDs, particularly in people who have impaired kidney function, can result in kidney failure.

DOs AND DON'Ts

On this page you will find a summary of the most important practical points concerning the management of your drug treatment. The advice is arranged under general headings, explaining the safest methods of storing drugs and following treatment, whether it is a prescribed medicine or an over-the-counter drug. This information is equally applicable whether you are taking medicine yourself or supervising the drug treatment of someone in your care.

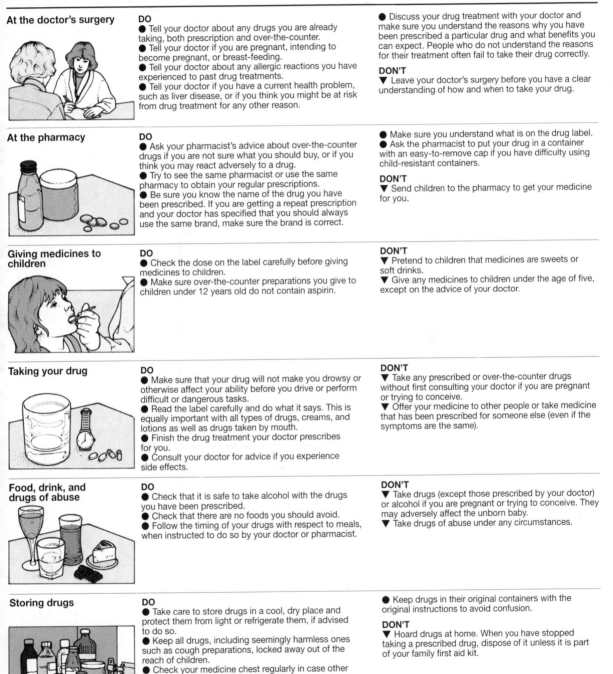

At the doctor's surgery

DO
● Tell your doctor about any drugs you are already taking, both prescription and over-the-counter.
● Tell your doctor if you are pregnant, intending to become pregnant, or breast-feeding.
● Tell your doctor about any allergic reactions you have experienced to past drug treatments.
● Tell your doctor if you have a current health problem, such as liver disease, or if you think you might be at risk from drug treatment for any other reason.

● Discuss your drug treatment with your doctor and make sure you understand the reasons why you have been prescribed a particular drug and what benefits you can expect. People who do not understand the reasons for their treatment often fail to take their drug correctly.
DON'T
▼ Leave your doctor's surgery before you have a clear understanding of how and when to take your drug.

At the pharmacy

DO
● Ask your pharmacist's advice about over-the-counter drugs if you are not sure what you should buy, or if you think you may react adversely to a drug.
● Try to see the same pharmacist or use the same pharmacy to obtain your regular prescriptions.
● Be sure you know the name of the drug you have been prescribed. If you are getting a repeat prescription and your doctor has specified that you should always use the same brand, make sure the brand is correct.

● Make sure you understand what is on the drug label.
● Ask the pharmacist to put your drug in a container with an easy-to-remove cap if you have difficulty using child-resistant containers.
DON'T
▼ Send children to the pharmacy to get your medicine for you.

Giving medicines to children

DO
● Check the dose on the label carefully before giving medicines to children.
● Make sure over-the-counter preparations you give to children under 12 years old do not contain aspirin.

DON'T
▼ Pretend to children that medicines are sweets or soft drinks.
▼ Give any medicines to children under the age of five, except on the advice of your doctor.

Taking your drug

DO
● Make sure that your drug will not make you drowsy or otherwise affect your ability before you drive or perform difficult or dangerous tasks.
● Read the label carefully and do what it says. This is equally important with all types of drugs, creams, and lotions as well as drugs taken by mouth.
● Finish the drug treatment your doctor prescribes for you.
● Consult your doctor for advice if you experience side effects.

DON'T
▼ Take any prescribed or over-the-counter drugs without first consulting your doctor if you are pregnant or trying to conceive.
▼ Offer your medicine to other people or take medicine that has been prescribed for someone else (even if the symptoms are the same).

Food, drink, and drugs of abuse

DO
● Check that it is safe to take alcohol with the drugs you have been prescribed.
● Check that there are no foods you should avoid.
● Follow the timing of your drugs with respect to meals, when instructed to do so by your doctor or pharmacist.

DON'T
▼ Take drugs (except those prescribed by your doctor) or alcohol if you are pregnant or trying to conceive. They may adversely affect the unborn baby.
▼ Take drugs of abuse under any circumstances.

Storing drugs

DO
● Take care to store drugs in a cool, dry place and protect them from light or refrigerate them, if advised to do so.
● Keep all drugs, including seemingly harmless ones such as cough preparations, locked away out of the reach of children.
● Check your medicine chest regularly in case other members of the family have left their unwanted drugs in it, and to make sure that none of the normal supplies are out of date.

● Keep drugs in their original containers with the original instructions to avoid confusion.
DON'T
▼ Hoard drugs at home. When you have stopped taking a prescribed drug, dispose of it unless it is part of your family first aid kit.

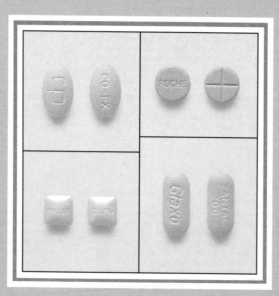

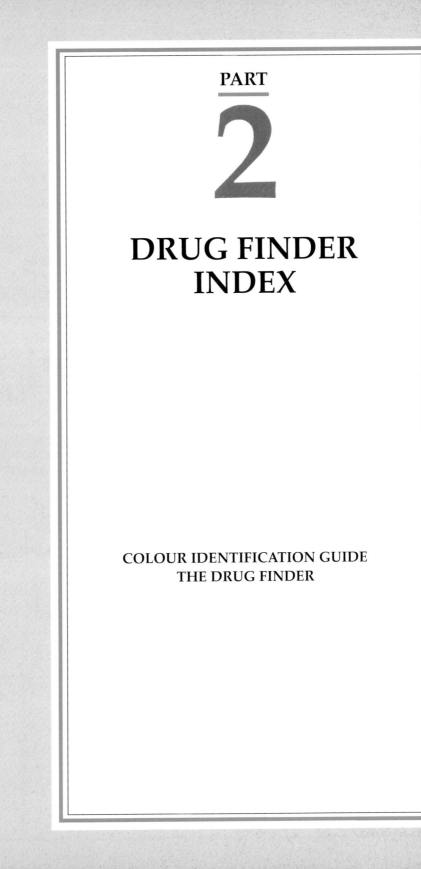

PART

2

DRUG FINDER
INDEX

COLOUR IDENTIFICATION GUIDE
THE DRUG FINDER

COLOUR IDENTIFICATION GUIDE

The following pages contain photographs of 240 brand-name drug products. The guide has seven sections – one-colour tablets, multicolour tablets, one-colour capsules, white capsules, multicolour capsules, white tablets, patches, and pens. Within each section the products are arranged according to their colour and size. The inclusion of a particular product in no way implies endorsement by the British Medical Association of that specific brand or product.

The products included on these pages represent a selection of the most popular brand names in use in Britain. Several dosage strengths of some of the more widely prescribed brand name products have been included. Each drug is photographed approximately life-size. Beneath each photograph you will find the name of the tablet, capsule, patch, or pen with details of its main generic ingredients and their amounts in grams (g), milligrams (mg), millimoles (mmols), micrograms (mcg), or international units (IU). The products are laid out in a grid format. Each entry can be located from the Drug Finder by reference to the page number and the letter in the top left-hand corner of each square of the grid.

To locate the photograph of a particular drug, consult the chart below, which will direct you to the relevant colour section. An example of an entry is also explained.

HOW TO LOCATE YOUR MEDICATION

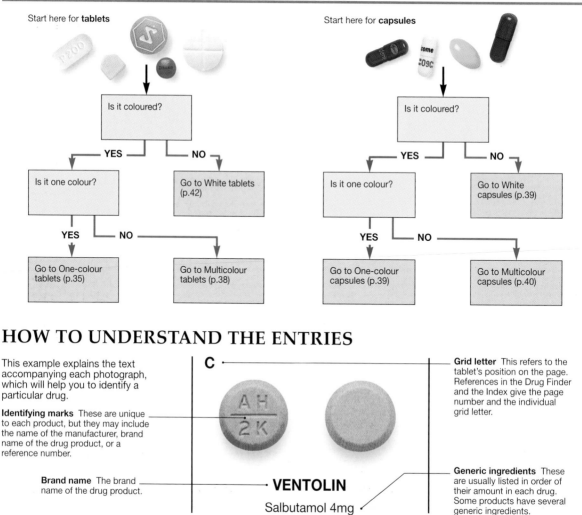

Start here for **tablets**

Is it coloured?
- YES → Is it one colour?
  - YES → Go to One-colour tablets (p.35)
  - NO → Go to Multicolour tablets (p.38)
- NO → Go to White tablets (p.42)

Start here for **capsules**

Is it coloured?
- YES → Is it one colour?
  - YES → Go to One-colour capsules (p.39)
  - NO → Go to Multicolour capsules (p.40)
- NO → Go to White capsules (p.39)

HOW TO UNDERSTAND THE ENTRIES

This example explains the text accompanying each photograph, which will help you to identify a particular drug.

Identifying marks These are unique to each product, but they may include the name of the manufacturer, brand name of the drug product, or a reference number.

Brand name The brand name of the drug product.

C

VENTOLIN

Salbutamol 4mg

Grid letter This refers to the tablet's position on the page. References in the Drug Finder and the Index give the page number and the individual grid letter.

Generic ingredients These are usually listed in order of their amount in each drug. Some products have several generic ingredients.

ONE-COLOUR TABLETS

A

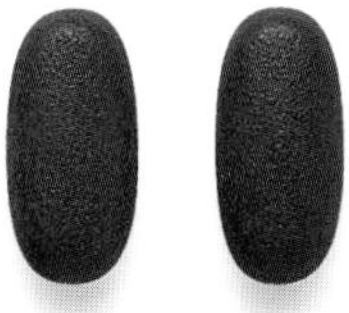

WELLDORM

Chloral hydrate 414mg

B

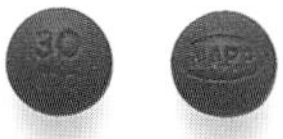

MST CONTINUS

Morphine sulphate 30mg

C

VENTOLIN

Salbutamol 4mg

D

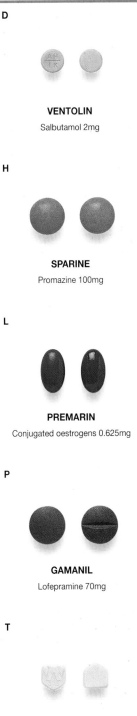

VENTOLIN

Salbutamol 2mg

E

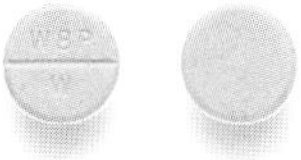

WARFARIN

Warfarin 5mg

F

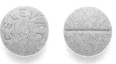

CELEVAC

Methyl cellulose 500mg

G

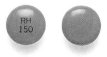

RIFINAH 150

Rifampicin 150mg
Isoniazid 100mg

H

SPARINE

Promazine 100mg

I

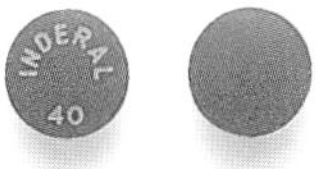

INDERAL

Propranolol 40mg

J

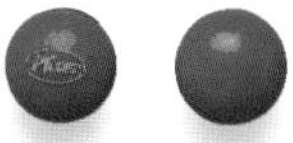

DELTACORTRIL ENTERIC

Prednisolone 5mg

K

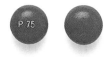

PROTHIADEN

Dothiepin 75mg

L

PREMARIN

Conjugated oestrogens 0.625mg

M

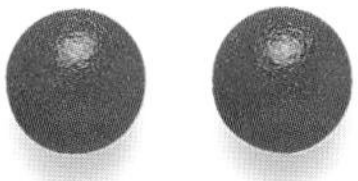

ERYTHROMID

Erythromycin 250mg

N

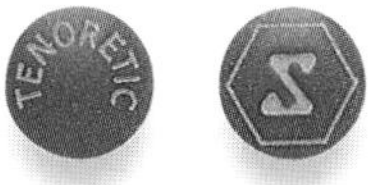

TENORETIC

Atenolol 100mg
Chlortalidone 25mg

O

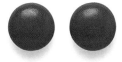

NYSTAN

Nystatin 500,000 units

P

GAMANIL

Lofepramine 70mg

Q

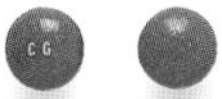

TOFRANIL

Imipramine 25mg

R

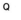

ZOCOR

Simvastatin 20mg

S

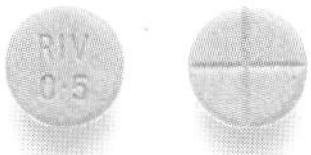

RIVOTRIL

Clonazepam 0.5mg

T

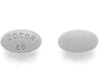

EFEXOR

Venlafaxine 37.5mg

ONE-COLOUR TABLETS continued

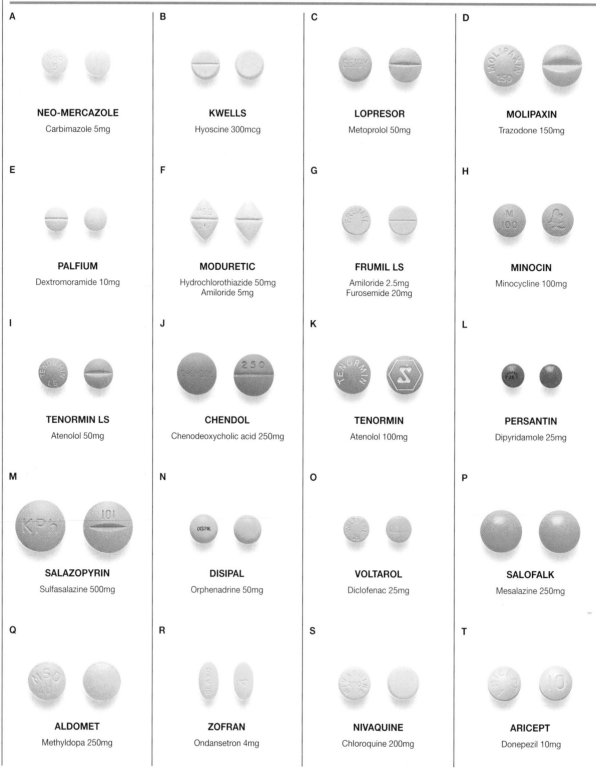

A

NEO-MERCAZOLE

Carbimazole 5mg

B

KWELLS

Hyoscine 300mcg

C

LOPRESOR

Metoprolol 50mg

D

MOLIPAXIN

Trazodone 150mg

E

PALFIUM

Dextromoramide 10mg

F

MODURETIC

Hydrochlorothiazide 50mg
Amiloride 5mg

G

FRUMIL LS

Amiloride 2.5mg
Furosemide 20mg

H

MINOCIN

Minocycline 100mg

I

TENORMIN LS

Atenolol 50mg

J

CHENDOL

Chenodeoxycholic acid 250mg

K

TENORMIN

Atenolol 100mg

L

PERSANTIN

Dipyridamole 25mg

M

SALAZOPYRIN

Sulfasalazine 500mg

N

DISIPAL

Orphenadrine 50mg

O

VOLTAROL

Diclofenac 25mg

P

SALOFALK

Mesalazine 250mg

Q

ALDOMET

Methyldopa 250mg

R

ZOFRAN

Ondansetron 4mg

S

NIVAQUINE

Chloroquine 200mg

T

ARICEPT

Donepezil 10mg

A

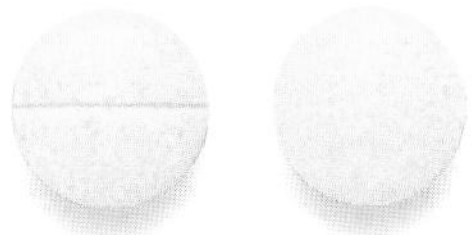

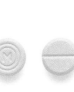

DROGENIL

Flutamide 250mg

B

CLOMID

Clomifene 50mg

C

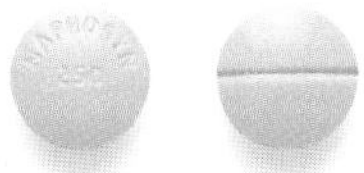

NAPROSYN

Naproxen 250mg

D

PIRITON

Chlorphenamine 4mg

E

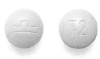

ZYDOL

Tramadol 150mg

F

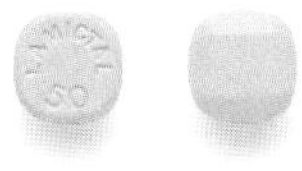

LAMICTAL

Lamotrigine 25mg

G

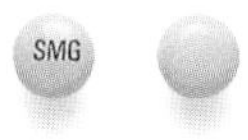

SANOMIGRAN

Pizotifen 500mcg

H

MIDAMOR

Amiloride 5mg

I

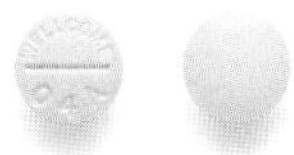

PURI-NETHOL

Mercaptopurine 50mg

J

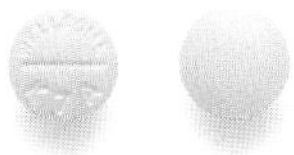

IMURAN

Azathioprine 50mg

K

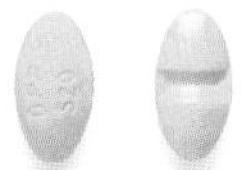

SINEMET 62.5

Carbidopa 12.5mg
Levodopa 50mg

L

MYAMBUTOL

Ethambutol 100mg

M

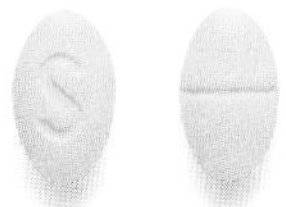

SORBITRATE

Isosorbide dinitrate 10mg

N

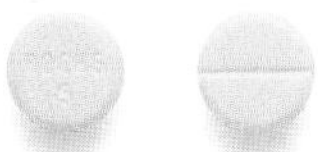

VALIUM

Diazepam 5mg

O

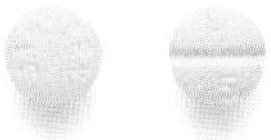

HALDOL

Haloperidol 1.5mg

P

VIOXX

Rofecoxib 12.5mg

Q

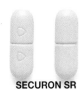

SECURON SR

Verapamil hydrochloride 240mg

R

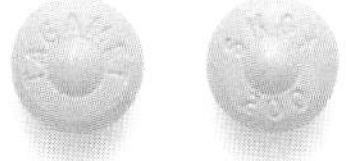

TAGAMET

Cimetidine 200mg

S

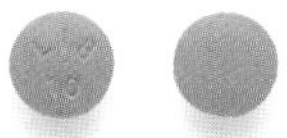

LIBRIUM

Chlordiazepoxide 10mg

T

CEDOCARD

Isosorbide dinitrate 40mg

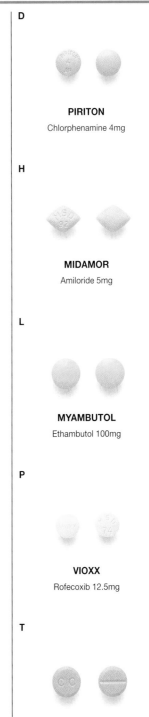

ONE-COLOUR TABLETS continued

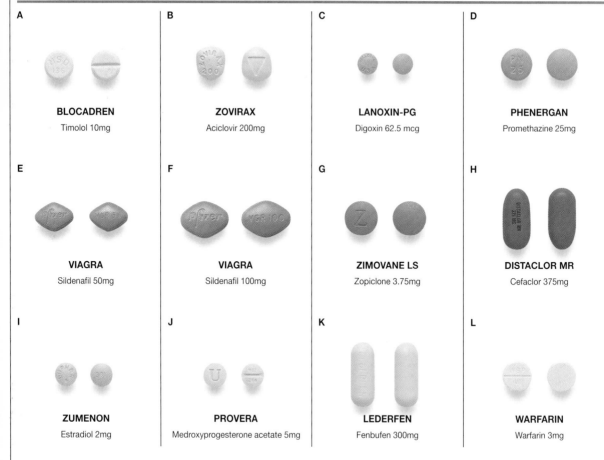

A

BLOCADREN

Timolol 10mg

B

ZOVIRAX

Aciclovir 200mg

C

LANOXIN-PG

Digoxin 62.5 mcg

D

PHENERGAN

Promethazine 25mg

E

VIAGRA

Sildenafil 50mg

F

VIAGRA

Sildenafil 100mg

G

ZIMOVANE LS

Zopiclone 3.75mg

H

DISTACLOR MR

Cefaclor 375mg

I

ZUMENON

Estradiol 2mg

J

PROVERA

Medroxyprogesterone acetate 5mg

K

LEDERFEN

Fenbufen 300mg

L

WARFARIN

Warfarin 3mg

MULTICOLOUR TABLETS

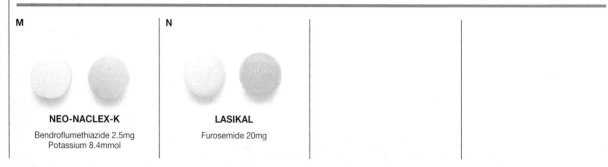

M

NEO-NACLEX-K

Bendroflumethiazide 2.5mg
Potassium 8.4mmol

N

LASIKAL

Furosemide 20mg

ONE-COLOUR CAPSULES

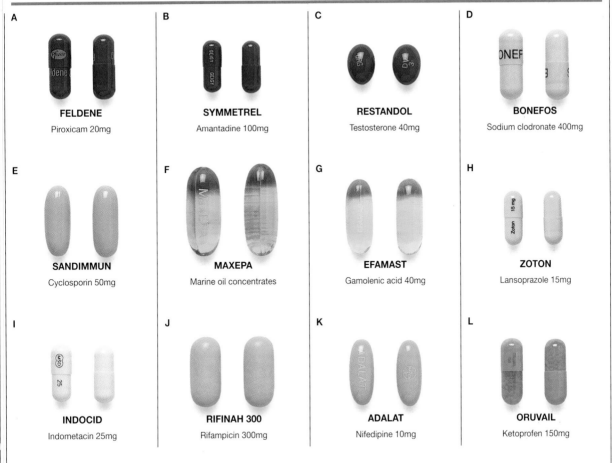

A

FELDENE

Piroxicam 20mg

B

SYMMETREL

Amantadine 100mg

C

RESTANDOL

Testosterone 40mg

D

BONEFOS

Sodium clodronate 400mg

E

SANDIMMUN

Cyclosporin 50mg

F

MAXEPA

Marine oil concentrates

G

EFAMAST

Gamolenic acid 40mg

H

ZOTON

Lansoprazole 15mg

I

INDOCID

Indometacin 25mg

J

RIFINAH 300

Rifampicin 300mg

K

ADALAT

Nifedipine 10mg

L

ORUVAIL

Ketoprofen 150mg

WHITE CAPSULES

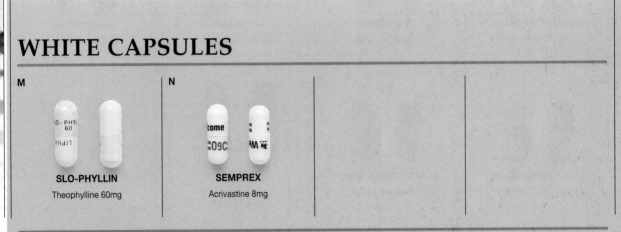

M

SLO-PHYLLIN

Theophylline 60mg

N

SEMPREX

Acrivastine 8mg

WHITE TABLETS

A

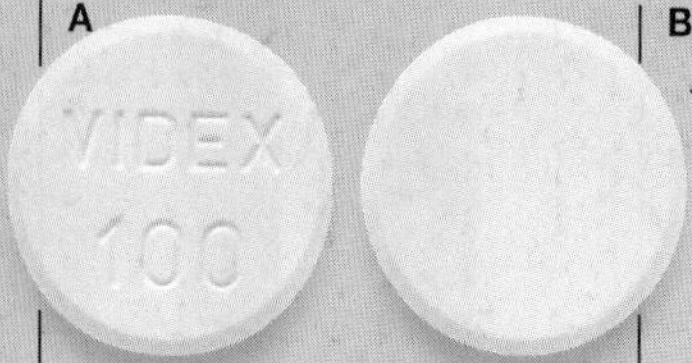

VIDEX

Aluminium hydroxide
Magnesium hydroxide
Didanosine 25mg

B

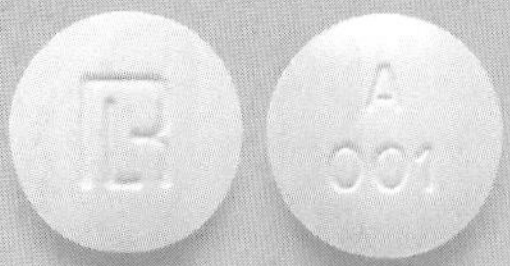

ALUMINIUM HYDROXIDE

Aluminium hydroxide 500mg

C

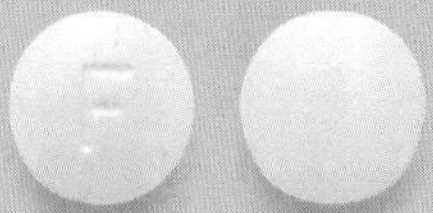

FULCIN

Griseofulvin 500mg

D

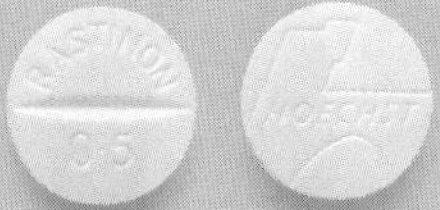

RASTINON

Tolbutamide 500mg

E

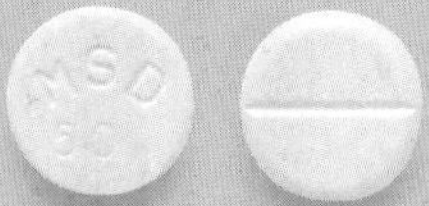

CALCICHEW

Calcium carbonate 500mg

F

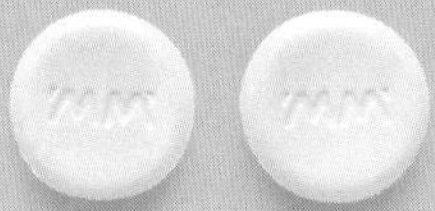

MILK OF MAGNESIA

Magnesium hydroxide 300mg

G

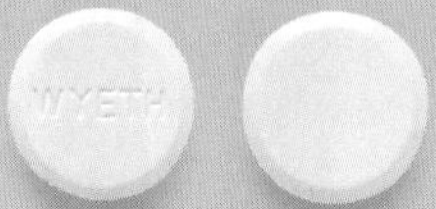

ALUDROX

Aluminium hydroxide 500mg

H

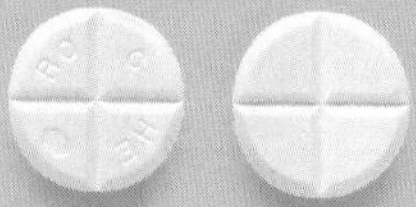

LARIAM

Mefloquine 250mg

I

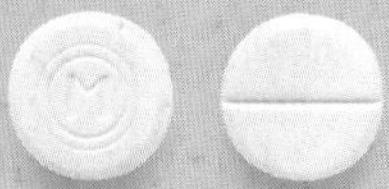

TRILUDAN

Terfenadine 60mg

J

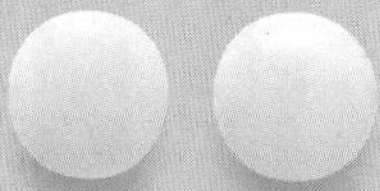

COLOFAC

Mebeverine 135mg

K

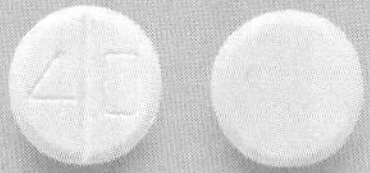

MEGACE

Megestrol 40mg

L

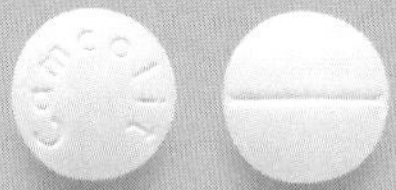

CAMCOLIT

Lithium 250mg

M

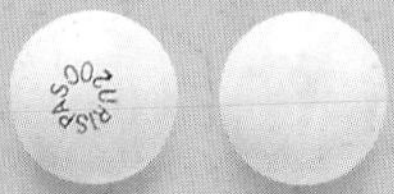

URISPAS

Flavoxate 200mg

N

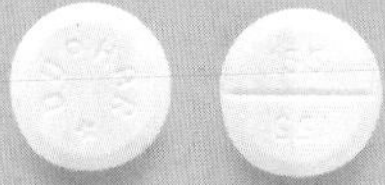

DUPHASTON

Dydrogesterone 10mg

O

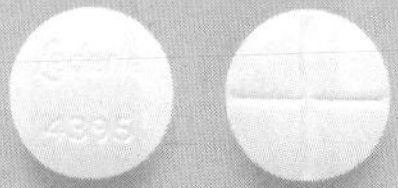

DIAMOX

Acetazolamide 250mg

P

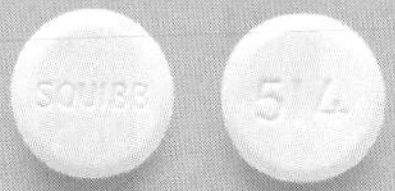

IPRAL

Trimethoprim 200mg

Q

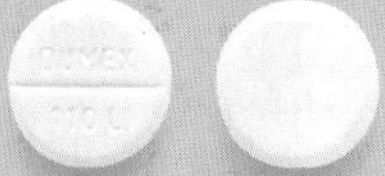

ANTABUSE

Disulfiram 200mg

R

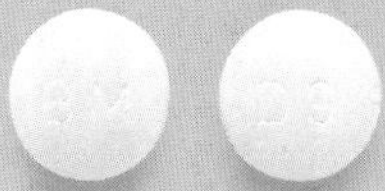

BEZALIP-MONO

Bezafibrate 400mg

S

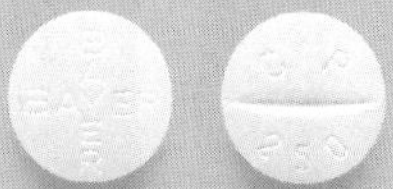

CIPROXIN

Ciprofloxacin 250mg

T

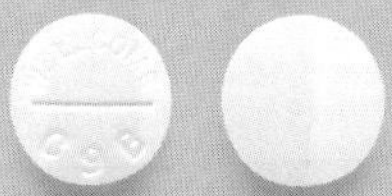

ZYLORIC

Allopurinol 300mg

A

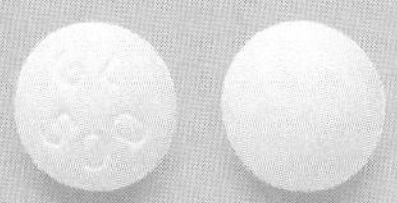

GLUCOPHAGE

Metformin 500mg

B

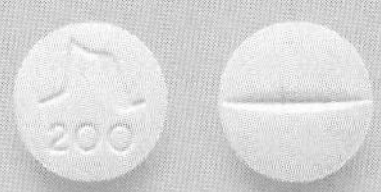

CORDARONE X

Amiodarone 200mg

C

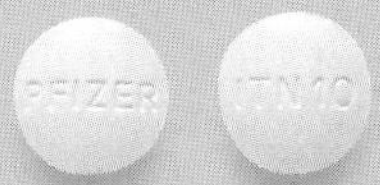

ISTIN

Amlodipine 5mg

D

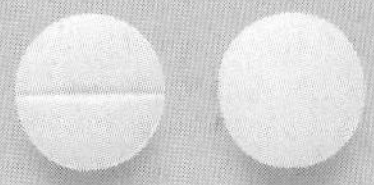

ASPIRIN

Aspirin 300mg

E

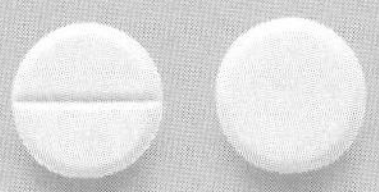

STABILLIN-VK

Phenoxymethylpenicillin 250mg

F

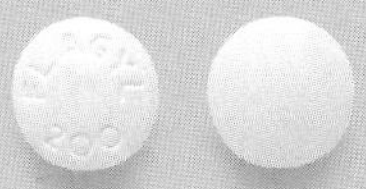

FLAGYL

Metronidazole 200mg

G

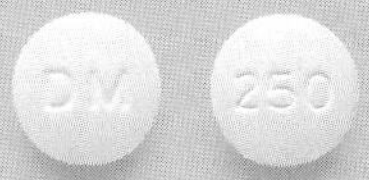

DISTAMINE

Penicillamine 250mg

H

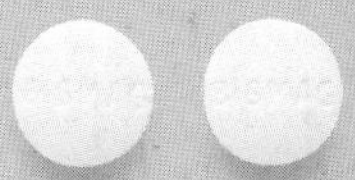

BISMAG

Sodium bicarbonate 149mg
Magnesium carbonate 156mg

I

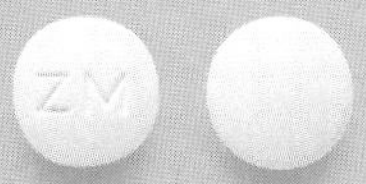

ZIMOVANE

Zopiclone 7.5mg

J

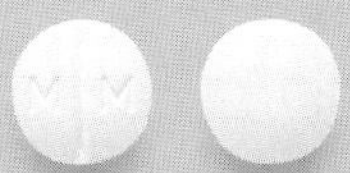

MYSOLINE

Primidone 250mg

K

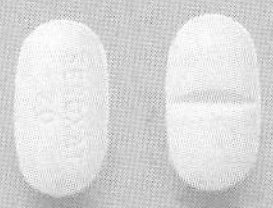

SEROXAT

Paroxetine 20mg

L

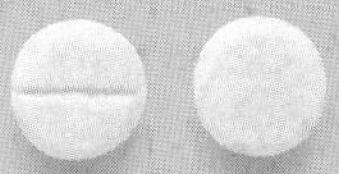

EPILIM

Sodium valproate 100mg

M

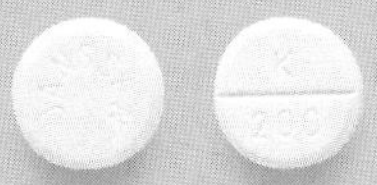

NIZORAL

Ketoconazole 200mg

N

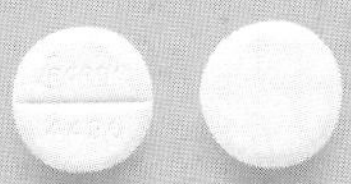

ARTANE

Trihexphenidyl 5mg

O

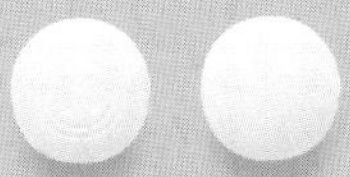

MERBENTYL

Dicycloverine 10mg

P

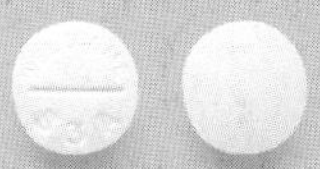

KEMADRIN

Procyclidine 5mg

Q

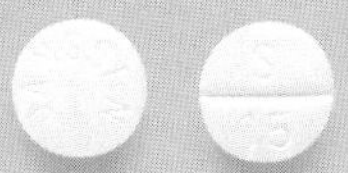

STUGERON

Cinnarizine 15mg

R

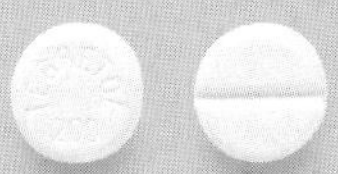

TEGRETOL

Carbamazepine 200mg

S

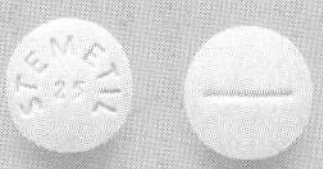

STEMETIL

Prochlorperazine 25mg

T

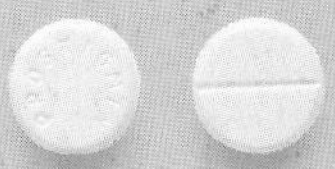

PROSTIGMIN

Neostigmine 15mg

WHITE TABLETS continued

A

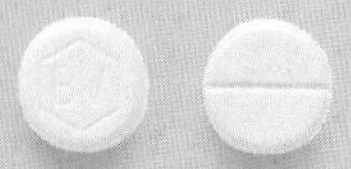

ANDROCUR

Cyproterone acetate 50mg

B

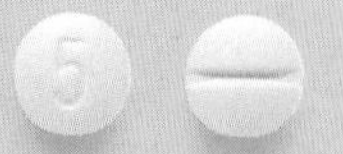

BRICANYL

Terbutaline 5mg

C

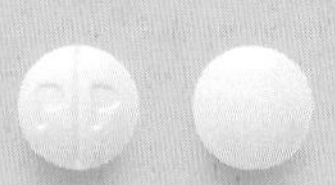

PALUDRINE

Proguanil 100mg

D

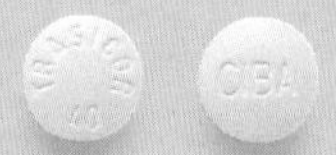

TRASICOR

Oxprenolol 40mg

E

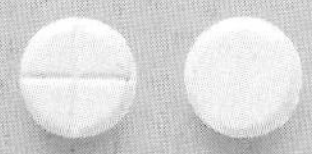

DIAMICRON

Gliclazide 80mg

F

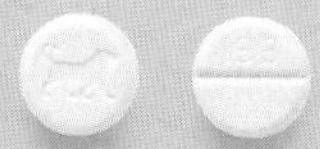

BURINEX

Bumetanide 1mg

G

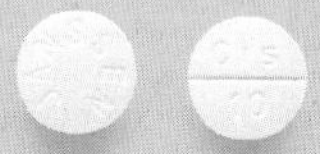

PREPULSID

Cisapride 10mg

H

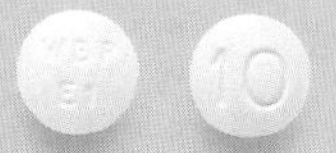

ENDOXANA

Cyclophosphamide 10mg

I

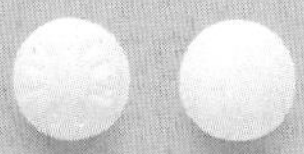

TILDIEM

Diltiazem 60mg

J

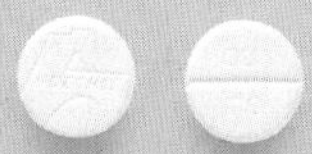

LASIX

Furosemide 40mg

K

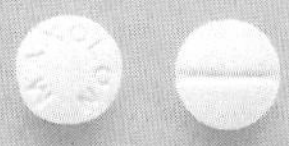

MAXOLON

Metoclopramide 10mg

L

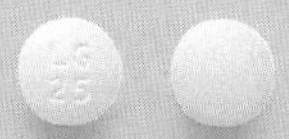

LARGACTIL

Chlorpromazine 25mg

M

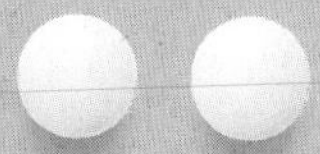

NATRILIX

Indapamide 2.5mg

N

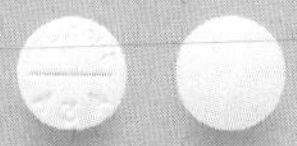

DARAPRIM

Pyrimethamine 25mg

O

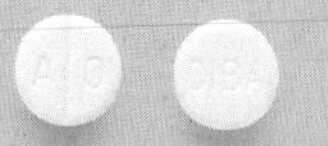

NAVIDREX

Cyclopenthiazide 500mcg

P

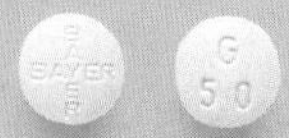

GLUCOBAY

Acarbose 50mg

Q

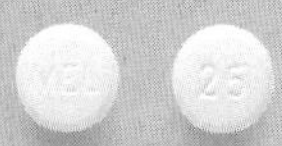

MELLERIL

Thioridazine 25mg

R

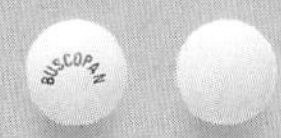

BUSCOPAN

Hyoscine 10mg

S

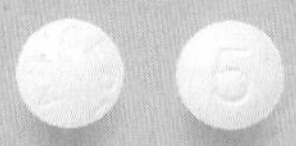

ARICEPT

Donepezil 5mg

T

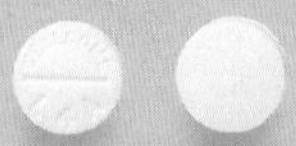

PHYSEPTONE

Methadone 5mg

A

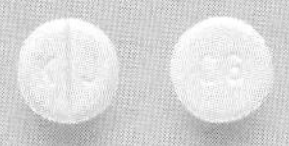

LIORESAL

Baclofen 10mg

B

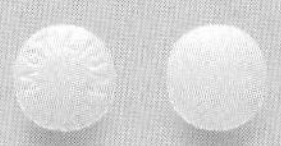

MOTILIUM

Domperidone 10mg

C

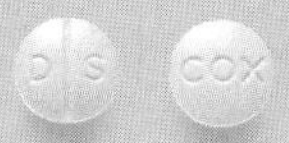

DAPSONE

Dapsone 100mg

D

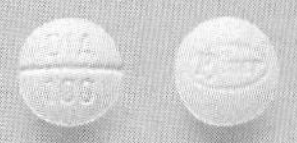

DIABINESE

Chlorpropamide 100mg

E

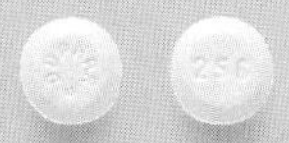

SERC

Betahistine 8mg

F

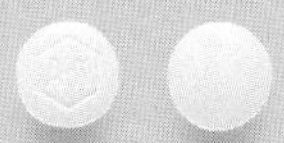

PRIMOLUT N

Norethisterone 5mg

G

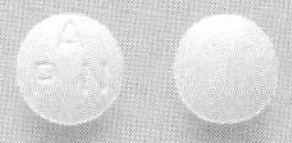

ACUPAN

Nefopam 30mg

H

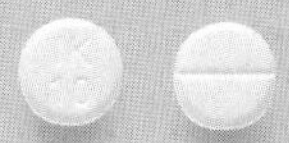

IKOREL

Nicorandil 10mg

I

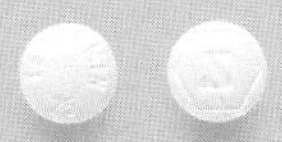

TENORMIN

Atenolol 25mg

J

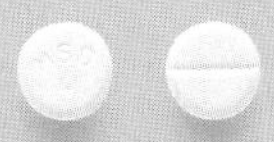

DECADRON

Dexamethasone 500mcg

K

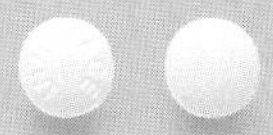

INNOVACE

Enalapril 2.5mg

L

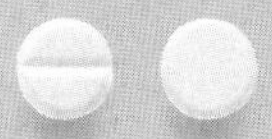

APRINOX

Bendroflumethiazide 5mg

M

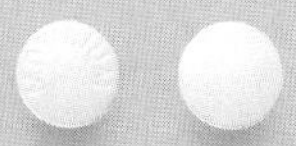

HYDROSALURIC

Hydrochlorothiazide 25mg

N

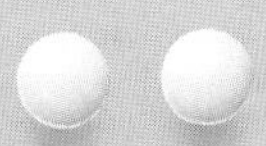

NATRILIX

Indapamide 1.5mg

O

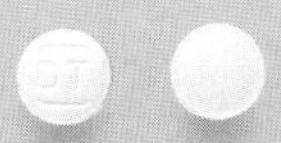

DETRUSITOL

Tolterodine 2mg

P

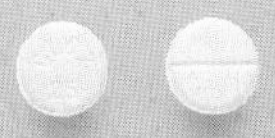

CLOZARIL

Clozapine 25mg

Q

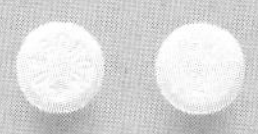

LIVIAL

Tibolone 2.5mg

R

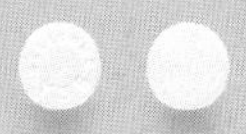

LANOXIN

Digoxin 125mcg

S

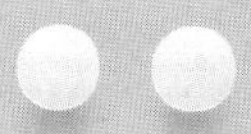

LOMOTIL

Diphenoxylate 2.5mg
Atropine 25mcg

T

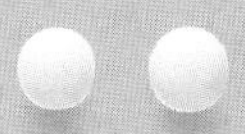

EUGYNON 30

Ethinylestradiol 30mcg
Levonorgestrel 250mcg

WHITE TABLETS continued

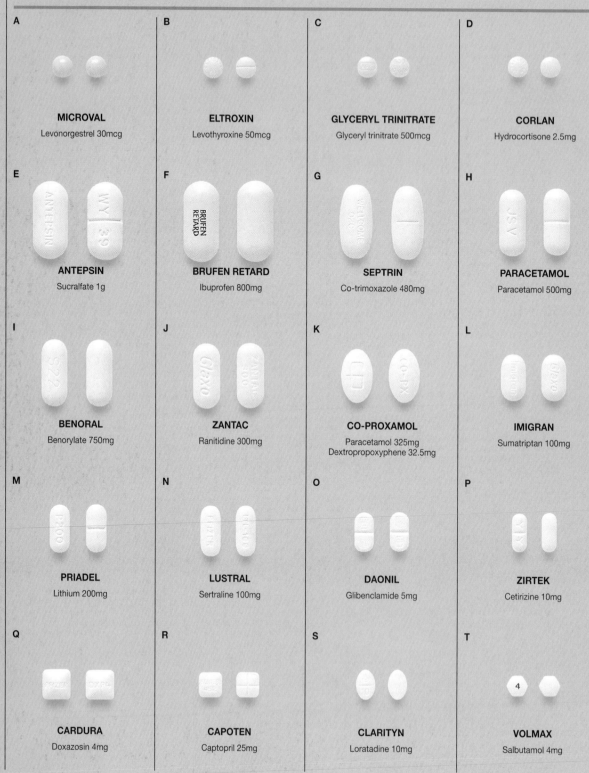

A

MICROVAL

Levonorgestrel 30mcg

B

ELTROXIN

Levothyroxine 50mcg

C

GLYCERYL TRINITRATE

Glyceryl trinitrate 500mcg

D

CORLAN

Hydrocortisone 2.5mg

E

ANTEPSIN

Sucralfate 1g

F

BRUFEN RETARD

Ibuprofen 800mg

G

SEPTRIN

Co-trimoxazole 480mg

H

PARACETAMOL

Paracetamol 500mg

I

BENORAL

Benorylate 750mg

J

ZANTAC

Ranitidine 300mg

K

CO-PROXAMOL

Paracetamol 325mg
Dextropropoxyphene 32.5mg

L

IMIGRAN

Sumatriptan 100mg

M

PRIADEL

Lithium 200mg

N

LUSTRAL

Sertraline 100mg

O

DAONIL

Glibenclamide 5mg

P

ZIRTEK

Cetirizine 10mg

Q

CARDURA

Doxazosin 4mg

R

CAPOTEN

Captopril 25mg

S

CLARITYN

Loratadine 10mg

T

VOLMAX

Salbutamol 4mg

PATCHES AND PENS

A

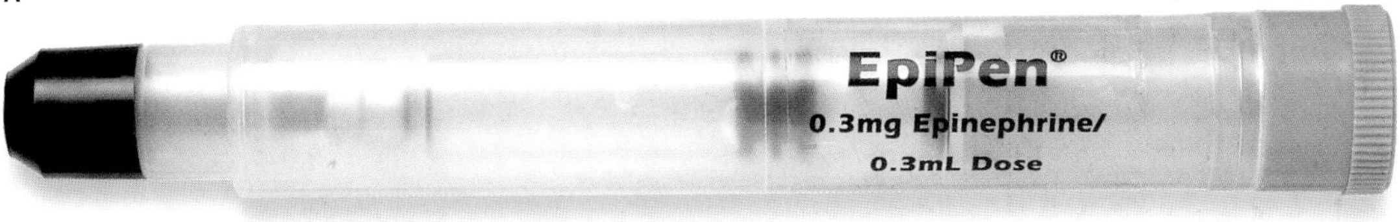

EPIPEN

Epinephrine 0.3mg

B

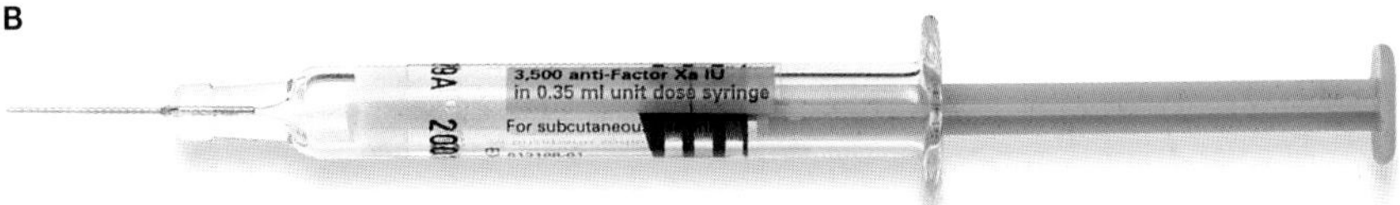

INNOHEP

Tinzaparin 3,500 IU

C

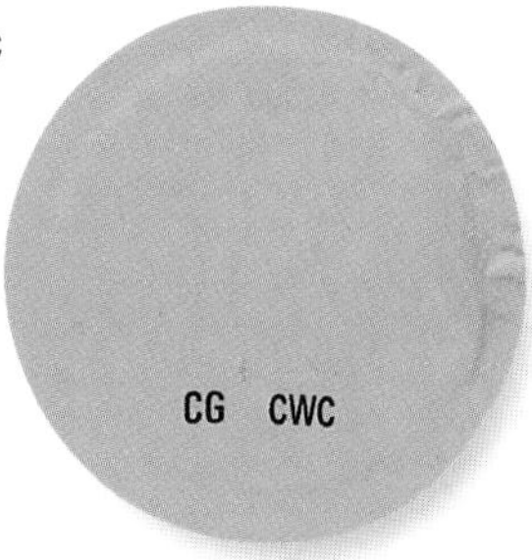

NICOTINELL

Nicotine 7mg

D

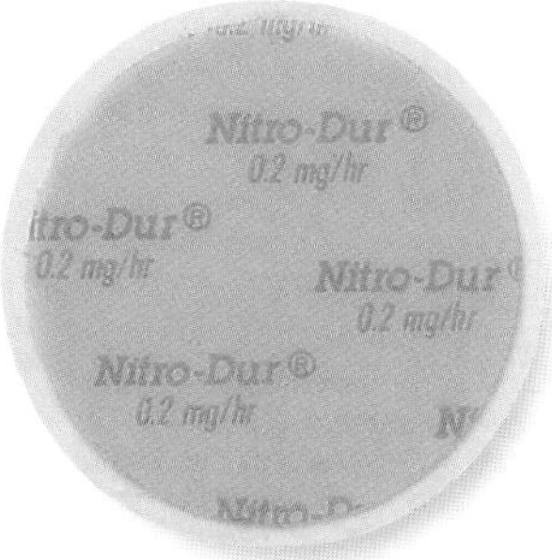

NITRO-DUR

Glyceryl trinitrate 5mg

E

NICOTINELL

Nicotine 14mg

F

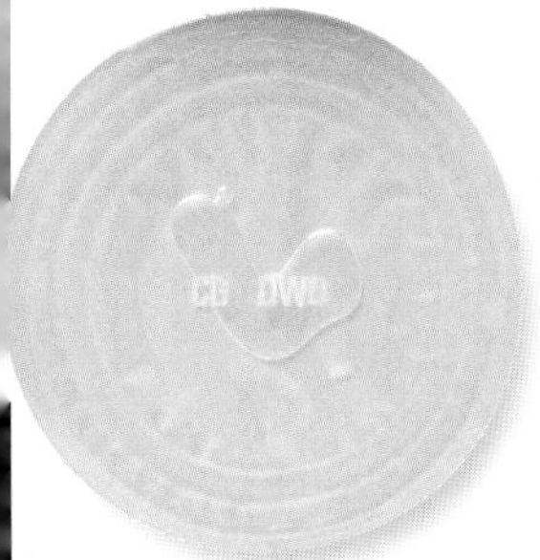

ESTRADERM TTS

Estradiol 25mcg

G

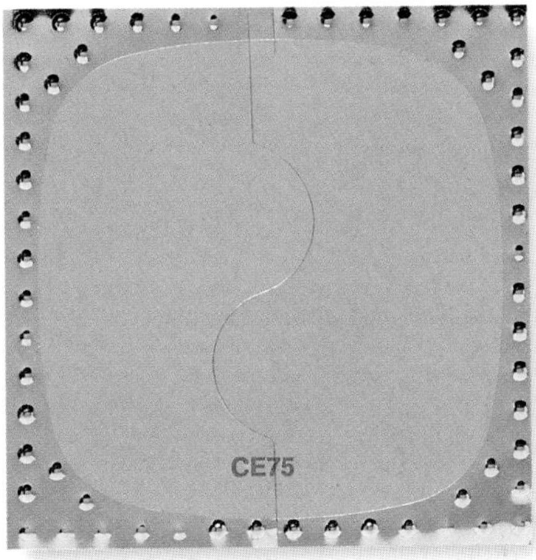

EVOREL

Estradiol 75mcg

H

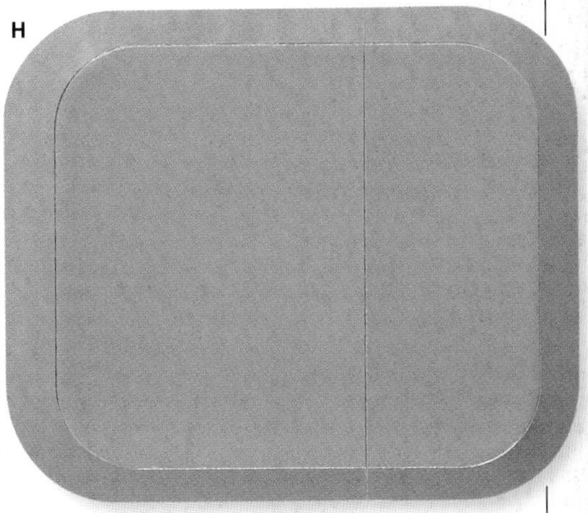

FEMATRIX

Estradiol 80mcg

THE DRUG FINDER

This section contains the names of approximately 2,500 individual drug products and substances. It provides a quick and easy reference for readers interested in learning about a specific drug or medication. There is no need for you to know whether the item is a brand name or a generic name, or whether it is a prescription or an over-the-counter drug; all types of drug are listed.

What it contains
The drugs are listed alphabetically and include all major generic drugs and many less widely used substances. A broad range of brand names, as well as many vitamins and minerals, are also included. This comprehensive selection reflects the wide diversity of products available for the treatment and prevention of disease. Inclusion of a drug or product does not imply BMA endorsement, nor does the exclusion of a particular drug or product indicate BMA disapproval.

How the references work
References are to the pages in Part 4, containing the drug profiles of each principal generic drug, and to the section in Part 3 that describes the relevant drug group, as appropriate. Some entries for generic drugs that do not have a full profile contain a brief description here. Certain technical terms within the entries are printed in italics to indicate that they are defined in the Glossary (pp.470–475).

Colour identification guide
Brand-name products pictured in the Colour Identification Guide (pp.34–47) contain a reference in italic type to the page and grid letter where the photograph of that product may be found.

A

abacavir an antiviral drug for HIV/AIDS 157

abciximab an antiplatelet drug 104

Abelcet a brand name for amphotericin 199 (an antifungal 138)

Abidec a brand-name multivitamin 149

acamprosate a drug for alcohol abuse 451, used in addition to counselling

acarbose an oral antidiabetic 142

Accolate a brand name for zafirlukast (a leukotriene *antagonist* for asthma 124 and bronchospasm 92)

Accupro a brand name for quinapril (an ACE inhibitor 98)

Accuretic a brand name for quinapril (an ACE inhibitor 98) with hydrochlorothiazide 300 (a diuretic 99)

acebutolol a beta blocker 97

aceclofenac a non-steroidal anti-inflammatory 116

acemetacin a non-steroidal anti-inflammatory 116

acenocoumarol previously known as nicoumalone (an anticoagulant 104)

Acepril a brand name for captopril 216 (an ACE inhibitor 98)

acetazolamide a carbonic anhydrase inhibitor diuretic 99 and drug for glaucoma 168

acetomenaphthone a vitamin K substance 449 used with nicotinic acid to treat chilblains

acetylcholine a chemical *neurotransmitter* that stimulates the parasympathetic nervous system 79 and is used as a *miotic* 170

acetylcysteine a *mucolytic* 94

Acezide a brand name for captopril 216 (an ACE inhibitor 98) with hydrochlorothiazide 300 (a thiazide diuretic 99)

Achromycin a brand name for tetracycline 418 (an antibiotic 128)

aciclovir 188 (an antiviral 133)

Aci-Jel a brand name for acetic acid (an *antiseptic*)

acipimox a lipid-lowering drug 103

Acitak a brand name for cimetidine 228 (an anti-ulcer drug 109)

acitretin a drug for psoriasis 178

aclarubicin an anticancer drug 154

Acnecide a brand name for benzoyl peroxide 208 (a drug for acne 177)

Acnidazil a brand name for benzoyl peroxide 208 (a drug for acne 177) with miconazole 347 (an antifungal 138)

Acnisal a brand name for salicylic acid (a drug for acne 177)

acrivastine an antihistamine 124

Actal a brand-name antacid containing alexitol (an antacid 108)

Actifed Compound a brand name for dextromethorphan (a cough suppressant 94) with pseudoephedrine (a decongestant 93) and triprolidine (an antihistamine 124)

Actifed Expectorant a brand name for guaifenesin (an *expectorant* 94) with pseudoephedrine (a decongestant 93) and triprolidine (an antihistamine 124)

Actinac a brand-name acne preparation 177 containing chloramphenicol 222, hydrocortisone 301, allantoin, butoxyethyl nicotinate, and sulphur

actinomycin D another name for dactinomycin (an anticancer drug 154)

activated charcoal a substance used in the emergency treatment of poisoning

Acular a brand name for ketorolac (a non-steroidal anti-inflammatory 116)

Acupan a brand name for nefopam (a non-*opioid* analgesic 80); *illus. 45G*

Adalat a brand name for nifedipine 359 (an anti-angina drug 101 and antihypertensive 102); *illus. 39K*

Adalat Retard a brand name for nifedipine 359 (an anti-angina drug 101 and antihypertensive 102)

adapalene a retinoid for acne 177

Adcortyl a brand name for triamcinolone (a corticosteroid 141)

adenosine an anti-arrhythmic 100

Adipine MR a brand name for nifedipine 359 (a calcium channel blocker 98)

Adizem-XL a brand name for diltiazem 259 (a calcium channel blocker 98); *illus. 41R, 41S*

adrenaline see epinephrine 273 (a bronchodilator 92 and drug for glaucoma 168 and anaphylactic shock 496)

AeroBec a brand name for beclometasone 206 (a corticosteroid 141)

Aerocrom a brand name for sodium cromoglicate 404 (an anti-allergy drug 124) with salbutamol 399 (a bronchodilator 92)

Aerolin a brand name for salbutamol 399 (a bronchodilator 92)

Afrazine a brand name for oxymetazoline (a *topical* decongestant 93)

Aggrastat a brand name for tirofiban (a drug for prevention of heart attacks 95)

Ailax a brand name for co-danthramer (a stimulant laxative 111)

Airomir a brand name for salbutamol 399 (a bronchodilator 92)

Akineton a brand name for biperiden (an *anticholinergic* for parkinsonism 87)

Aknemin a brand name for minocycline 348 (a tetracycline antibiotic 128)

albendazole an anthelmintic 139

alclometasone a topical corticosteroid 174

Alcobon a brand name for flucytosine (an antifungal 138)

Aldactide a brand name for spironolactone (a diuretic 99) with hydroflumethiazide (a diuretic 99)

Aldactone a brand name for spironolactone (a potassium-sparing diuretic 99)

Aldara a brand name for imiquimod (a drug to treat warts)

aldesleukin an anticancer drug 154

Aldomet a brand name for methyldopa 343 (an antihypertensive 102); *illus. 36Q*

alendronate a drug for the treatment of bone disorders 122

alexitol an antacid 108

alfacalcidol vitamin D 448 (a vitamin 149)

AlfaD a brand name for alfacalcidol (a vitamin 149)

alfentanil an *anaesthetic* 80

alfuzosin an alpha-*adrenergic* blocker for prostate disorders 166

Algesal a brand name for diethylamine salicylate (a *rubefacient*)

Algicon a brand name for aluminium hydroxide 191, magnesium carbonate, and potassium bicarbonate (all antacids 108) with magnesium alginate (an antifoaming agent 108)

alginic acid a binding agent in antacids 108

alimemazine previously known as trimeprazine (an antihistamine 124)

Alka-Seltzer a brand-name analgesic 80 and antacid 108 containing aspirin 200, sodium bicarbonate 403, and citric acid

Alkeran a brand name for melphalan (an anticancer drug 154)

allantoin a mild antibacterial 131

Allegron a brand name for nortriptyline (a tricyclic antidepressant 84)

Aller-eze a brand name for clemastine (an antihistamine 124)

allopurinol 189 (a drug for gout 119)

Almodan a brand name for amoxicillin 198 (a penicillin antibiotic 128)

Alomide a brand name for lodoxamide (an anti-allergy drug 124)

Alphaderm a brand name for hydrocortisone 301 (a corticosteroid 141) with urea (a hydrating agent)

Alphagan a brand name for brimonidine (a drug for glaucoma 168)

Alphaparin a brand name for certoparin (an anticoagulant 104)

alpha tocopheryl acetate vitamin E 448 (a vitamin 149)

Alphavase a brand name for prazosin (an antihypertensive 102)

Alphosyl a brand-name drug for eczema 179 and psoriasis 178 containing coal tar and allantoin (a mild antibacterial 131)

alprazolam a benzodiazepine anti-anxiety drug 83

alprostadil 190 a prostaglandin used for male impotence 146, 164

Altacite Plus a brand name for hydrotalcite (an antacid 108) with dimeticone (an antifoaming agent 108)

alteplase a thrombolytic 105 (also known as tissue plasminogen activator)

altretamine an anticancer drug 154

Alu-Cap a brand name for aluminium hydroxide 191 (an antacid 108)

Aludrox a brand name for aluminium hydroxide 191 (an antacid 108); illus. 42G

Aludrox-SA a brand name for ambutonium bromide (an antispasmodic for irritable bowel syndrome 110) with aluminium hydroxide 191 and magnesium hydroxide 329 (both antacids 108)

aluminium acetate an astringent used for inflammation of the skin or outer ear canal 175; also used in rectal preparations 113

aluminium chloride an antiperspirant

aluminium hydroxide 191 (an antacid 108); illus. 42B

Alupent a brand name for orciprenaline (a bronchodilator 92)

Alvedon a brand name for paracetamol 368 (a non-opioid analgesic 80)

Alvercol a brand name for sterculia (a bulking agent 110) and alverine (an antispasmodic 110)

alverine an antispasmodic for irritable bowel syndrome 110

amantadine 192 (an antiviral 133 and drug used for parkinsonism 87)

Amaryl a brand name for glimepiride (an oral antidiabetic 142)

AmBisome a brand name for amphotericin 199 (an antifungal 138)

amethocaine see tetracaine (a local anaesthetic 80)

Ametop a brand name for tetracaine (a local anaesthetic 80)

Amias a brand name for candesartan (an angiotensin II inhibitor, an antihypertensive 102)

amifostine a drug to reduce risk of infection in patients taking anticancer drugs 154

amikacin an aminoglycoside antibiotic 128

Amikin a brand name for amikacin (an aminoglycoside antibiotic 128)

Amil-Co a brand name for amiloride 193 with hydrochlorothiazide 300 (both diuretics 99)

Amilamont a brand name for amiloride (a potassium-sparing diuretic 99)

amiloride 193 (a potassium-sparing diuretic 99)

Amilospare a brand name for amiloride 193 (a potassium-sparing diuretic 99)

aminacrine a skin antiseptic 175

aminobenzoic acid an ingredient of sunscreens 181

aminoglutethimide a drug for advanced breast cancer 154 and Cushing's syndrome 141

aminophylline a bronchodilator 92 related to theophylline 419

amiodarone 194 (an anti-arrhythmic 100)

amisulpride 195 (an antipsychotic drug 85)

amitriptyline 196 (a tricyclic antidepressant 84)

Amix a brand name for amoxicillin 198 (a penicillin antibiotic 128)

amlodipine 197 (a calcium channel blocker 101)

ammonium chloride a drug that increases urine acidity 166 and speeds excretion of poisons, and is an expectorant 94

amobarbital a barbiturate sleeping drug 82

Amoram a brand name for amoxicillin 198 (a penicillin antibiotic 128)

amorolfine an antifungal 138

amoxapine a tricyclic antidepressant 84

amoxicillin 198 (a penicillin antibiotic 128)

Amoxil a brand name for amoxicillin 198 (a penicillin antibiotic 128); illus. 40A, 40B

Amphocil a brand name for amphotericin 199 (an antifungal 138)

amphotericin 199 (an antifungal 138)

ampicillin a penicillin antibiotic 128

amsacrine an anticancer drug 154

Amsidine a brand name for amsacrine (an anticancer drug 154)

Amytal a brand name for amobarbital (a barbiturate sleeping drug 82)

Anabact a brand name for metronidazole 346 (an antibacterial 131)

Anacal a brand-name preparation for haemorrhoids 113 containing heparinoid

Anadin 500 a brand-name analgesic 80 containing aspirin 200 and caffeine; illus. 41B

Anadin Extra a brand-name analgesic 80 containing aspirin 200, paracetamol 368, and caffeine

Anadin Paracetamol a brand name for paracetamol 368 (an analgesic 80)

Anaflex a brand name for polynoxylin (an antifungal 138 and antibacterial 131)

Anafranil, Anafranil SR brand names for clomipramine 236 (a tricyclic antidepressant 84); illus. 40 O

anastrozole an anticancer drug 154

Anbesol a brand-name topical liquid for mouth ulcers and teething pain, containing lidocaine (a local anaesthetic 80), cetylpyridinium, and chlorocresol (both topical antiseptics 175)

Andrews Antacid a brand name for calcium carbonate 438 and magnesium carbonate (both antacids 108)

Androcur a brand name for cyproterone acetate for the control of sexual deviation in males; illus. 44A

Anethaine a brand name for tetracaine (a local anaesthetic 80)

Angettes a brand-name antiplatelet drug 104 containing aspirin 200

Angilol a brand name for propranolol 386 (a beta blocker 97)

Angiopine MR a brand name for nifedipine 359 (a calcium channel blocker 101)

Angiozem a brand name for diltiazem 259 (a calcium channel blocker 101)

Angitil SR a brand name for diltiazem 259 (a calcium channel blocker 101)

Anhydrol Forte a brand name for aluminium chloride (an antiperspirant)

anistreplase a thrombolytic 105

Anodesyn a brand-name preparation for haemorrhoids 113 containing allantoin (a mild antibacterial 131), lidocaine (a local anaesthetic 80), and ephedrine 272

Anquil a brand name for benperidol (an antipsychotic 85)

Antabuse a brand name for disulfiram 262 (an alcohol abuse deterrent 24, 451); illus. 42Q

antazoline an antihistamine 124

Antepsin a brand name for sucralfate 408 (an ulcer-healing drug 109); illus. 46E

Anthisan a brand name for mepyramine (an antihistamine cream 124)

anti-D immunoglobulin a drug used to prevent sensitization to Rhesus antigen

antihaemophilic factor a blood protein used to promote blood clotting in haemophilia 104

Antipressan a brand name for atenolol 201 (a beta blocker 97)

Anturan a brand name for sulphinpyrazone (a drug for gout 119)

Antizol a brand name for fomepizole (an antidote for ethylene glycol poisoning)

Anugesic-HC a brand-name preparation for haemorrhoids 113 containing hydrocortisone 301, benzyl benzoate, bismuth, Peru balsam, pramocaine, and zinc oxide 449

Anusol a brand-name preparation for haemorrhoids 113 containing zinc oxide 449, bismuth, and Peru balsam

apomorphine a drug used to treat Parkinson's disease 87

APP a brand name for homatropine (an antispasmodic 110), with bismuth (an anti-ulcer drug 109), calcium carbonate 438, magnesium carbonate, magnesium trisilicate, and aluminium hydroxide 191 (all antacids108)

apraclonidine a drug for glaucoma 168

Apresoline a brand name for hydralazine (an antihypertensive 102)

APRINOX–CALCIFEROL

Aprinox a brand name for bendroflumethiazide 207 (a thiazide diuretic 99); *illus. 45L*

aprotinin an antifibrinolytic 104 used to promote blood clotting

Aprovel a brand name for irbesartan 310 (an angiotensin II inhibitor, an antihypertensive 102)

Apsin a brand name for phenoxymethylpenicillin 372 (a penicillin antibiotic 128)

Apsolol a brand name for propranolol 386 (a beta blocker 97 and anti-anxiety drug 83)

Apstil a brand name for diethylstilbestrol 257 (a female sex hormone 147)

AquaBan a brand name for caffeine with ammonium chloride as a mild diuretic 99

Aquadrate a brand name for urea (a hydrating agent)

Arava a brand name for leflunomide (an antirheumatic drug 117)

Aredia a brand name for pamidronate (a drug for bone disorders 122)

argipressin synthetic vasopressin (a drug for diabetes insipidus 145)

Aricept a brand name for donepezil 264 (a drug for Alzheimer's disease); *illus. 36T, 44S*

Aridil a brand name for amiloride 193 with furosemide 291 (both diuretics 99)

Arpicolin a brand name for procyclidine 382 (a drug for parkinsonism 87)

Arpimycin a brand name for erythromycin 276 (an antibiotic 128)

Arret a brand name for loperamide 326 (an antidiarrhoeal 110)

Artane a brand name for trihexyphenidyl (a drug for parkinsonism 87); *illus. 43N*

Arthrofen a brand name for ibuprofen 303 (an analgesic 80 and non-steroidal anti-inflammatory 116)

Arthrosin a brand name for naproxen 356 (a non-steroidal anti-inflammatory 116 and drug for gout 119)

Arthrotec a brand-name antirheumatic drug containing diclofenac 254 with misoprostol 350

Arthroxen a brand name for naproxen 356 (a non-steroidal anti-inflammatory 116 and drug for gout 119)

articaine a local anaesthetic 80

Arythmol a brand name for propafenone (an anti-arrhythmic 100)

Asacol a brand name for mesalazine 338 (a drug for ulcerative colitis 112)

Ascabiol a brand name for *topical* benzyl benzoate (an antiparasitic 176)

ascorbic acid vitamin C 447 (a vitamin 149)

Asendis a brand name for amoxapine (a tricyclic antidepressant 84)

Asilone a brand name for aluminium hydroxide 191 and magnesium oxide (both antacids 108) with dimeticone (an antifoaming agent 108)

Asmaven a brand name for salbutamol 399 (a bronchodilator 92)

asparaginase a drug for leukaemia 154

Aspav a brand-name analgesic 80 containing aspirin 200 and papaveretum

aspirin 200 (a non-*opioid* analgesic 80 and antiplatelet drug 104); *illus. 43D*

Aspro Clear a brand name for soluble aspirin 200 (a non-*opioid* analgesic 80)

Atarax a brand name for hydroxyzine (an anti-anxiety drug 83)

Atenix a brand name for atenolol 201 (a beta blocker 97)

atenolol 201 a beta blocker 97

Ativan a brand name for lorazepam (a benzodiazepine anti-anxiety drug 83 and sleeping drug 82)

atorvastatin 202 (a lipid-lowering drug 103)

atovaquone an antiprotozoal 136 and antimalarial 137

atracurium a drug used to relax the muscles in general *anaesthesia*

atropine 203 (an *anticholinergic* for irritable bowel syndrome 110 and a *mydriatic* 170)

Atrovent a brand name for ipratropium bromide 309 (a bronchodilator 92)

Audicort a brand-name anti-infective ear preparation 171 containing benzocaine, neomycin, and triamcinolone (a corticosteroid 141)

Augmentin a brand name for amoxicillin 198 (a penicillin antibiotic 128) with clavulanic acid (a substance that increases the effectiveness of amoxicillin)

auranofin an antirheumatic 117

Aureocort a brand name for chlortetracycline (a tetracycline antibiotic 128) with triamcinolone (a corticosteroid 141)

Aureomycin a brand name for chlortetracycline (a tetracycline antibiotic 128)

aurothiomalate an antirheumatic 117

Avloclor a brand name for chloroquine 224 (an antimalarial 137 and antirheumatic 117)

Avomine a brand name for promethazine 385 (an antihistamine 124 and anti-emetic 90)

Axid a brand name for nizatidine (an anti-ulcer drug 109)

Axsain a brand name for capsaicin (a *rubefacient*)

Azactam a brand name for aztreonam (an antibiotic 128)

Azamune a brand name for azathioprine 204 (an antirheumatic 117 and immunosuppressant 156)

azapropazone a non-steroidal anti-inflammatory 116

azatadine an antihistamine 124

azathioprine 204 (an antirheumatic 117 and immunosuppressant 156)

azelaic acid an antibacterial 131 (a drug for acne 177)

azelastine an antihistamine 124

azidothymidine zidovudine 435 (an antiviral for HIV infection and AIDS 157)

azithromycin an antibiotic 128

azlocillin a penicillin antibiotic 128

AZT zidovudine 435 (an antiviral for HIV infection and AIDS 157)

aztreonam an antibiotic 128

B

bacitracin an antibiotic 128

baclofen 205 (a muscle relaxant 120)

Baclospas a brand of baclofen 205 (a muscle relaxant 120)

Bactroban a brand name for mupirocin (an antibacterial for skin infections 175)

balsalazide a drug for ulcerative colitis 112

Bambec a brand name for bambuterol (a *sympathomimetic* bronchodilator 92)

bambuterol a *sympathomimetic* bronchodilator 92

Baratol a brand name for indoramin 306 (an antihypertensive 102)

basiliximab an immunosuppressant 156

Baxan a brand name for cefadroxil (a cephalosporin antibiotic 128)

Baycaron a brand name for mefruside (a thiazide-like diuretic 99)

Bazuka a brand-name preparation for verrucas containing salicylic acid (a keratolytic 177) and lactic acid

becaplermin a drug for healing skin ulcers

Beclazone a brand name for beclometasone 206 (a corticosteroid 141)

Becloforte a brand name for beclometasone 206 (a corticosteroid 141)

beclometasone 206 (a corticosteroid 141)

Becodisks a brand of beclometasone 206 (a corticosteroid 141)

Beconase a brand name for beclometasone 206 (a corticosteroid 141)

Becosym a brand-name vitamin B complex preparation (a vitamin 149)

Becotide Rotacaps a brand name for beclometasone 206 (a corticosteroid 141); *illus. 40Q, 40R*

Beechams Coughcaps a brand name for dextromethorphan (a cough suppressant 94); *illus. 40K*

Beechams Pills a brand name for aloin (a stimulant laxative 111)

Beechams Powders a brand name for paracetamol 368 (a non-*opioid* analgesic 80) and pseudoephedrine (a decongestant 93)

Beechams Powders Capsules a brand name for paracetamol 368 (a non-*opioid* analgesic 80) with phenylephrine (a decongestant 93) and caffeine (a stimulant 88)

belladonna an *antispasmodic anticholinergic* for irritable bowel syndrome 110

bendroflumethiazide 207 previously known as bendrofluazide (a thiazide diuretic 99)

Bendrofluazide see bendroflumethiazide 207

Benemid a brand name for probenecid (a drug for gout 119)

Benoral a brand name for benorilate (a non-steroidal anti-inflammatory 116); *illus. 46 I*

benorilate a non-steroidal anti-inflammatory 116

benperidol an antipsychotic 85

benserazide a drug used to enhance the effect of levodopa 320 (a drug for parkinsonism 87)

Benylin a brand name for diphenhydramine (an antihistamine 124) with menthol (an alcohol) and, in some preparations, codeine 241 (an *opioid* analgesic 80)

benzalkonium chloride a skin *antiseptic* 175

Benzamycin a brand name for erythromycin 276 (an antibiotic 128) and benzoyl peroxide 208 (a drug for acne 177)

benzhexol see trihexyphenidyl (a drug for parkinsonism 87)

benzocaine a local anaesthetic 80

benzoin tincture a resin used in inhalations for sinusitis and nasal congestion 93

benzoyl peroxide 208 (a drug for acne 177 and fungal skin infections 138)

benzthiazide a thiazide diuretic 99

benztropine an *anticholinergic* for parkinsonism 87

benzydamine an analgesic 80 used in mouthwash and throat spray

benzyl benzoate an antiparasitic 176

benzylpenicillin a penicillin antibiotic 128

beractant a drug to mature the lungs of premature babies

Berkatens a brand name for verapamil 431 (an anti-angina drug 101 and anti-arrhythmic 100)

Berkolol a brand name for propranolol 386 (a beta blocker 97)

Berkozide a brand name for bendroflumethiazide 207 (a thiazide diuretic 99)

Berotec a brand name for fenoterol (a *sympathomimetic* bronchodilator 92)

Beta-Adalat a brand name for nifedipine 359 (an anti-angina drug 101 and antihypertensive 102) with atenolol 201 (a beta blocker 97)

Betacap a brand name for betamethasone 210 (a corticosteroid 141)

Beta-Cardone a brand name for sotalol 406 (a beta blocker 97)

beta-carotene vitamin A 446 (a vitamin 149 and food additive)

Betadine a brand name for povidone-iodine (a skin *antiseptic* 175)

Betaferon a brand name for interferon beta 308 (a drug for multiple sclerosis 120)

Betagan a brand name for levobunolol (a beta blocker 97 and drug for glaucoma 168)

betahistine 209 (a drug for Ménière's disease 90)

Betaloc a brand name for metoprolol 345 (a beta blocker 97)

betamethasone 210 (a corticosteroid 141)

Beta-Prograne a brand name for propranolol 386 (a beta blocker 97)

betaxolol a beta blocker 97 also used in glaucoma 168

bethanechol a *parasympathomimetic* for urinary retention 166 and paralytic ileus

Betim a brand name for timolol 423 (a beta blocker 97)

Betnelan a brand name for betamethasone 210 (a corticosteroid 141)

Betnesol a brand name for betamethasone 210 (a corticosteroid 141)

Betnesol-N a brand name for betamethasone 210 (a corticosteroid 141) with neomycin (an aminoglycoside antibiotic 128)

Betnovate a brand name for betamethasone 210 (a corticosteroid 141)

Betnovate-C a brand name for betamethasone 210 (a corticosteroid 141) with clioquinol (an anti-infective 175)

Betnovate-N a brand name for betamethasone 210 (a corticosteroid 141) with neomycin (an aminoglycoside antibiotic 128)

Betnovate-Rectal a brand-name preparation for haemorrhoids containing betamethasone 210, lidocaine (a local anaesthetic 80), and phenylephrine (a decongestant 93)

Betoptic a brand-name drug for glaucoma 168 containing betaxolol

Bettamousse a brand name for betamethasone 210 (a corticosteroid 141)

bezafibrate 211 (a lipid-lowering drug 103)

Bezalip-Mono a brand name for bezafibrate 211 (a lipid-lowering drug 103); *illus. 42R*

bicalutamide an anticancer drug 154

BiNovum a brand-name oral contraceptive 161 containing ethinylestradiol 279 and norethisterone 360

Bioplex a brand-name drug for mouth ulcers containing carbenoxolone

Bioral a brand-name drug for mouth ulcers containing carbenoxolone

Biorphen a brand name for orphenadrine 366 (a drug for parkinsonism 87)

biotin 438 (a vitamin 149)

biperiden an *anticholinergic* for parkinsonism 87

bisacodyl a stimulant laxative 111

Bismag a brand name for sodium bicarbonate 403 with magnesium carbonate (both antacids 108)

bismuth a metal given in compound form for gastric and duodenal ulcers 109 and haemorrhoids 113

BiSoDol a brand name for sodium bicarbonate 403 with calcium carbonate 438 and magnesium carbonate (all antacids 108)

bisoprolol a beta blocker 97

Blemix a brand name for minocycline 348 (a tetracycline antibiotic 128)

bleomycin a *cytotoxic* antibiotic for cancer 154

Blocadren a brand name for timolol 423 (a beta blocker 97); *illus. 38A*

Bocasan a brand-name antimicrobial mouthwash 131 containing sodium perborate

Bonefos a brand name for sodium clodronate for low blood calcium 438 in cancer patients 154; *illus. 39D*

Bonjela a brand name for choline salicylate (a drug similar to aspirin 200)

Bonjela pastilles a brand name for pastilles for mouth ulcers containing lidocaine (a local anaesthetic 80) and aminacrine (a skin *antiseptic* 175)

Boots Nirolex Lozenges a cough suppressant containing dextromethorphan and menthol

Botox a brand name for botulinum *toxin* (a muscle relaxant 120)

botulinum toxin a muscle relaxant 120

Bradosol a brand name for benzalkonium chloride (an *antiseptic* 175)

Brasivol a brand-name abrasive paste for acne 177

bretylium tosilate an anti-arrhythmic 100

Brevinor a brand-name oral contraceptive 161 containing ethinylestradiol 279 and norethisterone 360

Bricanyl a brand name for terbutaline 415 (a bronchodilator 92 and drug used in premature labour 165); *illus. 44B*

brimonidine a drug for glaucoma 168

Britaject a brand name for apomorphine (a drug for Parkinson's disease 87)

Britlofex a brand name for lofexidine (a drug used to treat *opioid withdrawal* symptoms 24)

Broflex a brand name for trihexyphenidyl (a drug for parkinsonism 87)

Brolene a brand name for propamidine isethionate (an antibacterial 131) for eye infections

bromazepam a benzodiazepine anti-anxiety drug 83

bromocriptine 212 (a pituitary agent 145 and drug for parkinsonism 87)

brompheniramine an antihistamine 124

Bronchodil a brand name for reproterol (a bronchodilator 92)

Brufen, Brufen Retard brand names for ibuprofen 303 (a non-steroidal anti-inflammatory 116); *illus. 46F*

Buccastem a brand name for prochlorperazine 381 (an anti-emetic 90)

buclizine an antihistamine 124 and anti-emetic 90 used for motion sickness

budesonide 213 (a corticosteroid 141)

bumetanide 214 (a loop diuretic 99)

bupivacaine a long-lasting local anaesthetic 80 used in labour 165

buprenorphine an *opioid* analgesic 80

Burinex a brand name for bumetanide 214 (a loop diuretic 99); *illus. 44F*

Burinex A a brand name for bumetanide 214 (a loop diuretic 99) with amiloride 193 (a potassium-sparing diuretic 99)

Burinex K a brand name for bumetanide 214 (a loop diuretic 99) with potassium 443

BurnEze a brand name for benzocaine (a local anaesthetic 80)

Buscopan a brand name for hyoscine 302 (an *antispasmodic* for irritable bowel syndrome 110); *illus. 44R*

buserelin a drug for menstrual disorders 160

Buspar a brand name for buspirone (an anti-anxiety drug 83)

buspirone a non-benzodiazepine anti-anxiety drug 83

busulfan an alkylating agent for certain leukaemias 154

Butacote a brand name for phenylbutazone (a non-steroidal anti-inflammatory 116)

butobarbital a barbiturate sleeping drug 82

butoxyethyl nicotinate a vasodilator 98

C

cabergoline a drug to treat infertility 164 or to stop milk production in women who do not want to breast-feed

Cacit a brand name for calcium carbonate 438 (a mineral 150)

Cafergot a brand name for ergotamine 275 (a drug for migraine 89) with caffeine (a stimulant 88)

caffeine a stimulant 88 in coffee, tea, and cola, added to some analgesics 80

Calabren a brand name for glibenclamide 294 (an oral antidiabetic 142)

Caladryl a brand name for diphenhydramine (an antihistamine 124) with calamine lotion (an antipruritic 173)

calamine a substance containing zinc carbonate (an antipruritic 173) used to soothe irritated skin

Calcicard CR a brand of diltiazem 259 (an antihypertensive 102 and anti-angina drug 101)

Calcichew a brand name for calcium carbonate (calcium 438, a mineral 150); *illus. 42E*

calciferol vitamin D 448 (a vitamin 149)

CALCIJEX–CONCORDIN

Calcijex a brand name for calcitriol 448 (a vitamin 149)

Calciparine a brand of heparin 299 (an anticoagulant 104)

calcipotriol 215 (a drug for psoriasis 178)

calcitonin a drug for bone disorders 122

calcitonin (salmon) previously known as salcatonin (a drug for bone disorders 122)

calcitriol vitamin D 448 (a vitamin 149)

calcium 438 (a mineral 150)

calcium acetate calcium 438 (a mineral 150)

calcium carbonate a calcium salt 438 (a mineral 150) used as an antacid 108

calcium chloride calcium 438 (a mineral 150)

calcium folinate folinic acid salt used to reduce *side effects* of methotrexate 341

calcium gluconate calcium 438 (a mineral 150)

Calcium Resonium a drug to lower the amount of potassium 443 in the blood

Calcort a brand name for deflazacort (a corticosteroid 141, 174)

Calgel a brand-name teething gel containing lidocaine (a local anaesthetic 80) and cetylpyridinium (an antibacterial 131)

Calimal a brand name for chlorphenamine 225 (an antihistamine 124)

Calmurid HC a brand-name substance for eczema 179 containing hydrocortisone 301, lactic acid, and urea

Calpol a brand name for paracetamol 368 (a non-*opioid* analgesic 80)

Calsynar a brand name for calcitonin (salmon) (a drug for bone disorders 122)

CAM a brand name for ephedrine 272 (a bronchodilator 92)

Camcolit a brand name for lithium 324 (a drug for mania 85); *illus. 42L*

camphor a *topical* antipruritic 173

Campral EC a brand name for acamprosate (a drug for alcohol abuse 451)

Campto a brand name for irinotecan (an anticancer drug 154)

candesartan an angiotensin II inhibitor, an antihypertensive 102

Canesten a brand name for clotrimazole 239 (an antifungal 138)

Canesten HC a brand name for clotrimazole 239 (an antifungal 138) with hydrocortisone 301 (a corticosteroid 141)

canrenoate a potassium-sparing diuretic 99

Capastat a brand name for capreomycin sulphate (an antituberculous drug)

Capoten a brand name for captopril 216 (an ACE inhibitor 98); *illus. 46R*

Capozide a brand name for captopril 216 (an ACE inhibitor 98) with hydrochlorothiazide 300 (a thiazide diuretic 99)

capreomycin an antituberculous drug 132

Caprin a brand name for aspirin 200 (a non-*opioid* analgesic 80 and antiplatelet drug 104)

capsaicin a *rubefacient*

captopril 216 (an ACE inhibitor 98)

Carace a brand name for lisinopril 323 (an ACE inhibitor 98)

Carace Plus a brand-name preparation containing lisinopril 323 (an ACE inhibitor 98) and hydrochlorothiazide 300 (a thiazide diuretic 99)

carbachol a drug used for its *miotic* effect in glaucoma 168 and *parasympathomimetic* effect in urinary retention 166

Carbalax a brand name for sodium acid phosphate (a laxative 111) and sodium bicarbonate 403 (an antacid 108)

carbamazepine 217 (an anticonvulsant 86 and antipsychotic 85)

carbaryl 218 (an antiparasitic 176 for head lice infestation)

Carbellon a brand name for magnesium hydroxide 329 (an antacid 108 and laxative 111) with charcoal (an adsorbent) and peppermint oil (both substances for bowel spasm 110)

carbenoxolone an anti-ulcer drug 109

carbidopa a substance that enhances the therapeutic effect of levodopa 320 (a drug for parkinsonism 87)

carbimazole 219 (an anti-thyroid drug 144)

carbocisteine a *mucolytic* 93

Carbo-Dome a brand name for coal tar (a substance for psoriasis 178)

carboplatin an anticancer drug 154

carboprost a drug to control bleeding after childbirth 165

Cardene a brand name for nicardipine (a calcium channel blocker 101)

Cardilate MR a brand name for nifedipine 359 (a calcium channel blocker 101)

Cardinol a brand name for propranolol 386 (a beta blocker 97)

Cardura a brand name for doxazosin 267 (a *sympatholytic* antihypertensive 102); *illus. 46Q*

Carisoma a brand name for carisoprodol (a muscle relaxant 120 related to meprobamate, an anti-anxiety drug 83)

carisoprodol a muscle relaxant 120 related to meprobamate (an anti-anxiety drug 83)

carmustine an alkylating agent for Hodgkin's disease and solid tumours 154

carnitine an amino acid used as a nutritional supplement 148

Carnitor a brand name for carnitine (an amino acid used as a nutritional supplement 148)

carteolol a beta blocker 97 for glaucoma 168 and angina 101

carvedilol a beta blocker 97

Carylderm a brand name for carbaryl 218 (an antiparasitic 176 for head lice infestation)

cascara a stimulant laxative 111

castor oil a stimulant laxative 111

Catapres a brand name for clonidine (an antihypertensive 102 and drug for migraine 89)

Catarrh-Ex a brand-name decongestant 93 containing pseudoephedrine and paracetamol 368 (a non-*opioid* analgesic 80)

Caverject a brand name for alprostadil 190 (a prostaglandin used for male impotence 146, 164)

Cedocard a brand name for isosorbide dinitrate 312 (a nitrate vasodilator 98 and anti-angina drug 101); *illus. 37T*

cefaclor a cephalosporin antibiotic 128

cefadroxil a cephalosporin antibiotic 128

cefalexin 220 (a cephalosporin antibiotic 128)

cefamandole a cephalosporin antibiotic 128

cefazolin a cephalosporin antibiotic 128

cefixime a cephalosporin antibiotic 128

cefodizime a cephalosporin antibiotic 128

cefotaxime a cephalosporin antibiotic 128

cefoxitin a cephalosporin antibiotic 128

cefpirome a cephalosporin antibiotic 128

cefpodoxime a cephalosporin antibiotic 128

cefprozil a cephalosporin antibiotic 128

cefradine a cephalosporin antibiotic 128

Cefrom a brand name for cefpirome (a cephalosporin antibiotic 128)

ceftazidime a cephalosporin antibiotic 128

ceftriaxone a cephalosporin antibiotic 128

cefuroxime a cephalosporin antibiotic 128

Cefzil a brand name for cefprozil (a cephalosporin antibiotic 128)

Celance a brand name for pergolide (a drug for parkinsonism 87)

Celectol a brand name for celiprolol (a beta blocker 97)

Celevac a brand name for methylcellulose 342 (a laxative 111 and antidiarrhoeal 110); *illus. 35F*

celiprolol a beta blocker 97

Cellcept a brand name for mycophenolate mofetil (an immunosuppressant 156)

Ceporex a brand name for cefalexin 220 (a cephalosporin antibiotic 128)

Cerebrovase a brand name for dipyridamole 261 (an antiplatelet drug 104)

Cerezyme a brand name for imiglucerase (an *enzyme* for enzyme replacement therapy)

cerivastatin a lipid-lowering drug 103

certoparin an anticoagulant 104

Cerumol a brand-name preparation for ear-wax removal 171

cetirizine 221 (an antihistamine 124)

cetrimide a skin *antiseptic* 175

cetrorelix a drug for infertility 164

Cetrotide a brand name for cetrorelix (a drug for infertility 164)

cetylpyridinium (a *topical* skin *antiseptic* 175)

Chemotrim a brand name for co-trimoxazole 246 (an antibacterial 131)

Chendol a brand name for chenodeoxycholic acid (a drug for gallstones 114); *illus. 36J*

Chimax a brand name for flutamide 288 (an anticancer drug 154)

Chloractil a brand name for chlorpromazine 226 (a phenothiazine antipsychotic 85 and anti-emetic 90)

chloral hydrate a sleeping drug 82

chlorambucil an anticancer drug 154 used for chronic lymphocytic leukaemia and lymphatic and ovarian cancers, and as an immunosuppressant 156 for rheumatoid arthritis 117

chloramphenicol 222 (an antibiotic 128)

chlordiazepoxide 223 (a benzodiazepine anti-anxiety drug 83)

chlorhexidine a skin *antiseptic* 175

chlormethine previously known as mustine (a drug for Hodgkin's disease 154)

Chloromycetin a brand name for chloramphenicol 222 (an antibiotic 128)

chloroquine 224 (an antimalarial 137 and antirheumatic 117)

chlorothiazide a thiazide diuretic 99

chloroxylenol a skin *antiseptic* 175

chlorphenamine 225 previously known as chlorpheniramine (an antihistamine 124)

chlorpheniramine see chlorphenamine 225

chlorpromazine 226 (a phenothiazine antipsychotic 85 and anti-emetic 90)

chlorpropamide a drug for diabetes 142

chlortalidone a thiazide diuretic 99

chlortetracycline a tetracycline antibiotic 128

choline salicylate a drug similar to aspirin 200 used in pain-relieving mouth gels 80

choline theophyllinate a xanthine bronchodilator 92

chorionic gonadotrophin 227 (a drug for infertility 164)

chromium 439 (a mineral 150)

Cicatrin a brand name for bacitracin (an antibacterial 131) with neomycin (an antibiotic 128)

cidofovir an antiviral for cytomegalovirus 133 in AIDS 157

Cidomycin a brand name for gentamicin 293 (an aminoglycoside antibiotic 128)

cilastatin an *enzyme* inhibitor used to make imipenem (an antibiotic 128) more effective

cilazapril an ACE inhibitor 98

Cilest a brand-name oral contraceptive containing ethinylestradiol 279 and norgestimate

cimetidine 228 (an anti-ulcer drug 109)

Cinaziere a brand name for cinnarizine 229 (an antihistamine anti-emetic 90)

cinchocaine a local anaesthetic 80

cinnarizine 229 (an antihistamine anti-emetic 90)

Cinobac a brand name for cinoxacin (a urinary tract antibiotic 128)

cinoxacin a urinary tract antibiotic 128

Cipramil a brand name for citalopram 233 (an antidepressant 84)

ciprofibrate a lipid-lowering drug 103

ciprofloxacin 230 (an antibiotic 128)

Ciproxin a brand name for ciprofloxacin 230 (an antibacterial 131); *illus. 42S*

cisapride 231 (a gastrointestinal motility regulator 110)

cisatracurium a drug used to relax the muscles in general *anaesthesia*

cisplatin 232 (an anticancer drug 154)

citalopram 233 (an antidepressant 84)

Citanest a brand name for prilocaine (a local anaesthetic 80)

Citramag a brand name for magnesium citrate (an osmotic laxative 111)

cladribine an anticancer drug 154

clarithromycin a macrolide antibiotic 128

Clarityn a brand name for loratadine 327 (an antihistamine 124); *illus. 46S*

clavulanic acid a substance given with amoxicillin 198 (a penicillin antibiotic 128) to make it more effective

clemastine an antihistamine 124

Clexane a brand name for enoxaparin (a low-molecular-weight heparin 299, an anticoagulant 104)

Climagest a brand-name preparation for menopausal symptoms 147 containing estradiol 277 and norethisterone 360

Climaval a brand-name preparation for menopausal symptoms 147 containing estradiol 277

Climesse a brand-name preparation for menopausal symptoms 147 containing estradiol 277 and norethisterone 360

clindamycin a lincosamide antibiotic 128

Clinitar a brand name for coal tar (a substance used for psoriasis 178 and dandruff 180)

Clinoril a brand name for sulindac (a non-steroidal anti-inflammatory 116)

clioquinol an antibacterial 131 and antifungal 138 for outer-ear infections 171

clobazam a benzodiazepine anti-anxiety drug 83

clobetasol 234 (a topical corticosteroid 174)

clobetasone a topical corticosteroid 174

Cloburate a brand name for clobetasone (a topical corticosteroid 174)

clodronate an anticancer drug 154

clofazimine a drug for leprosy 131

clofibrate a lipid-lowering drug 103

clomethiazole a non-benzodiazepine, non-barbiturate sleeping drug 82

Clomid a brand name for clomifene 235 (a drug for infertility 164); *illus. 37B*

clomifene 235 (a drug for infertility 164)

clomipramine 236 (a tricyclic antidepressant 84)

clonazepam 237 (a benzodiazepine anticonvulsant 86)

clonidine an antihypertensive 102 and drug for migraine 89

clopamide a thiazide diuretic 99

clopidogrel 238 (an antiplatelet drug 104)

Clopixol a brand name for zuclopenthixol (an antipsychotic 85)

cloral betaine a sleeping drug 82

clorazepate a benzodiazepine anti-anxiety drug 83

Clotam a brand name for tolfenamic acid (a drug for migraine 89)

clotrimazole 239 (an antifungal 138)

clozapine 240 (an antipsychotic 85)

Clozaril a brand name for clozapine 240 (an antipsychotic 85); *illus. 45P*

coal tar a substance for psoriasis 178 and eczema 179

co-amilofruse a generic product containing amiloride 193 with furosemide 291 (both diuretics 99)

co-amilozide a generic product containing amiloride 193 with hydrochlorothiazide 300 (both diuretics 99)

co-amoxiclav a generic product containing amoxicillin 198 (a penicillin antibiotic 128) with clavulanic acid (a substance that increases the effectiveness of amoxicillin)

Cobadex a brand name for hydrocortisone 301 (a corticosteroid 141) and dimeticone (an anti-foaming agent 108)

Cobalin-H a brand name for hydroxocobalamin (a vitamin 149)

co-beneldopa a generic product containing levodopa 320 (a drug for parkinsonism 87) with benserazide (a drug that enhances the effect of levodopa)

Co-Betaloc a brand name for hydrochlorothiazide 300 (a thiazide diuretic 99) with metoprolol 345 (a beta blocker 97)

cocaine a local anaesthetic 80

co-careldopa a generic product containing carbidopa with levodopa 320 (both drugs for parkinsonism 87)

co-codamol a generic product containing codeine 241 with paracetamol 368 (both analgesics 80)

co-codaprin a generic product containing aspirin 200 with codeine 241 (both analgesics 80)

Codafen Continus a brand name for codeine 241 (an *opioid* analgesic 80) and ibuprofen 303 (a non-steroidal anti-inflammatory 116)

Codalax a brand name for co-danthramer (a stimulant laxative 111)

co-danthramer a generic product containing dantron with poloxamer (both stimulant laxatives 111)

co-danthrusate a generic product containing dantron with docusate (both stimulant laxatives 111)

codeine 241 (an *opioid* analgesic 80, cough suppressant 94, and antidiarrhoeal 110)

co-dergocrine mesylate a vasodilator 98 used to improve blood flow to the brain in senile dementia

Codis a brand name for aspirin 200 with codeine 241 (both analgesics 80)

co-dydramol a generic product containing paracetamol 368 with dihydrocodeine (both analgesics 80)

co-fluampicil a generic product containing flucloxacillin with ampicillin (both penicillin antibiotics 128)

co-flumactone a generic product containing hydroflumethiazide with spironolactone (both diuretics 99)

Cogentin a brand name for benztropine (an *anticholinergic* for parkinsonism 87)

Colazide a brand name for balsalazide (a drug for ulcerative colitis 112)

colchicine 242 (a drug for gout 119)

cold cream an antipruritic 173

colecalciferol vitamin D 448 (a vitamin 149)

colestipol a lipid-lowering drug 103

colestyramine 243 (a lipid-lowering drug 103)

colfosceril palmitate a drug to mature the lungs of premature babies

Colifoam a brand name for hydrocortisone 301 (a corticosteroid 141)

colistimethate the injection form of colistin (an antibiotic 128)

colistin an antibiotic 128

collodion a substance that dries to form a sticky film, protecting broken skin 175

Colofac a brand name for mebeverine 331 (an *antispasmodic* for irritable bowel syndrome 110); *illus. 42J*

Colomycin a brand name for colistin (an antibiotic 128)

Colpermin a brand name for peppermint oil (a substance for indigestion 108 and spasm of the bowel 110)

co-magaldrox a generic product containing aluminium hydroxide 191 with magnesium hydroxide 329 (both antacids 108)

Combivent a brand-name *inhaler* containing salbutamol 399 and ipratropium bromide 309 (both bronchodilators 92)

Combivir a brand-name preparation containing lamivudine 317 and zidovudine 435 (antivirals 133 used for HIV/AIDS 157)

co-methiamol a generic product containing paracetamol 368 and methionine (an *antidote* to paracetamol poisoning)

Comixco a brand name for co-trimoxazole 246 (an antibacterial 131 and antiprotozoal 136)

Compound W a brand-name keratolytic 177 for warts, containing salicylic acid

Comtess a brand name for entacapone (a drug for parkinsonism 87)

Concavit a brand-name multivitamin 149

Concordin a brand name for protriptyline (a tricyclic antidepressant 84)

CONDYLINE–DIPHENOXYLATE

Condyline a brand name for podophyllotoxin (a drug for genital warts 133)

conjugated oestrogens 244 (a female sex hormone 147 and drug for bone disorders 122)

Conotrane a brand name for benzalkonium chloride (a skin *antiseptic* 175) with dimeticone (a base for skin preparations 175)

Contac 400 a brand name for chlorphenamine 225 (an antihistamine 124) with phenyl-propanolamine 373 (a decongestant 93)

Contac Cough Caps a brand name for dextromethorphan (a cough suppressant 94)

Contimin a brand name for oxybutynin 367 (an *anticholinergic* and *antispasmodic* for urinary disorders 166)

Convulex a brand name for sodium valproate 405 (an anticonvulsant 86)

co-phenotrope a generic product containing diphenoxylate 260 with atropine 203

copper 439 (a mineral 150)

co-prenozide a generic product containing oxprenolol (a beta blocker 97) with cyclopenthiazide 247 (a thiazide diuretic 99)

co-proxamol 245 (an *opioid* analgesic 80); *illus. 46K*

Coracten a brand name for nifedipine 359 (an anti-angina drug 101 and antihypertensive 102)

Cordarone X a brand name for amiodarone 194 (an anti-arrhythmic 100); *illus. 43B*

Cordilox a brand name for verapamil 431 (an anti-angina drug 101 and anti-arrhythmic 100)

Corgard a brand name for nadolol (a beta blocker 97)

Corgaretic a brand name for bendroflumethiazide 207 (a thiazide diuretic 99) with nadolol (a beta blocker 97)

Corlan a brand name for hydrocortisone 301 (a corticosteroid 141); *illus. 46D*

Coro-Nitro a brand name for glyceryl trinitrate 296 (an anti-angina drug 101)

Corsodyl a brand-name mouthwash and oral gel containing chlorhexidine (an *antiseptic* 175)

corticotropin a pituitary *hormone* 145

cortisol an old name for hydrocortisone 301

cortisone a corticosteroid 141

Cortisyl a brand name for cortisone (a corticosteroid 141)

Cosalgesic a brand name for co-proxamol 245 (an *opioid* analgesic 80)

co-simalcite a generic product containing hydrotalcite (an antacid 108) with dimeticone (an antifoaming agent 108)

Cosopt a brand-name preparation containing dorzolamide 265 and timolol 423 (drugs for glaucoma 168)

co-tenidone a generic product containing atenolol 201 (a beta blocker 97) with chlortalidone (a thiazide diuretic 99)

co-triamterzide a generic product containing hydrochlorothiazide 300 with triamterene 428 (both diuretics 99)

co-trimoxazole 246 (an antibacterial 131 and antiprotozoal 136)

Coversyl a brand name for perindopril (an ACE inhibitor 98)

Cozaar a brand name for losartan 328 (an antihypertensive 102)

Cozaar-Comp a brand-name preparation containing losartan 328 and hydrochlorothiazide 300 (a product for high blood pressure 102)

Cream of Magnesia a brand-name for magnesium hydroxide 329 (an antacid 108 and laxative 111)

Cremalgin a brand name *topical* preparation for muscular pain relief containing glycol salicylate, methyl nicotinate, and capsicum oleoresin

Creon a brand name for pancreatin (a preparation of pancreatic *enzymes* 114)

crisantaspase an anticancer drug 154

Crixivan a brand name for indinavir (an antiviral for HIV/AIDS 157)

Cromogen a brand name for sodium cromoglicate 404 (an anti-allergy drug 124)

cromoglicate 404 an anti-allergy drug 124

crotamiton an antipruritic 173 and antiparasitic 176 for scabies

Crystapen a brand name for penicillin G (a penicillin antibiotic 128)

Cupanol a brand name for paracetamol 368 (a non-*opioid* analgesic 80)

Cuplex a brand-name wart preparation containing copper acetate, lactic acid, and salicylic acid

Cuprofen a brand name for ibuprofen 303 (a non-steroidal anti-inflammatory 116)

Curatoderm a brand name for tacalcitol (a drug for psoriasis 178)

Cutivate a brand name for fluticasone 289 (a corticosteroid 141)

cyanocobalamin vitamin B_{12} 447 (a vitamin 149)

Cyclimorph a brand name for morphine 353 (an *opioid* analgesic 80) with cyclizine (an anti-emetic 90)

cyclizine an antihistamine 124 used as an anti-emetic 90

cyclobenzaprine a muscle relaxant 120

Cyclodox a brand name for doxycycline 269 (a tetracycline antibiotic 128)

Cyclogest a brand name for progesterone (a female sex hormone 147)

cyclopenthiazide 247 (a thiazide diuretic 99)

cyclopentolate an *anticholinergic mydriatic* 170

cyclophosphamide 248 (an anticancer drug 154)

Cyclo-Progynova a brand name for estradiol 277 with levonorgestrel 322 (both female sex hormones 147)

cycloserine an antibiotic 128 for tuberculosis 132

cyclosporin 249 (an immunosuppressant 156)

Cyklokapron a brand name for tranexamic acid (an antifibrinolytic used to promote blood clotting 104)

Cymalon a brand-name preparation for cystitis 166 containing sodium bicarbonate 403, citric acid, sodium citrate, and sodium carbonate

Cymevene a brand name for ganciclovir (an antiviral 133)

cyproheptadine an antihistamine 124 used to stimulate the appetite 88

Cyprostat a brand name for cyproterone acetate (a synthetic sex hormone used for acne 177 and cancer of the prostate 154)

cyproterone a synthetic sex hormone used for acne 177, cancer of the prostate 154, and male sexual disorders 146

Cystoleve a brand name for sodium citrate (used for cystitis 166)

Cystopurin a brand name for potassium citrate 443 (used for cystitis 166)

Cystrin a brand name for oxybutynin 367 (an *anticholinergic* and *antispasmodic* for urinary disorders 166)

cytarabine a drug for leukaemia 154

Cytotec a brand name for misoprostol 350 (an anti-ulcer drug 109)

D

dacarbazine a drug for malignant melanoma and cancer of soft tissues 154

daclizumab an immunosuppressant 156

dactinomycin a *cytotoxic* antibiotic for cancer 154

Daktacort a brand name for hydrocortisone 301 (a corticosteroid 141) with miconazole 347 (an antifungal 138)

Daktarin a brand name for miconazole 347 (an antifungal 138)

Dalacin C a brand name for clindamycin (a lincosamide antibiotic 128)

dalfopristin an antibiotic 130

Dalivit a brand-name multivitamin 149

Dalmane a brand name for flurazepam (a benzodiazepine sleeping drug 82)

dalteparin a type of heparin 299 (an anticoagulant 104)

danaparoid an anticoagulant 104

danazol 250 (a drug for menstrual disorders 160)

Daneral-SA a brand name for pheniramine (an antihistamine 124)

Danol a brand name for danazol 250 (a drug for menstrual disorders 160); *illus. 40F*

Dantrium a brand name for dantrolene (a muscle relaxant 120)

dantrolene a muscle relaxant 120

dantron a stimulant laxative 111

Daonil a brand name for glibenclamide 294 (an oral antidiabetic 142); *illus. 46 O*

dapsone an antibacterial 131; *illus. 45C*

Daraprim a brand name for pyrimethamine 389 (an antimalarial 137); *illus. 44N*

daunorubicin a *cytotoxic* antibiotic (an anticancer drug 154)

Day Nurse a brand name for dextromethorphan (a cough suppressant 94) with paracetamol 368 (a non-*opioid* analgesic 80) and phenylpropanolamine 373 (a decongestant 93)

debrisoquine an antihypertensive 102

DDAVP a brand name for desmopressin 251 (a pituitary *hormone* 145)

Decadron a brand name for dexamethasone 252 (a corticosteroid 141); *illus. 45J*

Deca-Durabolin-100 a brand name for nandrolone (an anabolic steroid 154)

De-capeptyl sr a brand name for triptorelin (an anticancer drug 154)

deflazacort a corticosteroid 141, 174

Delfen a brand name for nonoxinol '9' (a spermicidal agent 161)

Deltacortril Enteric a brand name for prednisolone 379 (a corticosteroid 141); *illus. 35J*

Deltastab a brand name for prednisolone 379 (a corticosteroid 141)

demeclocycline a tetracycline antibiotic 128

Demix a brand of doxycycline 269 (a tetracycline antibiotic 128)

De-Nol a brand name for bismuth (a substance for gastric and duodenal ulcers 109)

Dentomycin a brand name for minocycline 348 (a tetracycline antibiotic 128)

Depixol a brand name for flupentixol 287 (an antipsychotic 85 and antidepressant 84)

Depo-Medrone a brand name for methyl-prednisolone (a corticosteroid 141)

Deponit a brand name for glyceryl trinitrate 296 (an anti-angina drug 101)

Depo-Provera a brand name for medroxyprogesterone 332 (a female sex hormone 147)

Depostat a brand name for gestonerone (a progestogen 147)

Dequacaine a brand name for benzocaine (a local anaesthetic 80) with dequalinium (an antibacterial 131)

Dequadin a brand name for dequalinium (an antibacterial 131)

dequalinium an antibacterial 131 used for mouth infections

Derbac-M a brand-name shampoo containing malathion 330 (an anti-parasitic 176)

Dermacort a brand-name preparation for hydrocortisone cream 301

Dermidex Cream a brand-name *topical* preparation for skin irritation containing chlorobutanol, lignocaine, cetrimide, and alcloxa

Dermovate a brand name for clobetasol 234 (a topical corticosteroid 174)

Dermovate-NN a brand name for nystatin 361 (an antifungal 138) with clobetasol 234 (a topical corticosteroid 174) and neomycin (an aminoglycoside antibiotic 128)

desferrioxamine an *antidote* for iron 441 overdose

desflurane a general *anaesthetic*

desirudin an anticoagulant 104

desmopressin 251 (a pituitary *hormone* 145 used for diabetes insipidus 142)

desogestrel a progestogen 147

desoxymetasone a topical corticosteroid 174

Destolit a brand name for ursodeoxycholic acid (a drug for gallstones 114)

Deteclo a brand name for tetracycline 418 with chlortetracycline and demeclocycline (all tetracycline antibiotics 128)

Detrunorm a brand name for propiverine (a drug for urinary frequency 166)

Detrusitol a brand name for tolterodine 425 (an *anticholinergic* and *antispasmodic* for urinary disorders 166); *illus. 45 O*

Dettol a brand-name liquid skin *antiseptic* 175 containing chloroxylenol

dexketoprofen a non-steroidal anti-inflammatory 116

dexamethasone 252 (a corticosteroid 141)

dexamfetamine an amfetamine 452

Dexa-Rhinaspray a brand name for dexamethasone 252 (a corticosteroid 141) with neomycin (an aminoglycoside antibiotic 128) and tramazoline (a nasal decongestant 93)

Dexedrine a brand name for dexamfetamine (an amfetamine 452)

dextromethorphan a cough suppressant 94

dextromoramide an *opioid* analgesic 80

dextropropoxyphene a constituent of co-proxamol 245 (an *opioid* analgesic 80)

DF 118 a brand name for dihydrocodeine (an *opioid* analgesic 80)

DHC Continus a brand name for dihydrocodeine (an *opioid* analgesic 80)

Diabetamide a brand name for glibenclamide 294 (an oral antidiabetic 142)

Diabinese a brand name for chlorpropamide (an oral antidiabetic 142); *illus. 45D*

Dialar a brand of diazepam 253 (a benzodiazepine anti-anxiety drug 83, muscle relaxant 120, and anticonvulsant 86)

Diamicron a brand name for gliclazide 295 (an oral antidiabetic 142); *illus. 44E*

diamorphine 353 (an *opioid* analgesic 80)

Diamox a brand name for acetazolamide (a carbonic anhydrase inhibitor diuretic 99); *illus. 42 O*

Dianette a brand name for cyproterone acetate (a synthetic sex hormone used for acne 177) with ethinylestradiol 279 (a female sex hormone 147)

Diarphen a brand name for diphenoxylate 260 (an *opioid* antidiarrhoeal 110) with atropine 203

Diarrest a brand-name antidiarrhoeal 110 containing dicycloverine 255 and codeine 241

Diasorb a brand name for loperamide 326 (an antidiarrhoeal 110)

Diazemuls a brand name for diazepam 253 (a benzodiazepine anti-anxiety drug 83, muscle relaxant 120, and anticonvulsant 86)

diazepam 253 (a benzodiazepine anti-anxiety drug 83, muscle relaxant 120, and anticonvulsant 86)

diazoxide an antihypertensive 102 also used for hypoglycaemia 142

diclofenac 254 (a non-steroidal anti-inflammatory 116)

Dicloflex a brand name for diclofenac 254 (a non-steroidal anti-inflammatory 116)

Diclomax Retard a brand name for diclofenac sodium 254 (a non-steroidal anti-inflammatory 116)

dicobalt edetate an *antidote* for cyanide poisoning

Diconal a brand name for dipipanone (an *opioid* analgesic 80)

dicyclomine see dicycloverine 255

dicycloverine 255 previously known as dicyclomine (a drug for irritable bowel syndrome 110)

Dicynene a brand name for etamsylate (an antifibrinolytic used to promote blood clotting 104)

didanosine 256 (an antiviral drug for HIV infection and AIDS 157)

Didronel a brand name for etidronate 281 (a drug for bone disorders 122)

Didronel PMO a brand name for etidronate 281 (a drug for bone disorders 122) and calcium carbonate 438

dienestrol a female sex hormone 147 applied as a cream for vaginal dryness

diethylamine salicylate a *rubefacient*

diethylcarbamazine an anthelmintic 139

diethylstilbestrol 257 previously known as stilboestrol (a female sex hormone 147)

diethyltoluamide (DEET) a mosquito repellent

Differin a brand name for adapalene a retinoid for acne 177

Difflam a brand name for benzydamine (an analgesic 80)

Diflucan a brand name for fluconazole 285 (an antifungal 138); *illus. 41G, 41P*

diflucortolone a topical corticosteroid 174

diflunisal a non-steroidal anti-inflammatory 116

Digibind an *antidote* for digoxin overdose

digitoxin a digitalis drug 96

digoxin 258 (a digitalis drug 96)

dihydrocodeine an *opioid* analgesic 80

dihydroergotamine a drug for migraine 89

dihydrotachysterol vitamin D 448 (a vitamin 149)

Dijex a brand name for didanosine 256 (an antiviral drug for HIV infection and AIDS 157)

diloxanide furoate an antiprotozoal 136 for amoebic dysentery

diltiazem 259 (an antihypertensive 102 and calcium channel blocker 101)

Dilzem a brand name for diltiazem 259 (a calcium channel blocker 101)

dimenhydrinate an antihistamine 124 used as an anti-emetic 90

dimercaprol an *antidote* for heavy metal poisoning

dimeticone a silicone-based substance used in barrier creams 175 and as an antifoaming agent 108

dimethyl sulfoxide a drug to treat bladder inflammation

Dimetriose a brand name for gestrinone (a drug for menstrual disorders 160)

Dimotane a brand name for brompheniramine (an antihistamine 124)

Dimotapp a brand name for phenylephrine with phenylpropanolamine 373 (both decongestants 93) and brompheniramine (an antihistamine 124)

Dindevan a brand name for phenindione (an oral anticoagulant 104)

dinoprost a prostaglandin used to terminate pregnancy 165

dinoprostone a prostaglandin used to terminate pregnancy 165

Diocalm a brand-name antidiarrhoeal 110 containing attapulgite and morphine 353

Diocalm Ultra a brand name for loperamide 326 (an antidiarrhoeal 110)

Dioctyl a brand name for docusate (a stimulant laxative 111)

Dioderm a brand name for hydrocortisone 301 (a corticosteroid 141)

Dioralyte a brand name for rehydration tablets containing sodium bicarbonate 403, glucose, potassium chloride 443, and sodium chloride 445

Dioralyte Relief a brand name for rehydration powder containing sodium chloride 445, potassium chloride 443, and sodium citrate

Diovol a brand-name antacid 108 containing aluminium hydroxide 191, magnesium hydroxide 329, and dimeticone

Dipentum a brand name for olsalazine (a drug for ulcerative colitis 112)

diphenhydramine an antihistamine 124, anti-emetic 90, and antipruritic 173

diphenoxylate 260 (an *opioid* antidiarrhoeal 110)

DIPHENYPYRALINE–FEMODENE

diphenylpyraline an antihistamine 124

dipipanone an *opioid* analgesic 80

dipivefrine a *sympathomimetic* for glaucoma 168

Diprobase a brand-name *emollient* preparation 173

Diprosalic a brand-name skin preparation containing betamethasone 210 (a corticosteroid 141) and salicylic acid (a keratolytic 177)

Diprosone a brand name for betamethasone 210 (a corticosteroid 141)

dipyridamole 261 (an antiplatelet drug 104)

Dirythmin SA a brand name for disopyramide (an anti-arrhythmic 100)

Disipal a brand name for orphenadrine 366 (a drug for parkinsonism 87); *illus. 36N*

disopyramide an anti-arrhythmic 100

Disprin a brand name for soluble aspirin 200 (a non-*opioid* analgesic 80)

Disprin Extra a brand-name soluble analgesic 80 containing aspirin 200 and paracetamol 368

Disprol a brand name for paracetamol 368 (a non-*opioid* analgesic 80)

Distaclor MR a brand name for cefaclor (a cephalosporin antibiotic 128); *illus. 38H*

Distalgesic a brand name for co-proxamol 245 (an *opioid* analgesic 80)

Distamine a brand name for penicillamine (an antirheumatic 117); *illus. 43G*

distigmine a *parasympathomimetic* for urinary retention 166 and myasthenia gravis 121

disulfiram 262 (an alcohol abuse deterrent 24, 451)

dithranol a drug for psoriasis 178

Dithrocream a brand name for dithranol (a drug for psoriasis 178)

Ditropan a brand name for oxybutynin 367 (an *anticholinergic* and *antispasmodic* for urinary disorders 166)

Diumide-K Continus a brand name for furosemide 291 (a loop diuretic 99 and antihypertensive 102) with potassium 443

Diurexan a brand name for xipamide (a thiazide diuretic 99)

Dixarit a brand name for clonidine (a drug for migraine 89)

dobutamine a drug for heart failure and shock

docetaxel an anticancer drug 154

docusate a faecal softener, stimulant laxative 111, and ear-wax softener 171

Do-Do tablets a brand-name bronchodilator 92 and decongestant 93 containing ephedrine 272, theophylline 419, and caffeine

Dolmatil a brand name for sulpiride 195 (an antipsychotic 85)

Dolobid a brand name for diflunisal (a non-steroidal anti-inflammatory 116)

Doloxene a brand name for dextropropoxyphene (an *opioid* analgesic 80)

Domical a brand name for amitriptyline 196 (a tricyclic antidepressant 84)

domperidone 263 (an anti-emetic 90)

donepezil 264 a drug for dementia 87

dopamine a drug for heart failure, kidney failure, and shock

dopexamine a drug for heart failure

Doralese a brand name for indoramin 306 (an antihypertensive 102)

dornase alfa a drug for cystic fibrosis 114

dorzolamide 265 a carbonic anhydrase inhibitor for glaucoma 168

Dostinex a brand name for cabergoline (a drug to treat infertility 164)

dosulepin 266 previously known as dothiepin (a tricyclic antidepressant 84)

Dothapax a brand name for dosulepin 266 (a tricyclic antidepressant 84)

dothiepin see dosulepin 266 (a tricyclic antidepressant 84)

Dovonex a brand name for calcipotriol 215 (a drug for psoriasis 178)

doxapram a respiratory stimulant 88

doxazosin 267 (a *sympatholytic* antihypertensive 102)

doxepin a tricyclic antidepressant 84

doxorubicin 268 (a *cytotoxic* anticancer drug 154)

doxycycline 269 (a tetracycline antibiotic 128)

doxylamine an antihistamine 124

Doxylar a brand name for doxycycline 269 (a tetracycline antibiotic 128)

Dozic a brand name for haloperidol 298 (a butyrophenone antipsychotic 85)

Dramamine a brand name for dimenhydrinate (an antihistamine 124 used as an anti-emetic 90)

Drapolene a brand name for benzalkonium chloride with cetrimide (both skin *antiseptics* 175)

Driclor a brand name for aluminium chloride (an *antiperspirant*)

Dristan Nasal Spray a brand name for oxymetazoline hydrochloride (a *topical* decongestant 93) with chlorphenamine 225 (an antihistamine 124)

Drogenil a brand name for flutamide 288 (an anticancer drug 154); *illus. 37A*

Droleptan a brand name for droperidol (a butyrophenone antipsychotic 85)

droperidol a butyrophenone antipsychotic 85

Dryptal a brand name for furosemide 291 (a loop diuretic 99 and antihypertensive 102)

Dulco-Lax a brand name for bisacodyl (a stimulant laxative 111)

Duofilm a brand-name wart preparation containing lactic acid, salicylic acid, and collodion 175

Duovent a brand name for fenoterol with ipratropium bromide 309 (both bronchodilators 92)

Duphalac a brand name for lactulose 316 (a laxative 111)

Duphaston, Duphaston HRT a brand name for dydrogesterone 270 (a female sex hormone 147); *illus. 42N*

Duragel a brand name for nonoxinol '11' (a spermicidal agent 161)

Durogesic a brand name for fentanyl (an *opioid* analgesic 80)

Duromine a brand name for phentermine (an appetite suppressant 88)

Dutonin a brand name for nefazodone (an antidepressant 84)

Dyazide a brand name for hydrochlorothiazide 300 with triamterene 428 (both diuretics 99)

dydrogesterone 270 (a female sex hormone 147)

Dynese a brand name for magaldrate (an antacid 108)

Dysman a brand name for mefenamic acid 333 (a non-steroidal anti-inflammatory 116)

Dyspamet a brand name for cimetidine 228 (an anti-ulcer drug 109)

Dysport a brand name for botulinum *toxin* (used as a muscle relaxant 120)

Dytac a brand name for triamterene 428 (a potassium-sparing diuretic 99)

Dytide a brand name for benzthiazide with triamterene 428 (both diuretics 99)

E

Earex a brand-name preparation for ear-wax removal 171

Ebufac a brand name for ibuprofen 303 (a non-steroidal anti-inflammatory 116)

Econacort a brand name for econazole (an antifungal 138) with hydrocortisone 301 (a corticosteroid 141)

econazole an antifungal 138

Economycin a brand name for tetracycline 418 (an antibiotic 128)

Ecostatin a brand name for econazole (an antifungal 138)

ecothiopate a drug for glaucoma 168

Edronax a brand name for reboxetine (an antidepressant 84)

edrophonium a drug for diagnosis of myasthenia gravis 121

Efalith a brand-name ointment for dermatitis 174, 179, containing lithium succinate 324 and zinc sulphate 449

Efamast a brand name for gamolenic acid 292 (a drug used to treat breast pain); *illus. 39G*

efavirenz an antiviral for HIV/AIDS 157

Efcortelan a brand name for hydrocortisone 301 (a corticosteroid 141)

Efcortesol a brand name for hydrocortisone 301 (a corticosteroid 141)

Efexor a brand name for venlafaxine 430 (an antidepressant 84); *illus. 35T*

Effercitrate a brand name for potassium 443 (a mineral 150)

eformoterol (formoterol) a *sympathomimetic* bronchodilator 92

Elantan a brand name for isosorbide mononitrate 312 (a nitrate vasodilator 98 and anti-angina drug 101)

Elavil a brand name for amitriptyline 196 (a tricyclic antidepressant 84)

Eldepryl a brand name for selegiline (a drug for parkinsonism 87)

Electrolade brand-name oral rehydration salts with potassium chloride 443, sodium chloride 445, sodium bicarbonate 403, and glucose

Elleste Duet a brand-name preparation for menopausal symptoms 147 containing estradiol 277 and norethisterone 360

Elleste Solo a brand name for estradiol 277 (an oestrogen 147)

Elocon a brand name for mometasone 351 (a topical corticosteroid 174)

Eloxatin a brand name for oxaliplatin an anticancer drug 154

Eltroxin a brand name for levothyroxine 421 (a thyroid *hormone* 144); *illus. 46B*

Eludril a brand name for chlorhexidine (an *antiseptic*)

Elyzol a brand name for metronidazole 346 (an antibacterial 131 and antiprotozoal 136)

Emblon a brand name for tamoxifen 411 (an anticancer drug 154)

Emcor a brand name for bisoprolol (a beta blocker 97)

Emeside a brand name for ethosuximide 280 (an anticonvulsant 86)

Emflex a brand name for acemetacin (a non-steroidal anti-inflammatory 116)

Eminase a brand name for anistreplase (a thrombolytic 105)

Emla a brand-name local anaesthetic 80 containing lidocaine and prilocaine

enalapril 271 (a vasodilator 98 and antihypertensive 102)

En-De-Kay a brand name for fluoride 440 (a mineral 150)

Endoxana a brand name for cyclophosphamide 248 (an anticancer drug 154); *illus. 44H*

enflurane a general *anaesthetic*

ENO's a brand-name antacid 108 containing sodium bicarbonate 403, sodium carbonate, and citric acid

enoxaparin a type of heparin 299 (an anticoagulant 104)

enoximone a drug for heart failure 95

entacapone a drug for parkinsonism 87

Entocort CR a brand name for budesonide 213 (a corticosteroid 141)

Epanutin a brand name for phenytoin 374 (an anticonvulsant 86); *illus. 40 I*

ephedrine 272 (a bronchodilator 92 and decongestant 93)

Epilim a brand name for sodium valproate 405 (an anticonvulsant 86); *illus. 43L*

epinephrine 273 (a bronchodilator 92 and drug for glaucoma 168 and anaphylactic shock 496). Also known as adrenaline

EpiPen a brand name for epinephrine 273 (an anti-allergy drug 124); *illus. 47A*

epirubicin a *cytotoxic* anticancer drug 154

Epivir a brand name for lamivudine 317 an antiviral 133 used for HIV/AIDS 157

epoetin 274 (a kidney *hormone* 140 used for *anaemia* due to kidney failure). Also known as erythropoietin

Epogam a brand name for gamolenic acid 292 (a drug for eczema 179)

epoprostenol a prostaglandin used for its vasodilator effects 98

Eppy a brand name for epinephrine 273 (a drug for glaucoma 168)

Eprex a brand name for epoetin 274 (a kidney *hormone* 140 used for *anaemia* due to kidney failure)

eptifibatide a drug for prevention of heart attacks 95

Equagesic a brand name for aspirin 200 with ethoheptazine (both analgesics 80) and meprobamate (an anti-anxiety drug 83)

ergocalciferol vitamin D 448 (a vitamin 149)

ergometrine a uterine stimulant 165

ergotamine 275 (a drug for migraine 89)

Erwinase a brand name for crisantaspase (an anticancer drug 154)

Erycen a brand name for erythromycin 276 (an antibiotic 128)

Erymax a brand name for erythromycin 276 (an antibiotic 128)

Erythrocin a brand name for erythromycin 276 (an antibiotic 128)

Erythromid a brand name for erythromycin 282 (an antibiotic 128); *illus. 35M*

erythromycin 276 (an antibiotic 128)

Erythroped a brand name for erythromycin 276 (an antibiotic 128)

erythropoietin 274 (a kidney *hormone* 140 used for *anaemia* due to kidney failure). Also known as epoetin

Eskamel a brand name for resorcinol (a drug for acne 177) with sulphur (a *topical* antibacterial 131 and antifungal 138)

Eskornade a brand name for phenylpropanolamine 373 (a decongestant 93) with diphenylpyraline (an antihistamine 124)

esmolol a beta blocker 97

Estracombi a brand-name preparation for menopausal symptoms 147 containing estradiol 277 and norethisterone 360

Estraderm TTS a brand name for estradiol 277 (an oestrogen 147); *illus. 47F*

estradiol 277 (an oestrogen 147)

estramustine an alkylating agent for cancer of the prostate 154

Estrapak a brand-name preparation for menopausal symptoms 147 containing estradiol 277 and norethisterone 360

Estring a brand-name vaginal ring for menopausal symptoms 147 containing estradiol 277

estriol an oestrogen 147

estrone an oestrogen 147

estropipate an oestrogen 147

etacrynic acid a loop diuretic 99

etamsylate an antifibrinolytic used to promote blood clotting 104

ethambutol 278 (an antituberculous drug 132)

ethinylestradiol 279 (a female sex hormone 147 and oral contraceptive 161)

ethoheptazine an *opioid* analgesic 80

ethosuximide 280 (an anticonvulsant 86)

etidronate 281 (a drug for bone disorders 122)

etodolac a non-steroidal anti-inflammatory 116

etomidate a drug for induction of general *anaesthesia*

etonorgestrel a progestogen 147

etoposide a drug for cancers of the lung, lymphatic system, and testes 154

etynodiol a progestogen (a female sex hormone 147)

Eucardic a brand name for carvedilol (an antihypertensive 102)

Euglucon a brand name for glibenclamide 294 (an oral antidiabetic 142)

Eugynon 30 a brand-name oral contraceptive 161 containing ethinylestradiol 279 and levonorgestrel 322; *illus. 45T*

Eumovate a brand name for clobetasone (a topical corticosteroid 174)

Eurax a brand name for crotamiton (an antipruritic 173)

Eurax-Hydrocortisone a brand name for hydrocortisone 301 (a corticosteroid 141) with crotamiton (an antipruritic 173)

Evista a brand name for raloxifene 392 (an anti-oestrogen sex hormone *antagonist* 147 for osteoporosis 122)

Evorel a brand name for estradiol 277 (an oestrogen 147); *illus. 47G*

Exelderm a brand name for sulconazole (an antifungal 138)

Exelon a brand name for rivastigmine 398 a drug for dementia 87

Ex-Lax a brand name for senna (a stimulant laxative 111)

Exocin a brand name for ofloxacin (an antibiotic 128)

Expulin a brand-name cough preparation 94 containing chlorphenamine 225, menthol, pholcodine, and pseudoephedrine

Expulin Decongestant a brand-name decongestant 93 with chlorphenamine 225, ephedrine 272, and menthol

Exterol brand-name ear drops for wax removal 171 containing urea

F

factor VIIa a blood extract to promote blood clotting 104

factor VIII a blood extract to promote blood clotting 104

factor IX a blood extract to promote blood clotting 104

famciclovir an antiviral 133

famotidine an anti-ulcer drug 109

Famvir a brand name for famciclovir (an antiviral 133)

Fansidar a brand-name antimalarial 137 containing pyrimethamine 389 and sulfadoxine

Farlutal a brand name for medroxyprogesterone 332 (a female sex hormone 147)

Fasigyn a brand name for tinidazole (an antibacterial 131)

Faverin a brand name for fluvoxamine (an antidepressant 84)

Fectrim a brand name for co-trimoxazole 246 (an antibacterial 131)

Fefol a brand name for folic acid 440 (a vitamin 149) with iron 441 (a mineral 150)

felbinac 282 a non-steroidal anti-inflammatory 116

Feldene a brand name for piroxicam 376 (a non-steroidal anti-inflammatory 116 and drug for gout 119); *illus. 39A*

felodipine a calcium channel blocker 101

felypressin a *vasoconstrictor* 95 used in dentistry

Femapak a brand-name preparation for menopausal symptoms 147 containing estradiol 277 and dydrogesterone 270

Femara a brand name for letrozole (an anticancer drug 154)

Fematrix a brand name for estradiol 277 (an oestrogen 147); *illus. 47H*

Femeron a brand name for miconazole 347 (an antifungal 142)

Femigraine a brand-name drug for migraine containing aspirin 200 (a non-*opioid* analgesic 80) with cyclizine (an anti-emetic 90)

Feminax a brand-name analgesic 80 for dysmenorrhoea containing paracetamol 368, codeine 241, hyoscine 302, and caffeine

Femodene a brand-name oral contraceptive 161 containing ethinylestradiol 279 and gestodene

FEMODETTE–HEMINEVRIN

Femodette a brand-name oral contraceptive 161 containing gestodene and ethinylestradiol 279

Femoston a brand-name preparation for menopausal symptoms 147 containing estradiol 277 and dydrogesterone 270

FemSeven a brand name for estradiol 277 (an oestrogen 147)

Femulen a brand-name oral contraceptive 161 containing etynodiol diacetate

Fenbid a brand name for ibuprofen 303 (a non-steroidal anti-inflammatory 116)

fenbufen a non-steroidal anti-inflammatory 116

Fenbuzip a brand name for fenbufen (a non-steroidal anti-inflammatory 116)

fenofibrate a lipid-lowering drug 103

Fenoket a brand name for ketoprofen 315 (a non-steroidal anti-inflammatory 116)

fenoprofen a non-steroidal anti-inflammatory 116

Fenopron a brand name for fenoprofen (a non-steroidal anti-inflammatory 116)

fenoterol a *sympathomimetic* bronchodilator 92

Fentamox a brand name for tamoxifen 411 (an anticancer drug 154)

fentanyl an *opioid* analgesic 80 used in general *anaesthesia* and labour 165

Fentazin a brand name for perphenazine (an antipsychotic 85 and anti-emetic 90)

fenticonazole an antifungal drug 138

Feospan a brand name for iron 441 (a mineral 150)

Ferfolic SV a brand name for folic acid 440 (a vitamin 149) and ferrous gluconate (a mineral 150)

ferric ammonium citrate iron 441 (a mineral 150)

Ferrograd a brand name for iron 441 (a mineral 150)

Ferrograd C a brand name for iron 441 (a mineral 150) with vitamin C 447 (a vitamin 149)

Ferrograd Folic a brand name for folic acid 440 (a vitamin 149) with iron 441 (a mineral 150)

ferrous fumarate iron 441 (a mineral 150)

ferrous gluconate iron 441 (a mineral 150)

ferrous glycine sulphate iron 441 (a mineral 150)

ferrous sulphate iron 441 (a mineral 150)

Fersaday a brand name for iron 441 (a mineral 150)

Fersamal a brand name for iron 441 (a mineral 150)

fexofenadine an antihistamine 124

fibrinolysin a thrombolytic *enzyme* used to break down blood clots 104 and to aid healing of skin ulcers 109

Fibro-vein a brand name for sodium tetradecyl sulphate (a drug for varicose veins)

Filair a brand name for beclometasone 206 (a corticosteroid 141)

filgrastim 283 (a blood growth stimulant)

finasteride 284 (a drug for benign prostatic hypertrophy, a urinary disorder 166)

Flagyl a brand name for metronidazole 346 (an antibacterial 131 and antiprotozoal 136); *illus. 43F*

Flamatrol a brand name for piroxicam 376 (a non-steroidal anti-inflammatory 116 and drug for gout 119)

Flamazine a brand name for silver sulfadiazine (a *topical* antibacterial 131)

flavoxate a urinary *antispasmodic* 166

flecainide an anti-arrhythmic 100

Flexin Continus a brand name for indometacin (a non-steroidal anti-inflammatory 116)

Flixonase a brand name for fluticasone 289 (a corticosteroid 141)

Flixotide a brand name for fluticasone 289 (a corticosteroid 141)

Flomax MR a brand name for tamsulosin 412 (an alpha-blocking drug for prostate disorders 166)

Florinef a brand name for fludrocortisone (a corticosteroid 141)

Floxapen a brand name for flucloxacillin (a penicillin antibiotic 128); *illus. 40N*

Fluanxol a brand name for flupentixol 287 (an antipsychotic 85 used in depression 84)

flucloxacillin a penicillin antibiotic 128

fluconazole 285 (an antifungal 138)

flucytosine an antifungal 138

fludarabine an anticancer drug 154

fludrocortisone a corticosteroid 141

fludroxycortide previously known as flurandrenolone (a topical corticosteroid 174)

flumazenil an *antidote* for benzodiazepine overdose

flumetasone a corticosteroid 141

flunisolide a corticosteroid 141

flunitrazepam a benzodiazepine sleeping drug 82

fluocinolone a topical corticosteroid 174

fluocinonide a topical corticosteroid 174

fluocortolone a topical corticosteroid 174

Fluor-a-day a brand name for fluoride 440 (a mineral 150)

fluorescein a drug used to stain the eye before examination

fluoride 440 (a mineral 150)

Fluorigard a brand name for fluoride 440 (a mineral 150)

fluorometholone a corticosteroid 141 for eye disorders

fluorouracil an anticancer drug 154

fluoxetine 286 (an antidepressant 84)

flupentixol 287 (an antipsychotic 85 used in depression 84)

fluphenazine an antipsychotic 85 used in depression 84

flurandrenolone see fludroxycortide (a topical corticosteroid 174)

flurazepam a benzodiazepine sleeping drug 82

flurbiprofen a non-steroidal anti-inflammatory 116

Flurex a brand name for paracetamol 368 (a non-*opioid* analgesic 80) with phenylephrine (a decongestant 93) and dextromethorphan (a cough suppressant 94)

flutamide 288 an anticancer drug 154

fluticasone 289 (a corticosteroid 141)

fluvastatin a lipid-lowering drug 102

fluvoxamine an antidepressant 84

FML a brand name for fluorometholone (a corticosteroid 141)

folate sodium folic acid 440 (a vitamin 149)

folic acid 440 (a vitamin 149)

folinic acid a vitamin 149

follicle-stimulating hormone (FSH) a natural *hormone* for infertility 164

follitropin alfa a drug for infertility 164

follitropin beta a drug for infertility 164

fomepizole an *antidote* for ethylene glycol poisoning

Foradil a brand name for formoterol (a bronchodilator 92)

formoterol previously known as eformoterol (a bronchodilator 92)

formestane a drug for breast cancer 154

Fortagesic a brand name for pentazocine (an *opioid* analgesic 80) and paracetamol 368

Fortovase a brand name for saquinavir (an antiviral for HIV/AIDS 157)

Fortral a brand name for pentazocine (an *opioid* analgesic 80)

Fortum a brand name for ceftazidime (a cephalosporin antibiotic 128)

Fosamax a brand name for alendronate (a drug for bone disorders 122)

foscarnet an antiviral 133

Foscavir a brand name for foscarnet (an antiviral 133)

fosfestrol a female sex hormone 147 and anticancer drug 154

fosinopril 290 an ACE inhibitor 98

Fragmin a brand name for dalteparin (a low-molecular-weight heparin 299 used as an anticoagulant 104)

framycetin a *topical* aminoglycoside antibiotic 128 for ear, eye, and skin infections

frangula a mild stimulant laxative 111

Franol a brand-name bronchodilator 92 containing ephedrine 272 and theophylline 419

Frisium a brand name for clobazam (a benzodiazepine anti-anxiety drug 83)

Froben a brand name for flurbiprofen (a non-steroidal anti-inflammatory drug 116)

Froop a brand name for furosemide 291 (a loop diuretic 99)

Fru-Co a brand name for amiloride 193 with furosemide 291 (both diuretics 99)

Frumil a brand name for amiloride 193 with furosemide 291 (both diuretics 99); *illus. 36G*

frusemide see furosemide 291

Frusene a brand name for furosemide 291 with triamterene 428 (both diuretics 99)

FSH follicle-stimulating *hormone* (a natural hormone for infertility 164)

Fucibet a brand name for betamethasone 210 (a corticosteroid 141) with fusidic acid (an antibiotic 128)

Fucidin a brand name for fusidic acid (an antibiotic 128)

Fucidin H a brand name for fusidic acid (an antibiotic 128) and hydrocortisone 301 (a corticosteroid 141)

Fucithalmic a brand name for fusidic acid (an antibiotic 128)

Fulcin a brand name for griseofulvin (an antifungal 138); *illus. 42C*

Full Marks a brand name for phenothrin (a *topical* antiparasitic 176)

Fungilin a brand name for amphotericin 199 (an antifungal 138)

Fungizone a brand name for amphotericin 199 (an antifungal 138)

Furadantin a brand name for nitrofurantoin (an antibacterial 131)

Furamide a brand name for diloxanide furoate (an antiprotozoal 136)

furosemide previously known as frusemide 291 (a loop diuretic 99)

fusidic acid an antibiotic 128

Fybogel a brand name for ispaghula (a bulk-forming agent used as a laxative 111 and antidiarrhoeal 110)

Fynnon Calcium Aspirin a brand name for aspirin 200 (an analgesic 80), calcium carbonate 438 (a mineral 150), and sodium sulphate (an osmotic laxative 111)

G

gabapentin an anticonvulsant 86

Gabitril a brand name for tiagabine (an anticonvulsant 86)

Galcodine a brand name for codeine 241 (a cough suppressant 94)

Galenphol a brand name for pholcodine (a cough suppressant 94)

Galfer a brand name for iron 441 (a mineral 150)

Galfer FA a brand name for folic acid 440 (a vitamin 149) with iron 441 (a mineral 150)

gallamine a drug used to relax the muscles in general *anaesthesia*

Galpseud a brand name for pseudoephedrine (a *sympathomimetic* decongestant 93)

Gamanil a brand name for lofepramine 325 (a tricyclic antidepressant 84); *illus. 35P*

gamma globulin an immune globulin 134

gamolenic acid 292 (an extract of evening primrose used for breast pain and eczema 179)

ganciclovir an antiviral 133

Ganda a brand-name preparation for glaucoma 168 containing epinephrine 273 and guanethidine

Garamycin a brand name for gentamicin 293 (an aminoglycoside antibiotic 128)

Gardenal a brand name for phenobarbital 371 (a barbiturate anticonvulsant 86)

Gastrobid Continus a brand name for metoclopramide 344 (a gastrointestinal motility regulator and anti-emetic 90)

Gastrocote a brand-name antacid 108 containing aluminium hydroxide 191, sodium bicarbonate 403, magnesium trisilicate, and alginic acid

Gastroflux a brand name for metoclopramide 344 (a gastrointestinal motility regulator and anti-emetic 90)

Gastromax a brand name for metoclopramide 344 (a gastrointestinal motility regulator and anti-emetic 90)

Gaviscon a brand-name antacid 108 containing aluminium hydroxide 191, sodium bicarbonate 403, magnesium trisilicate, and alginic acid

Gelcosal a brand-name preparation for eczema 179 and psoriasis 178 containing coal tar and salicylic acid

Gelcotar a brand name for coal tar (used for dandruff 180, eczema 179, and psoriasis 178)

gemcitabine an anticancer drug 154

gemeprost a drug used in labour 165

gemfibrozil a lipid-lowering drug 103

Genotropin a brand name for somatropin (a synthetic pituitary *hormone* 145)

gentamicin 293 (an aminoglycoside antibiotic 128)

gentian mixture, acid and alkaline an appetite stimulant 88

Genticin a brand name for gentamicin 293 (an aminoglycoside antibiotic 128)

Gentisone HC a brand name for gentamicin 293 (an aminoglycoside antibiotic 128) with hydrocortisone 301 (a corticosteroid 141)

gestodene a progestogen 147 and oral contraceptive 161

Gestone a brand name for progesterone (a female sex hormone 147)

gestonerone previously known as gestronol (a progestogen 147)

gestrinone a drug for menstrual disorders 160

Glandosane a brand name for artificial saliva

glibenclamide 294 (an oral antidiabetic 142)

Glibenese a brand name for glipizide (an oral antidiabetic 142)

gliclazide 295 (an oral antidiabetic 142)

glimepiride an oral antidiabetic 142

glipizide an oral antidiabetic 142

gliquidone an oral antidiabetic 142

GlucaGen a brand name for glucagon (a drug for hypoglycaemia 142)

glucagon a pancreatic *hormone* for hypoglycaemia 142

Glucamet a brand name for metformin 339 (an oral antidiabetic 142)

Glucobay a brand name for acarbose (an oral antidiabetic 142); *illus. 44P*

Glucophage a brand name for metformin 339 (an oral antidiabetic 142); *illus. 43A*

Glurenorm a brand name for gliquidone (an oral antidiabetic 142)

glutaraldehyde a *topical* preparation for treating warts

Glutarol a brand name for glutaraldehyde (a *topical* wart preparation)

glycerol a drug used to reduce pressure inside the eye 168, and an ingredient in cough mixtures 94, skin preparations 175, laxative *suppositories* 111, and ear-wax softening drops 171

glyceryl trinitrate 296 (an anti-angina drug 101); *illus. 46C*

glycopyrronium bromide an *anticholinergic* used in general *anaesthesia*

Glytrin a brand name for glyceryl trinitrate 296 (an anti-angina drug 101)

gold a metal used medically for rheumatoid arthritis 117

Golden Eye a brand name for propamidine isethionate (an antibacterial 131)

gonadorelin a drug for infertility 164

gonadotrophin, chorionic 227 (a drug for infertility 164)

Gopten a brand name for trandolapril (an antihypertensive 102); *illus. 40E*

goserelin 297 (a female sex hormone 147 and anticancer drug 154, also used for menstrual disorders 160 and infertility 164)

gramicidin an aminoglycoside antibiotic 128 for eye, ear, and skin infections

Graneodin a brand name for gramicidin with neomycin (both aminoglycoside antibiotics 128)

granisetron an anti-emetic 90

Gregoderm a brand name for hydrocortisone 301 (a corticosteroid 141) with nystatin 361 (an antifungal 138), neomycin (an aminoglycoside antibiotic 128), and polymyxin B (an antibiotic 128)

griseofulvin an antifungal 138

Grisovin a brand name for griseofulvin (an antifungal 138)

growth hormone somatropin (a pituitary *hormone* 145)

GTN 300mcg a brand name for glyceryl trinitrate 296 (an anti-angina drug 101)

guaifenesin an *expectorant* 94

guanethidine an antihypertensive 102 also used for glaucoma 168

Guanor Expectorant a brand-name cough preparation 94 containing diphenhydramine, ammonium chloride, and menthol

Guarem a brand name for guar gum (a drug used to control blood sugar levels 142)

guar gum a drug used to control blood sugar levels 142

Gyno-Daktarin a brand name for miconazole 347 (an antifungal 138)

Gynol II a brand name for nonoxinol '9' (a spermicidal agent 161)

Gyno-Pevaryl a brand name for econazole (an antifungal 138)

H

Haelan a brand name for fludroxycortide (a topical corticosteroid 174)

haem arginate a drug to treat porphyria

Halciderm Topical a brand name for halcinonide (a topical corticosteroid 174)

halcinonide a topical corticosteroid 174

Haldol a brand name for haloperidol 298 (a butyrophenone antipsychotic 85); *illus. 37 O*

Halfan a brand name for halofantrine (an antimalarial 137)

halibut liver oil a natural fish oil rich in vitamin A 446 and vitamin D 448 (both vitamins 149)

halofantrine an antimalarial 137

haloperidol 298 (a butyrophenone antipsychotic 85)

halothane a gas used to induce general *anaesthesia*

Halycitrol a brand name for vitamin A 446 with vitamin D 448 (both vitamins 149)

hamamelis an *astringent* in rectal preparations 113

Harmogen a brand name for piperazine oestrogen sulphate (a drug for hormone replacement therapy 147)

Hay-Crom a brand name for sodium cromoglicate 404 (an anti-allergy drug 124)

Haymine a brand name for chlorphenamine 225 (an antihistamine 124) with ephedrine 272 (a bronchodilator 92 and decongestant 93)

HCG human chorionic gonadotrophin 227 (a drug for infertility 164)

Hedex a brand name for paracetamol 368 (a non-*opioid* analgesic 80)

Hedex Extra a brand name for paracetamol 368 (a non-*opioid* analgesic 80) with caffeine

Heliclear a brand-name preparation containing lansoprazole 319, amoxicillin 198, and clarithromycin 128 (an anti-ulcer product 109)

Heminevrin a brand name for clomethiazole (a non-benzodiazepine, non-barbiturate sleeping drug 82)

HEPARIN–LACTIC ACID

heparin 299 (an anticoagulant 104)

heparinoid a drug applied *topically* to reduce inflammation of the skin 174

Hep-Flush a brand name for heparin 299 (an anticoagulant 104)

heroin diamorphine (an *opioid* 458 and analgesic 80)

Herpid a brand name for idoxuridine (an antiviral 133)

hexachlorophene a skin *antiseptic* 175

Hexalen a brand name for altretamine (an anticancer drug 154)

hexamine another name for methenamine (a drug for urinary tract infections 166)

hexetidine an *antiseptic* 175

Hexopal a brand name for nicotinic acid (a vasodilator 98)

Hibitane a brand name for chlorhexidine (a skin *antiseptic* 175)

Hioxyl a brand name for hydrogen peroxide (an *antiseptic* 175)

Hiprex a brand name for hexamine (a drug for urinary tract infections 166)

Hirudoid a brand name for heparinoid (a *topical* anti-inflammatory 174)

Histafen a brand name for terfenadine 416 (an antihistamine 124)

Histalix a brand-name cough preparation 94 containing diphenhydramine, ammonium chloride, and menthol

Hivid a brand name for zalcitabine 433 (an antiviral for HIV infection and AIDS 157)

homatropine a *mydriatic* 170

Honvan a brand name for fosfestrol (a female sex hormone 147 and anticancer drug 154)

Hormonin a brand name for estradiol 277 (a female sex hormone 147)

Humalog a brand name for insulin 307 lispro (a very quick-acting drug for diabetes 142)

Human Actrapid a brand name for insulin 307 (a drug for diabetes 142)

Human Insulatard a brand name for insulin 307 (a drug for diabetes 142)

human menopausal gonadotrophins also known as menotrophin (a drug for infertility 164)

Human Mixtard a brand name for insulin 307 (a drug for diabetes 142)

Human Monotard a brand name for insulin 307 (a drug for diabetes 142)

Human Ultratard a brand name for insulin 307 (a drug for diabetes 142)

Human Velosulin a brand name for insulin 307 (a drug for diabetes 142)

Humatrope a brand name for somatropin (a pituitary *hormone* 145, a synthetic pituitary hormone 145)

Humulin a brand name for insulin 307 (a drug for diabetes 142)

Hyalase a brand name for hyaluronidase (helps injections to penetrate tissues)

hyaluronidase helps injections to penetrate tissues

Hycamtin a brand name for topotecan (an anticancer drug 154)

Hydergine a brand name for co-dergocrine mesylate (a vasodilator 98)

hydralazine an antihypertensive 102

hydrochlorothiazide 300 (a thiazide diuretic 99)

hydrocortisone 301 (a corticosteroid 141 and antipruritic 173)

Hydrocortistab a brand name for hydrocortisone 301 (a corticosteroid 141)

Hydrocortone a brand name for hydrocortisone 301 (a corticosteroid 141)

hydroflumethiazide a thiazide diuretic 99

hydrogen peroxide an *antiseptic* mouthwash 175

hydromorphone an *opioid* analgesic 80

HydroSaluric a brand name for hydrochlorothiazide 300 (a thiazide diuretic 99); *illus. 45M*

hydrotalcite an antacid 108

hydroxocobalamin vitamin B_{12} 447 (a vitamin 149)

hydroxyapatite a drug to treat bone disorders 122

hydroxycarbamide previously known as hydroxyurea (a drug for chronic myeloid leukaemia 154)

hydroxychloroquine an antimalarial 137 and antirheumatic drug 117

hydroxyprogesterone a progestogen 147 used to prevent miscarriage

hydroxyurea see hydroxycarbamide (a drug for leukaemia 154

hydroxyzine an anti-anxiety drug 83

Hygroton a brand name for chlortalidone (a thiazide diuretic 99)

hyoscine 302 (a drug for irritable bowel syndrome 110 and a drug for affecting the pupil 170)

Hypotears a brand name for polyvinyl alcohol (artificial tears 170)

Hypovase a brand name for prazosin (an antihypertensive 102)

hypromellose a substance in artificial tear preparations 170

Hypurin a brand name for insulin 307 (a drug for diabetes 142)

Hytrin a brand name for terazosin (an alpha blocker 102)

I

Ibugel a brand name for ibuprofen 303 (a non-steroidal anti-inflammatory 116)

Ibuleve a brand-name gel for muscular pain relief containing ibuprofen 303 (a non-steroidal anti-inflammatory 116)

ibuprofen 303 (a non-*opioid* analgesic 80 and non-steroidal anti-inflammatory 116)

Ibuspray a brand name for ibuprofen 303 (a non-steroidal anti-inflammatory 116)

ichthammol a substance used in skin preparations for eczema 179

idarubicin a *cytotoxic* antibiotic (an anticancer drug 154)

idoxuridine an antiviral 133

ifosfamide an anticancer drug 154

Ikorel a brand name for nicorandil (an anti-angina drug 101); *illus. 45H*

Ilosone a brand name for erythromycin 276 (an antibiotic 128)

Ilube a brand name for acetylcysteine (a *mucolytic* 94) with hypromellose (a substance in artificial tear preparations 170)

Imbrilon a brand name for indometacin (a non-steroidal anti-inflammatory 116 and drug for gout 119)

Imdur a brand name for isosorbide mononitrate 312 (a nitrate vasodilator 98 and anti-angina drug 101)

imidapril an ACE inhibitor 98

imiglucerase an *enzyme* for enzyme replacement therapy

Imigran a brand name for sumatriptan 410 (a drug for migraine 89); *illus. 46L*

imipenem an antibiotic 128

imipramine 304 (a tricyclic antidepressant 84 and drug for urinary disorders 166)

imiquimod a drug to treat warts

Immukin a brand name for interferon gamma 308 (an antiviral 133)

immunoglobulin a preparation injected to prevent infectious diseases 134

Immunoprin a brand name for azathioprine 204 (an antirheumatic 117 and immunosuppressant 156)

Imodium a brand name for loperamide 326 (an antidiarrhoeal 110); *illus. 40T*

Implanon a brand name for etonorgestrel (a progestogen 147)

Imuran a brand name for azathioprine 204 (an antirheumatic 117 and immunosuppressant 156); *illus. 37J*

indapamide 305 (a thiazide-like diuretic 99)

Inderal a brand name for propranolol 386 (a beta blocker 97); *illus. 35 I*

Inderal-LA a brand name for propranolol 386 (a beta blocker 97); *illus. 40G*

Inderetic a brand name for bendroflumethiazide 207 (a thiazide diuretic 99) with propranolol 386 (a beta blocker 97)

Inderex a brand name for bendroflumethiazide 207 (a thiazide diuretic 99) with propranolol 386 (a beta blocker 97)

indinavir an antiviral for HIV/AIDS 157

Indocid a brand name for indometacin (a non-steroidal anti-inflammatory 116 and drug for gout 119); *illus. 39 I*

Indocid-R a brand name for indometacin (a non-steroidal anti-inflammatory 116 and drug for gout 119); *illus. 41D*

Indolar a brand name for indometacin (a non-steroidal anti-inflammatory 116 and drug for gout 119)

indometacin a non-steroidal anti-inflammatory 116 and drug for gout 119

Indomod a brand name for indometacin (a non-steroidal anti-inflammatory 116 and drug for gout 119)

indoramin 306 an antihypertensive 102 and drug for urinary disorders 166

Infacol a brand name for dimeticone (an antifoaming agent 108)

Infadrops a brand name for paracetamol 368 (a non-*opioid* analgesic 80)

Innohep a brand name for tinzaparin (a low-molecular-weight heparin 299 used as an anticoagulant 104); *illus. 47B*

Innovace a brand name for enalapril 271 (a vasodilator 98 and antihypertensive 102); *illus. 45K*

Innozide a brand name for enalapril 271 (a vasodilator 98 and antihypertensive 102)

inosine pranobex an antiviral 133

inositol a drug related to nicotinic acid (a vasodilator 98, lipid-lowering drug 103, and vitamin supplement 442)

Inoven a brand name for ibuprofen 303 (an analgesic 80 and non-steroidal anti-inflammatory 116)

Insulatard a brand name for insulin 307 (a drug for diabetes 142)

insulin 307 (a drug for diabetes 142)

insulin lispro a type of insulin 307 (a drug for diabetes 142)

Intal a brand name for sodium cromoglicate 404 (an anti-allergy drug 124); *illus. 40L*

integrilin a brand name for eptifibatide (a drug for prevention of heart attacks 95)

interferon 308 (an antiviral 133 and anticancer drug 154)

Intralgin a brand-name *topical* gel containing benzocaine (a local anaesthetic 80) for muscle strains and sprains

Intron-A a brand name for interferon 308 (an antiviral 133 and anticancer drug 154)

Invirase a brand name for saquinavir (an antiviral for HIV/AIDS 157)

iodine 441 (a mineral 150)

Ionamin a brand name for phentermine (an appetite suppressant 88)

Ionax a brand-name treatment for acne 177

Ionil T a brand-name dandruff shampoo 180 containing benzalkonium chloride, coal tar, and salicylic acid

Iopidine a brand name for apraclonidine (a drug for glaucoma 168)

ipecacuanha a drug used to induce vomiting in drug overdose and poisoning, also used as an *expectorant* 94

Ipral a brand name for trimethoprim 429 (an antibacterial 131); *illus. 42P*

ipratropium bromide 309 (a bronchodilator 92)

irbesartan 310 (an angiotensin II inhibitor, an antihypertensive 102)

irinotecan an anticancer drug 154

iron 441 (a mineral 150)

Ismelin a brand name for guanethidine (an antihypertensive 102 also used for glaucoma 168)

Ismo a brand name for isosorbide mononitrate 312 (a nitrate vasodilator 98 and anti-angina drug 101)

isocarboxazid an MAOI antidepressant 84

isoconazole an antifungal 138

isoflurane a volatile liquid inhaled as a general *anaesthetic*

Isogel a brand name for ispaghula (a laxative 111 and antidiarrhoeal 110)

Isoket a brand name for isosorbide dinitrate 312 (a nitrate vasodilator 98 and anti-angina drug 101)

isometheptene mucate a drug for migraine 89

isoniazid 311 (an antituberculous drug 132)

isophane insulin a type of insulin 307 (a drug for diabetes 142)

isoprenaline a bronchodilator 92

Isopto Alkaline a brand name for hypromellose (a substance in artificial tear preparations 170)

Isopto Atropine a brand name for atropine 203 (an *anticholinergic mydriatic* 170) with hypromellose (a substance in artificial tear preparations 170)

Isopto Carbachol a brand name for carbachol eye drops (a *miotic* for glaucoma 168)

Isopto Carpine a brand name for pilocarpine 375 (a *miotic* for glaucoma 168) with hypromellose (a substance in artificial tear preparations 170)

Isopto Frin brand-name eye drops containing phenylephrine and hypromellose (a substance in artificial tear preparations 170) for minor eye irritation and redness

Isopto Plain a brand name for hypromellose eye drops (a substance in artificial tear preparations 170)

Isordil a brand name for isosorbide dinitrate 312 (a nitrate vasodilator 98 and anti-angina drug 101)

isosorbide dinitrate 312 (a nitrate vasodilator 98 and anti-angina drug 101)

isosorbide mononitrate 312 (a nitrate vasodilator 98 and anti-angina drug 101)

Isotrate a brand name for isosorbide mononitrate 312 (a nitrate vasodilator 98 and anti-angina drug 101)

isotretinoin 313 (a drug for acne 177)

Isotrex a brand name for isotretinoin 313 (a drug for acne 177)

ispaghula a bulk-forming agent for constipation 111 and diarrhoea 110

isradipine a calcium channel blocker 101

Istin a brand name for amlodipine 197 (a calcium channel blocker 101); *illus. 43C*

itraconazole an antifungal 138

ivermectin an anthelmintic 139

J

Jectofer a brand name for iron 441 (a mineral 150)

Joy-rides a brand name for hyoscine 302 (used to prevent motion sickness 90)

K

Kabikinase a brand name for streptokinase 407 (a thrombolytic 105)

Kalspare a brand name for triamterene 428 with chlortalidone (both diuretics 99)

Kalten a brand name for amiloride 193 with hydrochlorothiazide 300 (both diuretics 99) and atenolol 201 (a beta blocker 97)

Kamillosan an ointment 175 containing chamomile used for treating nappy rash, sore nipples, and chapped skin

kanamycin an aminoglycoside antibiotic 128

Kannasyn a brand name for kanamycin (an aminoglycoside antibiotic 128)

kaolin an adsorbent used as an antidiarrhoeal 110

Kapake a brand name for paracetamol 368 (a non-*opioid* analgesic 80)

Karvol a brand name for menthol (a decongestant inhalant 93)

Kay-Cee-L a brand name for potassium 443 (a mineral 150)

Kefadol a brand name for cefamandole (a cephalosporin antibiotic 128)

Keflex a brand name for cefalexin 220 (a cephalosporin antibiotic 128); *illus. 41C*

Kefzol a brand name for cefazolin (a cephalosporin antibiotic 128)

Kelfizine W a brand name for sulfametopyrazine (a sulphonamide antibacterial 131)

Kemadrin a brand name for procyclidine 382 (an *anticholinergic* for parkinsonism 87); *illus. 43P*

Kemicetine a brand name for chloramphenicol 222 (an antibiotic 128)

Kenalog a brand name for triamcinolone (a corticosteroid 141)

Kentene a brand name for piroxicam 376 (a non-steroidal anti-inflammatory 116 and drug for gout 119)

Keral a brand name for dexketoprofen (a non-steroidal anti-inflammatory 116)

Kerlone a brand name for betaxolol (a beta blocker 97)

ketamine a drug used to induce general *anaesthesia*

Ketocid a brand name for ketoprofen 315 (a non-steroidal anti-inflammatory 116)

ketoconazole 314 (an antifungal 138)

ketoprofen 315 (a non-steroidal anti-inflammatory 116)

ketorolac a non-steroidal anti-inflammatory 116 used as an analgesic 80

ketotifen a drug similar to sodium cromoglicate 404 for allergies and asthma 124

Ketovail a brand name for ketoprofen 315 (a non-steroidal anti-inflammatory 116)

Ketovite a brand-name vitamin supplement 149

Ketozip XL a brand name for ketoprofen 315 (a non-steroidal anti-inflammatory 116)

Klaricid a brand name for clarithromycin (an antibiotic 128)

Klean-prep a brand-name osmotic laxative 111

Kliofem a brand-name product for menopausal symptoms 147 containing estradiol 277 and norethisterone 360

Kloref a brand-name potassium supplement 443 (a mineral 150)

Kolanticon a brand name for aluminium hydroxide 191 and magnesium oxide (both antacids 108) with dicycloverine 255 (an *anticholinergic antispasmodic* 110) and dimeticone (an antifoaming agent 108)

Konakion a brand name for phytomenadione (vitamin K 449)

Konsyl a brand name for ispaghula (a bulk-forming agent for constipation 111 and diarrhoea 110)

Kwells a brand name for hyoscine 302 (used to prevent motion sickness 90); *illus. 36B*

Kytril a brand name for granisetron (an anti-emetic 90)

L

labetalol a beta blocker 97

Labosept brand-name throat pastilles containing dequalinium (an antibacterial 131)

lacidipine a calcium channel blocker 101

Lacri-Lube a brand-name eye ointment for dry eyes 170

lactic acid an ingredient in preparations for warts, *emollients* 175, and pessaries

LACTITOL–METROLYL

lactitol an osmotic laxative 111

Lactugal a brand name for lactulose 316 (an osmotic laxative 111)

lactulose 316 (an osmotic laxative 111)

Ladropen a brand name for flucloxacillin (a penicillin antibiotic 128)

Lamictal a brand name for lamotrigine 318 (an anticonvulsant 86); *illus. 37F*

Lamisil a brand name for terbinafine 414 (an antifungal 138)

lamivudine 317 (an antiviral 133 used for HIV/AIDS 157)

lamotrigine 318 (an anticonvulsant 86)

Lamprene a brand name for clofazimine (a drug for leprosy 131)

Lanoxin a brand name for digoxin 258 (a digitalis drug 96); *illus. 45R*

Lanoxin-PG a brand name for digoxin 258 (a digitalis drug 96); *illus. 38C*

lanreotide an anticancer drug 154

lansoprazole 319 an anti-ulcer drug 109

Laractone a brand name for spironolactone (a potassium-sparing diuretic 99)

Larafen a brand name for ketoprofen 315 (a non-steroidal anti-inflammatory 116)

Larapam a brand name for piroxicam 376 (a non-steroidal anti-inflammatory 116 and drug for gout 119)

Largactil a brand name for chlorpromazine 226 (a phenothiazine antipsychotic 85 and anti-emetic 90); *illus. 44L*

Lariam a brand name for mefloquine 334 (an antimalarial 137); *illus. 42H*

Lasikal a brand name for furosemide 291 (a loop diuretic 99) with potassium 443 (a mineral 150); *illus. 38N*

Lasilactone a brand name for furosemide 291 with spironolactone (both diuretics 99)

Lasix a brand name for furosemide 291 (a loop diuretic 99); *illus. 44J*

Lasma a brand name for theophylline 419 (a bronchodilator 92)

Lasonil a brand name for heparinoid (a *topical* anti-inflammatory 174)

Lasoride a brand name for amiloride 193 (a potassium-sparing diuretic 99) with furosemide 291 (a loop diuretic 99 and antihypertensive 102)

Lassar's Paste a skin preparation for psoriasis 178 containing dithranol, zinc oxide 449, and salicylic acid

latanoprost a drug for glaucoma 168

Laxoberal a brand name for sodium picosulfate (a stimulant laxative 111)

Laxose a brand name for lactulose 316 (an osmotic laxative 111)

Ledclair a brand name for sodium calcium edetate (an *antidote* for poisoning with lead and heavy metals)

Lederfen a brand name for fenbufen (a non-steroidal anti-inflammatory 116); *illus. 38K*

Lederfolin a brand name for folinic acid (a vitamin 149)

Ledermycin a brand name for demeclocycline (a tetracycline antibiotic 128)

Lederspan a brand name for triamcinolone (a corticosteroid 141)

leflunomide an antirheumatic drug 117

Lemsip a brand name for paracetamol 368 (a non-*opioid* analgesic 80) with phenylephrine (a decongestant 93), chlorphenamine 225 (an antihistamine 124), and caffeine

Lenium a brand-name dandruff shampoo 180 containing selenium 445 (a mineral 150)

lenograstim a blood growth stimulant

Lentard MC a brand name for insulin 307 (a drug for diabetes 142)

Lentaron a brand name for formestane (a drug for breast cancer 154)

Lentizol a brand name for amitriptyline 196 (a tricyclic antidepressant 84)

lepirudin an anticoagulant 104

lercanidipine a calcium channel blocker 101

Lescol a brand name for fluvastatin (a lipid-lowering drug 103)

letrozole an anticancer drug 154

Leucovorin see calcium folinate 149

Leukeran a brand name for chlorambucil (an anticancer drug 154)

leuprorelin a drug for menstrual disorders 160

levamisole an anthelmintic 139

levobunolol a beta blocker 97 and drug for glaucoma 168

levocabastine a *topical* antihistamine 174

levodopa 320 (a drug for parkinsonism 87)

levofloxacin 321 (an antibacterial 131)

levomepromazine previously known as methotrimeprazine (an antipsychotic 85)

levonorgestrel 322 (a female sex hormone 147 and oral contraceptive 161)

levothyroxine previously known as thyroxine 421 (a thyroid *hormone* 144)

Librium a brand name for chlordiazepoxide 223 (a benzodiazepine anti-anxiety drug 83); *illus. 37S*

lidocaine previously known as lignocaine (a local anaesthetic 80, anti-arrhythmic 100, and antipruritic 173)

lignocaine see lidocaine

Li-liquid a brand name for lithium 324 (a drug for mania 85)

lindane a *topical* antiparasitic 176

Lingraine a brand name for ergotamine 275 (a drug for migraine 89)

Lioresal a brand name for baclofen 205 (a muscle relaxant 120); *illus. 45A*

liothyronine a thyroid *hormone* 144

Lipantil a brand name for fenofibrate (a lipid-lowering drug 103)

Lipitor a brand name for atorvastatin 202 (a lipid-lowering drug 103)

Lipobay a brand name for cerivastatin (a lipid-lowering drug 103)

Lipostat a brand name for pravastatin 378 (a cholesterol-lowering agent 103)

liquid paraffin a lubricating agent used as a laxative 111 and in artificial tear preparations 170

Liquifilm Tears brand-name eye drops containing polyvinyl acetate (artificial tears 170)

liquorice a substance for peptic ulcers 109

lisinopril 323 (an ACE inhibitor 98)

Liskonum a brand name for lithium 324 (a drug for mania 85)

lisuride a drug for parkinsonism 87

Litarex a brand name for lithium 324 (a drug for mania 85)

lithium 324 (a drug for mania 85)

Livial a brand name for tibolone 422 (a female sex hormone 147); *illus. 45Q*

Livostin a brand name for levocabastine (an antihistamine 124)

Locabiotal a brand name for fusafungine (an antibacterial 131 and anti-inflammatory agent 116)

Loceryl a brand name for amorolfine (an antifungal 138)

Locoid a brand name for hydrocortisone 301 (a corticosteroid 141)

Locorten-Vioform a brand name for clioquinol (an anti-infective skin preparation 175) with flumetasone (a corticosteroid 141)

Lodine SR a brand name for etodolac (a non-steroidal anti-inflammatory 116)

Iodoxamide an anti-allergy drug 124

Loestrin 20 a brand-name oral contraceptive 161 containing ethinylestradiol 279 and norethisterone 360

lofepramine 325 (a tricyclic antidepressant 84)

lofexidine a drug to treat *opioid withdrawal* symptoms 24

Logynon a brand-name oral contraceptive 161 containing ethinylestradiol 279 and levonorgestrel 322

Lomexin a brand name for fenticonazole (an antifungal 138)

Lomotil a brand-name antidiarrhoeal 110 containing atropine 203 and diphenoxylate 260; *illus. 45S*

lomustine an alkylating agent for Hodgkin's disease 154

Loniten a brand name for minoxidil 349 (an antihypertensive 102)

Loperagen a brand name for loperamide 326 (an antidiarrhoeal 110)

loperamide 326 (an antidiarrhoeal 110)

Lopid a brand name for gemfibrozil (a lipid-lowering drug 103)

loprazolam a benzodiazepine sleeping drug 82

Lopresor a brand name for metoprolol 345 (a cardioselective beta blocker 97); *illus. 36C*

loratadine 327 (an antihistamine 124)

lorazepam a benzodiazepine anti-anxiety drug 83 and sleeping drug 82

lormetazepam a benzodiazepine sleeping drug 82

losartan 328 (an antihypertensive 102)

Losec a brand name for omeprazole 363 (an anti-ulcer drug 109); *illus. 40C*

Lotriderm a brand-name product containing betamethasone 210 (a corticosteroid 141) and clotrimazole 239 (an antifungal 138)

Loxapac a brand name for loxapine (an antipsychotic 85)

loxapine an antipsychotic 85

Luborant a brand name for artificial saliva

Ludiomil a brand name for maprotiline (an antidepressant 84)

Lugol's solution an iodine 441 solution for an overactive thyroid gland 144

Lustral a brand name for sertraline (an antidepressant 84); *illus. 46N*

luteinizing hormone (LH) an infertility drug 164

Lyclear a brand name for permethrin 370 (a *topical* antiparasitic 176)

lymecycline a tetracycline antibiotic 128

M

Maalox a brand-name antacid containing aluminium hydroxide 191 and magnesium hydroxide 329

Maalox Plus a brand-name antacid containing aluminium hydroxide 191, magnesium hydroxide 329, and dimeticone

Mabthera a brand name for rituximab (an anticancer drug 154)

Macrobid a brand name for nitrofurantoin (an antibacterial 131); *illus. 41M*

Macrodantin a brand name for nitrofurantoin (an antibacterial 131)

Madopar a brand name for levodopa 320 (a drug for parkinsonism 87) with benserazide (a drug that enhances the effect of levodopa)

Magnapen a brand name for ampicillin with flucloxacillin (both penicillin antibiotics 128); *illus. 40S*

magnesium 442 (a mineral 150)

magnesium alginate an antifoaming agent 108

magnesium carbonate an antacid 108

magnesium citrate an osmotic laxative 111

magnesium hydroxide 329 (an antacid 108 and laxative 111)

magnesium oxide an antacid 108

magnesium sulphate an osmotic laxative 111

magnesium trisilicate an antacid 108

malathion 330 (an antiparasitic 176 for head lice and scabies infestation)

Malix a brand name for glibenclamide 294 (an oral antidiabetic 142)

Maloprim a brand-name antimalarial 137 containing dapsone and pyrimethamine 389

Manerix a brand name for moclobemide (a reversible MAOI antidepressant 84)

Manevac a brand name for ispaghula (a bulk-forming agent 108) with senna (a stimulant laxative 111)

mannitol an osmotic diuretic 99

maprotiline an antidepressant 84

Marcain a brand name for bupivacaine (a local anaesthetic 80 used in labour 165)

Marevan a brand name for warfarin 432 (an anticoagulant 104)

Marvelon a brand-name oral contraceptive 161 containing ethinylestradiol 279 and desogestrel

Masnoderm a brand name for clotrimazole 239 (an antifungal 138)

Maxalt a brand name for rizatriptan (a drug for migraine 89)

Maxepa a brand name for concentrated fish oils (used to reduce fats in the blood 103); *illus. 39F*

Maxidex a brand name for dexamethasone 252 (a corticosteroid 141) with hypromellose (a substance in artificial tear preparations 170)

Maxitrol a brand name for dexamethasone 252 (a corticosteroid 141) with hypromellose (a substance used in artificial tear preparations 170) and neomycin and polymyxin B (both antibiotics 128)

Maxivent a brand name for salbutamol 399 (a bronchodilator 92)

Maxolon a brand name for metoclopramide 344 (a gastrointestinal motility regulator and anti-emetic 90); *illus. 44 K*

Maxtrex a brand name for methotrexate 341 (an antimetabolite anticancer drug 154)

MCR-50 a brand name for isosorbide mononitrate 312 (a nitrate vasodilator 98 and anti-angina drug 101)

MCT Oil used to treat cystic fibrosis

mebendazole an anthelmintic 139

mebeverine 331 (an *antispasmodic* for irritable bowel syndrome 110)

meclozine an antihistamine 124 used for travel sickness

mecysteine a *mucolytic* for coughs 94

Medijel a brand name for a pain-relieving mouth gel containing lidocaine (a local anaesthetic 80) and aminacrine (a skin *antiseptic* 175)

Medinex a brand name for diphenhydramine (an antihistamine 124)

Medinol a brand name for paracetamol 368 (a non-*opioid* analgesic 80)

Medised a brand name for paracetamol 368 (a non-*opioid* analgesic 80) with promethazine 385 (an antihistamine 124 and anti-emetic 90)

Medrone a brand name for methylprednisolone (a corticosteroid 141)

medroxyprogesterone 332 (a female sex hormone 147 and anticancer drug 154)

mefenamic acid 333 (a non-steroidal anti-inflammatory 116)

mefloquine 334 (an antimalarial 137)

Mefoxin a brand name for cefoxitin (a cephalosporin antibiotic 128)

mefruside a thiazide-like diuretic 99

Megace a brand name for megestrol 335 (a female sex hormone 147 and anticancer drug 154); *illus. 42K*

megestrol 335 (a female sex hormone 147 and anticancer drug 154)

melatonin a *hormone* 140

Melleril a brand name for thioridazine 420 (a phenothiazine antipsychotic 85); *illus. 44Q*

meloxicam 336 a non-steroidal anti-inflammatory drug 116 and non-*opioid* analgesic 80

melphalan an alkylating agent for multiple myeloma 154

menadiol vitamin K 449 (a vitamin 149)

Menorest a brand name for estradiol 277 (an oestrogen 147)

menotrophin also known as human menopausal gonadotrophins (a drug for infertility 164)

menthol an alcohol from mint oils used as an inhalation and *topical* antipruritic 173

mepacrine an antiprotozoal 136 (for giardiasis)

mepivacaine a local anaesthetic 80

meprobamate an anti-anxiety drug 83

meptazinol an *opioid* analgesic 80

Meptid a brand name for meptazinol (an *opioid* analgesic 80)

mequitazine an antihistamine 124

Merbentyl a brand name for dicycloverine 255 (a drug for irritable bowel syndrome 110); *illus. 43 O*

mercaptopurine 337 (an anticancer drug 154)

Mercilon a brand-name oral contraceptive 161 containing ethinylestradiol 279 and desogestrel

Merocaine Lozenges a brand-name preparation for sore throat and minor mouth infections, containing benzocaine (a local anaesthetic 80) and cetylpyridinium (a *topical antiseptic* 175)

Merocet a brand name for cetylpyridinium (a *topical antiseptic* 175)

mesalazine 338 (a drug for ulcerative colitis 112)

mesna a drug used to protect the urinary tract from damage caused by some anticancer drugs 154

mesterolone a male sex hormone 146

Mestinon a brand name for pyridostigmine 388 (a drug for myasthenia gravis 121)

mestranol an oestrogen 147 and oral contraceptive 161

metaraminol a drug used to treat hypotension (low blood pressure)

Metenix-5 a brand name for metolazone (a thiazide-like diuretic 99)

metformin 339 (a drug for diabetes 142)

methadone 340 (an *opioid* 458 used as an analgesic 80 and to treat heroin *dependence*)

Methadose a brand name for methadone 340 (an *opioid* 458 used as an analgesic 80 and to ease heroin *withdrawal*)

Metharose a brand name for methadone 340 (an *opioid* 458 used as an analgesic 80 and to ease heroin *withdrawal*)

methenamine a drug for urinary tract infections 166

Methex a brand name for methadone 340 (an *opioid* 458 used as an analgesic 80 and to ease heroin *withdrawal*)

methionine an *antidote* for paracetamol 368 poisoning

methocarbamol a muscle relaxant 120

methohexital a barbiturate used to induce general anaesthesia

methotrexate 341 (an antimetabolite anticancer drug 154)

methotrimeprazine see levomepromazine, an antipsychotic 85

methoxamine a drug used to treat hypotension (low blood pressure)

methoxsalen a drug for psoriasis 178

methylcellulose 342 (a laxative 111, antidiarrhoeal 110, and artificial tear preparation 170)

methyldopa 343 (an antihypertensive 102)

methylphenidate a drug used to treat hyperactivity in children

methylphenobarbital a barbiturate anticonvulsant 86

methylprednisolone a corticosteroid 141

methyl salicylate a *topical* analgesic 80 for muscle and joint pain

methysergide a drug to prevent migraine 89

metipranolol a beta blocker 97 for glaucoma 168

metirosine a drug for phaeochromocytoma (a tumour of the adrenal glands 154)

metoclopramide 344 (a gastrointestinal motility regulator and anti-emetic 90)

metolazone a thiazide-like diuretic 99

Metopirone a brand name for metyrapone (a diuretic 142)

metoprolol 345 a beta blocker 97

Metosyn a brand name for fluocinonide (a topical corticosteroid 174)

Metrodin a brand name for urofollitropin (a drug for pituitary disorders 145)

Metrogel a brand name for *topical* metronidazole 346 (an antibacterial 131)

Metrolyl a brand name for metronidazole 346 (an antibacterial 131 and antiprotozoal 136)

METRONIDAZOLE–NOREPINEPHRINE

metronidazole 346 (an antibacterial 131 and antiprotozoal 136)

Metrotop a brand name for *topical* metronidazole 346 (an antibacterial 131)

metyrapone a diuretic 99 used to reduce fluid retention in Cushing's disease

mexiletine an anti-arrhythmic 100

Mexitil a brand name for mexiletine (an anti-arrhythmic 100)

mianserin an antidepressant 84

miconazole 347 (an antifungal 134)

Microgynon 30 a brand-name oral contraceptive 161 containing ethinylestradiol 279 and levonorgestrel 322

Micronor a brand-name oral contraceptive 161 containing norethisterone 360

Microval a brand-name oral contraceptive 161 containing levonorgestrel 322; *illus. 46A*

Mictral a brand-name drug for urinary tract infections 166 containing nalidixic acid (an antibacterial 131) and sodium bicarbonate 403 (an antacid 108)

Midamor a brand name for amiloride 193 (a potassium-sparing diuretic 99); *illus. 37H*

midazolam a benzodiazepine 82 used as *premedication*

Midrid a brand-name drug for migraine 89 containing paracetamol 368 and isometheptene mucate

mifepristone a drug used during labour 165

Migraleve a brand-name drug for migraine 89 containing codeine 241, paracetamol 368, and buclizine

Migranal a brand name for dihydroergotamine (a drug for migraine 89)

Migravess a brand-name drug for migraine 89 containing aspirin 200 and metoclopramide 344

Migril a brand-name drug for migraine 89 containing ergotamine 275, caffeine, and cyclizine

Milk of Magnesia a brand name for magnesium hydroxide 329 (an antacid 108 and laxative 111); *illus. 42F*

Milpar a brand-name laxative 111 containing magnesium hydroxide 329 and liquid paraffin

milrinone a drug used for its vasodilator effects 98

Minihep a brand name for heparin 299 (an anticoagulant 104)

Minims Atropine a brand name for atropine 203 (a *mydriatic* 170)

Minims Chloramphenicol a brand name for chloramphenicol 222 (an antibiotic 128)

Minims Cyclopentolate a brand name for cyclopentolate (an *anticholinergic mydriatic* 170)

Minims Gentamicin a brand name for gentamicin 293 (an aminoglycoside antibiotic 128)

Minims Phenylephrine a brand name for phenylephrine (a decongestant 93)

Minims Pilocarpine a brand name for pilocarpine 375 (a *miotic* for glaucoma 168)

Minims Prednisolone a brand name for prednisolone 379 (a corticosteroid 141)

Minitran a brand name for glyceryl trinitrate 296 (an anti-angina drug 101)

Minocin a brand name for minocycline 348 (a tetracycline antibiotic 128); *illus. 36H*

minocycline 348 (a tetracycline antibiotic 128)

Minodiab a brand name for glipizide (an oral antidiabetic 142)

minoxidil 349 (an antihypertensive 102)

Mintec a brand name for peppermint oil (a substance for irritable bowel syndrome 110)

Mintezol a brand name for tiabendazole (an anthelmintic 139)

Minulet a brand-name oral contraceptive 161 containing ethinylestradiol 279 and gestodene

Mirapexin a brand name for pramipexole (a drug for parkinsonism 87)

Mirena an intrauterine contraceptive device 161 containing levonorgestrel 322 (a female sex hormone 147)

mirtazapine an antidepressant 84

misoprostol 350 (an anti-ulcer drug 109)

Mistamine a brand name for mizolastine an antihistamine 124

mitobronitol an anticancer drug 154

mitomycin a *cytotoxic* antibiotic for breast and stomach cancer 154

mitoxantrone previously known as mitozantrone (an anticancer drug 154)

mitozantrone see mitoxantrone

mivacurium a drug used to relax muscles during general *anaesthesia*

Mixtard a brand name for insulin 307 (a drug for diabetes 142)

mizolastine an antihistamine 124

Mizollen a brand name for mizolastine (an antihistamine 124)

Mobic a brand name for meloxicam 336 (a non-steroidal anti-inflammatory drug 116 and non-*opioid* analgesic 80)

Mobiflex a brand name for tenoxicam (a non-steroidal anti-inflammatory 116)

moclobemide a reversible MAOI antidepressant 84

modafinil a drug for narcolepsy 88

Modalim a brand name for ciprofibrate (a lipid-lowering drug 103)

Modaplate a brand name for dipyridamole 261 (an antiplatelet drug 104)

Modecate a brand name for fluphenazine (an antipsychotic 85)

Moditen a brand name for fluphenazine (an antipsychotic 85)

Modrasone a brand name for alclometasone (a topical corticosteroid 174)

Modrenal a brand name for trilostane (an adrenal *antagonist* used for Cushing's syndrome (an adrenal disorder 141) and for breast cancer 154)

Moducren a brand-name antihypertensive 102 containing amiloride 193, hydrochlorothiazide 300, and timolol 423

Moduret-25 a brand name for amiloride 193 with hydrochlorothiazide 300 (both diuretics 99)

Moduretic a brand name for amiloride 193 with hydrochlorothiazide 300 (both diuretics 99); *illus. 36F*

moexipril an ACE inhibitor 98

Mogadon a brand name for nitrazepam (a benzodiazepine sleeping drug 82); *illus. 41 O*

molgramostim a blood growth stimulant

Molipaxin a brand name for trazodone 427 (an antidepressant 84); *illus. 36D*

molybdenum a mineral 150 required in minute amounts in the diet, poisonous if ingested in large quantities

mometasone 351 a topical corticosteroid 174

Monit a brand name for isosorbide mononitrate 312 (a nitrate vasodilator 98 and anti-angina drug 101)

Mono-Cedocard a brand name for isosorbide mononitrate 312 (a nitrate vasodilator 98 and anti-angina drug 101)

Monoclate-P a brand name for factor VIII (a blood extract used to promote blood clotting 104)

Monocor a brand name for bisoprolol (a beta blocker 97)

Monoparin, Monoparin CA brand names for heparin 299 (an anti-coagulant 104)

monosulfiram an antiparasitic 176 for scabies

Monotrim a brand name for trimethoprim 429 (an antibacterial 131)

Monovent a brand name for terbutaline 415 (a bronchodilator 92 and drug for premature labour 165)

Monozide 10 a brand name for bisoprolol (a beta blocker 97) with hydrochlorothiazide 300 (a thiazide diuretic 99)

Monphytol a brand-name antifungal 138 for athlete's foot

montelukast 352 a leukotriene *antagonist* for asthma 124 and bronchospasm 92

morphine 353 (an *opioid* analgesic 80)

Motens a brand name for lacidipine (a calcium channel blocker 101)

Motifene a brand name for diclofenac 254 (a non-steroidal anti-inflammatory drug 116)

Motilium a brand name for domperidone 263 (an anti-emetic 90); *illus. 45B*

Motipress a brand name for fluphenazine (an antipsychotic 85) with nortriptyline (a tricyclic antidepressant 84)

Motival a brand name for fluphenazine (an antipsychotic 85) with nortriptyline (a tricyclic antidepressant 84)

Motrin a brand name for ibuprofen 303 (a non-steroidal anti-inflammatory 116)

Movelat a brand-name *topical* anti-inflammatory 175 containing mucopolysaccharide and salicylic acid

Movicol an osmotic laxative 111

moxisylyte previously known as thymoxamine (a drug used to reduce pupil size after examination 170 and as a vasodilator 98 to improve blood supply to the limbs)

moxonidine 354 (a centrally acting antihypertensive 102)

MST Continus a brand name for morphine 353 (an *opioid* analgesic 80); *illus. 35B*

Mucaine a brand-name antacid 108 containing aluminium hydroxide 191, magnesium hydroxide 329, and oxetacaine

Mucodyne a brand name for carbocisteine (a *mucolytic* decongestant 94)

Mucogel a brand-name antacid 108 containing aluminium hydroxide 191 and magnesium hydroxide 329

Mu-Cron Tablets a brand name for phenylpropanolamine 373 (a decongestant 93) with paracetamol 368 (a non-*opioid* analgesic 80)

Multiparin a brand name for heparin 299 (an anticoagulant 104)

mupirocin an antibacterial for skin infections 175

mustine see chlormethine (a drug for Hodgkin's disease 154)

MXL a brand name for morphine sulphate 353 (an *opioid* analgesic 116)

Myambutol a brand name for ethambutol 278 (an antituberculous drug 132); *illus. 37L*

Mycil Gold a brand name for clotrimazole 239 (an antifungal 138)

Mycobutin a brand name for rifabutin (an antituberculous drug 132)

mycophenolate mofetil an immunosuppressant drug 156

Mycota a brand name for undecanoate acid (an antifungal 138)

Mydriacyl a brand name for tropicamide (a *mydriatic* 170)

Mydrilate a brand name for cyclopentolate (an *anticholinergic mydriatic* 170)

Myelobromol a brand name for mitobronitol (an anticancer drug 154)

Myocrisin a brand name for sodium aurothiomalate (an antirheumatic 117)

Myotonine a brand name for bethanechol (a *parasympathomimetic* for urinary retention 166)

Mysoline a brand name for primidone 380 (an anticonvulsant 86); *illus. 43J*

N

nabilone an anti-emetic 90 derived from marijuana for nausea and vomiting induced by anticancer drugs 154

nabumetone a non-steroidal anti-inflammatory 116

nadolol a beta blocker 97

nafarelin a drug for menstrual disorders 160

naftidrofuryl 355 a vasodilator 98

nalbuphine an *opioid* analgesic 80

Nalcrom a brand name for sodium cromoglicate 404 (an anti-allergy drug 124)

nalidixic acid an antibacterial 131

Nalorex a brand name for naltrexone (a drug for *opioid withdrawal* 24)

naloxone an *antidote* for *opioid* 458 poisoning

naltrexone a drug for *opioid withdrawal* 24

nandrolone an anabolic steroid 146

Napratec a brand name for an antirheumatic drug containing naproxen 356 (a non-steroidal anti-inflammatory 116 and drug for gout 119) and misoprostol 350 (an anti-ulcer drug 109)

Naprosyn a brand name for naproxen 356 (a non-steroidal anti-inflammatory 116 and drug for gout 119); *illus. 37C*

naproxen 356 (a non-steroidal anti-inflammatory 116 and drug for gout 119)

Naramig a brand name for naratriptan (a drug for migraine 89)

naratriptan a drug for migraine 89

Narcan a brand name for naloxone (an *antidote* for *opioid* 458 poisoning)

Nardil a brand name for phenelzine (an MAOI antidepressant 84)

Naropin a brand name for ropivacaine (local anaesthetic 80)

Narphen a brand name for phenazocine (an *opioid* analgesic 80)

Naseptin a brand name for chlorhexidine (a skin *antiseptic* 175) with neomycin (an aminoglycoside antibiotic 128)

Nasonex a brand name for mometasone 351 (a topical corticosteroid 174)

Natrilix a brand name for indapamide 305 (a thiazide-like diuretic 99); *illus. 44M, 45N*

Navidrex a brand name for cyclopenthiazide 247 (a thiazide diuretic 99); *illus. 44 O*

Navispare a brand name for cyclopenthiazide 247 with amiloride 193 (both diuretics 99)

Navoban a brand name for tropisetron (an anti-emetic 90)

Nebcin a brand name for tobramycin (an aminoglycoside antibiotic 128)

Nebilet a brand name for nebivolol (a beta blocker 97 antihypertensive 102)

nebivolol a beta blocker 97 antihypertensive 102

nedocromil a drug similar to sodium cromoglicate 404 used to prevent asthma attacks

nefazodone an antidepressant 84

nefopam a non-*opioid* analgesic 80

Negram a brand name for nalidixic acid (an antibacterial 131)

nelfinavir an antiviral for HIV/AIDS 157

Neo-Bendromax a brand of bendroflumethiazide 207 (a thiazide diuretic 99)

Neogest a brand name for norgestrel (a female sex hormone 147)

Neo-Mercazole a brand name for carbimazole 219 (an antithyroid drug 144); *illus. 36A*

neomycin an aminoglycoside antibiotic 128 used in ear drops 171

Neo-NaClex a brand name for bendroflumethiazide 207 (a thiazide diuretic 99)

Neo-NaClex-K a brand name for bendroflumethiazide 207 (a thiazide diuretic 99) with potassium 443; *illus. 38M*

Neoral a brand name for cyclosporin 249 (an immunosuppressant 156)

NeoRecormon a brand name for epoetin 274 (a kidney *hormone* 140)

Neosporin a brand name for gramicidin with neomycin and polymyxin B (all antibiotics 128)

neostigmine a drug for myasthenia gravis 121

Neotigason a brand name for acitretin (a drug for psoriasis 178)

Nephril a brand name for polythiazide (a thiazide diuretic 99)

Nericur a brand name for benzoyl peroxide 208 (a drug for acne 177)

Nerisone a brand name for diflucortolone (a topical corticosteroid 174)

Netillin a brand name for netilmicin (an aminoglycoside antibiotic 128)

netilmicin an aminoglycoside antibiotic 128

Neulactil a brand name for pericyazine (an antipsychotic 85)

Neupogen a brand name for filgrastim 283 (a blood growth stimulant)

Neurontin a brand name for gabapentin (an anticonvulsant 86)

Neutrexin a brand name for trimetrexate (an antimicrobial for pneumocystis pneumonia in AIDS 136)

niacin nicotinic acid 442 (a vitamin 149)

niacinamide also known as nicotinamide 442 (a vitamin 149)

nicardipine a calcium channel blocker 101

niclosamide an anthelmintic 139 for tapeworm infestation

nicorandil 357 (an anti-angina drug 101)

Nicorette a brand name for nicotine given as a drug for relief of smoking *withdrawal* symptoms

nicotinamide a B vitamin 442 (a vitamin 149)

nicotine 358 (a nervous system stimulant 88)

Nicotinell a brand name for nicotine given as a drug for relief of smoking *withdrawal* symptoms; *illus. 47C, 47E*

nicotinic acid a vasodilator 98, lipid-lowering drug 103, and vitamin 149

nicotinyl alcohol tartrate niacin 442 (a vitamin 149)

nicoumalone see acenocoumarol (an anticoagulant 104)

nifedipine 359 (a calcium channel blocker 101)

Niferex a brand name for iron 441 (a mineral 150)

Night Nurse a brand-name preparation for relief of cold symptoms, containing paracetamol 368 (a non-*opioid* analgesic 80) with promethazine 385 (an antihistamine 124 and anti-emetic 90)

nikethamide a respiratory stimulant 88

nimodipine a calcium channel blocker 101

Nindaxa a brand name for indapamide 305 (a thiazide-like diuretic 99)

Nipent a brand name for pentostatin (an anticancer drug 154)

nisoldipine a calcium channel blocker 101

nitrazepam a benzodiazepine sleeping drug 82

Nitrocine a brand name for glyceryl trinitrate 296 (an anti-angina drug 101)

Nitro-Dur a brand name for glyceryl trinitrate 296 (an anti-angina drug 101); *illus. 47G*

nitrofurantoin an antibacterial 131

Nitrolingual a brand name for glyceryl trinitrate 296 (an anti-angina drug 101)

Nitronal a brand name for glyceryl trinitrate 296 (an anti-angina drug 101)

nitroprusside antihypertensive 102

nitrous oxide an *anaesthetic* gas

Nivaquine a brand name for chloroquine 224 (an antimalarial 137 and antirheumatic 117); *illus. 36S*

Nivemycin a brand name for neomycin (an aminoglycoside antibiotic 128)

nizatidine an anti-ulcer drug 109

Nizoral a brand name for ketoconazole 314 (an antifungal 138); *illus. 43M*

Nolvadex a brand name for tamoxifen 411 (an anticancer drug 154)

Nolvadex Forte a brand name for tamoxifen 411 (an anticancer drug 154)

nonoxinol '9' (a spermicidal agent 161)

nontocog alfa a synthetic form of factor IX to promote blood clotting 104

Nootropil a brand name for piracetam (an anticonvulsant 86)

noradrenaline see norepinephrine

Norditropin a brand name for somatropin (a synthetic pituitary *hormone* 145)

norepinephrine previously known as noradrenaline (a drug similar to epinephrine 273 used to raise blood pressure during anaphylactic shock 496)

NORETHISTERONE–PILOCARPINE

norethisterone 360 (a female sex hormone 147 and oral contraceptive 161)

norfloxacin an antibiotic 128

Norgalax a brand name for docusate (a stimulant laxative 111)

norgestimate an oral contraceptive 161

Norgeston a brand-name oral contraceptive 161 containing levonorgestrel 322

norgestrel a progestogen 147

Noriday a brand-name oral contraceptive 161 containing norethisterone 360

Norimin a brand-name oral contraceptive 161 containing ethinylestradiol 279 and norethisterone 360

Norimode a brand name for loperamide 326 (an antidiarrhoeal 110)

Norinyl-1 a brand-name oral contraceptive 161 containing norethisterone 360 and mestranol

Noristerat a brand-name injectable contraceptive 161 containing norethisterone 360 (a female sex hormone 147)

Normacol Plus a brand name for frangula with sterculia (both laxatives 111)

Normax a brand name for dantron and docusate (both laxatives 111)

Normosang a brand name for haem arginate (a drug to treat porphyria)

Norplant a brand name for levonorgestrel 322 (a female sex hormone 147)

Norprolac a brand name for quinagolide (a drug used for infertility 164)

nortriptyline a tricyclic antidepressant 84

Norvir a brand name for ritonavir (an antiviral for HIV/AIDS 157)

NovoNorm a brand name for repaglinide 395 an oral antidiabetic 142

Nozinan a brand name for methotrimeprazine (an antipsychotic 85)

Nubain a brand name for nalbuphine (an *opioid* analgesic 80)

Nuelin a brand name for theophylline 419 (a bronchodilator 92)

Nulacin a brand-name antacid 108 containing calcium carbonate 438, magnesium carbonate, magnesium trisilicate, and magnesium oxide

Nupercainal a brand name for cinchocaine (a local anaesthetic 80)

Nurofen a brand name for ibuprofen 303 (a non-*opioid* analgesic 80 and non-steroidal anti-inflammatory 116)

Nurofen Plus a brand name for ibuprofen 303 (a non-steroidal anti-inflammatory drug 116) with codeine 241 (an *opioid* analgesic 80)

Nu-Seals Aspirin a brand name for aspirin 200 (a non-*opioid* analgesic 80 and antiplatelet drug 104)

Nutraplus a brand name for urea (an *emollient*)

Nutrizym GR a brand name for pancreatin (a preparation of pancreatic *enzymes* 114)

Nuvelle a brand name for estradiol 277 and levonorgestrel 322 (both female sex hormones 147)

Nycopren a brand name for naproxen 356 (a non-steroidal anti-inflammatory 116 and drug for gout 119)

Nylax a brand-name stimulant laxative 111

Nystadermal a brand name for nystatin 361 (an antifungal 138) with triamcinolone (a corticosteroid 141)

Nystaform a brand name for nystatin 361 (an antifungal 138) with chlorhexidine (a skin *antiseptic* 175)

Nystaform-HC a brand name for hydrocortisone 301 (a corticosteroid 141) with nystatin 361 (an antifungal 138) and chlorhexidine (a skin *antiseptic* 175)

Nystamont a brand name for nystatin 361 (an antifungal 138)

Nystan a brand name for nystatin 361 (an antifungal 138); *illus. 35 O*

nystatin 361 (an antifungal 138)

Nytol a brand-name preparation for sleep disturbance containing diphenhydramine (an antihistamine 124)

O

Occlusal a brand name for salicylic acid (a wart remover)

Octapressin a brand name for felypressin (a *vasoconstrictor* 95 used in dentistry)

octocog alfa a synthetic form of factor VIII to promote blood clotting 104

octoxinol a spermicidal agent 161

octreotide a synthetic pituitary *hormone* 145 used to relieve symptoms of cancer of the pancreas 154

Ocufen a brand name for flurbiprofen (a non-steroidal anti-inflammatory 116)

Ocusert Pilo a brand name for pilocarpine 375 (a *miotic* for glaucoma 168)

Odrik a brand name for trandolapril (an ACE inhibitor 98)

Oestrifen a brand name for tamoxifen 411 (an anticancer drug 154)

Oestrogel a brand name for estradiol 277 (an oestrogen 147)

oestrogen a female sex hormone 147

ofloxacin an antibiotic 128

Oilatum Emollient a brand-name bath additive containing liquid paraffin for dry skin conditions

Oilatum Gel a brand name for a shower gel containing liquid paraffin for dry skin conditions

olanzapine 362 (an antipsychotic 85)

Olbetam a brand name for acipimox (a lipid-lowering drug 103)

olsalazine a drug for ulcerative colitis 112

omeprazole 363 (an anti-ulcer drug 109)

Oncovin a brand name for vincristine (an anticancer drug 154)

ondansetron 364 (an anti-emetic 90)

One-Alpha a brand name for alfacalcidol 448 (a vitamin 149)

Opilon a brand name for moxisylyte (a vasodilator 98)

opium tincture morphine 353 (an *opioid* analgesic 80)

Opticrom a brand name for sodium cromoglicate 404 (an anti-allergy drug 124)

Optimine a brand name for azatadine (an antihistamine 124)

Optrex Eye Lotion a brand-name preparation containing witch hazel (an *astringent*)

Opumide a brand name for indapamide 305 (a thiazide-like diuretic 99)

Orabase a brand-name ointment to protect the skin or mouth from damage

Orabet a brand name for metformin 339 (a drug for diabetes 142)

Oraldene a brand name *antiseptic* mouthwash containing hexetidine

Oramorph a brand name for morphine 353 (an *opioid* analgesic 80)

Orap a brand name for pimozide (an antipsychotic 85)

orciprenaline a *sympathomimetic* used as a bronchodilator 92

Orelox a brand name for cefpodoxime (a cephalosporin antibiotic 128)

Orgaran a brand name for danaparoid (an anticoagulant 104)

Orimeten a brand name for aminoglutethimide (an anticancer drug 154)

Orlept a brand name for sodium valproate 405 (an anticonvulsant 86)

orlistat 365 (an anti-obesity drug 148)

Orovite a brand-name multivitamin 149

orphenadrine 366 (an *anticholinergic* muscle relaxant 120 and drug for parkinsonism 87)

Ortho-Creme a brand name for nonoxinol '9' (a spermicidal agent 161)

Ortho-Dienoestrol a brand name for dienestrol (a female sex hormone 147)

Orthoforms a brand name for nonoxinol '9' (a spermicidal agent 161)

Ortho-Gynest a brand name for estriol (an oestrogen 147)

Orudis a brand name for ketoprofen 315 (a non-steroidal anti-inflammatory 116)

Oruvail a brand name for ketoprofen 315 (a non-steroidal anti-inflammatory 116); *illus. 39L*

Osmolax a brand name for lactulose 316 (an osmotic laxative 111)

Ossopan a brand name for hydroxyapatite (a calcium supplement 438 used to treat bone disorders 122)

Ostram a brand name for calcium phosphate (a mineral 150)

Otomize a brand name for dexamethasone 252 (a corticosteroid 141) and neomycin (an aminoglycoside antibiotic 128)

Otosporin a brand name for hydrocortisone 301 (a corticosteroid 141) with neomycin and polymyxin B (both antibiotics 128)

Otrivine a brand name for xylometazoline (a decongestant 93)

Otrivine-Antistin a brand name for antazoline (an antihistamine 124) with xylometazoline (a decongestant 93)

Ovestin a brand name for estriol (an oestrogen 147)

Ovex a brand name for mebendazole (an anthelmintic 139)

Ovran a brand-name oral contraceptive 161 containing ethinylestradiol 279 and levonorgestrel 322

Ovranette a brand-name oral contraceptive 161 containing ethinylestradiol 279 and levonorgestrel 322

Ovysmen a brand-name oral contraceptive 161 containing ethinylestradiol 279 and norethisterone 360

oxaliplatin an anticancer drug 154

oxazepam a benzodiazepine anti-anxiety drug 83

oxerutin a drug used to treat peripheral vascular disease 98

oxetacaine a local anaesthetic 80 used with antacids 108 for reflux oesophagitis

oxitropium a bronchodilator 92

Oxivent a brand name for oxitropium (a bronchodilator 92)

oxpentifylline see pentoxifylline (a vasodilator 98 used to improve blood flow to the limbs in peripheral vascular disease)

oxprenolol a beta blocker 97

oxybenzone a sunscreen 181

oxybuprocaine a local anaesthetic 80

oxybutynin 367 (an *anticholinergic* and *antispasmodic* for urinary disorders 166)

oxycodone an *opioid* analgesic 80

oxymetazoline a *topical* decongestant 93 also used for ear disorders 171

Oxymycin a brand name for oxytetracycline (a tetracycline antibiotic 128)

oxypertine an antipsychotic 85

oxytetracycline a tetracycline antibiotic 128

oxytocin a uterine stimulant 165

P

paclitaxel an anticancer drug 154

Paldesic a brand name for paracetamol 368 (a non-*opioid* analgesic 80)

Palfium a brand name for dextromoramide (an *opioid* analgesic 80); *illus. 36E*

palivizumab an antiviral drug 133

Palladone a brand name for hydromorphone (an *opioid* analgesic 80)

Paludrine a brand name for proguanil 383 (an antimalarial 137); *illus. 44C*

Pamergan P100 a brand name for pethidine (an *opioid* analgesic 80) with promethazine 385 (an antihistamine 124 and anti-emetic 90)

pamidronate a drug for bone disorders 122

Panadeine a brand name for paracetamol 368 (a non-*opioid* analgesic 80) with codeine 241

Panadol a brand name for paracetamol 368 (a non-*opioid* analgesic 80)

Panadol Extra a brand name for paracetamol 368 (a non-*opioid* analgesic 80) with caffeine

Panadol Ultra a brand name for paracetamol 368 with codeine 241 (both analgesics 80)

Panaleve a brand name for paracetamol 368 (a non-*opioid* analgesic 80)

Pancrease a brand name for pancreatin (a preparation of pancreatic *enzymes* 114)

pancreatin a preparation of pancreatic *enzymes* 114

Pancrex a brand name for pancreatin (a preparation of pancreatic *enzymes* 114)

pancuronium a muscle relaxant 120 used during general *anaesthesia*

Panoxyl a brand name for benzoyl peroxide 208 (a drug for acne 177)

panthenol pantothenic acid 443 (a vitamin 149)

pantoprazole an ulcer healing drug 109

pantothenic acid 443 (a vitamin 149)

papaveretum an *opioid* analgesic 80

papaverine a muscle relaxant 120

Papulex a brand name for nicotinamide (a drug for acne 177)

paracetamol 368 (a non-*opioid* analgesic 80); *illus. 46H*

Paracodol a brand-name analgesic 80 containing codeine 241 and paracetamol 368

Paradote a brand-name analgesic 80 containing paracetamol 368 and methionine (an *antidote* for paracetamol poisoning)

Parake a brand-name analgesic 80 containing codeine 241 and paracetamol 368

paraldehyde an anticonvulsant 86 used for status epilepticus

Paramax a brand-name migraine drug 89 containing paracetamol 368 and metoclopramide 344

Paramol a brand name for paracetamol 368 with dihydrocodeine (both analgesics 80)

Paraplatin a brand name for carboplatin (an anticancer drug 154)

Pariet a brand name for rabeprazole (an anti-ulcer drug 109)

Parlodel a brand name for bromocriptine 212 (a pituitary agent 145 and drug for parkinsonism 87); *illus. 41H*

Parmid a brand name for metoclopramide 344 (a gastrointestinal motility regulator and anti-emetic 90)

Parnate a brand name for tranylcypromine (an MAOI antidepressant 84)

paromomycin an antiprotozoal 136

Paroven a brand name for oxerutin (a drug used to treat peripheral vascular disease 98)

paroxetine 369 (an antidepressant 84)

Partobulin a brand name for anti-D immunoglobulin (a drug used to prevent sensitization to Rhesus antigen)

Parvolex a brand name for acetylcysteine (a *mucolytic* 94)

Pavacol-D a brand name for pholcodine (a cough suppressant 94)

Penbritin a brand name for ampicillin (a penicillin antibiotic 128)

penciclovir an antiviral drug 133

Pendramine a brand name for penicillamine (an antirheumatic 117)

penicillamine (an antirheumatic 117)

penicillin antibiotics 128

penicillin G see benzylpenicillin (a penicillin antibiotic 128)

penicillin V see phenoxymethylpenicillin 372 (a penicillin antibiotic 128)

Pentacarinat a brand name for pentamidine (an antiprotozoal 136)

pentamidine an antiprotozoal 136

Pentasa a brand name for mesalazine 338 (a drug for ulcerative colitis 112)

pentazocine an *opioid* analgesic 80

pentostatin an anticancer drug 154

pentoxifylline previously known as oxpentifylline (a vasodilator 98 used to improve blood flow to the limbs in peripheral vascular disease)

Pepcid a brand name for famotidine (an anti-ulcer drug 109)

peppermint oil a substance for indigestion and bowel spasm 110

Peptimax a brand name for cimetidine 228 (an anti-ulcer drug 109)

Pepto-Bismol a brand-name preparation for diarrhoea 110 and upset stomach 108 containing bismuth

Percutol a brand name for glyceryl trinitrate 296 (an anti-angina drug 101)

Perdix a brand name for moexipril (an ACE inhibitor 98)

Perfan a brand name for enoximone (a drug for heart failure 95)

pergolide a drug for parkinsonism 87

Pergonal a brand name for menotrophin (a drug for infertility 164)

Periactin a brand name for cyproheptadine (an antihistamine 124 used as an appetite stimulant 88)

pericyazine an antipsychotic 85

Perinal a brand name for hydrocortisone 301 (a corticosteroid 141) with lidocaine (a local anaesthetic 80)

perindopril an ACE inhibitor 98

permethrin 370 a *topical* antiparasitic 176

Peroxyl a brand of hydrogen peroxide *antiseptic* mouthwash 175

perphenazine an antipsychotic 85 and anti-emetic 90

Persantin a brand name for dipyridamole 261 (an antiplatelet drug 104); *illus. 36L*

Peru balsam an *antiseptic* 175 for haemorrhoids 113

pethidine an *opioid* analgesic 80 and drug used in labour 165

Pevaryl a brand name for econazole (an antifungal 138)

phenazocine an *opioid* analgesic 80

phenelzine an MAOI antidepressant 84

Phenergan a brand name for promethazine 385 (an antihistamine 124 and anti-emetic 90); *illus. 38D*

phenindione an oral anticoagulant 104

pheniramine an antihistamine 124

phenobarbital 371 (a barbiturate anticonvulsant 86)

phenol an *antiseptic* used in throat lozenges and sprays 175

phenothrin a *topical* antiparasitic 176 for head and pubic lice infestation

phenoxybenzamine a drug for phaeochromocytoma (a tumour of the adrenal glands 154)

phenoxymethylpenicillin 372 (a penicillin antibiotic 128)

Phensic a brand-name analgesic 80 containing aspirin 200 and caffeine

phentermine an appetite suppressant 88

phentolamine an antihypertensive 102

phenylbutazone a non-steroidal anti-inflammatory 116

phenylephrine a decongestant 93

phenylpropanolamine 373 (a decongestant 93)

phenytoin 374 (an anticonvulsant 86)

Phimetin a brand name for cimetidine 228 (an anti-ulcer drug 109)

pHiso-Med a brand name for chlorhexidine (a skin *antiseptic* 175)

pholcodine a cough suppressant 94

phosphorus a mineral 150

Phyllocontin Continus a brand name for aminophylline 419 (a bronchodilator 92)

Physeptone a brand name for methadone 340 (an *opioid* 458 used as an analgesic 80 and to ease heroin *withdrawal*); *illus. 44T*

Physiotens a brand name for moxonidine 354 (a centrally acting antihypertensive 102)

Phytex a brand-name antifungal 138 containing salicylic acid

phytomenadione natural vitamin K 449 (a vitamin 149)

Picolax a brand name for sodium picosulfate and magnesium citrate (both laxatives 111)

pilocarpine 375 (a *miotic* for glaucoma 168)

PIMOZIDE–RIMACTAZID

pimozide an antipsychotic 85

pindolol a beta blocker 97

piperacillin a penicillin antibiotic 128

piperazine an anthelmintic 139

piperonal a head-lice repellent

pipotiazine palmitate an antipsychotic 85

Pipril a brand name for piperacillin (a penicillin antibiotic 128)

piracetam an anticonvulsant 86

pirenzepine an *anticholinergic* for peptic ulcers 109

Piriton a brand name for chlorphenamine 225 (an antihistamine 124); *illus. 37D*

piroxicam 376 (a non-steroidal anti-inflammatory 116 and drug for gout 119)

Pirozip a brand name for piroxicam 376 (a non-steroidal anti-inflammatory 116 and drug for gout 119)

pizotifen 377 (a drug for migraine 89)

Plaquenil a brand name for hydroxychloroquine (an antimalarial 137 and antirheumatic 117)

Plavix a brand name for clopidogrel 238 (an antiplatelet drug 104)

Plendil a brand name for felodipine (a calcium channel blocker 101)

podophyllin a *topical* treatment for genital warts

podophyllotoxin a *topical* treatment for genital warts

podophyllum a *topical* treatment for warts

poloxamer a stimulant laxative 111

Polyfax a brand name for bacitracin with polymyxin B (both antibiotics 128)

polymyxin B an antibiotic 128

polynoxylin an antifungal 138 and antibacterial 131

polystyrene sulphonate a drug to remove excess potassium 443 from the blood

Polytar a brand name for coal tar (a substance used for eczema 179, psoriasis 178, and dandruff 180)

polythiazide a thiazide diuretic 99

Polytrim a brand-name antibacterial 131 containing trimethoprim 429 and polymyxin B

polyvinyl alcohol an ingredient of artificial tear preparations 170

Ponstan a brand name for mefenamic acid 333 (a non-steroidal anti-inflammatory 116); *illus. 41F*

Poractant alfa a drug to mature the lungs of premature babies

Pork Insulatard a brand name for insulin 307 (a drug for diabetes 142)

Pork Mixtard a brand name for insulin 307 (a drug for diabetes 142)

Posalfilin a brand name for podophyllum with salicylic acid (both drugs for warts)

potassium 443 (a mineral 150)

potassium bicarbonate an antacid 108

potassium chloride potassium 443 (a mineral 150)

potassium citrate a drug for cystitis that reduces the acidity of urine 166, 443

potassium clavulanate a preparation of clavulanic acid (a substance given with amoxicillin 198 to make it more effective)

potassium hydroxyquinolone sulphate an agent with antibacterial 131, antifungal 138, and deodorant properties, used for skin infections 175 and acne 177

potassium iodide a drug used for an overactive thyroid before surgery 144

potassium permanganate a skin *antiseptic* 175

povidone-iodine a skin *antiseptic* 175

Pragmatar a brand-name preparation for eczema 179, psoriasis 178, and dandruff 180 containing coal tar, salicylic acid, and sulphur

pralidoxime mesylate an *antidote* for organophosphorus poisoning

pramipexole a drug for parkinsonism 87

pramocaine a local anaesthetic 80

pravastatin 378 a cholesterol-lowering agent 103

Praxilene a brand name for naftidrofuryl 355 (a vasodilator 98)

praziquantel an anthelmintic 139 for tapeworm infestation

prazosin an antihypertensive 102 also used to relieve urinary obstruction 166

Precortisyl a brand name for prednisolone 379 (a corticosteroid 141)

Predenema a brand name for prednisolone 379 (a corticosteroid 141)

Predfoam a brand name for prednisolone 379 (a corticosteroid 141)

Prednesol a brand name for prednisolone 379 (a corticosteroid 141)

prednisolone 379 (a corticosteroid 141)

Predsol a brand name for prednisolone 379 (a corticosteroid 141)

Predsol-N a brand name for prednisolone 379 (a corticosteroid 141) with neomycin (an aminoglycoside antibiotic 128)

Pregaday a brand name for folic acid 440 (a vitamin 149) with iron 441 (a mineral 150)

Pregnyl a brand name for chorionic gonadotrophin 227 (a drug for infertility 164)

Premarin a brand name for conjugated oestrogens 244 (a female sex hormone 147); *illus. 35L*

Premique a brand-name preparation for menopausal symptoms 147 containing conjugated oestrogens 244 with medroxyprogesterone 332

Prempak-C a brand-name drug for menopausal symptoms 147 containing conjugated oestrogens 244 and norgestrel

Prepadine a brand name for dosulepin 266 (a tricyclic antidepressant 84)

Prepulsid a brand name for cisapride 231 (a motility stimulant laxative 111 and antacid 108); *illus. 44G*

Prescal a brand name for isradipine (a calcium channel blocker 101)

Preservex a brand name for aceclofenac (a non-steroidal anti-inflammatory 116)

Prestim a brand name for bendroflumethiazide 207 (a thiazide diuretic 99) with timolol 423 (a beta blocker 97)

Priadel a brand name for lithium 324 (a drug for mania 85); *illus. 46M*

prilocaine a local anaesthetic 80

Primalan a brand name for mequitazine (an antihistamine 124)

primaquine an antimalarial 137 and antiprotozoal 136

Primaxin a brand name for imipenem (an antibiotic 128) with cilastatin (used to make imipenem more effective)

primidone 380 (an anticonvulsant 86)

Primolut N a brand name for norethisterone 360 (a female sex hormone 147); *illus. 45F*

Primoteston Depot a brand name for testosterone 417 (a male sex hormone 146)

Primperan a brand name for metoclopramide 344 (a gastrointestinal motility regulator and anti-emetic 90)

Prioderm a brand name for malathion 330 (a *topical* antiparasitic 176)

Pripsen a brand name for piperazine (an anthelmintic 139) with senna (a stimulant laxative 111)

Pro-Banthine a brand name for propantheline (an *anticholinergic antispasmodic* for irritable bowel syndrome 110 and urinary incontinence 166)

probenecid a uricosuric for gout 119

procainamide an anti-arrhythmic 100

procaine a local anaesthetic 80

procaine benzylpenicillin a penicillin antibiotic 128

procarbazine a drug for lymphatic cancers and small-cell cancer of the lung 154

prochlorperazine 381 (a phenothiazine anti-emetic 90 and antipsychotic 85)

Proctofoam HC a brand name for hydrocortisone 301 (a corticosteroid 141) with pramocaine (a local anaesthetic 80)

Proctosedyl a brand name for hydrocortisone 301 (a corticosteroid 141) with cinchocaine (a local anaesthetic 80)

procyclidine 382 (an *anticholinergic* for parkinsonism 87)

Profasi a brand name for chorionic gonadotrophin 227 (a drug for infertility 164)

Proflex a brand name for ibuprofen 303 (a non-steroidal anti-inflammatory 116); *illus. 40H*

progesterone a female sex hormone 147

Prograf a brand name for tacrolimus (an immunosuppressant 156)

proguanil 383 (an antimalarial 137)

Progynova a brand name for estradiol 277 (an oestrogen 147)

Progynova TS a brand name for estradiol 277 (an oestrogen 147)

Proluton Depot a brand name for hydroxyprogesterone (a progestogen 147 used to prevent miscarriage)

promazine 384 (a phenothiazine antipsychotic 85)

promethazine 385 (an antihistamine 124 and anti-emetic 90)

Prominal a brand name for methylphenobarbital (a barbiturate anticonvulsant 86)

Propaderm a brand name for beclometasone 206 (a corticosteroid 141)

propafenone an anti-arrhythmic 100

Propain a brand-name analgesic 80 containing codeine 241, diphenhydramine, paracetamol 368, and caffeine

propamidine isethionate an antibacterial 131 for eye infections

Propanix a brand name for propranolol 386 (a beta blocker 97 and anti-anxiety drug 83)

propantheline an *anticholinergic* antispasmodic for irritable bowel syndrome 110 and urinary incontinence 166

Propine a brand name for dipivefrine (a *sympathomimetic* for glaucoma 168)

propiverine a drug for urinary frequency 166

Pro-Plus a brand name for caffeine (a stimulant 88)
propofol an anaesthetic agent 80
propranolol 386 (a beta blocker 97 and anti-anxiety drug 83)
propylthiouracil 387 (an antithyroid drug 144)
Proscar a brand name for finasteride 284 (a drug for benign prostatic hypertrophy)
Prostap SR a brand name for leuprorelin (a drug for menstrual disorders 160)
Prostigmin a brand name for neostigmine (a drug for myasthenia gravis 121); *illus. 43T*
protamine an *antidote* for heparin 299
Prothiaden a brand name for dosulepin 266 (a tricyclic antidepressant 84); *illus. 35K*
protirelin a drug to test thyroid function 144
Protium a brand name for pantoprazole (an ulcer healing drug 109)
protriptyline a tricyclic antidepressant 84
Provera a brand name for medroxyprogesterone 332 (a female sex hormone 147); *illus. 38J*
Provigil a brand name for modafinil (a drug for narcolepsy 88)
Pro-Viron a brand name for mesterolone (a male sex hormone 146)
proxymetacaine a local anaesthetic 80
Prozac a brand name for fluoxetine 286 (an antidepressant 84); *illus. 41E*
Proziere a brand name for prochlorperazine 381 (a phenothiazine anti-emetic 90)
pseudoephedrine a *sympathomimetic* decongestant 93
Psorin a brand-name drug for psoriasis 178 containing dithranol, coal tar, and salicylic acid
Pulmicort a brand name for budesonide 213 (a corticosteroid 141)
Pulmozyme a brand name for dornase alfa (a drug for cystic fibrosis 94)
pumactant a drug to mature the lungs of premature babies
Puri-Nethol a brand name for mercaptopurine 337 (an anticancer drug 154); *illus. 37 I*
Pylorid a brand name for ranitidine bismuth citrate (an anti-ulcer drug 109)
Pyralvex an anti-inflammatory drug for mouth ulcers
pyrazinamide an antituberculous drug 132
pyridostigmine 388 (a drug for myasthenia gravis 121)
pyridoxine 444 (a vitamin 149)
pyrimethamine 389 (an antimalarial 137)
pyrithione zinc an antimicrobial for dandruff 180
Pyrogastrone a brand name for aluminium hydroxide 191, magnesium trisilicate, and sodium bicarbonate 403 (all antacids 108), carbenoxolone (an anti-ulcer drug 109) and alginic acid (an antifoaming agent 108)

Q

Quellada M a brand name for malathion 330 (an antiparasitic 176)
Questran a brand name for colestyramine 243 (a lipid-lowering drug 103)
quetiapine 390 (an antipsychotic drug 85)
quinagolide a drug for infertility 164
quinapril an ACE inhibitor 98

quinidine an anti-arrhythmic drug 100
quinine 391 (an antimalarial 137 and muscle relaxant 120)
Quinocort a brand name for hydrocortisone 301 (a corticosteroid 141) with potassium hydroxyquinoline sulphate (an agent for skin infections 175)
Quinoderm a brand-name preparation for acne 177 containing benzoyl peroxide 208 and potassium hydroxyquinoline sulphate (an agent for skin infections 175)
Quinoped a brand-name antifungal 138 containing benzoyl peroxide 208 and potassium hydroxyquinoline sulphate (an agent for skin infections 175)
quinupristin an antibiotic 130

R

rabeprazole an anti-ulcer drug 109
Radian B a brand-name *topical* preparation for muscle aches and sprains
raloxifene 392 (an anti-oestrogen sex hormone *antagonist* 147 used for osteoporosis 122)
raltitrexed an anticancer drug 154
ramipril 393 (an ACE inhibitor 98)
ranitidine 394 (an anti-ulcer drug 109)
ranitidine bismuth citrate an anti-ulcer drug 109
Rapilysin a brand name for reteplase (a thrombolytic 105)
Rapitard MC a brand name for insulin 307 (a drug for diabetes 142)
Rapitil a brand name for nedocromil (an anti-allergy drug 124)
Rappell a brand name for piperonal (a head-lice repellent)
Rastinon a brand name for tolbutamide 424 (a drug for diabetes 142); *illus. 42D*
razoxane a *cytotoxic* anticancer drug 154
reboxetine an antidepressant 84
Redoxon a brand name for vitamin C 447 (a vitamin 149)
Refludan a brand name for lepirudin (an anticoagulant 104)
Refolinon a brand name for folinic acid (a vitamin 149)
Regaine a brand name for minoxidil 349 (for treatment of male pattern baldness 180)
Regranex a brand name for beclapermin (a drug for healing skin ulcers)
Regulan a brand name for ispaghula (a bulk-forming agent used as a laxative 111)
Regulose a brand of lactulose 316 (an osmotic laxative 111)
Rehidrat a brand name for oral rehydration salts containing potassium 443, sodium chloride 445, sodium bicarbonate 403, and glucose
Relaxit a brand-name lubricant laxative 111
Relenza a brand name for zanamivir 434 (an antiviral drug 133)
Relifex a brand name for nabumetone (a non-steroidal anti-inflammatory 116)
Remedeine a brand name for paracetamol 368 (a non-*opioid* analgesic 80) with dihydrocodeine (an opioid analgesic 80)
remifentanil a drug used in *anaesthesia*

Rennie Digestif a brand-name antacid 108 containing calcium carbonate 438 with magnesium carbonate
repaglinide 395 an oral antidiabetic 142
reproterol a bronchodilator 92
Requip a brand name for ropinirole (a drug for parkinsonism 87)
Resolve a brand-name analgesic 80 and antacid 108 with paracetamol 368, sodium bicarbonate 403, potassium bicarbonate, calcium carbonate 438, citric acid, and vitamin C 447
Resonium A a brand name for polystyrene sulphonate (a drug to remove excess potassium 443 from the blood)
resorcinol a keratolytic mainly for acne 177
Restandol a brand name for testosterone 417 (a male sex hormone 146); *illus. 39C*
reteplase a thrombolytic 105
Retin-A a brand name for tretinoin (a drug for acne 177)
retinoic acid vitamin A 446 (a vitamin 149)
retinoids vitamin A 446 (a vitamin 149)
retinol vitamin A 446 (a vitamin 149)
Retinova a brand name for tretinoin (a drug for acne 177)
Retrovir a brand name for zidovudine 435 (an antiviral for HIV infection and AIDS 157); *illus. 41J*
Revanil a brand name for lisuride (a drug for parkinsonism 87)
Revasc a brand name for desirudin (an anticoagulant 104)
Rheumacin LA a brand name for indometacin (a non-steroidal anti-inflammatory 116 and drug for gout 119)
Rheumox a brand name for azapropazone (a non-steroidal anti-inflammatory 116)
Rhinocort a brand name for budesonide 213 (a corticosteroid 141)
Rhinolast a brand name for azelastine (an antihistamine 124)
Rhumalgan a brand name for diclofenac 254 (a non-steroidal anti-inflammatory 116)
ribavirin see tribavirin, an antiviral 133 used for certain lung infections in infants and children
riboflavin 444 (a vitamin 149)
Ridaura a brand name for auranofin (an antirheumatic 117)
Rideril a brand name for thioridazine 420 (a phenothiazine antipsychotic 85)
rifabutin an antituberculous drug 132
Rifadin a brand name for rifampicin 396 (an antituberculous drug 132); *illus. 41Q*
rifampicin 396 (an antituberculous drug 132)
Rifater a brand name for isoniazid 311 with rifampicin 396 and pyrazinamide (all antituberculous drugs 132)
Rifinah a brand name for isoniazid 311 with rifampicin 396 (both antituberculous drugs 132); *illus. 35G, 39J*
Rilutek a brand name for riluzole (a glutamate inhibitor used to help patients who have sclerosis)
riluzole a glutamate inhibitor used to help patients with sclerosis
Rimactane a brand name for rifampicin 396 (an antituberculous drug 132)
Rimactazid a brand name for isoniazid 311 with rifampicin 396 (both antituberculous drugs 132)

RIMAPAM–SUPRAX

Rimapam a brand name for diazepam 253 (a benzodiazepine anti-anxiety drug 83, muscle relaxant 120, and anticonvulsant 86)

rimexolone a corticosteroid 141

Rimoxallin a brand name for amoxicillin 198 (a penicillin antibiotic 128)

Rimso-50 a brand name for dimethyl sulfoxide (a drug for urinary infection 166)

Rinatec a brand name for ipratropium bromide 309 (a bronchodilator 92)

Rinstead pastilles a brand name for pastilles for mouth ulcers containing chloroxylenol

Risperdal a brand name for risperidone 397 (an antipsychotic 85)

risperidone 397 (an antipsychotic 85)

Ritalin a brand name for methylphenidate (a drug for hyperactivity)

ritodrine a uterine muscle relaxant 165

ritonavir an antiviral for HIV/AIDS 157

rituximab an anticancer drug 154

rivastigmine 398 (a drug for dementia 87)

Rivotril a brand name for clonazepam 237 (a benzodiazepine anticonvulsant 86); *illus. 35S*

rizatriptan a drug for migraine 89

Roaccutane a brand name for isotretinoin 313 (a drug for acne 177); *illus. 40D*

Robaxin a brand name for methocarbamol (a muscle relaxant 120)

Robinul a brand name for glycopyrronium bromide (an *anticholinergic* used in general *anaesthesia*)

Robinul-Neostigmine a brand name for neostigmine (a drug for myasthenia gravis 121)

Robitussin Dry Cough a brand name for guaifenesin (an *expectorant* 94)

Rocaltrol a brand name for calcitriol 448 (a vitamin 149)

rocuronium a drug to relax the muscles during general *anaesthesia*

rofecoxib a non-steroidal anti-inflammatory drug 116

Roferon-A a brand name for interferon 308 (an antiviral 133 and anticancer drug 154)

Rohypnol a brand name for flunitrazepam (a benzodiazepine sleeping drug 82)

Rommix a brand name for erythromycin 276 (an antibiotic 128)

Ronicol a brand name for nicotinyl alcohol (a form of niacin 442)

ropinirole a drug for parkinsonism 87

ropivacaine a local anaesthetic 80

Roter a brand-name antacid 108 containing sodium bicarbonate 403, magnesium carbonate, frangula, and bismuth

Rowachol a brand-name preparation of essential oils for gallstones 114

Rowatinex a brand-name preparation to dissolve kidney stones 119 and to treat kidney infections

Rozex a brand name for metronidazole 346 (an antibacterial 131)

Rusyde a brand name for furosemide 291 (a loop diuretic 99)

Rynacrom a brand name for sodium cromoglicate 404 (an anti-allergy drug 124)

Rynacrom Compound a brand name for sodium cromoglicate 404 (an anti-allergy drug 124) with xylometazoline (a decongestant 93)

Rythmodan a brand name for disopyramide (an anti-arrhythmic 100); *illus. 41A*

S

Sabril a brand name for vigabatrin (an anticonvulsant 86)

Saizen a brand name for somatropin (a synthetic pituitary *hormone* 145)

Salactol a brand-name wart preparation containing salicylic acid, lactic acid, and collodion 175

Salagen a brand name for pilocarpine 375 (a *miotic* for glaucoma 168)

Salamol a brand name for salbutamol 399 (a bronchodilator 92)

Salatac a brand-name wart preparation containing salicylic acid, lactic acid, and collodion 175

Salazopyrin a brand name for sulfasalazine 409 (a drug for inflammatory bowel disease 110 and an antirheumatic 117); *illus. 36M*

Salbulin a brand name for salbutamol 399 (a bronchodilator 92)

salbutamol 399 (a bronchodilator 92 and drug used in labour 165)

salcatonin see calcitonin (salmon) (a drug used for bone disorders 122)

salicylic acid a keratolytic for acne 177, dandruff 180, psoriasis 178, and warts

Salivace a brand name for artificial saliva

Saliva Orthana a brand name for artificial saliva

Saliveze a brand name for artificial saliva

Salivix a brand name for artificial saliva

salmeterol 400 (a bronchodilator 92)

Salofalk a brand name for mesalazine 338 (a drug for ulcerative colitis 112); *illus. 36P*

Salzone a brand name for paracetamol 368 (a non-*opioid* analgesic 80)

Sandimmun a brand name for cyclosporin 249 (an immunosuppressant 156); *illus. 39E*

Sandocal a brand name for calcium 438 (a mineral 150)

Sando-K a brand name for potassium 443 (a mineral 150)

Sandostatin a brand name for octreotide (a synthetic pituitary *hormone* 145 used for symptoms of cancer of the pancreas 154)

Sanomigran a brand name for pizotifen 377 (a drug for migraine 89); *illus. 37G*

saquinavir an antiviral for HIV/AIDS 157

Saventrine a brand name for isoprenaline (a bronchodilator 92)

Savlon a brand name for chlorhexidine with cetrimide (both skin *antiseptics* 175)

Schering PC4 a brand-name postcoital contraceptive containing ethinylestradiol 279 and levonorgestrel 322

Scheriproct a brand name for prednisolone 379 (a corticosteroid 141) with cinchocaine (a local anaesthetic 80)

Scopoderm TTS a brand-name anti-emetic 90 containing hyoscine 302

Sea-Legs a brand name for meclozine (an antihistamine 124 used to prevent motion sickness 90)

Secadrex a brand name for hydrochlorothiazide 300 (a thiazide diuretic 99) with acebutolol (a beta blocker 97)

secobarbital a barbiturate sleeping drug 82

Seconal Sodium a brand name for secobarbital (a barbiturate sleeping drug 82)

Sectral a brand name for acebutolol (a beta blocker 97)

Securon SR a brand name for verapamil 431 (an anti-angina drug 101 and anti-arrhythmic 100); *illus. 37Q*

Securopen a brand name for azlocillin (a penicillin antibiotic 128)

selegiline a drug for severe parkinsonism 87

selenium 445 (a mineral 150)

selenium sulphide 444 (a substance for skin inflammation 175 and dandruff 180)

Selsun a brand-name dandruff shampoo 180 containing selenium sulphide 444

Semi-Daonil a brand name for glibenclamide 294 (an oral antidiabetic 142)

Semprex a brand name for acrivastine (an antihistamine 124); *illus. 39N*

senna a stimulant laxative 111

Senokot a brand name for senna (a stimulant laxative 111)

Septanest a brand name for articaine (a local anaesthetic 80)

Septrin a brand name for co-trimoxazole 246 (an antibacterial 131); *illus. 46G*

Serc a brand name for betahistine 209 (a drug for Ménière's disease 90); *illus. 45E*

Serdolect a brand name for sertindole (an antipsychotic 85)

Serenace a brand name for haloperidol 298 (a butyrophenone antipsychotic 85)

Serevent a brand name for salmeterol 400 (a bronchodilator 92)

sermorelin a drug for growth disorders 145

Serophene a brand name for clomifene 235 (a drug for infertility 164)

Seroquel a brand name for quetiapine 390 (an antipsychotic drug 85)

Seroxat a brand name for paroxetine 369 (an antidepressant 84); *illus. 43K*

sertindole an antipsychotic 85

sertraline an antidepressant 84

Setlers a brand-name antacid 108 containing calcium carbonate 438 and magnesium hydroxide 329

Sevoflurane a general *anaesthetic*

Sevredol a brand name for morphine 353 (an *opioid* analgesic 80)

sildenafil 401 (a drug for impotence 146, 164)

silver nitrate a skin disinfectant 175

silver sulfadiazine a *topical* antibacterial 131 used to prevent infection in burns 175

Simeco a brand-name antacid 108 containing aluminium hydroxide 191, dimeticone, magnesium carbonate, and magnesium hydroxide 329

Simplene a brand name for epinephrine 273 (a drug for glaucoma 168)

Simulect a brand name for basiliximab (an immunosuppressant 156)

simvastatin 402 (a lipid-lowering drug 103)

Sinemet 62.5 a brand name for levodopa 320 with carbidopa (both drugs for parkinsonism 87); *illus. 37K*

Sinequan a brand name for doxepin (a tricyclic antidepressant 84)

Singulair a brand name for montelukast 352 (a leukotriene *antagonist* for asthma 124 and bronchospasm 92)

Sinthrome a brand name for acenocoumarol (an anticoagulant 104)

Sinutab a brand name for paracetamol 368 (a non-*opioid* analgesic 80) with phenylpropanolamine 373 (a decongestant 93)

Siopel a brand-name barrier cream containing cetrimide and dimeticone

Skelid a brand name for tiludronic acid (a drug for bone disorders 122)

Skinoren a brand name for azelaic acid (an antibacterial 131, drug for acne 177)

Slo-Indo a brand name for indometacin (a non-steroidal anti-inflammatory 116 and drug for gout 119)

Slo-Phyllin a brand name for theophylline 419 (a bronchodilator 92); *illus. 39M*

Slow-Fe a brand name for iron 441 (a mineral 150)

Slow-Fe Folic a brand name for folic acid 440 (a vitamin 149) with iron 441 (a mineral 150)

Slow-K a brand name for potassium 443 (a mineral 150)

Slow-Sodium a brand name for sodium chloride 445 (a mineral 150)

Slozem a brand name for diltiazem 259 (a calcium channel blocker 98)

Sno Phenicol a brand name for eye drops containing chloramphenicol 222 (an antibiotic 128)

Sno Tears a brand name for polyvinyl alcohol (used in artificial tear preparations 170)

soda mint tablets sodium bicarbonate 403 (an antacid 108)

sodium 445 (a mineral 150)

sodium acid phosphate a laxative 111

sodium aurothiomalate a substance containing gold, an antirheumatic 117

sodium bicarbonate 403 (an antacid 108)

sodium calcium edetate an *antidote* for poisoning by lead and other heavy metals

sodium cellulose phosphate an agent used to reduce levels of calcium 438 in the blood

sodium chloride common salt, contains sodium 445 (a mineral 150)

sodium citrate a drug for urinary tract infections 166

sodium clodronate an agent used to treat low blood calcium 438 in cancer patients 154

sodium cromoglicate 404 (an anti-allergy drug 124)

sodium feredetate iron 441 (a mineral 150)

sodium fluoride 440 (a mineral 150)

sodium fusidate an antibiotic 128

sodium nitroprusside a vasodilator 98

sodium perborate an *antiseptic* 175

sodium picosulfate a stimulant laxative 111

sodium stibogluconate an antiprotozoal 136

sodium tetradecyl sulphate a drug for treating varicose veins

sodium valproate 405 (an anticonvulsant 86)

Sofradex a brand name for dexamethasone 252 (a corticosteroid 141) with framycetin and gramicidin (both antibiotics 128)

Solarcaine a brand name for benzocaine (a local anaesthetic 80) with triclosan (an antimicrobial 175)

Solian a brand name for amisulpride 195, an antipsychotic 85

Solpadeine a brand-name analgesic 80 containing codeine 241, paracetamol 368, and caffeine

Solpadol a brand name for paracetamol 368 (a non-*opioid* analgesic 80) with codeine 241 (an opioid analgesic 80)

Soltamox a brand name for tamoxifen 411 (an antioestrogen anticancer drug 154)

Solu-Cortef a brand name for hydrocortisone 301 (a corticosteroid 141)

Solu-Medrone a brand name for methylprednisolone (a corticosteroid 141)

Solvazinc a brand name for zinc 449 (a mineral 150)

somatropin a synthetic pituitary *hormone* 145

Somatuline a brand name for lanreotide (an anticancer drug 154)

Sominex a brand-name sleeping drug 82 containing promethazine 385

Soneryl a brand name for butobarbital (a benzodiazepine sleeping drug 82)

Sorbichew a brand name for isosorbide dinitrate 312 (a nitrate vasodilator 98 and anti-angina drug 101)

Sorbid SA a brand name for isosorbide dinitrate 312 (a nitrate vasodilator 98 and anti-angina drug 101)

sorbitol a sweetening agent used in diabetic foods and included in skin creams as a moisturizer 175

Sorbitrate a brand name for isosorbide dinitrate 312 (a nitrate vasodilator 98 and anti-angina drug 101); *illus. 37M*

Sotacor a brand name for sotalol 406 (a beta blocker 97)

sotalol 406 (a beta blocker 97)

Sparine a brand name for promazine 384 (a phenothiazine antipsychotic 85); *illus. 35H*

Spasmonal a brand name for alverine citrate (an *antispasmodic* for irritable bowel syndrome 110)

spectinomycin an aminoglycoside antibiotic 128

Spectraban a brand name for aminobenzoic acid with padimate-O (both sunscreens 181)

Spiro-Co a brand name for spironolactone and hydroflumethiazide (both diuretics 99)

Spirolone a brand name for spironolactone (a potassium-sparing diuretic 99)

spironolactone a potassium-sparing diuretic 99

Spirospare a brand name for spironolactone (a potassium-sparing diuretic 99)

Sporanox a brand name for itraconazole (an antifungal 138); *illus. 41K*

Sprilon a brand-name skin preparation containing dimeticone and zinc oxide 175, 449

Stabillin-VK a brand name for phenoxymethylpenicillin 372 (a penicillin antibiotic 128); *illus. 43E*

stanozolol an anabolic steroid 146

Staril a brand name for fosinopril 290 (an ACE inhibitor 98)

stavudine an antiviral used to treat HIV infection and AIDS 157

Stelazine a brand name for trifluoperazine (a phenothiazine antipsychotic 85 and anti-emetic 90)

Stemetil a brand name for prochlorperazine 381 (a phenothiazine anti-emetic 90 and antipsychotic 85); *illus. 43S*

sterculia a bulk-forming agent used as an antidiarrhoeal 110 and laxative 111

Ster-Zac a brand name for triclosan (an antimicrobial 175)

Stesolid a brand name for diazepam 253 (a benzodiazepine anti-anxiety drug 83, muscle relaxant 120, and anticonvulsant 86)

Stiedex a brand name for desoxymetasone (a topical corticosteroid 174)

Stiemycin a brand name for erythromycin 276 (an antibiotic 128)

stilboestrol see diethylstilbestrol 257 (a female sex hormone 147)

Stilnoct a brand name for zolpidem (a sleeping drug 82)

Stimlor a brand name for naftidrofuryl 355 (a vasodilator 98)

Strefen a brand name for flurbiprofen (a non steroidal antinflammatory drug 116)

Strepsils a brand-name preparation for mouth and throat infections containing amylmetacresol and dichlorobenzyl alcohol (both *antiseptics* 175)

Streptase a brand name for streptokinase 407 (a thrombolytic 105)

streptokinase 407 (a thrombolytic 105)

streptomycin an antituberculous drug 132 and aminoglycoside antibiotic 128

Stromba a brand name for stanozolol (an anabolic steroid 146)

Stugeron a brand name for cinnarizine 236 (an antihistamine anti-emetic 90); *illus. 43Q*

Stugeron Forte a brand name for cinnarizine 236 (an antihistamine anti-emetic 90); *illus. 40M*

sucralfate 408 (an ulcer-healing drug 109)

Sudafed a brand name for pseudoephedrine (a decongestant 93)

Sudafed-Co a brand name for paracetamol 368 (a non-*opioid* analgesic 80) and pseudoephedrine (a decongestant 93)

Sudafed Expectorant a brand name for guaifenesin (an *expectorant* 94) with pseudoephedrine (a decongestant 93)

Sudafed SA a brand name for pseudoephedrine (a decongestant 93)

Sudocrem a brand-name skin preparation containing benzyl benzoate and zinc oxide 449

sulconazole an antifungal 138

Suleo-M a brand name for malathion 330 (a *topical* antiparasitic 176)

sulfacetamide a sulphonamide antibacterial 131

sulfadiazine a sulphonamide antibacterial 131

sulfadimidine a sulphonamide antibacterial 131

sulfadoxine a drug used with pyrimethamine 389 for malaria 137

sulfamethoxazole a sulphonamide antibacterial 131 combined with trimethoprim in co-trimoxazole 246

sulfametopyrazine a sulphonamide antibacterial 131

sulfasalazine 409 (a drug for inflammatory bowel disease 112 and an antirheumatic 117)

sulfathiazole a sulphonamide antibacterial 131

sulfinpyrazone a drug for gout 119

sulindac a non-steroidal anti-inflammatory 116

Sulparex a brand name for sulpiride 195 (an antipsychotic 85)

sulphur a *topical* antibacterial 131 and anti-fungal 138 for acne 177 and dandruff 180

sulpiride 195 (an antipsychotic 85)

Sulpitil a brand name for sulpiride 195 (an antipsychotic 85)

sumatriptan 410 (a drug for migraine 89)

Suprane a brand name for desflurane (a general *anaesthetic*)

Suprax a brand name for cefixime (a cephalosporin antibiotic 128)

SUPRECUR–TULOBUTEROL

Suprecur a brand name for buserelin (a drug for menstrual disorders 160)

Suprefact a brand name for buserelin (a drug for menstrual disorders 160)

Surgam a brand name for tiaprofenic acid (a non-steroidal anti-inflammatory 116)

Surmontil a brand name for trimipramine (a tricyclic antidepressant 84)

Suscard a brand name for glyceryl trinitrate 296 (an anti-angina drug 101)

Sustac a brand name for glyceryl trinitrate 296 (an anti-angina drug 101)

Sustanon a brand name for testosterone 417 (a male sex hormone 146)

Sustiva a brand name for efavirenz (an antiviral for HIV/AIDS 157)

suxamethonium a muscle relaxant used during general *anaesthesia*

Symmetrel a brand name for amantadine 192 (an antiviral 133 and drug for parkinsonism 87); *illus. 39B*

Synacthen a brand name for tetracosactide (a drug to assess adrenal gland function 145)

Synagis a brand name for palvizumab, an antiviral drug 133

Synalar a brand name for fluocinolone (a topical corticosteroid 174)

Synalar C a brand name for fluocinolone (a topical corticosteroid 174) with clioquinol (an *antiseptic* 175)

Synalar N a brand name for fluocinolone (a topical corticosteroid 174) with neomycin (an aminoglycoside antibiotic 128)

Synarel a brand name for nafarelin (a drug for menstrual disorders 160)

Syndol a brand name for codeine 241 and paracetamol 368 (both analgesics 80), with caffeine (a stimulant 88) and doxylamine (an antihistamine 124)

Synflex a brand name for naproxen 356 (a non-steroidal anti-inflammatory 116 and drug for gout 119)

Synphase a brand-name oral contraceptive 161 containing ethinylestradiol 279 and norethisterone 360

Syntaris a brand name for flunisolide (a corticosteroid 141)

Syntocinon a brand name for oxytocin (a uterine stimulant 165)

Syntometrine a brand name for ergometrine with oxytocin (both uterine stimulants 165)

Syscor MR a brand name for nisoldipine (a calcium channel blocker 101)

Sytron a brand name for sodium feredetate (iron 441, a mineral 150)

T

tacalcitol a drug for psoriasis 178

tacrolimus an immunosuppressant 156

Tagamet a brand name for cimetidine 228 (an anti-ulcer drug 109); *illus. 37R*

Tambocor a brand name for flecainide (an anti-arrhythmic 100)

Tamofen a brand name for tamoxifen 411 (an anticancer drug 154)

tamoxifen 411 (an anticancer drug 154)

Tampovagan a brand name for diethylstilbestrol 257 (a female sex hormone 147) and lactic acid

tamsulosin 412 (an alpha-blocking drug for prostate disorders 166)

Tanatril a brand name for imidapril (an ACE inhibitor 98)

Targocid a brand name for teicoplanin (an antibiotic 128)

Tarivid a brand name for ofloxacin (an antibiotic 128)

Tavanic a brand name for levofloxacin 321 (an antibacterial 131)

Tavegil a brand name for clemastine (an antihistamine 124)

tazarotene a retinoid 446 for psoriasis 178

tazobactam an antibiotic 128

Tazocin a brand name for piperacillin (an antibiotic 128) with tazobactam (a substance that increases the effectiveness of piperacillin)

TCP Liquid a brand-name *antiseptic* 175 containing phenol, chlorophenol, and 2-iodophenol

Tears Naturale a brand-name artificial tear preparation 170 containing hypromellose

Tegretol a brand name for carbamazepine 217 (an anticonvulsant 86); *illus. 43R*

teicoplanin an antibiotic 128

Telfast a brand name for fexofenadine (an antihistamine 124)

temazepam 413 (a benzodiazepine sleeping drug 82)

Temgesic a brand name for buprenorphine (an *opioid* analgesic 80)

Temodal a brand name for temozolomide (an anticancer drug 154)

temozolomide an anticancer drug 154

Tenchlor a brand name for atenolol 201 (a beta blocker 97) with chlortalidone (a thiazide diuretic 99)

Tenif a brand name for atenolol 201 (a beta blocker 97) with nifedipine 359 (an anti-angina drug 101 and antihypertensive 102)

Tenkicin a brand name for phenoxymethylpenicillin 372 (a penicillin antibiotic 128)

Tenoret-50 a brand name for atenolol 201 (a beta blocker 97) with chlortalidone (a thiazide diuretic 99)

Tenoretic a brand name for atenolol 201 (a beta blocker 97) with chlortalidone (a thiazide diuretic 99); *illus. 35N*

Tenormin a brand name for atenolol 201 (a beta blocker 97); *illus. 36 I, 36K, 45 I*

tenoxicam a non-steroidal anti-inflammatory 116

Tensipine MR a brand name for nifedipine 359 (a calcium channel blocker 101)

Tensium a brand name for diazepam 253 (a benzodiazepine anti-anxiety drug 83 and muscle relaxant 120)

Teoptic a brand name for carteolol (a beta blocker 97 used for glaucoma 168)

terazosin a *sympatholytic* antihypertensive 102

terbinafine 414 (an antifungal 138)

terbutaline 415 (a *sympathomimetic* bronchodilator 92 and uterine muscle relaxant 165)

terfenadine 416 (an antihistamine 124)

Terfinax a brand name for terfenadine 416 (an antihistamine 124)

terlipressin a drug similar to vasopressin (a pituitary *hormone* 145) used to stop bleeding

Terra-Cortril a brand name for hydrocortisone 301 (a corticosteroid 141) with oxytetracycline (a tetracycline antibiotic 128)

Terra-Cortril Nystatin a brand name for hydrocortisone 301 (a corticosteroid 141) with nystatin 361 (an antifungal 138) and oxytetracycline (a tetracycline antibiotic 128)

Terramycin a brand name for oxytetracycline (a tetracycline antibiotic 128)

Tertroxin a brand name for liothyronine (a thyroid *hormone* 144)

testosterone 417 (a male sex hormone 146)

tetrabenazine a drug for tremor

Tetrabid a brand name for tetracycline 410 (an antibiotic 128 and antimalarial 137); *illus 41N*

tetracaine previously known as amethocaine (a local anaesthetic 80)

tetracosactide a drug similar to corticotropin used to assess adrenal gland function 145

tetracycline 418 (an antibiotic 128 and antimalarial 137)

Tetralysal 300 a brand name for lymecycline (a tetracycline antibiotic 128)

T-Gel a brand name for coal tar (an agent for dandruff 180 and psoriasis 178)

thalidomide a drug used for Hansen's disease (leprosy) 131

Theo-Dur a brand name for theophylline 419 (a bronchodilator 92)

theophylline 419 (a bronchodilator 92)

Thephorin a brand name for phenindamine (an antihistamine 124)

thiamine 446 (a vitamin 149)

thiopental a fast-acting barbiturate used to induce general *anaesthesia*

thioridazine 420 (a phenothiazine antipsychotic 85)

thiotepa an anticancer drug 154

thymoxamine see moxisylyte (a drug used to reduce pupil size after examination 170 and as a vasodilator 98 to improve blood supply to the limbs)

thyroid hormones synthetic thyroid *hormones* used for hypothyroidism 144

thyroxine see levothyroxine 421 (a thyroid *hormone* 144)

tiabendazole an anthelmintic 139

tiagabine an anti-epileptic 86

tiaprofenic acid a non-steroidal anti-inflammatory 116

tibolone 422 (a female sex hormone 147)

ticarcillin a penicillin antibiotic 128

Ticlid a brand name for ticlopidine (an antiplatelet drug 104)

ticlopidine an antiplatelet drug 104

Tilade a brand name for nedocromil (a bronchodilator 92)

Tildiem a brand name for diltiazem 259 (an anti-angina drug 101); *illus. 44 I*

Tiloryth a brand name for erythromycin 276 (an antibiotic 128)

tiludronic acid a drug for bone disorders 122

Timecef a brand name for cefodizime (a cephalosporin antibiotic 128)

Timentin a brand name for ticarcillin (a penicillin antibiotic 128) with clavulanic acid (a substance that increases the effectiveness of ticarcillin)

Timodine a brand name for hydrocortisone 301 (a corticosteroid 141) with nystatin 361 (an antifungal 138), benzalkonium chloride (an *antiseptic* 175), and dimeticone (a base for skin preparations 175)

timolol 423 (a beta blocker 97 and drug for glaucoma 168)

Timoptol a brand name for timolol 423 (a beta blocker 97 and drug for glaucoma 168)

Timpron a brand name for naproxen 356 (a non-steroidal anti-inflammatory 116 and drug for gout 119)

Tinaderm-M a brand name for nystatin 361 with tolnaftate (both antifungals 138)

tinidazole an antibacterial 131 and antiprotozoal 136

tinzaparin a type of heparin 299 (an anticoagulant 104)

tioconazole an antifungal 138

tioguanine an anticancer drug for acute leukaemia 154

tirofiban a drug for prevention of heart attacks 95

tissue plasminogen activator see alteplase (a thrombolytic 105)

Titralac a brand name for calcium carbonate 438 (a substance used to reduce blood phosphate levels) and glycine

Tixylix a brand name for promethazine 385 (an antihistamine 124) with pholcodine (a cough suppressant 94)

Tixylix Cough and Cold a brand-name cough suppressant 94 and decongestant 93 containing chlorphenamine 225, pseudoephedrine, and pholcodine

tobramycin an aminoglycoside antibiotic 128

tocainide an anti-arrhythmic 100

tocopherol vitamin E 448 (a vitamin 149)

tocopheryl vitamin E 448 (a vitamin 149)

Tofranil a brand name for imipramine 304 (a tricyclic antidepressant 84); *illus. 35Q*

Tolanase a brand name for tolazamide (an oral antidiabetic 142)

tolazamide an oral antidiabetic 142

tolbutamide 424 (a drug for diabetes 142)

tolfenamic acid a drug for migraine 89

tolnaftate an antifungal 138

tolterodine 425 (an *anticholinergic* and *antispasmodic* for urinary disorders 166)

Tonocard a brand name for tocainide (an anti-arrhythmic 100)

Topal a brand-name antacid 108 containing aluminium hydroxide 191, magnesium carbonate, and alginic acid

Topamax a brand name for topiramate (an anticonvulsant 86)

Topicycline a brand name for tetracycline 418 (an antibiotic 128)

topiramate an anticonvulsant 86

topotecan an anticancer drug 154

Toradol a brand name for ketorolac (a non-steroidal anti-inflammatory 116 used as an analgesic 80)

torasemide a loop diuretic 99

Torem a brand name for torasemide (a loop diuretic 99)

toremifene an anticancer drug 154

Totamol a brand name for atenolol 201 (a beta blocker 97)

Totaretic a brand name for atenolol 201 (a beta blocker 97) with chlortalidone (a thiazide diuretic 99)

tramadol 426 (an analgesic related to codeine 241, an *opioid* analgesic 80)

Tramake a brand name for tramadol 426 (an *opioid* analgesic 80)

tramazoline a nasal decongestant 93

Tramil a brand name for paracetamol 368 and caffeine (a stimulant 88)

Tramil 500 a brand name for paracetamol 368 (a non-*opioid* analgesic 80)

Trandate a brand name for labetalol (a beta blocker 97)

trandolapril an ACE inhibitor 98

tranexamic acid an antifibrinolytic used to promote blood clotting 104

Transiderm-Nitro a brand name for glyceryl trinitrate 296 (an anti-angina drug 101)

Transvasin a *topical* treatment for muscle aches and sprains 120

Tranxene a brand name for clorazepate (a benzodiazepine anti-anxiety drug 83)

tranylcypromine an MAOI antidepressant 84

Trasicor a brand name for oxprenolol (a beta blocker 97); *illus. 44D*

Trasidrex a brand name for cyclopenthiazide 247 (a thiazide diuretic 99) with oxprenolol (a beta blocker 97)

Travogyn a brand name for isoconazole (an antifungal 138)

Traxam a brand name for felbinac 282 (a non-steroidal anti-inflammatory 116)

trazodone 427 (an antidepressant 84)

Trental a brand name for pentoxifylline (a vasodilator 98)

treosulfan a drug for ovarian cancer 154

tretinoin a drug for acne 177

Tri-Adcortyl a brand name for nystatin 361 (an antifungal 138) with gramicidin and neomycin (both aminoglycoside antibiotics 128) and triamcinolone (a corticosteroid 141)

Triadene a brand-name oral contraceptive 161 containing ethinylestradiol 279 and gestodene

TriamaxCo a brand-name diuretic 99 containing triamterene 428 and hydrochlorothiazide 300

triamcinolone a corticosteroid 141 also used for ear disorders 171

Triam-Co a brand name for hydrochlorothiazide 300 with triamterene 428 (both diuretics 99)

triamterene 428 (a potassium-sparing diuretic 99)

Triapin a brand-name preparation containing felodipine (a calcium channel blocker 101) and ramipril (an ACE inhibitor 98)

tribavirin previously known as ribavirin (an antiviral 133 used for some lung infections in infants and children)

triclofos a non-benzodiazepine, non-barbiturate sleeping drug 82

triclosan a *topical* antimicrobial 175

Tridestra a brand-name preparation for menopausal symptoms 147 containing estradiol 277 and medroxyprogesterone acetate 332

trientine a drug to eliminate copper 439 from the liver in Wilson's disease

trifluoperazine a phenothiazine antipsychotic 85 and an anti-emetic 90

Trifyba a brand name for a bulk-forming laxative 111 containing bran

trihexyphenidyl previously known as benzhexol (a drug for parkinsonism 87)

tri-iodothyronine see liothyronine (a thyroid *hormone* 144)

trilostane an adrenal *antagonist* used for Cushing's syndrome (an adrenal disorder 141) and breast cancer 154

Triludan a brand name for terfenadine 416 (an antihistamine 124); *illus. 42 I*

trimeprazine see alimemazine (an antihistamine 124)

tremetaphan a camsylate drug used to lower blood pressure below normal in surgery

trimethoprim 429 (an antibacterial 131)

trimetrexate an antimicrobial for pneumocystis pneumonia in AIDS 136

Tri-Minulet a brand-name oral contraceptive 161 containing ethinylestradiol 279 and gestodene

trimipramine a tricyclic antidepressant 84

Trimogal a brand name for trimethoprim 429 (an antibacterial 131)

Trimopan a brand name for trimethoprim 429 (an antibacterial 131)

Trimovate a brand name for clobetasone (a topical corticosteroid 174) with nystatin 361 (an antifungal 138) and oxytetracycline (a tetracycline antibiotic 128)

Trinordiol a brand-name oral contraceptive 161 containing ethinylestradiol 279 and levonorgestrel 322

TriNovum a brand-name oral contraceptive 161 containing ethinylestradiol 279 with norethisterone 360

Triogesic a brand name for paracetamol 368 (a non-*opioid* analgesic 80) with phenyl-propanolamine 373 (a decongestant 93)

Triominic a brand name for phenylpropanolamine 373 (a decongestant 93) with pheniramine (an antihistamine 124)

tripotassium dicitratobismuthate a bismuth compound used to treat peptic ulcer 109

Triprimix a brand name for trimethoprim 429 (an antibacterial 131)

triprolidine an antihistamine 124

Triptafen a brand name for amitriptyline 196 (a tricyclic antidepressant 84) with perphenazine (an antipsychotic 85)

triptorelin an anticancer drug 154

Trisequens a brand name for estradiol 277 and estriol (both female sex hormones 147)

trisodium edetate a drug to remove excess calcium 438 from the blood

Tritace a brand name for ramipril 393 (an ACE inhibitor 98); *illus. 40J, 41 I*

Trobicin a brand name for spectinomycin (an aminoglycoside antibiotic 128)

Tropergen a brand name for diphenoxylate 260 (an antidiarrhoeal 110) and atropine 203

tropicamide a *mydriatic* 170

tropisetron an anti-emetic 90

Tropium a brand name for chlordiazepoxide 223 (a benzodiazepine anti-anxiety drug 83)

Trosyl a brand name for tioconazole (an antifungal 138)

Trusopt a brand name for dorzolamide 265 (a drug for glaucoma 168)

tryptophan an antidepressant 84

Tuinal a brand name for amobarbital with secobarbital (both barbiturate sleeping drugs 82)

tulobuterol a bronchodilator 92

TYLEX–ZYOMET

Tylex a brand-name analgesic 80 containing codeine 241 and paracetamol 368

Tyrozets a brand name for benzocaine (a local anaesthetic 80) with tyrothricin (an antibiotic 128)

U

Ubretid a brand name for distigmine (a *parasympathomimetic* for urinary retention 166 and myasthenia gravis 121)

Ucerax a brand name for hydroxyzine (an anti-anxiety drug 83)

Ukidan a brand name for urokinase (a thrombolytic 105)

Ultec a brand name for cimetidine 228 (an anti-ulcer drug 109)

Ultiva a brand name for remifentanil (a drug used in *anaesthesia*)

Ultralanum Plain a brand name for fluocortolone (a topical corticosteroid 174)

Ultraproct a brand name for fluocortolone (a topical corticosteroid 174) with cinchocaine (a local anaesthetic 80)

undecenoic acid an antifungal 138 for athlete's foot

Uniflu a brand name for codeine 241 (an *opioid* analgesic 80 and cough suppressant 94) with diphenhydramine (an antihistamine 128), paracetamol 368 (a non-*opioid* analgesic 80), phenylephrine (a decongestant 93), and caffeine (a stimulant 88)

Unigest a brand name for aluminium hydrochloride (an antacid 108) with dimeticone (an antifoaming agent 108)

Unihep a brand name for heparin 299 (an anticoagulant 104)

Uniparin, Uniparin Calcium a brand name for heparin 299 (an anticoagulant 104)

Uniphyllin Continus a brand name for theophylline 419 (a bronchodilator 92)

Uniroid HC a brand name for hydrocortisone 301 (a corticosteroid 141) with cinchocaine (a local anaesthetic 80)

Univer a brand name for verapamil 431 (an anti-angina drug 101 and anti-arrhythmic 100)

urea a *topical* treatment to moisturize dry skin 173 and soften ear wax 171

Uriben a brand name for nalidixic acid (an antibacterial 131)

Urispas a brand name for flavoxate (a urinary *antispasmodic* 166); *illus. 42M*

urofollitropin a drug for pituitary disorders 145

urokinase a thrombolytic 105

ursodeoxycholic acid a drug for gallstones 114

Ursofalk a brand name for ursodeoxycholic acid (a drug for gallstones 114)

Utinor a brand name for norfloxacin (an antibiotic 128)

Utovlan a brand name for norethisterone 360 (a female sex hormone 147)

V

Vagifem a brand name for estradiol 277 (a female sex hormone 147)

Vaginyl a brand name for metronidazole 346 (an antibacterial 131 and antiprotozoal 136)

valaciclovir an antiviral 133

Valclair a brand name for diazepam 253 (a benzodiazepine anti-anxiety drug 83, muscle relaxant 120, and anticonvulsant 86)

Valderma Cream a brand-name preparation for minor skin problems, containing potassium hydroxyquinoline sulphate (an antibacterial 131 and antifungal 138), and chlorocresol (a *topical antiseptic* 175)

Valium a brand name for diazepam 253 (a benzodiazepine anti-anxiety drug 83, muscle relaxant 120, and anticonvulsant 86); *illus. 37N*

Vallergan a brand name for trimeprazine (an antihistamine 124)

Valoid a brand name for cyclizine (an antiemetic 117)

valproate an anticonvulsant 86

valproic acid an anticonvulsant 86

valsartan an antihypertensive 102

Valtrex a brand name for valaciclovir (an antiviral 133)

Vancocin a brand name for vancomycin (an antibiotic 128 for serious infections)

vancomycin an antibiotic 128 for serious infections

Vaqta a brand-name *vaccine* to protect against viral hepatitis

Varidase a brand-name preparation containing streptokinase 407 (a thrombolytic 105), and streptodornase (a fibrinolytic *enzyme*) used to treat leg ulcers

Vascace a brand name for cilazapril (an ACE inhibitor drug 98)

Vaseline Petroleum Jelly an ointment used to treat dry skin 172

Vasogen a brand name barrier cream 175 containing calamine, dimeticone, and zinc oxide 449

vasopressin a pituitary *hormone* 145 used to treat diabetes insipidus 142

Vasoxine a brand name for methoxamine (a *vasoconstrictor*)

Vectavir a brand name for penciclovir (an antiviral 133 used in the treatment of AIDS 157)

vecuronium a muscle-relaxant 120 used in general *anaesthesia*

Veganin a brand name analgesic containing aspirin 200, paracetamol 368, and codeine 241

Veil a brand name skin preparation 172 to hide scars

Velbe a brand name for vinblastine (an anticancer drug 154)

Velosef a brand name for cefradine (a cephalosporin antibiotic 128; *illus. 41T*)

Velosulin a brand name for insulin 307 (a drug for diabetes 142)

venlafaxine 430 (an antidepressant 84)

Venofer a brand-name iron supplement 441

Ventmax SR a brand name for salbutamol 399 (a bronchodilator 92 and drug used in labour 165)

Ventodisks a brand name for salbutamol 399 (a bronchodilator 92 and drug used in labour 165)

Ventolin a brand name for salbutamol 399 (a bronchodilator 92 and drug used in labour 165); *illus. 35C, 35D*

Vepesid a brand name for etoposide (an anticancer drug 154)

Veracur a brand name for formaldehyde (a substance for warts)

verapamil 431 (a calcium channel blocker for angina 101 and arrhythmias 100)

Vermox a brand name for mebendazole (an anthelmintic 139)

Verrugon a brand name for salicylic acid (a keratolytic for warts)

Vesagex a brand name *antiseptic* 175 containing cetrimide

Vesanoid a brand name for tretinoin (a drug for acne 177)

Vexol a brand name for rimexolone (a corticosteroid 141)

Viagra a brand name for sildenafil 401 (a drug for impotence 146, 164); *illus. 38E, 38F*

Viazem XL a brand name for diltiazem (a calcium channel blocker 101 and antihypertensive 102)

Vibramycin, Vibramycin-D brand names for doxycycline 269 (a tetracycline antibiotic 128)

Vicks Cold Care a brand name cold remedy containing paracetamol 368 (a non-*opioid* analgesic 80), dextromethorphan (a cough suppressant 94), and phenylpropanolamine 373 (a decongestant 93)

Vicks Medinite a brand name cold remedy containing paracetamol 368 (a non-*opioid* analgesic 80), dextromethorphan (a cough suppressant 94) and pseudoephedrine (a decongestant 93)

Videne a brand name for povidone-iodine (a skin *antiseptic* 175)

Videx a brand name for didanosine 256 (an antiviral 133 for HIV infection and AIDS 157); *illus. 42A*

vigabatrin an anticonvulsant 86

Vigam a brand name for human normal immune globulin injection 134

Vigranon B a brand name for vitamin B complex preparation (a vitamin 149)

viloxazine a tricyclic antidepressant 84

vinblastine an anticancer drug 154

vincristine an anticancer drug 154

vindesine an anticancer drug 154

vinorelbine an anticancer drug 154

Vioform-Hydrocortisone a brand name for hydrocortisone 301 (a corticosteroid 141) and clioquinol (an antimicrobial 175)

Vioxx a brand name for rofecoxib (a non-steroidal anti-inflammatory drug 116); *illus. 37P*

Viracept a brand name for nelfinavir (an antiviral 133 used to treat HIV and AIDS 157)

Viraferon a brand name for interferon alfa 308 (an antiviral 133 used to treat viral hepatitis)

Viramune a brand name for nevirapine (an antiviral 133 used to treat HIV and AIDS 157)

Virazid a brand name for tribavirin (an antiviral 133)

Viridal, Viridal Duo brand names for alprostadil 190 (a prostaglandin used for impotence 146, 164)

Virormone a brand name for testosterone 417 (a male sex hormone 146)

Visclair a brand name for mecysteine (a *mucolytic* for coughs 94)

Viscotears a brand-name artificial tears preparation

Viskaldix a brand name for pindolol (a beta blocker 97) and clopamide (a thiazide diuretic 99)

Visken a brand name for pindolol (a beta blocker 97)

Vista-Methasone a brand name for betamethasone 210 (a corticosteroid 141)

Vistide a brand name for cidofovir (an antiviral 133 used for Cytomegalovirus infections in AIDS 157)

vitamin A 446 (a vitamin 149)

vitamin B Complex (see vitamins 149)

vitamin B₁ another name for thiamine 446 (a vitamin 149)

vitamin B₂ another name for riboflavin 444 (a vitamin 149)

vitamin B₆ another name for pyridoxine 444 (a vitamin 149)

vitamin B₁₂ 447 (a vitamin 149)

vitamin C another name for ascorbic acid 447 (a vitamin 149)

vitamin D 448 (a vitamin 149)

vitamin E 448 (a vitamin 149)

vitamin K 449 (a vitamin 149)

Vivalan a brand name for viloxazine (a tricyclic antidepressant 84)

Vivapryl a brand name for selegiline (a drug for Parkinsonism 87)

Vivotif a brand name *vaccine* 134 to protect against typhoid fever

Volmax a brand name for salbutamol 399 (a bronchodilator 92); *illus. 46T*

Volraman a brand name for diclofenac 254 (a non-steroidal anti-inflammatory 116)

Volsaid Retard a brand name for diclofenac 254 (a non-steroidal anti-inflammatory 116)

Voltarol a brand name for diclofenac 254 (a non-steroidal anti-inflammatory 116); *illus. 36 O*

Voltarol Retard a brand name for diclofenac 254 (a non-steroidal anti-inflammatory 116)

W

warfarin 432 (an anticoagulant 104); *illus. 35E, 38L*

Warticon a brand name for podophyllotoxin (a drug for genital warts)

WaspEze a brand-name aerosol preparation for insect bites and stings containing benzocaine (a local anaesthetic 80) and mepyramine (an antihistamine 124)

Waxsol a brand name for docusate (an ear-wax softener 171)

Welldorm Elixir a brand name for chloral hydrate (non-benzodiazepine, non-barbiturate sleeping drug 82)

Welldorm Tablets a brand name for cloral betaine (a non-benzodiazepine, non-barbiturate sleeping drug 82); *illus. 35A*

Wellferon a brand name for interferon 308 (an anticancer drug 154)

Wellvone a brand name for atovaquone (an antiprotozoal 136 and antimalarial 137)

Windcheaters a brand-name preparation containing dimeticone (an antifoaming agent 108)

witch hazel an *astringent* used in *topical* 175 and rectal preparations 113

Woodward's Gripe Water a brand-name preparation for wind pain in infants containing sodium bicarbonate 403 and dill seed oil

X

Xalatan a brand name for latanoprost (a drug for glaucoma 168)

xamoterol a drug for mild heart failure

Xanax a brand name for alprazolam (a benzodiazepine anti-anxiety drug 83)

Xatral a brand name for alfuzosin (a drug for prostate disorders 166)

Xenical a brand name for orlistat 365 (an anti-obesity drug 148)

xipamide a thiazide-like diuretic 99

Xylocaine a brand name for lidocaine (a local anaesthetic 80)

xylometazoline a decongestant 93

Xyloproct a brand-name anal preparation 113 containing hydrocortisone 301, aluminium acetate, lidocaine, and zinc oxide 449

Y

Yomesan a brand name for niclosamide (an anthelmintic 139 for tapeworm infestation)

Yutopar a brand name for ritodrine (a uterine muscle relaxant 165)

Z

Zaditen a brand name for ketotifen (a drug used to prevent asthma 92)

zafirlukast a leukotriene *antagonist* for asthma 124 and bronchospasm 92

zalcitabine 433 (an antiviral for HIV infection and AIDS 157)

Zamadol a brand name for tramadol 426 (an *opioid* analgesic 80)

zanamivir 434 an antiviral drug 133

Zanidip a brand name for lercanidipine (a calcium channel blocker 101)

Zantac a brand name for ranitidine 394 (an anti-ulcer drug 109); *illus. 46J*

Zarontin a brand name for ethosuximide 280 (an anticonvulsant 86)

Zenapax a brand name for daclizumab (an immunosuppressant 156)

Zerit a brand name for stavudine (an antiviral for HIV infection and AIDS 157)

Zestoretic a brand name for lisinopril 323 (an ACE inhibitor 98) and hydrochlorothiazide 300 (a diuretic 99)

Zestril a brand name for lisinopril 323 (an ACE inhibitor 98)

Ziagen a brand name for abacavir (an antiviral for HIV/AIDS 157)

zidovudine (AZT) 435 (an antiviral for HIV infection and AIDS 157)

Zimovane LS a brand name for zopiclone 436 (a sleeping drug 82); *illus. 38G, 43 I*

Zinacef a brand name for cefuroxime (a cephalosporin antibiotic 128)

Zinamide a brand name for pyrazinamide (an antituberculous drug 132)

zinc 449 (a mineral 150)

Zincomed a brand name for zinc 449 (a mineral 150)

zinc oxide 449 (a soothing agent 175)

zinc pyrithione an antimicrobial with antibacterial 131 and antifungal 138 properties used for dandruff 180

zinc sulphate zinc 449 (a mineral 150)

Zineryt a brand-name acne preparation 177 containing erythromycin 276 (an antibiotic 128) and zinc 449 (a mineral 150)

Zinga a brand name for nizatidine (an anti-ulcer drug 109)

Zinnat a brand name for cefuroxime (a cephalosporin antibiotic 128)

Zirtek a brand name for cetirizine 221 (an antihistamine 124); *illus. 46P*

Zispin a brand name for mirtazapine (an antidepressant 84)

Zita a brand name for cimetidine 228 (an anti-ulcer drug 109)

Zithromax a brand name for azithromycin (an antibiotic 128)

Zocor a brand name for simvastatin 402 (a lipid-lowering drug 103); *illus. 35R*

Zofran a brand name for ondansetron 364 (an anti-emetic 90); *illus. 36R*

Zoladex a brand name for goserelin 297 (a female sex hormone 147 and anticancer drug 154)

Zoleptil a brand name for zotepine (an antipsychotic 85)

zolmitriptan a drug for migraine 89

zolpidem a sleeping drug 82

Zomacton a brand name for somatropin (a synthetic pituitary *hormone* 145)

Zomig a brand name for zolmitriptan (a drug for migraine 89)

zopiclone 436 a sleeping drug 82

zotepine antipsychotic 85

Zoton a brand name for lansoprazole 319 (an anti-ulcer drug 109); *illus. 39H, 41L*

Zovirax a brand name for aciclovir 188 (an antiviral 133; *illus. 38B*

Z Span a brand name for zinc 449 (a mineral 150)

zuclopenthixol an antipsychotic 85

Zumenon a brand name for estradiol 277 (a female sex hormone 147); *illus. 38 I*

Zydol a brand name for tramadol 426 (an *opioid* analgesic 80); *illus. 37E, 40P*

Zyloric a brand name for allopurinol 189 (a drug for gout 119); *illus. 42T*

Zyprexa a brand name for olanzapine 362 (an antipsychotic 85)

Zyomet a brand name for metronidazole 346

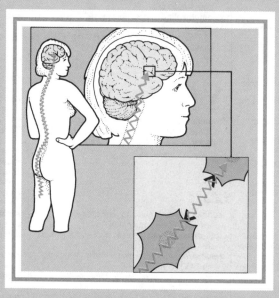

BRAIN AND NERVOUS SYSTEM

The human brain contains over 100 billion nerve cells (neurons). These nerve cells receive electro-chemical impulses from everywhere in the body. They interpret these impulses and send responsive signals back to various glands and muscles. The brain functions continuously as a switchboard for the human communications system. At the same time, it serves as the seat of emotions and mood, of memory, personality, and thought. Extending from the brain is an additional cluster of nerve cells that forms the spinal cord. Together, these two elements comprise the central nervous system.

Radiating from the central nervous system is the peripheral nervous system, which has three parts. One branches off the spinal cord and extends to skin and muscles throughout the body. Another, in the head, links the brain to the eyes, ears, nose, and taste buds. The third is a semi-independent network called the autonomic, or involuntary, nervous system. This is the part of the nervous system that controls unconscious body functions such as breathing, digestion, and glandular activity (see facing page).

Signals traverse the nervous system by electrical and chemical means. Electrical impulses carry signals from one end of a neuron to the other. To cross the gap between neurons, chemical *neurotransmitters* are released from one cell to bind on to the *receptor* sites of nearby cells. *Excitatory* transmitters stimulate action; *inhibitory* transmitters reduce it.

What can go wrong
Disorders of the brain and nervous system may manifest as illnesses that show themselves as physical impairments, such as epilepsy or strokes, or as mental and emotional impairments (for example, schizophrenia or depression).

Illnesses causing physical impairments can result from different types of disorder of the brain and nervous system. Death of nerve cells resulting from poor circulation can result in paralysis, while electrical disturbances of certain nerve cells cause the fits of epilepsy. Temporary changes in blood circulation within and around the brain are thought to cause migraine. Parkinson's disease is caused by a lack of dopamine, a neurotransmitter that is produced by specialized brain cells.

The causes of disorders that trigger mental and emotional impairment are not known, but these illnesses are thought to result from the defective functioning of nerve cells and neurotransmitters. The nerve cells may be underactive, overactive, or poorly coordinated. Alternatively, mental and

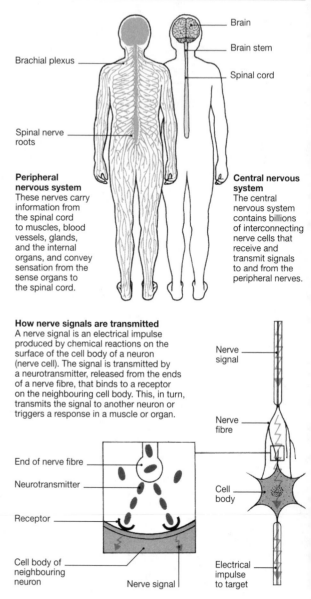

Brain
Brain stem
Brachial plexus
Spinal cord
Spinal nerve roots

Peripheral nervous system
These nerves carry information from the spinal cord to muscles, blood vessels, glands, and the internal organs, and convey sensation from the sense organs to the spinal cord.

Central nervous system
The central nervous system contains billions of interconnecting nerve cells that receive and transmit signals to and from the peripheral nerves.

How nerve signals are transmitted
A nerve signal is an electrical impulse produced by chemical reactions on the surface of the cell body of a neuron (nerve cell). The signal is transmitted by a neurotransmitter, released from the ends of a nerve fibre, that binds to a receptor on the neighbouring cell body. This, in turn, transmits the signal to another neuron or triggers a response in a muscle or organ.

Nerve signal
Nerve fibre
End of nerve fibre
Neurotransmitter
Cell body
Receptor
Cell body of neighbouring neuron
Nerve signal
Electrical impulse to target

emotional impairment may be due to too much or too little neurotransmitter in one area of the brain.

Why drugs are used
By and large, the drugs described in this section do not eliminate nervous system disorders. Their function is to correct or modify the communication of the signals that traverse the nervous system. By doing so they can relieve symptoms or restore normal functioning and behaviour. In some cases, such as anxiety and insomnia, drugs are used to

AUTONOMIC NERVOUS SYSTEM

The autonomic, or involuntary, nervous system governs the actions of the muscles of the organs and glands. Such vital functions as heart beat, salivation, and digestion continue without conscious direction, whether we are awake or asleep.

The autonomic system is divided into two parts, the effects of one generally balancing those of the other. The *sympathetic* nervous system has an *excitatory* effect. It widens the airways to the lungs, for example, and increases the flow of blood to the arms and legs. The *parasympathetic* system, by contrast, has an opposing effect. It slows the heart rate and redirects blood from the limbs to the gut.

Although the functional pace of most organs results from the interplay between the two systems, the muscles surrounding the blood vessels respond only to the signals of the sympathetic system. Whether a vessel is dilated or constricted is determined by the relative stimulation of two sets of receptor sites: alpha sites and beta sites.

Neurotransmitters

The parasympathetic nervous system depends on the neurotransmitter acetylcholine to transmit signals from one cell to another. The sympathetic nervous system relies on adrenaline and noradrenaline, products of the adrenal glands and neurons that act as both hormones and neurotransmitters.

Drugs that act on the sympathetic nervous system

The drugs that stimulate the sympathetic nervous system are called adrenergics (or sympathomimetics, see chart). They either promote the release of adrenaline and noradrenaline or mimic their effects. Drugs that interfere with the action of the sympathetic nervous system are called sympatholytics. Alpha blockers act on alpha receptors; beta blockers act on beta receptors (see also Beta blockers, p.97).

Drugs that act on the parasympathetic nervous system

Drugs that stimulate the parasympathetic nervous system are called cholinergics (or parasympathomimetics), and drugs that oppose its action are called anticholinergics. Many prescribed drugs have anticholinergic properties (see chart, right).

Effects of stimulation of the autonomic nervous system

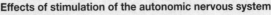

	Sympathetic	Parasympathetic
Heart	The rate and strength of the heart beat are increased.	The rate and strength of the heart beat are reduced.
Blood vessels in skin	These are constricted by stimulation of alpha receptors.	No effect.
Pupils	The pupils are dilated.	The pupils are constricted.
Airways	The bronchial muscles relax and widen the airways.	The bronchial muscles contract and narrow the airways.
Intestines	Activity of the muscles of the intestinal wall is reduced.	Activity of the muscles of the intestinal wall is increased.
Bladder	The bladder wall relaxes and the sphincter muscle contracts.	The bladder wall contracts and the sphincter muscle relaxes.
Salivary glands	Secretion of thick saliva increases.	Secretion of watery saliva increases.
Pancreas	Insulin secretion is increased (beta receptors) or reduced (alpha receptors).	Insulin secretion is increased.

Drugs that act on the autonomic nervous system

	Sympathetic	Parasympathetic
Stimulated by		
Natural neurotransmitters	Epinephrine (adrenaline) Norepinephrine (noradrenaline)	Acetylcholine
Drugs	Adrenergic drugs (including alpha agonists, beta agonists) Sympathomimetics	Cholinergic drugs Parasympathomimetics
Blocked by		
Drugs	Alpha blockers (antagonists) Beta blockers (antagonists)	Anticholinergic drugs

lower the level of activity in the brain. In other disorders – depression, for example – drugs are given to encourage the opposite effect, increasing the level of activity.

Drugs that act on the nervous system are also used for conditions that outwardly have nothing to do with nervous system disorders. Migraine headaches, for example, are often treated with drugs that cause the autonomic nervous system to send out signals constricting the dilated blood vessels that cause the migraine.

MAJOR DRUG GROUPS

Analgesics
Sleeping drugs
Anti-anxiety drugs
Antidepressant drugs
Antipsychotic drugs
Anticonvulsant drugs

Drugs for parkinsonism
Drugs for dementia
Nervous system stimulants
Drugs for migraine
Anti-emetics

ANALGESICS

Analgesics (painkillers) are drugs that relieve pain. Since pain is not a disease but a symptom, long-term relief depends on treatment of the underlying cause. For example, the pain of toothache can be relieved by drugs but can be cured only by appropriate dental treatment. If the underlying disorder is irreversible, such as some rheumatic conditions, long-term analgesic treatment may be necessary.

Damage to body tissues as a result of disease or injury is detected by nerve endings that transmit signals to the brain. The interpretation of these sensations can be affected by the psychological state of the individual, so that pain is worsened by anxiety and fear, for example. Often a reassuring explanation of the cause of discomfort can make pain easier to bear and may even relieve it altogether. Anti-anxiety drugs (see p.83) are helpful when pain is accompanied by anxiety, and some of these drugs are also used to reduce painful muscle spasms. Antidepressant drugs (see p.84) act to block the transmission of impulses signalling pain and are particularly useful for nerve pains (neuralgia), which do not always respond to analgesics.

Types of analgesics

Analgesics are divided into the opioids (with similar properties to drugs derived from opium, such as morphine) and non-opioids. Non-opioids include all the other analgesics, including paracetamol,

nefopam, and also the non-steroidal anti-inflammatory drugs (NSAIDs), the most well known of which is aspirin. The non-opioids are all less powerful as painkillers than the opioids. Local anaesthetics are also used to relieve pain (see below).

Opioid drugs and paracetamol act directly on the brain and spinal cord to alter the perception of pain. Opioids act like the endorphins, hormones naturally produced in the brain that stop the cell-to-cell transmission of pain sensation. NSAIDs prevent stimulation of the nerve endings at the site of the pain.

When pain is treated under medical supervision, it is common to start with paracetamol or an NSAID; if neither provides adequate pain relief, they may be combined. A mild opioid (for example, codeine) may also be used. If the less powerful drugs are ineffective, a strong opioid such as morphine may be given. As there is now a wide variety of oral analgesic formulations, injections are seldom necessary to control even the most severe pain.

When treating pain with an over-the-counter preparation, for example, taking aspirin for a headache, you should seek medical advice if pain persists for longer than 48 hours, recurs, or is worse or different from previous pain.

Non-opioid analgesics

Paracetamol

This analgesic is believed to act by reducing the production of chemicals called prostaglandins in the brain. However, paracetamol does not affect prostaglandin production in the rest of the body, so it does not reduce inflammation, although it can reduce fever. Paracetamol can be used for everyday aches and pains, such as headaches, toothache, and joint pains. It is given as a liquid to treat pain and reduce fever in children.

As well as being the most widely used analgesic, it is one of the safest when taken correctly. It does not usually irritate the stomach and allergic reactions are rare. However, an overdose can cause severe and possibly fatal liver or kidney

SITES OF ACTION

Paracetamol and the opioid drugs act on the brain and spinal cord to reduce pain perception. Non-steroidal anti-inflammatory drugs (NSAIDs) act at the site of pain to prevent the stimulation of nerve endings.

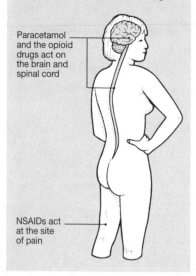

Paracetamol and the opioid drugs act on the brain and spinal cord

NSAIDs act at the site of pain

NSAIDs AND DIGESTIVE TRACT IRRITATION

NSAIDs can cause irritation, even ulceration and bleeding, of the stomach and duodenum, so they are best taken after a meal. NSAIDs are not usually given to people with stomach ulcers. An NSAID may be combined with an anti-ulcer drug (see p.109).

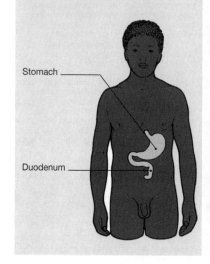

Stomach

Duodenum

damage. Its toxic potential may be increased in heavy drinkers.

Non-steroidal anti-inflammatory drugs (NSAIDs): aspirin

Used for many years to relieve pain and reduce fever, aspirin also acts to reduce inflammation by blocking the production of prostaglandins, which contribute to the swelling and pain in inflamed tissue (see Action of analgesics, facing page). Aspirin is useful for headaches, toothaches, mild rheumatic pain, sore throat, and discomfort caused by feverish illnesses. Given regularly, it can also relieve the pain and inflammation of chronic rheumatoid arthritis (see Antirheumatic drugs, p.117).

LOCAL ANAESTHETICS

These drugs are used to prevent pain, usually in minor surgical procedures, for example, dental treatment and stitching cuts. They can also be injected into the space around the spinal cord to numb the lower half of the body. This use is called spinal or epidural anaesthesia and can be used for some major operations in people who are not fit for a general anaesthetic. Local anaesthetics are also used for childbirth.

Local anaesthetics block the passage of nerve impulses at the site of administration, deadening all feeling conveyed by the nerves they come into contact with. They do not,

however, interfere with consciousness. Local anaesthetics are usually given by injection, but they can also be applied to the skin, the mouth and other areas lined with mucous membrane (such as the vagina), or the eye to relieve pain. Some local anaesthetics are formulated for injection together with epinephrine (adrenaline). Epinephrine constricts the blood vessels and prevents the local anaesthetic from being removed. This action prolongs the anaesthetic's effect.

Local anaesthetic creams are often used to numb the skin before injections in children and people with a fear of needles.

Aspirin is often found in combination with other substances in a variety of medicines (see Cold cures, p.94). It is also used in the treatment of some blood disorders, since aspirin helps to prevent abnormal clotting of blood (see Drugs that affect blood clotting, p.104). For this reason, it is not suitable for people whose blood does not clot normally.

Aspirin in the form of soluble tablets, dissolved in water before being taken, is absorbed into the bloodstream more quickly, thereby relieving pain faster than tablets. Soluble aspirin is not, however, less irritating to the stomach lining.

Aspirin is available in many forms, all of which have a similar effect, but because the amount of aspirin in a tablet of each type varies, it is important to read the packet for the correct dosage. It is not recommended for children aged under 12 years because its use has been linked to Reye's syndrome, a rare but potentially fatal liver and brain disorder.

Other non-steroidal anti-inflammatory drugs (NSAIDs)

These drugs can relieve both pain and inflammation. NSAIDs are related to aspirin and also work by blocking the production of *prostaglandins*. They are most commonly used to treat muscle and joint pain and may also be prescribed for menstrual period pain. For further information on these drugs, see p.116.

Combined analgesics

Mild opioids, such as codeine, are often found in combination preparations with non-opioids, such as paracetamol or NSAIDs. The prefix "co-" is used to denote a drug combination. These mixtures may add the advantages of analgesics that act on the brain to the benefits of those acting at the site of pain. Another advantage of combining analgesics is that the reductions in dose of the components may reduce the side effects of the preparation. Combinations can be helpful in reducing the number of tablets taken during long-term treatment.

Opioid analgesics

These drugs are related to opium, an extract of poppy seeds. They act directly on several sites in the central nervous system involved in pain perception, and block the transmission of pain signals (see Action of analgesics, above). Because they act directly on the parts of the brain where pain is perceived, opioids are the strongest analgesics and are therefore used to treat the pain arising from surgery, serious injury, and cancer. These drugs are particularly valuable for relieving severe pain during terminal illnesses. In addition, their ability to produce a state of relaxation and euphoria is often of help in relieving the stress that accompanies severe pain.

ACTION OF ANALGESICS

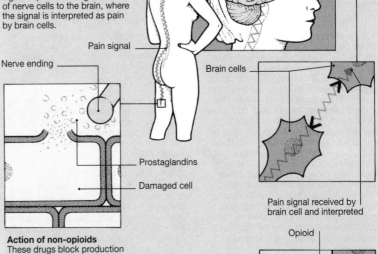

Cause of pain
Damage to tissue (due to injury or infection, for example) leads to the production of chemicals, called prostaglandins, which act on nerve endings so that a signal is passed along a series of nerve cells to the brain, where the signal is interpreted as pain by brain cells.

Brain

Pain signal

Nerve ending

Brain cells

Prostaglandins

Damaged cell

Pain signal received by brain cell and interpreted

Action of non-opioids
These drugs block production of prostaglandins. As a result, the nerve endings cannot be stimulated, so no pain signal passes to the brain.

Opioid

Opioid receptor

Pain signal blocked

Action of opioids
Normally the pain signal is transmitted between brain cells. Opioids combine with receptors on brain cells (opioid receptors), blocking transmission of pain signals within the brain and also in the spinal cord.

Brain cell

Morphine is the best known opioid analgesic. Others include diamorphine (heroin) and pethidine. The use of these powerful opioids is strictly controlled because the euphoria produced can lead to abuse and addiction. When these opioids are given under medical supervision to treat severe pain, the risk of addiction is negligible.

Opioid analgesics may prevent clear thought and cloud consciousness. Other possible adverse effects include nausea, vomiting, constipation, drowsiness, and depressed breathing. When they are taken in overdose, these drugs may induce a deep coma and lead to fatal breathing difficulties.

In addition to the powerful opioids, there are some less powerful drugs in this group that are used to relieve mild to moderate pain. They include dextropropoxyphene, dihydrocodeine, and codeine. Their normally unwanted side effects of depressing respiration and causing constipation make them useful as cough suppressants (p.94) and as anti-diarrhoeal drugs (p.110).

COMMON DRUGS

Opioids	NSAIDs (see p.116)
Co-codamol	Aspirin ✱
Co-codaprin	Diclofenac ✱
Codeine ✱	Etodolac
Co-dydramol	Fenbufen ✱
Co-proxamol ✱	Fenoprofen
Diamorphine (heroin) ✱	Ibuprofen ✱
Dipipanone	Indomethacin ✱
Fentanyl	Ketoprofen ✱
Meptazinol	Ketorolac
Methadone ✱	Mefenamic acid ✱
Morphine ✱	Naproxen ✱
Pentazocine	Piroxicam ✱
Pethidine	
Phenazocine	**Other non-opioids**
Tramadol ✱	Nefopam ✱
	Paracetamol ✱

✱ See Part 4

SLEEPING DRUGS

Difficulty in getting to sleep or staying asleep (insomnia) has many causes. Most people suffer from sleepless nights from time to time, usually as a result of a temporary worry or discomfort from a minor illness. Persistent sleeplessness can be caused by psychological problems including anxiety or depression, or by pain and discomfort arising from a physical disorder.

Why they are used

For occasional bouts of sleeplessness, simple, common remedies to promote relaxation – for example, taking a warm bath or a hot milk drink before bedtime – are usually the best form of treatment. Sleeping drugs (also known as hypnotics) are normally prescribed only when these self-help remedies have failed, and when lack of sleep is beginning to affect your general health. These drugs are used to re-establish the habit of sleeping. They should be used in the smallest dose and for the shortest possible time (not more than three weeks). It is best not to use sleeping tablets every night (see Risks and precautions). Do not use alcohol to get to sleep as it can cause disturbed sleep and insomnia. Long-term treatment of sleeplessness depends on resolving the underlying cause of the problem.

How they work

Most sleeping drugs promote sleep by depressing brain function. The drugs interfere with chemical activity in the brain and nervous system by reducing communication between nerve cells. This

TYPES OF SLEEPING DRUGS

Benzodiazepines These are the most commonly used class of sleeping drugs as they have comparatively few *adverse effects* and are relatively safe in overdose. They are also used to treat anxiety (see facing page).

Barbiturates These are now rarely used because of the risks of abuse, dependence, and *toxicity* in overdose. There is also a risk of prolonged sedation ("hangover").

Chloral derivatives These drugs are sometimes prescribed for the elderly. They may irritate the stomach, causing nausea and vomiting.

Other non-benzodiazepine sleeping drugs Zopiclone and zolpidem work in a similar way to benzodiazepines. They are not intended for long-term use and withdrawal symptoms have been reported.

Antihistamines Widely used to treat allergic symptoms (see p.124), antihistamines also cause drowsiness. They are sometimes used to promote sleep in children and the elderly.

Antidepressant drugs Some of these drugs may be used to promote sleep in depressed people (see p.84), as well as being effective in treating underlying depressive illness.

leads to reduced brain activity, allowing you to fall asleep more easily, but the nature of the sleep is affected by the drug. The main class of sleeping drugs, the benzodiazepines, is described on the facing page.

How they affect you

A sleeping drug rapidly produces drowsiness and slowed reactions. Some people find that the drug makes them appear to be drunk, their speech slurred, especially if they delay going to bed after taking their dose. Most people find they usually fall asleep within one hour of taking the drug.

Because the sleep induced by drugs is not the same as normal sleep, many people find they do not feel as well rested by it as by a night of natural sleep. This is the result of suppressed brain activity.

Sleeping drugs also suppress the sleep during which dreams occur, and both dream sleep and non-dream sleep are essential components of a good night's sleep (see The effects of drugs on sleep patterns, below).

Some people experience a variety of "hangover" effects the following day. Some benzodiazepines may produce minor side effects, such as daytime drowsiness, dizziness, and unsteadiness, that can impair the ability to drive or operate machinery. Elderly people are especially likely to become confused; for them, selection of an appropriate drug is particularly important.

Risks and special precautions

Sleeping drugs become less effective after the first few nights and there may be a temptation to increase the dose. Apart from the antihistamines, most sleeping drugs can produce psychological and physical dependence (see p.23) when taken regularly for more than a few weeks, especially if they are taken in larger-than-normal doses.

When sleeping drugs are suddenly withdrawn, anxiety, convulsions, and hallucinations sometimes occur. Nightmares and vivid dreams may be a problem because the time spent in dream sleep increases. Sleeplessness will recur and may lead to a temptation to use sleeping drugs again. Anyone who wishes to stop taking sleeping drugs, particularly after prolonged use, should seek his or her doctor's advice to prevent these withdrawal symptoms from occurring.

THE EFFECTS OF DRUGS ON SLEEP PATTERNS

Normal sleep can be divided into three types: light sleep, deep sleep, and dream sleep. The proportion of time spent in each type of sleep changes with age and is altered by sleeping drugs. Dramatic changes in sleep patterns also occur in the first few days following abrupt withdrawal of sleeping drugs after regular, prolonged use.

Normal sleep Young adults spend most sleep time in light sleep with roughly equal proportions of dream and deep sleep.

Drug-induced sleep has less dream sleep and less deep sleep with relatively more light sleep.

Sleep following drug withdrawal There is a marked increase in dream sleep, causing nightmares, following withdrawal of drugs used regularly for a long time.

○ Dream sleep

● Deep sleep

● Light sleep

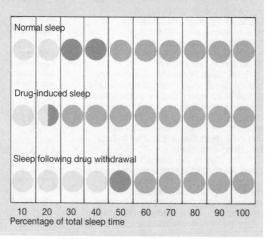

Normal sleep

Drug-induced sleep

Sleep following drug withdrawal

10　20　30　40　50　60　70　80　90　100
Percentage of total sleep time

COMMON DRUGS

Benzodiazepines	Chloral derivatives
Loprazolam	Chloral betaine
Lormetazepam	Chloral hydrate
Nitrazepam	
Temazepam *	**Other non-benzodiazepine sleeping drugs**
Barbiturate	Chlormethiazole
Amobarbital	Zolpidem
	Zopiclone *

* See Part 4

ANTI-ANXIETY DRUGS

A certain amount of stress can be beneficial, providing a stimulus to action. But too much will often result in anxiety, which might be described as fear or apprehension not caused by real danger.

Clinically, anxiety arises when the balance of certain chemicals in the brain is disturbed. The fearful feelings increase brain activity, stimulating the sympathetic nervous system (see p.79), and often triggers physical symptoms, for example, breathlessness, shaking, palpitations, digestive distress, and headaches.

Why they are used
Anti-anxiety drugs (also called anxiolytics or minor tranquillizers) are prescribed to alleviate persistent feelings of tension and nervousness caused by stress or other psychological problems. But these drugs cannot resolve the causes. Tackling the underlying problem through counselling and perhaps psychotherapy offer the best hope of a long-term solution. Anti-anxiety drugs are also used in hospitals to calm and relax people who are undergoing uncomfortable medical procedures.

There are two main classes of drugs for relieving anxiety: benzodiazepines and beta blockers. Benzodiazepines are the most widely used, given as a regular treatment for short periods to promote relaxation. Most benzodiazepines have a strong sedative effect, helping to relieve the insomnia that accompanies anxiety (see also Sleeping drugs, facing page).

Beta blockers are mainly used to reduce physical symptoms of anxiety, such as shaking and palpitations. These drugs are commonly prescribed for people who feel excessively anxious in certain situations, such as interviews or public appearances.

When anxiety occurs in a person with depression, the anxiety can be treated with an antidepressant drug (see p.84).

How they work
Benzodiazepines and related drugs
These drugs depress activity in the part of the brain that controls emotion by promoting the action of the *neurotransmitter* gamma-aminobutyric acid (GABA) which binds to neurons, blocking transmission of electrical impulses and thus reducing communication between brain cells. Benzodiazepines increase the inhibitory effect of GABA on brain cells (see Action of benzodiazepines and related drugs, above), preventing the excessive brain activity that causes anxiety.

Buspirone is different from other anti-anxiety drugs; it binds mainly to serotonin (another neurotransmitter) receptors and does not cause drowsiness. Its effect is not felt for at least two weeks after starting treatment.

Beta blockers
The physical symptoms of anxiety are produced by an increase in the activity

ACTION OF BENZODIAZEPINES AND RELATED DRUGS

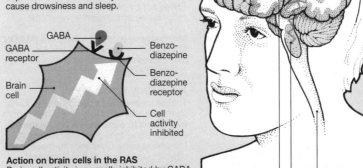

Action on the brain
The reticular activating system (RAS) in the brain stem controls the level of mental activity by stimulating higher centres of the brain controlling consciousness. Benzodiazepines and related drugs depress the RAS, relieving anxiety. In larger doses they depress the RAS sufficiently to cause drowsiness and sleep.

Higher centres of brain

GABA
GABA receptor
Brain cell
Benzodiazepine
Benzodiazepine receptor
Cell activity inhibited

Stimulation of brain — RAS — Brain stem

Action on brain cells in the RAS
Brain cell activity is normally inhibited by GABA, a chemical that binds to specialized cell *receptors*. Brain cells also have receptors for benzodiazepines. The drug binds to its receptor and promotes the inhibitory effect of GABA, thereby depressing brain cell activity in the RAS.

of the sympathetic nervous system. Sympathetic nerve endings release a chemical transmitter called norepinephrine (noradrenaline) that stimulates the heart, digestive system, and other organs. Beta blockers block the action of noradrenaline in the body, reducing the physical symptoms of anxiety. For more information on beta blockers, see p.97.

How they affect you
Benzodiazepines and related drugs reduce feelings of restlessness and agitation, slow mental activity, and often produce drowsiness. They are said to reduce motivation and, if they are taken in large doses, may lead to apathy. They also have a relaxing effect on the muscles, and some benzodiazepines are used specifically for that purpose (see Muscle relaxants, p.120).

Minor *adverse effects* of these drugs include dizziness and forgetfulness. People who need to drive or operate potentially dangerous machinery should be aware that their reactions may be slowed. Because the brain soon becomes tolerant to their effects, benzodiazepines are usually effective for only a few weeks at a time.

Beta blockers reduce the physical symptoms associated with anxiety. This in turn may promote greater mental calmness. Because they do not cause drowsiness they are safer for people who need to drive.

Risks and special precautions
The benzodiazepines are safe for most people and are not likely to be fatal in overdose. The main risk is psychological and physical dependence, especially for regular users or when larger-than-average doses have been used. For this reason, they are usually given for courses of two weeks or less. If they have been used for a longer period, they should be withdrawn gradually under medical supervision. If they are stopped suddenly, withdrawal symptoms, such as excessive anxiety, nightmares, and restlessness, may occur.

Benzodiazepines have been abused for their sedative effect, and are therefore prescribed with caution for people with a history of drug or alcohol abuse.

COMMON DRUGS

Benzodiazepines
Chlordiazepoxide ✳
Diazepam ✳
Lorazepam
Oxazepam

Beta blockers
Atenolol ✳
Oxprenolol
Propranolol ✳

Other non-benzodiazepines
Buspirone

✳ See Part 4

ANTIDEPRESSANT DRUGS

Occasional moods of discouragement or sadness are normal and usually pass quickly. But more severe depression, accompanied by despair, lethargy, loss of sex drive, and often poor appetite, may call for medical attention. Such depression can arise from life stresses such as the death of someone close, an illness, or sometimes from no apparent cause.

Three main types of drug are used to treat depression: tricyclic antidepressants (TCAs), selective serotonin re-uptake inhibitors (SSRIs), and monoamine oxidase inhibitors (MAOIs) (see Types of antidepressant, below). Lithium, a metallic element, is used to treat manic depression (see Antimanic drugs, facing page). In some cases, it is used with an anti-depressant drug for treating resistant depression. Several other antidepressants may be prescribed, including venlafaxine, nefazodone, maprotiline, mianserin, and trazodone.

Why they are used

Minor depression does not usually require drug treatment. Support and help in coming to terms with the cause of the depression is often all that is needed. Moderate or severe depression usually requires drug treatment, which is effective in most cases. Antidepressants may have to be taken for many months. Treatment should not be stopped too soon because symptoms are likely to reappear. When treatment is stopped, the dose should be gradually reduced over several weeks because withdrawal symptoms may occur if they are stopped suddenly.

How they work

Depression is thought to be caused by a reduction in the level of certain chemicals in the brain called *neurotransmitters*, which affect mood by stimulating brain cells. Antidepressants increase the level

of these *excitatory* neurotransmitters. See Action of antidepressants (right).

Tricyclics (TCAs)

TCAs and venlafaxine block the re-uptake of the neurotransmitters serotonin and norepinephrine (noradrenaline), thereby increasing the neurotransmitter levels at receptors.

Selective serotonin re-uptake inhibitors (SSRIs)

SSRIs act by blocking the re-uptake of only one neurotransmitter, serotonin.

Monoamine oxidase inhibitors (MAOIs)

MAOIs act by blocking the breakdown of neurotransmitters, mainly serotonin and norepinephrine (noradrenaline).

How they affect you

The antidepressant effect of these drugs starts after 10 to 14 days treatment and it may be six to eight weeks before the full effect is seen. However, side effects may happen at once. *Tolerance* to these side effects usually occurs and treatment should be continued.

Risks and special precautions

Overdose can be dangerous: tricyclics can produce coma, fits, and disturbed heart rhythm, which may be fatal; MAOIs can also cause muscle spasms and even death. Both are prescribed with caution for people with heart problems or epilepsy.

Monoamine oxidase inhibitors taken with certain drugs or foods rich in tyramine (for example, cheese, meat, yeast extracts, and red wine) can produce a dramatic rise in blood pressure, with headache or vomiting. People taking MAOIs are given a card that lists prohibited drugs and foods. Because of this adverse interaction, MAOIs are used much less frequently today and SSRIs or tricyclics are prescribed in preference to them.

ACTION OF ANTIDEPRESSANTS

Normally, the brain cells release sufficient quantities of excitatory chemicals (known as neurotransmitters) to stimulate neighbouring cells. The neurotransmitters are constantly reabsorbed into the brain cells where they are broken down by an enzyme called monoamine oxidase. In depression, fewer neurotransmitters are released. The levels of neurotransmitters in the brain are raised by antidepressant drugs.

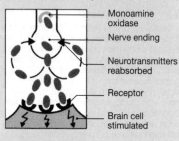

- Monoamine oxidase
- Nerve ending
- Neurotransmitters reabsorbed
- Receptor
- Brain cell stimulated

Normal brain activity
In a normal brain neurotransmitters are constantly being released, reabsorbed, and broken down.

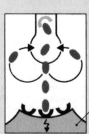

Brain activity in depression
The brain cells release fewer neurotransmitters than normal, leading to reduced stimulation.

- Brain cell poorly stimulated

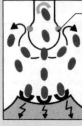

- Drug blocks reabsorption of neurotransmitter

Action of TCAs and SSRIs
TCA and SSRI drugs increase the levels of neurotransmitters by blocking their reabsorption.

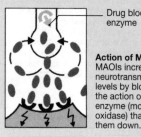

- Drug blocks enzyme

Action of MAOIs
MAOIs increase the neurotransmitter levels by blocking the action of the enzyme (monoamine oxidase) that breaks them down.

TYPES OF ANTIDEPRESSANT

Treatment usually begins with either a TCA or an SSRI. Both groups of drugs are equally effective.

Tricyclic antidepressants (TCAs)
Some TCAs, such as amitriptyline, cause drowsiness, which is useful for sleep problems in depression. TCAs also cause *anticholinergic* effects, including blurred vision, a dry mouth, and difficulty urinating.

Selective serotonin re-uptake inhibitors (SSRIs)
The SSRIs generally have fewer *side effects* than TCAs. The main unwanted effects of the SSRIs are nausea and vomiting. Anxiety, headache, and restlessness may also occur.

Monoamine oxidase inhibitors (MAOIs)
These are especially effective in people who are anxious as well as depressed, or who suffer from phobias.

COMMON DRUGS

Tricyclics
Amitriptyline ✱
Amoxapine
Clomipramine ✱
Dosulepin ✱
Doxepin
Imipramine ✱
Lofepramine ✱
Nortriptyline
Protriptyline
Trimipramine

SSRIs
Citalopram ✱
Fluoxetine ✱
Fluvoxamine
Paroxetine ✱
Sertraline

MAOIs
Moclobemide
Phenelzine
Isocarboxazid

Other drugs
Flupentixol ✱
Maprotiline
Mianserin ✱
Mirtazepine
Nefazodone
Reboxetine
Trazodone ✱
Venlafaxine ✱
Viloxazine

✱ See Part 4

ANTIPSYCHOTIC DRUGS

Psychosis is a term used to describe mental disorders that prevent the sufferer from thinking clearly, recognizing reality, and acting rationally. These disorders include schizophrenia, manic depression, and paranoia. The precise causes of these disorders are unknown, although a number of factors, including stress, heredity, and brain injury, may be involved. Temporary psychosis can also arise as a result of alcohol withdrawal or the abuse of mind-altering drugs (see Drugs of abuse, p.450). A variety of drugs is used to treat psychotic disorders (see Common drugs, below), most of which have similar actions and effects. One exception is lithium, which is particularly useful for manic depression (see Antimanic drugs, right).

Why they are used

A person with a psychotic illness may recover spontaneously, and so a drug will not always be prescribed. Long-term treatment is started only when normal life is seriously disrupted. Antipsychotic drugs (also called major tranquillizers or neuroleptics) do not cure the disorder, but they do help to control symptoms.

By controlling the symptoms of psychosis, antipsychotic drugs make it possible for most sufferers to live in the community and only be admitted to hospital for acute episodes.

The drug given to a particular individual depends on the nature of his or her illness and the expected *adverse effects* of that drug. Drugs differ in the amount of sedation produced; the need for sedation also influences the choice of drug.

Antipsychotics may also be given to calm or sedate a highly agitated or aggressive person, whatever the cause. Some antipsychotic drugs also have a powerful action against nausea and vomiting (see p.90), and are therefore sometimes used as premedication before a person has surgery

How they work

It is thought that some forms of mental illness are caused by an increase in communication between brain cells due to overactivity of an *excitatory* chemical called dopamine. This may disturb normal thought processes and produce abnormal behaviour. Dopamine combines with *receptors* on the brain cells. Antipsychotic drugs reduce the transmission of nerve signals by binding to these receptors, thereby making the brain cells less sensitive to dopamine (see Action of antipsychotics, below). Some new antipsychotic drugs, such as clozapine, risperidone, and sertindole, also bind to receptors for the chemical serotonin.

How they affect you

Because antipsychotics depress the action of dopamine, they can disturb its balance with another chemical in the brain, acetylcholine. If an imbalance occurs, extrapyramidal side effects (EPSE) may appear. These include restlessness, disorders of movement, and parkinsonism (see Drugs for parkinsonism, p.87).

In these circumstances, a change in medication to a different type of antipsychotic may be necessary. If this is not possible, an anticholinergic drug (see p.87) may be prescribed.

Antipsychotics may also block the action of noradrenaline, another neurotransmitter in the brain. This lowers the blood pressure, especially when you stand up, causing dizziness. It may also prevent ejaculation.

Risks and special precautions

It is important to continue taking these drugs even if all symptoms have gone, because the symptoms are controlled only by taking the prescribed dose.

Because antipsychotic drugs can have permanent as well as temporary side effects, the minimum necessary dosage is used. This minimum dose is found by

ANTIMANIC DRUGS

Changes in mood are normal, but when a person's mood swings become grossly exaggerated, with peaks of elation or mania alternating with troughs of depression, it becomes an illness known as manic depression. It is usually treated with lithium, a drug that reduces the intensity of the mania, lifts the depression, and lessens the frequency of mood swings. Because it may take three weeks before the lithium starts to work, an antipsychotic may be prescribed with lithium at first to give immediate relief of symptoms.

Lithium can be toxic if levels of the drug in the blood rise too high. Regular checks on the blood concentration of lithium should therefore be carried out during treatment. Symptoms of lithium poisoning include blurred vision, twitching, vomiting, and diarrhoea (see p.324).

starting with a low dose and increasing it until the symptoms are controlled. Sudden withdrawal after more than a few weeks can cause nausea, sweating, headache, and restlessness. Therefore, the dose is reduced gradually when treatment needs to be stopped.

The most serious long-term risk of antipsychotic treatment is a disorder known as *tardive dyskinesia*, which may develop after one to five years. This consists of repeated jerking movements of the mouth, tongue, and face, and sometimes of the hands and feet.

The condition is less common during treatment with the new antipsychotic drugs than with phenothiazine and butyrophenone drugs.

How they are administered

Antipsychotics may be given by mouth as tablets, capsules, or syrup, or by injection. They can also be given in the form of a *depot injection* which releases the drug slowly over several weeks. This is helpful for people who might forget to take their drugs or who might take an overdose.

ACTION OF ANTIPSYCHOTICS

Brain activity is partly governed by the action of a chemical called dopamine, which transmits signals between brain cells. In psychotic illness the brain cells release too much dopamine, resulting in excessive stimulation. The antipsychotic drugs help to reduce the adverse effects of excess dopamine.

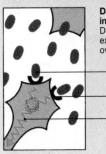

Dopamine activity in psychosis
Dopamine activity is excessive, causing overstimulation.

- Dopamine
- Dopamine receptor
- Stimulation

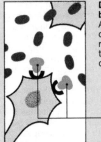

Dopamine activity blocked by drugs
Antipsychotic drugs occupy dopamine receptors and prevent the effects of excess dopamine being felt.

- Drugs

COMMON DRUGS

Phenothiazine antipsychotics	Other antipsychotics
Chlorpromazine ✻	Amisulpride/
Fluphenazine	sulpiride ✻
Methotrimeprazine	Clozapine ✻
Perphenazine	Flupentixol ✻
Pipotiazine	Olanzapine ✻
Thioridazine ✻	Oxypertine
Trifluoperazine	Pericyazine
	Pimozide
Butyrophenone antipsychotics	Quetiapine ✻
Benperidol	Risperidone ✻
Droperidol	Zotepine
Haloperidol ✻	Zuclopenthixol

	Antimanic drug
✻ See Part 4	Carbamazepine ✻
	Lithium ✻

ANTICONVULSANT DRUGS

Electrical signals from nerve cells in the brain are normally finely coordinated to produce smooth movements of arms and legs, but these signals can become irregular and chaotic, and trigger the disorderly muscular activity and mental changes that are characteristic of a fit (also called a seizure or convulsion). The most common cause of fits is the disorder known as epilepsy, as a result of brain disease or injury. In epileptics, a fit may be triggered by an outside stimulus such as a flashing light. Fits can also result from the *toxic* effects of certain drugs and, in young children, by a high temperature.

Anticonvulsant drugs are used both to reduce the risk of an epileptic fit and to stop one that is in progress.

Why they are used

Isolated convulsions seldom require drug treatment, but anticonvulsant drugs are the usual treatment for controlling epileptic fits. These drugs permit people with epilepsy to lead a normal life and reduce the possibility of brain damage, which can result from recurrent fits.

ACTION OF ANTICONVULSANTS

Normally, there is a relatively low level of electrical activity in the brain. In an epileptic fit, excessive electrical activity builds up, causing uncontrolled stimulation of the brain. Anticonvulsant drugs have an inhibitory effect, which neutralizes excessive electrical activity in the brain.

Normal brain activity

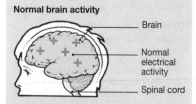

- Brain
- Normal electrical activity
- Spinal cord

Brain activity in a fit

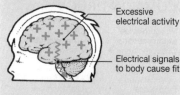

- Excessive electrical activity
- Electrical signals to body cause fit

Drug action on brain activity

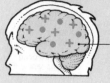

- Anticonvulsant neutralizes excess electrical activity

Most people with epilepsy need to take anticonvulsants on a regular basis to prevent fits. Usually a single drug is used, and treatment continues until there have been no attacks for at least two years. The particular drug that is prescribed depends on the kind of epilepsy (see Types of epilepsy, right).

If one drug is not effective, then a different anticonvulsant will be tried. Occasionally, it is necessary to take a combination of drugs. Even when receiving treatment, a person can suffer fits. A prolonged fit can be halted by injection of diazepam or a similar drug.

How they work

Brain cells bring about body movement by electrical activity that passes through the nerves to the muscles. In an epileptic fit, excessive electrical activity starts in one part of the brain and spreads to other parts, causing uncontrolled stimulation of brain cells. Most of the anticonvulsants have an *inhibitory* effect on brain cells and damp down electrical activity, preventing the excessive build-up that causes epileptic fits (see Action of anticonvulsants, left).

How they affect you

Ideally, the only effect an anticonvulsant should have is to reduce or prevent epileptic fits. Unfortunately, no drug prevents fits without potentially affecting normal brain function, leading to poor memory, inability to concentrate, lack of coordination, and lethargy. It is important, therefore, to find a dosage sufficient to prevent fits without causing unacceptable side effects. The dose has to be carefully tailored to the individual. It is usual to start with a low dose of a selected drug and to increase it gradually until a balance is achieved between the effective control of fits and the occurrence of side effects, many of which wear off after the first few weeks of treatment.

Blood tests are used to monitor levels of some anticonvulsants in the body as an aid to dose adjustment. Finding the correct dose may take several months.

Risks and special precautions

Each anticonvulsant drug has its own specific *adverse effects* and risks. In addition, most of them affect the liver's ability to break down other drugs (see Drug interactions, p.16) and so may influence the action of other drugs you are taking. Doctors try to prescribe no more than the minimum number of anticonvulsants needed to control the person's fits in order to reduce the risk of such interactions.

Most anticonvulsants have risks for a developing baby – if you are hoping to become pregnant, you should discuss the risks, and whether your medication should be changed, with your doctor. People taking anticonvulsants need to be careful

TYPES OF EPILEPSY

The selection of anticonvulsant drug depends on the type of epilepsy, although the age and particular response to drug treatment of the individual are also important.

Tonic/clonic (grand mal) seizures This type of fit is characterized by a warning sensation, such as flashing lights or a sound, which is followed by a sudden loss of consciousness during which convulsions occur, and the sufferer may lose bowel or bladder control, bite the tongue, or foam at the mouth. The fit usually lasts for a few minutes only but it can occasionally last longer. Prolonged attacks that last for over 50 minutes are called status epilepticus and can be fatal without emergency treatment.

The principal drugs used to prevent tonic/clonic seizures are phenytoin, sodium valproate, and carbamazepine. Doctors try to avoid prescribing phenytoin for young children because of its unpleasant side effects, which include overgrowth of the gums, acne, and increased body hair. These effects are less prominent in adults. If the patient is still having convulsions when medical help arrives, a benzodiazepine drug such as diazepam is given by injection or enema.

Absence (petit mal) seizures This form of epilepsy most commonly affects children. The fits consist of a momentary loss of consciousness, during which the child may stare off into space. Convulsions do not occur. Ethosuximide, sodium valproate, and, less commonly, clonazepam are used for the prevention of this type of fit.

Partial seizures There are a number of different variations of this form of epilepsy. Most partial seizures cause a sudden severe disturbance of the senses and/or muscle spasm without loss of consciousness. Phenytoin and carbamazepine are the medicines most commonly prescribed to prevent partial seizures.

to take their medicine regularly as prescribed. If the anticonvulsant levels in the body are allowed to fall suddenly, fits are very likely to occur. The dose should not be reduced or the treatment stopped, except on the advice of a doctor.

If, for any reason, anticonvulsant drug treatment needs to be stopped, the dose should be reduced gradually. People on anticonvulsant therapy are advised to carry an identification tag giving full details of their condition and treatment (see p.29).

COMMON DRUGS

Carbamazepine ✳	Lamotrigine ✳
Clobazam	Lorazepam
Clomethiazole	Phenobarbital ✳
Clonazepam ✳	Phenytoin ✳
Diazepam ✳	Piracetam
Ethosuximide ✳	Primidone ✳
Gabapentin	Sodium valproate ✳
	Tiagabine
	Topiramate
	Vigabatrin

✳ See Part 4

DRUGS FOR PARKINSONISM

Parkinsonism is a general term used to describe shaking of the head and limbs, muscular stiffness, an expressionless face, and inability to control or initiate movement. It is caused by an imbalance of chemicals in the brain; the effect of acetylcholine is increased by a reduction in the action of dopamine.

Parkinsonism has a variety of causes, but the most common is Parkinson's disease, degeneration of the dopamine-producing cells in the brain. Other causes include the *side effects* of certain drugs, notably antipsychotics (see p.85), and narrowing of the blood vessels in the brain.

Why they are used

Drugs can relieve the symptoms of parkinsonism but, unfortunately, the degeneration of brain cells in Parkinson's disease cannot be halted, although drugs can minimize symptoms for many years.

How they work

Drugs to treat parkinsonism restore the balance between the chemicals dopamine and acetylcholine. They fall into two main groups: those that reduce the effect of acetylcholine (*anticholinergic* drugs) and those that boost the effect of dopamine.

Anticholinergics combine with *receptors* on brain cells, preventing acetylcholine from binding to them. This action reduces acetylcholine's relative overactivity and restores the balance with dopamine.

Dopamine cannot pass from the blood to the brain, and therefore cannot be given to boost its levels in the brain. Levodopa (L-dopa), the chemical from which it is naturally produced in the brain, is combined with carbidopa or benserazide to prevent it from being converted to dopamine before it reaches the brain. Amantadine (also used as an antiviral, see p.133) boosts levels of dopamine in the brain by stimulating its release. The action

ACTION OF DRUGS FOR PARKINSONISM

Normal movement depends on a balance in the brain between dopamine and acetylcholine, which combine with receptors on brain cells. In parkinsonism, there is less dopamine present, with the result that acetylcholine is relatively overactive. The balance between acetylcholine and dopamine may be restored by anticholinergic drugs, which combine with the receptor for acetylcholine to block the action of acetylcholine on the brain cell, or by dopamine-boosting drugs, which increase the level of dopamine activity in the brain.

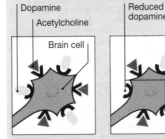

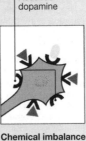

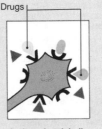

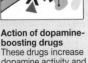

Normal chemical balance
Normally dopamine and acetylcholine are balanced.

Chemical imbalance in parkinsonism
If dopamine activity is low, acetylcholine is overactive.

Action of anticholinergic drugs
Anticholinergic drugs displace acetylcholine and restore balance.

Action of dopamine-boosting drugs
These drugs increase dopamine activity and restore balance.

of dopamine can also be boosted by other drugs, including bromocriptine, lisuride, pergolide, or apomorphine (injection only), which mimic the action of dopamine.

Choice of drug

Anticholinergics are often effective in the early stages of Parkinson's disease and are used to treat parkinsonism due to antipsychotic drugs, which have dopamine-blocking properties. L-dopa is usually given when the disease impairs walking. Its effectiveness usually wanes after two to five years, in which case other dopamine-boosting drugs may also be prescribed.

COMMON DRUGS

Anticholinergic drugs
Benzhexol
Benztropine
Biperiden
Orphenadrine *
Procyclidine *

Dopamine-boosting drugs
Amantadine *
Apomorphine
Bromocriptine *
Cabergoline
Levodopa *
Lisuride
Pergolide
Pramipexole
Ropinirole
Selegiline

* See Part 4

DRUGS FOR DEMENTIA

Dementia is a decline in mental function that is severe enough to affect normal social or occupational activities. It can be sudden and irreversible, for example due to a stroke or a head injury. It can also develop gradually and may be a feature of a number of disorders, including poor circulation in the brain, multiple sclerosis, and Alzheimer's disease. Much research is in progress on the cause of Alzheimer's disease, which is the single most common cause of dementia.

Why they are used

Drugs called acetylcholinesterase inhibitors have been found to improve the symptoms of dementia in Alzheimer's disease, although they do not prevent its long-term progression.

How they work

In healthy people, acetylcholinesterase (an enzyme in the brain) breaks down the *neurotransmitter* acetylcholine, balancing its levels and limiting its effects. In Alzheimer's disease, there is a deficiency of acetylcholine. Acetylcholinesterase inhibitors block the action of the enzyme acetylcholinesterase, raising brain levels of acetylcholine, thus increasing the patient's alertness and slowing the rate of deterioration.

How they affect you

Drug treatment is started at a low dose following an assessment of mental function by a specialist. The dosage is then increased gradually to minimize *side effects*. Any improvements should begin to appear in about 3 weeks. Assessment is repeated after 3 months to see if the treatment has been beneficial. About half of those people treated show some improvement.

Risks and special precautions

It is important to continue taking these drugs because there is a gradual loss of improvement after they are stopped. Side effects include urinary difficulties, nausea, vomiting, and diarrhoea.

COMMON DRUGS

Acetylcholinesterase inhibitors
Donepezil *
Rivastigmine *

NERVOUS SYSTEM STIMULANTS

A person's state of mental alertness varies throughout the day and is under the control of chemicals in the brain, some of which are depressant, causing drowsiness, and others that are stimulant, heightening awareness.

It is thought that an increase in the activity of the depressant chemicals may be responsible for a condition called narcolepsy, which is a tendency to fall asleep during the day for no obvious reason. In this case, the nervous system stimulants are administered to increase wakefulness. These drugs include the amphetamines (usually dexamfetamine), the related drug methylphenidate, and modafinil. Apart from their use in treating narcolepsy, amphetamines are no longer used because of the risk of dependence. The most common home remedy for increasing alertness is caffeine, a mild stimulant present in coffee, tea, and cola. Respiratory stimulants related to caffeine are used to improve breathing (see right).

Why they are used

In adults who suffer from narcolepsy, some of these drugs prevent excessive drowsiness during the day. Stimulants do not cure narcolepsy and, since the disorder usually lasts throughout the sufferer's lifetime, may have to be taken indefinitely. Methylphenidate is also occasionally given to children suffering from Attention Deficit Disorder. Stimulants have also been used as part of the treatment for obesity because reduced appetite is a *side effect* of amphetamines. Phentermine is a drug related to amfetamine but with a more modest stimulant action. It is used (for a maximum of 3 months) to promote weight loss in severe cases of obesity.

Caffeine is added to some analgesics to counteract the effects of caffeine withdrawal which can cause headaches, but no clear medical justification exists for this.

Apart from their use in narcolepsy, nervous system stimulants are not useful in the long term because the brain soon develops *tolerance* to them.

How they work

The level of wakefulness is controlled by a part of the brain stem called the reticular activating system (RAS). Activity in this area depends on the balance between chemicals, some of which are *excitatory* (including norepinephrine (noradrenaline)) and some *inhibitory,* such as gamma aminobutyric acid (GABA). Stimulants promote release of noradrenaline increasing activity in the RAS and other parts of the brain, so raising alertness.

How they affect you

In adults, the central nervous system stimulants taken in the prescribed dose for narcolepsy increase wakefulness, thereby allowing normal concentration and thought processes to occur. They may

RESPIRATORY STIMULANTS

Some stimulants (for example, aminophylline, theophylline, and doxapram) act on the part of the brain – the respiratory centre – that controls respiration. They are sometimes used in hospitals to help people who have difficulty breathing, mainly very young babies and adults with severe chest infections.

also reduce appetite and cause tremors. In hyperactive children, they reduce the general level of activity to a more normal level and increase the attention span.

Risks and special precautions

Some people, especially the elderly or those with previous psychiatric problems, are particularly sensitive to stimulants and may experience adverse effects, even when the drugs are given in comparatively low doses. They need to be used with caution in children because they can retard growth if taken for prolonged periods. An excess of these drugs given to a child may depress the nervous system, producing drowsiness or even loss of consciousness. Palpitations may also occur.

These drugs reduce the level of natural stimulants in the brain, so after regular use for a few weeks a person may become physically dependent on them for normal function. If they are abruptly withdrawn, the excess of natural inhibitory chemicals in the brain depresses central nervous system activity, producing withdrawal symptoms. These may include lethargy, depression, increased appetite, and difficulty staying awake.

Stimulants can produce overactivity in the brain if used inappropriately or in excess, resulting in extreme restlessness, sleeplessness, nervousness, or anxiety. They also stimulate the sympathetic branch of the autonomic nervous system (see p.79), causing shaking, sweating, and palpitations. More serious risks of exceeding the prescribed dose are fits and a major disturbance in mental functioning that may result in delusions and hallucinations. Because these drugs have been abused, amphetamines and methylphenidate are classified as controlled drugs (see pp.13 and 452).

ACTION OF NERVOUS SYSTEM STIMULANTS

Wakefulness is controlled by a part of the brain stem called the reticular activating system (RAS).

Normal brain activity
When the brain is functioning normally, signals from the RAS stimulate the upper parts of the brain, which control thought processes and alertness.

Brain activity in narcolepsy
In narcolepsy, the level of signals from the RAS is greatly reduced.

Normal brain activity restored
Central nervous system stimulants act on the RAS to increase the level of stimulatory signals to the brain.

COMMON DRUGS

Respiratory stimulants
Doxapram
Theophylline/ aminophylline ✳

Other drugs
Caffeine
Methylphenidate
Modafinil

✳ See Part 4

DRUGS USED FOR MIGRAINE

Migraine is a term applied to recurrent severe headaches affecting only one side of the head and caused by changes in the blood vessels around the brain and scalp. They may be accompanied by nausea and vomiting and preceded by warning signs, usually an impression of flashing lights or numbness and tingling in the arms. Occasionally, speech may be impaired, or the attack may be disabling. The cause of migraine is unknown, but an attack may be triggered by a blow to the head, physical exertion, certain foods and drugs, or emotional factors such as excitement, tension, or shock. A family history of migraine also increases the chance of an individual suffering from it.

Why they are used
Drugs are used either to relieve symptoms or to prevent attacks. Different drugs are used in each approach, but none cures the underlying disorder. However, a susceptibility to migraine headaches can clear up spontaneously, and if you are taking drugs regularly, your doctor may recommend that you stop them after a few months to see if this has happened.

In most people, migraine headaches can be relieved by a mild analgesic (painkiller), for example, paracetamol or aspirin, or a stronger one like codeine (see Analgesics, p.80). If nausea and vomiting accompany the migraine, tablets may not be absorbed sufficiently from the gut. Absorption can be increased if drugs are taken as soluble tablets in water or with an anti-emetic.

Some drugs used to relieve attacks can be given by injection, inhaler, nasal spray, or suppository. Preparations that contain caffeine should be avoided since headaches may be caused by excessive use or on stopping treatment. Ergotamine or 5HT$_1$ *agonist* drugs (such as sumatriptan) are used if analgesics are not effective.

The factors that trigger an individual's attacks should be identified, so that they can be avoided. Anti-anxiety drugs are not usually prescribed if stress is a precipitating factor because of the potential for dependence. If the attacks occur more often than once a month, drugs to prevent migraine may be taken every day. Drugs used to prevent migraine are propranolol (a beta blocker, see p.97) or pizotifen (an antihistamine and serotonin blocker). Other drugs that have been used include amitriptyline (an antidepressant, see p.84), clonidine, methysergide (which is given under hospital supervision), cyproheptadine, nifedipine, and verapamil.

How they work
A migraine attack begins when blood vessels surrounding the brain constrict (become narrower), producing the typical migraine warning signs. The constriction is thought to be caused by certain

ACTION OF DRUGS USED FOR MIGRAINE

Migraine is caused by the action of chemicals in the bloodstream on blood vessels surrounding the brain and in the scalp. In the first stage of a migraine attack, the blood vessels surrounding the brain constrict, causing warning signs (below left). In the second stage, the blood vessels in the scalp dilate, causing a severe headache (below right).

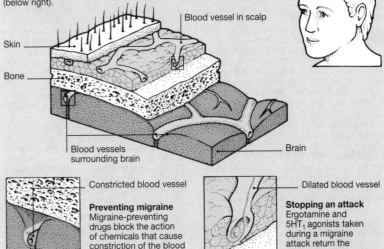

Skin
Bone
Blood vessel in scalp
Blood vessels surrounding brain
Brain

Constricted blood vessel

Preventing migraine
Migraine-preventing drugs block the action of chemicals that cause constriction of the blood vessels surrounding the brain.

Dilated blood vessel

Stopping an attack
Ergotamine and 5HT$_1$ agonists taken during a migraine attack return the dilated blood vessels in the scalp to their normal size.

chemicals found in food or produced by the body. The neurotransmitter serotonin causes large blood vessels in the brain to constrict. Pizotifen and propranolol block the effect of chemicals on blood vessels and thereby prevent attacks (see Action of drugs used for migraine, above).

The next stage of a migraine attack occurs when blood vessels in the scalp and around the eyes dilate (widen). As a result, chemicals called prostaglandins are released, producing pain. Aspirin and paracetamol relieve this pain by blocking prostaglandins. Codeine acts directly on the brain, altering pain perception (see Action of analgesics, p.80). Ergotamine and 5HT$_1$ agonists relieve pain by narrowing dilated blood vessels in the scalp.

How they affect you
Each drug has its own *adverse effects*. 5HT$_1$ agonists may cause chest tightness and drowsiness. Ergotamine may cause drowsiness, tingling sensations in the skin (paraesthesia), cramps, and weakness in the legs, and vomiting may be made worse. Pizotifen may cause drowsiness and weight gain. Clonidine may disturb sleep. For the effects of propranolol, see p.97, and for analgesics, see p.80.

Risks and special precautions
5HT$_1$ agonists should not usually be used by those with high blood pressure, angina,

or coronary heart disease. Ergotamine can damage blood vessels by prolonged overconstriction so it should be used with caution by those with poor circulation. Excessive use can lead to dependence and many adverse effects, including headache. You should not take more than your doctor advises in any one week.

How they are administered
These drugs are usually taken by mouth as tablets or capsules. Sumatriptan can also be taken as an injection or a nasal spray. Ergotamine can be taken by aerosol inhalation, as suppositories, or as tablets that dissolve under the tongue.

COMMON DRUGS

Drugs to prevent migraine
Amitriptyline ✱
Clonidine ✱
Cyproheptadine
Methysergide
Nifedipine ✱
Pizotifen ✱
Propranolol ✱
Verapamil ✱

5HT$_1$ agonists
Naratriptan
Rizatriptan
Sumatriptan ✱
Zolmitriptan

Other drugs to relieve migraine
Aspirin ✱
Codeine ✱
Dihydroergotamine
Ergotamine ✱
Isometheptene
Paracetamol ✱
Tolfenamic acid

✱ See Part 4

ANTI-EMETICS

Drugs used to treat or prevent vomiting or the feeling of sickness (nausea) are known as anti-emetics. Vomiting is a reflex action for getting rid of harmful substances, but it may also be a symptom of disease. Vomiting and nausea are often caused by a digestive tract infection, travel sickness, pregnancy, or vertigo (a balance disorder involving the inner ear). They can also occur as a *side effect* of some drugs, especially those used for cancer, radiation therapy, or general anaesthesia.

Commonly used anti-emetics include metoclopramide, domperidone, cyclizine, haloperidol, ondansetron, granisetron, prochlorperazine, promethazine, and cinnarizine. The phenothiazine and butyrophenone drug groups are also used as antihistamines (see p.124) and to treat some types of mental illness (see Antipsychotic drugs, p.85).

Why they are used

Doctors usually diagnose the cause of vomiting before prescribing an anti-emetic because vomiting may be due to an infection of the digestive tract or some other condition of the abdomen that might require treatment such as surgery. Treating only the vomiting and nausea might delay diagnosis, correct treatment, and recovery. Anti-emetics may be taken to prevent travel sickness (using one of the antihistamines), vomiting resulting from anticancer (see p.154) and other drug treatments (metoclopramide, haloperidol, domperidone, ondansetron, and prochlorperazine) to help the nausea in vertigo (see right), and occasionally to relieve cases of severe vomiting during pregnancy. You should not take an anti-emetic during pregnancy except on medical advice.

No anti-emetic drug should be taken for longer than a couple of days without consulting your doctor.

How they work

Nausea and vomiting occur when the vomiting centre in the brain is stimulated by signals from three places in the body: the digestive tract, the part of the inner ear controlling balance, and the brain itself via thoughts and emotions and via

VERTIGO AND MÉNIÈRE'S DISEASE

Vertigo is a spinning sensation in the head, which is often accompanied by nausea and vomiting. It is usually caused by a disease affecting the organ of balance in the inner ear. Anti-emetic drugs are prescribed to relieve the symptoms.

Ménière's disease is a disorder in which excess fluid builds up in the inner ear, causing vertigo, noises in the ear, and gradual deafness. It is usually treated with betahistine, prochlorperazine, or an anti-anxiety drug (see p.83). A diuretic (see p.99) may also be given in order to reduce the excess fluid in the ear.

its chemoreceptor trigger zone, which responds to harmful substances in the blood. Anti-emetic drugs may act at one or more of these places (see Action of anti-emetics, left). Some help the stomach to empty its contents into the intestine. A combination may be used that works at different sites and has an additive effect.

How they affect you

As well as to treating vomiting and nausea, many anti-emetic drugs may make you feel drowsy. However, for preventing travel sickness on long journeys, a sedating antihistamine may be an advantage.

Some anti-emetics (in particular, the phenothiazines and antihistamines) can block the parasympathetic nervous system (see p.79), causing dry mouth, blurred vision, or difficulty in passing urine. The phenothiazines may also lower blood pressure, leading to dizziness or fainting.

Risks and special precautions

Because some antihistamines can make you drowsy, it may be advisable not to drive while taking them. Phenothiazines, butyrophenones, and metoclopramide can produce uncontrolled movements of the face and tongue, so they are used with caution in people with *parkinsonism*.

ACTION OF ANTI-EMETICS

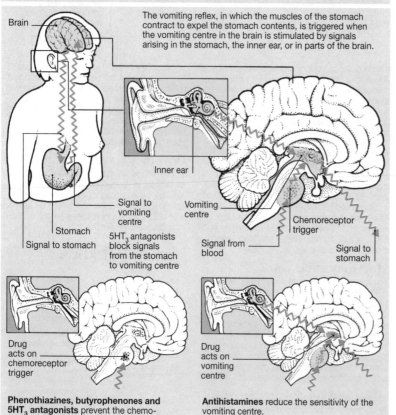

The vomiting reflex, in which the muscles of the stomach contract to expel the stomach contents, is triggered when the vomiting centre in the brain is stimulated by signals arising in the stomach, the inner ear, or in parts of the brain.

Brain

Inner ear

Stomach

Signal to vomiting centre

Signal to stomach

5HT₃ antagonists block signals from the stomach to vomiting centre

Vomiting centre

Signal from blood

Chemoreceptor trigger

Signal to stomach

Drug acts on chemoreceptor trigger

Drug acts on vomiting centre

Phenothiazines, butyrophenones and 5HT₃ antagonists prevent the chemoreceptor trigger from stimulating vomiting.

Antihistamines reduce the sensitivity of the vomiting centre.

COMMON DRUGS

Antihistamines
Cinnarizine ✳
Cyclizine ✳
Dimenhydrinate
Meclozine
Promethazine ✳

Phenothiazines
Chlorpromazine ✳
Perphenazine
Prochlorperazine ✳

5HT₃ antagonists
Granisetron
Ondansetron ✳
Tropisetron

Butyrophenones
Haloperidol ✳

Other drugs
Betahistine ✳
Domperidone ✳
Hyoscine hydrobromide ✳
Metoclopramide ✳
Nabilone

✳ See Part 4

RESPIRATORY SYSTEM

The respiratory system consists of the lungs and the passageways, such as the trachea and bronchi, by which air reaches them. Through the process of inhaling and exhaling air – breathing – the body is able to obtain the oxygen necessary for survival, and to expel carbon dioxide, which is the waste product of the basic human biological process.

What can go wrong

Difficulty in breathing may be due to narrowing of the air passages, from spasm, as in asthma and bronchitis, or from swelling of the linings of the air passages, as in bronchiolitis and bronchitis. Breathing difficulties may also be due to an infection of the lung tissue, as in pneumonia and bronchitis, or to damage to the small air sacs (alveoli) from emphysema or from inhaled dusts or moulds, which cause pneumoconiosis and farmer's lung. Smoking and air pollution can affect the respiratory system in many ways, leading to diseases such as lung cancer and bronchitis.

Sometimes difficulty in breathing may be due to congestion of the lungs from heart disease, to an inhaled object such as a peanut, or to infection or inflammation of the throat. Symptoms of breathing difficulties often include a cough and a tight feeling in the chest.

Why drugs are used

Drugs with a variety of actions are used to clear the air passages, soothe inflammation, and reduce the production of mucus. Some can be bought without a prescription as single-ingredient or combined-ingredient preparations, often with an analgesic.

Decongestants (p.93) reduce the swelling inside the nose, thereby making it possible to breathe more freely. If the cause of the congestion is an allergic response, an antihistamine (p.124) is often recommended to relieve symptoms or to prevent attacks. Infections of the respiratory tract are usually treated with antibiotics (p.128).

Bronchodilators are drugs that widen the bronchi (p.92). They are used to relieve or prevent asthma attacks. This group includes drugs that relax the muscles around the airways, and corticosteroids (p.141) that reduce both inflammation and the narrowing of airways. Other drugs, such as sodium cromoglycate, may be used for treating allergies and preventing asthma attacks but they are not effective once an asthma attack has begun.

A variety of drugs are used to relieve a cough, depending on the type of cough involved. Some drugs make it easier to eliminate phlegm; others suppress the cough by inhibiting the cough reflex.

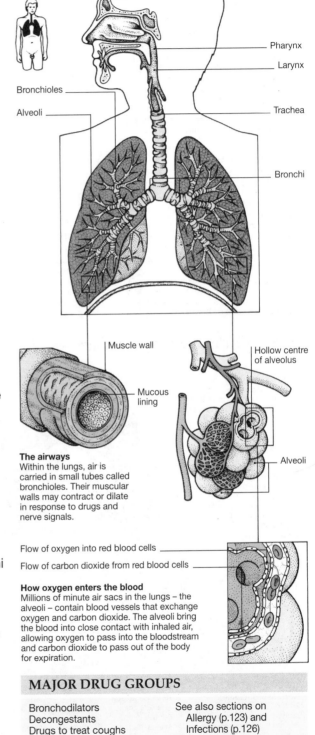

Pharynx

Larynx

Bronchioles

Alveoli

Trachea

Bronchi

Muscle wall

Hollow centre of alveolus

Mucous lining

Alveoli

The airways
Within the lungs, air is carried in small tubes called bronchioles. Their muscular walls may contract or dilate in response to drugs and nerve signals.

Flow of oxygen into red blood cells

Flow of carbon dioxide from red blood cells

How oxygen enters the blood
Millions of minute air sacs in the lungs – the alveoli – contain blood vessels that exchange oxygen and carbon dioxide. The alveoli bring the blood into close contact with inhaled air, allowing oxygen to pass into the bloodstream and carbon dioxide to pass out of the body for expiration.

MAJOR DRUG GROUPS

Bronchodilators
Decongestants
Drugs to treat coughs

See also sections on
Allergy (p.123) and
Infections (p.126)

BRONCHODILATORS

Air entering the lungs passes through narrow tubes called bronchioles. In asthma and bronchitis the bronchioles become narrower, either as a result of contraction of the muscles in their walls, or as a result of mucus congestion. This narrowing of the bronchioles obstructs the flow of air into and out of the lungs and causes breathlessness.

Bronchodilators are prescribed to widen the bronchioles and improve breathing. There are three main groups of bronchodilators: *sympathomimetics*, *anticholinergics*, and xanthine drugs, which are related to caffeine.

Why they are used

Bronchodilators help to dilate the bronchioles of people suffering from asthma and bronchitis. However, they are of little benefit to those suffering from severe chronic bronchitis.

Bronchodilators can either be taken when they are needed in order to relieve an attack of breathlessness that is in progress, or on a regular basis to prevent such attacks from occurring. Some people find it helpful to take an extra dose of their bronchodilator immediately before undertaking any activity likely to provoke an attack of breathlessness. A

INHALERS

Inhaling a bronchodilator drug directly into the lungs is the best way of getting benefit without excessive side effects. Devices for delivering the drug into the airways are described below.

Inhalers or **puffers** release a small dose when they are pressed, but require some skill to use effectively. A large hollow plastic "spacer" can help you to inhale your drug more easily.

patient who requires treatment with a sympathomimetic inhaler more than once daily should see his or her doctor about preventative treatment with an inhaled corticosteroid. Sympathomimetic drugs are mainly used for the rapid relief of breathlessness; anticholinergic and xanthine drugs are used long term.

How they work

Bronchodilator drugs act by relaxing the muscles surrounding the bronchioles. Sympathomimetic and anticholinergic drugs achieve this by interfering with nerve signals passed to the muscles through the autonomic nervous system (see p.79). Xanthine drugs are thought

Insufflation cartridges deliver larger amounts of drug than inhalers and are easier to use because the drug is taken in as you breathe normally.

Nebulizers pump compressed air through a solution of drug to produce a fine mist which is inhaled through a face mask. They deliver large doses of the drug to the lungs, rapidly relieving breathing difficulty.

to relax the muscle in the bronchioles by a direct effect on the muscle fibres, but their precise action is not known.

Bronchodilator drugs usually improve breathing within a few minutes of administration. Corticosteroids usually start to increase the sufferer's capacity for exercise within a few days, and most people find that the frequency of their attacks of breathlessness is reduced.

Because sympathomimetic drugs stimulate a branch of the autonomic nervous system that controls heart rate, they may sometimes cause palpitations and trembling. Typical side effects of anticholinergic drugs include dry mouth, blurred vision, and difficulty in passing urine. Xanthine drugs may cause headaches and nausea.

Risks and special precautions

Since most bronchodilators are not taken by mouth, but inhaled (see above), they do not commonly cause serious side effects. However, because of their possible effect on heart rate, xanthine and sympathomimetic drugs need to be prescribed with caution to people with heart problems, high blood pressure, or an overactive thyroid gland. The anticholinergic drugs may not be suitable for people with urinary retention or those who have a tendency to glaucoma.

ACTION OF BRONCHODILATORS

When the bronchioles are narrowed following contraction of the muscle layer and swelling of the mucous lining, the passage of air is impeded. Bronchodilators act on the nerve signals that govern muscle activity. Sympathomimetics enhance the action of neurotransmitters that encourage muscle relaxation. Anticholinergics block the neurotransmitters that trigger muscle contraction and reduce production of mucus. Xanthines promote muscle relaxation by a direct effect on the muscles.

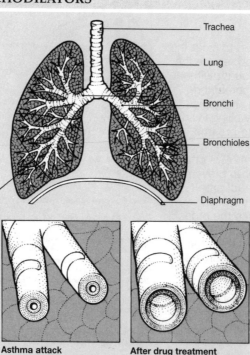

Trachea

Lung

Bronchi

Bronchioles

Diaphragm

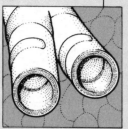

Normal bronchioles
The muscle surrounding the bronchioles is relaxed, thus leaving the airway open.

Asthma attack
The bronchiole muscle contracts and the lining swells, narrowing the airway.

After drug treatment
The muscles relax, thereby opening the airway, but the lining remains swollen.

COMMON DRUGS

Sympathomimetics	Xanthines
Bambuterol	Theophylline/
Eformoterol	aminophylline ✳
Ephedrine ✳	
Epinephrine ✳	**Corticosteroids**
Fenoterol	Beclometasone ✳
Reproterol	Budesonide ✳
Salbutamol ✳	Fluticasone ✳
Salmeterol ✳	Prednisolone ✳
Terbutaline ✳	
Tulobuterol	**Other drugs**
	Antihistamines (see
Anticholinergics	p.124)
Ipratropium	Ketotifen
bromide ✳	Nedocromil
Oxitropium	Sodium
	cromoglicate ✳

✳ See Part 4

DECONGESTANTS

The usual cause of a blocked nose is swelling of the delicate mucous membrane that lines the nasal passages and excessive production of mucus as a result of inflammation. This may be caused by an infection (for example, a common cold) or it may be caused by an allergy – for example, to pollen – a condition known as allergic rhinitis or hay fever. Congestion can also occur in the sinuses (the air spaces in the skull), resulting in sinusitis. Decongestants are drugs that reduce swelling of the mucous membrane and suppress the production of mucus, helping to clear blocked nasal passages and sinuses. Antihistamines counter the allergic response in allergy-related conditions (see p.124). If the symptoms are persistent, either topical corticosteroids (see p.141) or sodium cromoglycate (p.404) may be preferred.

Why they are used

Most common colds and blocked noses do not need to be treated with decongestants. Simple home remedies, for example, steam inhalation, possibly with the addition of an aromatic oil – such as menthol or eucalyptus – are often effective. Decongestants are used when such measures are ineffective or when there is a particular risk from untreated congestion – for example, in people who suffer from recurrent middle-ear or sinus infections.

Decongestants are available in the form of drops or sprays applied directly into the nose (*topical* decongestants), or they can be taken by mouth. Small quantities of decongestant drugs are added to many over-the-counter cold remedies (see p.94).

How they work

When the mucous membrane lining the nose is irritated by infection or allergy, the blood vessels supplying the membrane become enlarged. This leads to fluid accumulation in the surrounding tissue and encourages the production of larger-than-normal amounts of mucus.

Most decongestants belong to the *sympathomimetic* group of drugs that stimulate the sympathetic branch of the autonomic nervous system (see p.79).

ACTION OF DECONGESTANTS

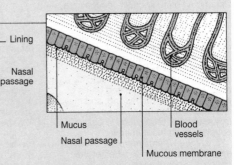

Normal nasal passages
The lining of the nasal passages consists of a layer of mucus-producing cells (the mucous membrane) supplied by blood vessels. The walls of the blood vessels contain nerve endings that, when stimulated, cause the vessels to constrict.

Sinus

Lining

Nasal passage

Mucus

Nasal passage

Blood vessels

Mucous membrane

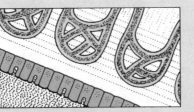

Congested nasal lining
When the blood vessels enlarge in response to infection or irritation, increased amounts of fluid pass into the mucous membrane, which swells and produces more mucus.

Effect of decongestants
Decongestants enhance the action of chemicals that stimulate constriction of the blood vessels. Narrowing of the blood vessels reduces swelling and mucus production.

One effect of this action is to constrict the blood vessels, so reducing swelling of the lining of the nose and sinuses.

How they affect you

When applied topically in the form of drops or sprays, these drugs start to relieve congestion within a few minutes. Decongestants by mouth take a little longer to act, but their effect may also last longer. Used in moderation, topical decongestants have few *adverse effects*, because they are not absorbed by the body in large amounts.

Used for too long or in excess, topical decongestants can, after giving initial relief, do more harm than good, causing a "rebound congestion" (see left). This effect can be prevented by taking the minimum effective dose and by using decongestant preparations only when absolutely necessary. Decongestants taken by mouth do not cause rebound congestion but are more likely to cause other side effects.

REBOUND CONGESTION

This can happen when decongestant nose drops and sprays are withdrawn or overused. The result is a sudden increase in congestion due to widening of the blood vessels in the nasal lining because blood vessels are no longer constricted by the decongestant.

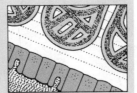

Congestion before drug treatment

Congestion after stopping drug treatment

COMMON DRUGS

Used topically	Taken by mouth
Ephedrine ✳	Ephedrine
Ipratropium ✳	Phenylephrine
Xylometazoline	Phenylpropanol-
Oxymetazoline	amine ✳
Phenylephrine ✳	Pseudoephedrine

✳ See Part 4

DRUGS TO TREAT COUGHS

Coughing is a natural response to irritation of the lungs and air passages, designed to expel harmful substances from the respiratory tract. Common causes of coughing include infection of the respiratory tract (for example, bronchitis or pneumonia), inflammation of the airways caused by asthma, or exposure to certain irritant substances such as smoke or chemical fumes. Depending on their cause, coughs may be productive – that is, phlegm-producing – or they may be dry.

In most cases coughing is a helpful reaction that assists the body in ridding itself of excess phlegm and substances that irritate the respiratory system; suppressing the cough may actually delay recovery. However, repeated bouts of coughing can be distressing, and may increase irritation of the air passages. In such cases, medication to ease the cough may be recommended.

There are two main groups of cough remedies, according to whether the cough is productive or dry.

Productive coughs

Mucolytics and expectorants are sometimes recommended for productive coughs when simple home remedies such as steam inhalation have failed to "loosen" the cough and make it easier to cough up phlegm. Mucolytics alter the consistency of the phlegm, making it less sticky and easier to cough up. These are often given by inhalation. However, there

is little evidence that they are effective. Dornase alfa may be given to people who suffer from cystic fibrosis; the drug, given by inhalation via a nebulizer, is an enzyme that improves lung function by thinning the mucus. Expectorant drugs are taken by mouth to loosen a cough. There is some evidence that guaifenesin is effective. Expectorants are included in many over-the-counter cough remedies.

Dry coughs

In dry coughs there is no advantage to be gained from promoting the expulsion of phlegm. Drugs used for dry coughs are given to suppress the coughing mechanism by calming the part of the brain that governs the coughing reflex. Antihistamines are often given for mild coughs, particularly in children. A demulcent, such as a simple linctus, can be used to soothe a dry, irritating cough. For persistent coughs, mild opioid drugs such as codeine may be prescribed (see also Analgesics, p.80). All cough suppressants have a generally sedating effect on the brain and nervous system and commonly cause drowsiness and other *side effects*.

Selecting a cough medication

There is a bewildering variety of over-the-counter medications available for treating coughs. Most consist of a syrupy base to which active ingredients and flavourings are added. Many contain a number of different active ingredients,

(see p.124)

COLD CURES

Many preparations are available over the counter to treat different symptoms of the common cold. The main ingredient in most preparations is a mild analgesic such as aspirin or paracetamol, accompanied by a decongestant (p.93), an antihistamine (p.124), and sometimes caffeine. Often the dose of each added ingredient is too low to provide any benefit. There is no evidence that vitamin C (see p.447) speeds recovery, but zinc supplements (see p.449) may be effective in shortening the cold's duration.

While some people find these drugs help to relieve symptoms, over-the-counter "cold cures" do not alter the course of the illness. Most doctors recommend using a product with a single analgesic, as the best way of alleviating symptoms. Other decongestants or antihistamines may be taken if needed. These medicines are not harmless: take care to avoid overdose if using different brands.

sometimes with contradictory effects: it is not uncommon to find an expectorant (for a productive cough) and a cough suppressant (for a dry cough) included in the same preparation.

It is important to select the correct type of medication for your cough to avoid the risk that you may make your condition worse. For example, using a cough suppressant for a productive cough may prevent you getting rid of excess infected phlegm and may delay your recovery. It is best to choose a preparation with a single active ingredient that is appropriate for your type of cough. Diabetics may need to select a sugar-free product. If you are in any doubt, ask your doctor or pharmacist for advice. Since there is a danger that use of over-the-counter cough remedies to alleviate symptoms may delay the diagnosis of a more serious underlying disorder, it is important to seek medical advice for any cough that persists for longer than a few days or if a cough is accompanied by additional symptoms such as fever or blood in the phlegm.

ACTION OF COUGH REMEDIES

Cough remedies are divided into two main groups: those that alter the consistency or production of phlegm (mucolytics and expectorants); and those that suppress the coughing reflex (opioid and non-opioid cough suppressants). Mucolytics are usually given by inhalation and act directly on the lungs and airways. Expectorants are taken by mouth, and are supposed to help bring up phlegm. Cough suppressants are taken by mouth and they act on the coughing centre in the brain.

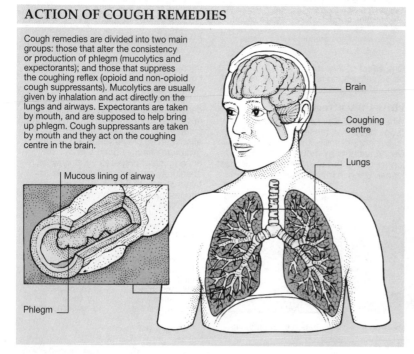

Brain

Coughing centre

Lungs

Mucous lining of airway

Phlegm

COMMON DRUGS

Expectorants
Ammonium chloride
Guaifenesin

Mucolytics
Carbocysteine
Dornase alfa
Mecysteine

Steam inhalation
Eucalyptus
Menthol

Opioid cough suppressants
Codeine ✳
Dextromethorphan
Pholcodine

Non-opioid cough suppressants
Antihistamines (see p.124)

✳ See Part 4

HEART AND CIRCULATION

The blood transports oxygen, nutrients, and heat, contains chemical messages in the form of drugs and hormones, and carries away waste products for excretion by the kidneys. It is pumped by the heart to and from the lungs, and then in a separate circuit to the rest of the body, including the brain, digestive organs, muscles, kidneys, and skin.

What can go wrong

The efficiency of the circulation may be impaired by weakening of the heart's pumping action (heart failure) or irregularity of heart rate (arrhythmia). In addition, the blood vessels may be narrowed and clogged by fatty deposits (atherosclerosis). This may reduce blood supply to the brain, the extremities (peripheral vascular disease), or the heart muscle (coronary heart disease), causing angina. These last disorders can be complicated by the formation of clots that may block a blood vessel. A clot in the arteries supplying the heart muscle is known as coronary thrombosis; a clot in an artery inside the brain is the most frequent cause of stroke.

One common circulatory disorder is abnormally high blood pressure (hypertension), in which the pressure of circulating blood on the vessel walls is increased for reasons not yet fully understood. One factor may be loss of elasticity of the vessel walls (arteriosclerosis). Several other conditions, such as migraine and Raynaud's disease, are caused by temporary alterations to blood vessel size.

Why drugs are used

Because those suffering from heart disease often have more than one problem, several drugs may be prescribed at once. Many act directly on the heart to alter the rate and rhythm of the heart beat. These are known as anti-arrhythmics and include beta blockers and digoxin.

Other drugs affect the diameter of the blood vessels, either dilating them (vasodilators) to improve blood flow and reduce blood pressure, or constricting them (vasoconstrictors).

Drugs may also reduce blood volume and fat levels, and alter clotting ability. Diuretics (used in the treatment of hypertension and heart failure) increase the body's excretion of water. Lipid-lowering drugs reduce blood cholesterol levels, thereby minimizing the risk of atherosclerosis. Drugs to reduce blood clotting are administered if there is a risk of abnormal blood clots forming in the heart, veins, or arteries. Drugs that increase clotting are given when the body's natural clotting mechanism is defective.

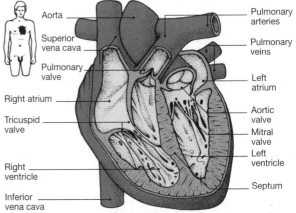

The heart
The heart is a pump with four chambers. The atrium and ventricle on the left side pump oxygenated blood to the body, while the chambers on the right pump deoxygenated blood to the lungs. Backflow of blood is stopped by valves at the chamber exits.

How blood circulates
Deoxygenated blood is carried to the heart from all parts of the body. It is then pumped to the lungs, where it becomes oxygenated. The oxygenated blood returns to the heart and from there is pumped throughout the body.

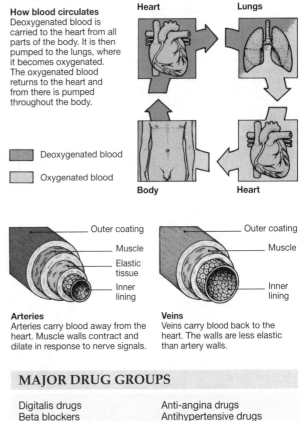

▨ Deoxygenated blood

▨ Oxygenated blood

Arteries
Arteries carry blood away from the heart. Muscle walls contract and dilate in response to nerve signals.

Veins
Veins carry blood back to the heart. The walls are less elastic than artery walls.

MAJOR DRUG GROUPS

Digitalis drugs	Anti-angina drugs
Beta blockers	Antihypertensive drugs
Vasodilators	Lipid-lowering drugs
Diuretics	Drugs that affect blood
Anti-arrhythmics	clotting

DIGITALIS DRUGS

Digitalis is the collective term for the naturally occurring substances (also called cardiac glycosides) that are found in the leaves of plants of the foxglove family and used to treat certain heart disorders. The principal drugs in this group are digoxin and digitoxin. Digoxin is more commonly used because it is shorter acting and dosage is easier to adjust (see also Risks and special precautions, below).

Why they are used

Digitalis drugs do not cure heart disease but improve the heart's pumping action and so relieve many of the symptoms that result from poor heart function. They are useful for treating conditions in which the heart beats irregularly or too rapidly (notably in atrial fibrillation, see Anti-arrhythmic drugs, p.100), when it pumps too weakly (in congestive heart failure), or when the heart muscle is damaged and weakened following a heart attack.

Digitalis drugs can be used for a short period when the heart is working poorly, but in many cases they have to be taken indefinitely. Their effect does not diminish with time. In heart failure, digitalis drugs are often given together with a diuretic drug (see p.99).

How they work

The normal heart beat results from electrical impulses generated in nerve tissue within the heart. These cause the heart muscle to contract and pump blood. By reducing the flow of electrical impulses in the heart, digitalis makes the heart beat more slowly.

The force with which the heart muscle contracts depends on chemical changes in the heart muscle. By promoting these chemical changes, digitalis increases the force of muscle contraction each time the heart is stimulated. This compensates for the loss of power that occurs when some of the muscle is damaged following a heart attack. The stronger heart beat increases blood flow to the kidneys. This increases urine production and helps to remove the excess fluid that often accumulates as a result of heart failure.

How they affect you

Digitalis relieves the symptoms of heart failure – fatigue, breathlessness, and swelling of the legs – and increases your capacity for exercise. The frequency with which you need to pass urine is also increased initially.

Risks and special precautions

Digitalis drugs can be *toxic* and, if blood levels rise too high, they may produce symptoms of digitalis poisoning. These include excessive tiredness, confusion, loss of appetite, nausea, vomiting, visual disturbances, and diarrhoea. If such symptoms occur, it is important to report them to your doctor promptly.

Digoxin is normally removed from the body by the kidneys; if kidney function is impaired, the drug is more likely to accumulate in the body and cause toxic effects. Digitoxin, which is broken down in the liver, is sometimes preferred in such cases. Digitoxin can accumulate after repeated dosage if liver function is severely impaired.

Both digoxin and digitoxin are more toxic when blood potassium levels are low. Potassium deficiency is commonly caused by diuretic drugs, so that people taking these along with digitalis drugs need to have the effects of both drugs and blood potassium levels carefully monitored. Potassium supplements may be required.

ACTION OF DIGITALIS DRUGS

The heart beat is triggered by electrical impulses that are generated by the pacemaker, a small mass of nerve tissue in the right atrium. Electrical signals are passed from the pacemaker to the atrio-ventricular node. From here a wave of impulses spreads throughout the heart muscle, causing it to contract and pump blood to the body. The pumping action of the heart can become weak if the heart muscle is damaged or if the heart beat is too fast, as in atrial fibrillation. In this condition (shown right), rapid signals from the pacemaker trigger fast and inefficient contractions of both the atria and the ventricles.

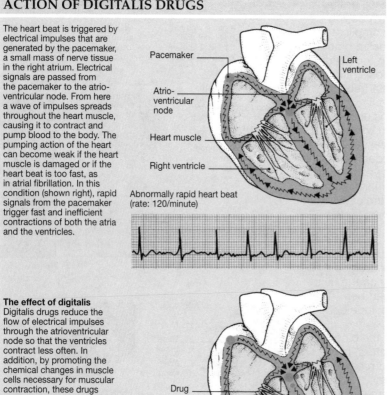

Pacemaker
Atrio-ventricular node
Heart muscle
Right ventricle
Left ventricle

Abnormally rapid heart beat (rate: 120/minute)

The effect of digitalis
Digitalis drugs reduce the flow of electrical impulses through the atrioventricular node so that the ventricles contract less often. In addition, by promoting the chemical changes in muscle cells necessary for muscular contraction, these drugs increase the force with which the heart muscle contracts and thereby improve the efficiency of each heart beat.

Drug

Slowed heart beat (rate: 80/minute)

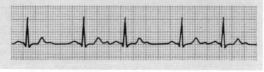

COMMON DRUGS

Digitoxin
Digoxin *

* See Part 4

BETA BLOCKERS

Beta blockers are drugs that interrupt the transmission of stimuli through the beta *receptors* of the body. Since the actions they block originate in the adrenal glands (and elsewhere) they are also sometimes called beta adrenergic blocking agents. Used mainly in heart disorders, these drugs are occasionally prescribed for other conditions.

Why they are used

Beta blockers are used for treating angina (see p.101), hypertension (see p.102), and irregular heart rhythms (see p.100). They are sometimes given after a heart attack to reduce the likelihood of abnormal heart rhythms or further damage to the heart muscle. These drugs are also prescribed to improve heart function in heart muscle disorders, known as cardiomyopathies.

Beta blockers may also be given to prevent migraine headaches (see p.89), or to reduce the physical symptoms of anxiety (see p.83). These drugs may be given to control symptoms of an overactive thyroid gland. A beta blocker is sometimes given in the form of eye drops in glaucoma to lower the fluid pressure inside the eye (see p.168).

How they work

By occupying the beta receptors, beta blockers nullify the stimulating action of norepinephrine (noradrenaline), the main "fight or flight" hormone. As a result, they reduce the force and speed of the heart

BETA RECEPTORS

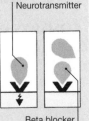

Signals from the sympathetic nervous system are carried by noradrenaline, a *neurotransmitter* produced in the adrenal glands and at the ends of the sympathetic nerve fibres. Beta blockers stop the signals from the neurotransmitter.

Neurotransmitter

Beta blocker

Types of beta receptor
There are two types of beta receptor: beta 1 and beta 2. Beta 1 receptors are located mainly in the heart muscle; beta 2 receptors are found both in the airways and blood vessels. Cardioselective drugs act mainly on beta 1 receptors; non-cardioselective drugs act on both types of receptor.

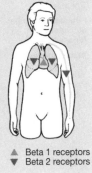

▲ Beta 1 receptors
▼ Beta 2 receptors

THE USES AND EFFECTS OF BETA BLOCKERS

Blocking the transmission of signals through beta receptors in different parts of the body produces a wide variety of benefits and side effects depending on the disease being treated. The illustration (right) shows the main areas and body systems affected by the action of beta blockers.

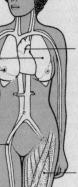

Brain
Dilation of the blood vessels surrounding the brain is inhibited, so preventing migraine.

Eye
Beta blocker eye drops reduce fluid production and so lower pressure inside the eye.

Heart
Slowing of the heart rate and reduction of the force of the heart beat reduces the workload of the heart, helping to prevent angina and abnormal heart rhythms. But this action may worsen heart failure.

Lungs
Constriction of the airways may provoke breathlessness in asthmatics or those with chronic bronchitis.

Blood vessels
Constriction of the blood vessels may cause coldness of the hands and feet.

Blood pressure
This is lowered because the rate and force at which the heart pumps blood into the circulatory system is reduced.

Muscles
Muscle tremor due to anxiety or to overactivity of the thyroid gland is reduced.

beat and prevent the dilation of the blood vessels surrounding the brain and leading to the extremities. The effect of this "beta blockade" in a variety of disorders is shown in the box above.

How they affect you

Beta blockers are taken to treat angina. They reduce the frequency and severity of attacks. As part of the treatment for hypertension, beta blockers help to lower blood pressure and thus reduce the risks that are associated with this condition. Beta blockers help to prevent severe attacks of arrhythmia, in which the heart beat is wild and uncontrolled.

Because beta blockers affect many parts of the body, they often produce minor *side effects*. By reducing heart rate and air flow to the lungs, they may reduce capacity for strenuous exercise, although this is unlikely to be noticed by somebody whose physical activity was previously limited by heart problems. Many people experience cold hands and feet while taking these drugs as a result of the reduction in the blood supply to the limbs. Reduced circulation can also lead to temporary impotence during treatment.

Risks and special precautions

The main risk of beta blockers is that of provoking breathing difficulties as a result of their blocking effect on beta receptors in the lungs. Cardioselective beta blockers, which act principally on the heart, are thought to be less likely than non-cardioselective ones to cause such problems. But all beta blockers are prescribed with caution for people who

have asthma, bronchitis, or other forms of respiratory disease.

Beta blockers are not commonly prescribed for people who have poor circulation in the limbs because they reduce the flow of blood and may aggravate such conditions. They are not normally given to people who are subject to heart failure because they may further reduce the force of the heart beat. Diabetics who need to take beta blockers should be aware that they may notice a change in the warning signs of low blood sugar; in particular, they may find that symptoms such as palpitations and tremor are suppressed.

Beta blockers should not be stopped suddenly after prolonged use; this may provoke a sudden and severe recurrence of symptoms of the original disorder, even a heart attack. The blood pressure may also rise markedly. When treatment with beta blockers needs to be stopped, it should be withdrawn gradually under medical supervision.

COMMON DRUGS

Cardioselective	Non-cardioselective
Atenolol ✱	Acebutolol
Betaxolol	Carvedilol
Bisoprolol	Labetalol
Celiprolol	Nadolol
Metoprolol ✱	Pindolol
	Propranolol ✱
	Sotalol ✱
	Timolol ✱

✱ See Part 4

VASODILATORS

Vasodilators are drugs that widen blood vessels. Their most obvious use is to reverse narrowing of the blood vessels when this leads to reduced blood flow and, consequently, a lower oxygen supply to parts of the body. This problem occurs in angina, when narrowing of the coronary arteries reduces blood supply to the heart muscle. Vasodilators are often used to treat high blood pressure (hypertension).

Why they are used

Vasodilators improve the blood flow and thus the oxygen supply to areas of the body where they are most needed. In angina, dilation of the blood vessels throughout the body reduces the force with which the heart needs to pump and thereby eases its workload (see also Anti-angina drugs, p.101). This also may be helpful in treating congestive heart failure when other treatments are not effective.

Because blood pressure is dependent partly on the diameter of blood vessels, vasodilators are often helpful in treating hypertension (see p.102).

In peripheral vascular disease, narrowed blood vessels in the legs cannot supply sufficient blood to the extremities, often leading to pain in the legs during exercise. Unfortunately, because the vessels are narrowed by atherosclerosis, vasodilators have little effect.

Vasodilator drugs have also been used to treat senile dementia, in the hope of increasing the supply of oxygen to the brain. The benefits of this treatment have not yet been proved.

How they work

Vasodilators widen the blood vessels by relaxing the muscles surrounding them. They achieve this either by affecting the action of the muscles directly (nitrates, hydralazine, and calcium channel blockers) or by interfering with the nerve signals that govern contraction of the

ACTION OF VASODILATORS

The diameter of blood vessels is governed by the contraction of the surrounding muscle. The muscle contracts in response to signals from the sympathetic nervous system (p.79). Vasodilators encourage the muscles to relax, thus increasing the size of blood vessels.

Constricted blood vessel   **Dilated blood vessel**

Muscle band

Where they act
Each type of vasodilator acts on a different part of the mechanism controlling blood vessel size in order to prevent contraction of the surrounding layer of muscles.

Nerves – Alpha blockers interfere with nerve signals to the muscles.

Muscle layer – Nitrates and calcium channel blockers act directly on the muscle to inhibit contraction.

Blood – ACE inhibitors block enzyme activity in the blood (see box below).

blood vessels (alpha blockers). ACE inhibitors act by blocking the activity of an enzyme in the blood. The enzyme is responsible for producing angiotensin II, a powerful vasoconstrictor (see box below).

How they affect you

As well as relieving the symptoms of the disorders for which they are taken, vasodilators can have many minor *side effects* related to their action on the circulation. Flushing and headaches are common at the start of treatment. Dizziness and fainting may also occur as a result of lowered blood pressure. Dilation of the blood vessels can also

cause fluid build-up, leading to swelling, particularly of the ankles.

Risks and special precautions

The major risk is that blood pressure may fall too low. Therefore vasodilator drugs are prescribed with caution for people with unstable blood pressure. It is also advisable to sit or lie down after taking the first dose of a vasodilator drug.

COMMON DRUGS

ACE inhibitors Captopril * Cilazapril Enalapril * Fosinopril Lisinopril Moexipril Perindopril Quinapril Ramipril * Trandolapril	**Calcium channel blockers** Amlodipine * Diltiazem * Felodipine Isradipine Lacidipine Lercanidipine Nicardipine Nifedipine * Verapamil *
Potassium channel activators Nicorandil *	**Angiotensin II blockers** Candesartan Irbesartan Valsartan
Alpha blockers Doxazosin * Indoramin Prazosin * Terazosin	**Nitrates** Glyceryl trinitrate * Isosorbide dinitrate/ mononitrate *
	Other drugs Hydralazine Minoxidil *

* See Part 4

ACE INHIBITORS

The ACE (angiotensin-converting enzyme) inhibitors are powerful vasodilators. They act by blocking the action of an enzyme in the bloodstream that is responsible for converting a chemical called angiotensin I into angiotensin II. Angiotensin II encourages constriction of the blood vessels, and its absence permits them to dilate (see right).

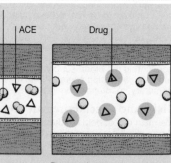

Angiotensin II

Angiotensin I | ACE   Drug

Before drug
Angiotensin I is converted by the enzyme into angiotensin II. The blood vessel constricts.

Drug action
ACE inhibitors block enzyme activity, thereby preventing the formation of angiotensin II. The blood vessel dilates.

DIURETICS

Diuretic drugs help to turn excess body water into urine. As the urine is expelled, two disorders are relieved: the tissues become less water-swollen (oedema) and the heart action improves because it has to pump a smaller volume of blood. There are several classes of diuretics, each of which has different uses, modes of action, and effects (see Types of diuretic, below). But all diuretics act on the kidneys, the organs that govern the water content of the body.

Why they are used

Diuretics are most commonly used in the treatment of high blood pressure (hypertension). By removing a larger amount of water than usual from the bloodstream, the kidneys reduce the total volume of blood circulating. This drop in volume causes a reduction of the pressure within the blood vessels (see Antihypertensive drugs, p.102).

Diuretics are also widely used to treat heart failure in which the heart's pumping mechanism has become weak. In the treatment of this disorder, they remove fluid that has accumulated in the tissues and lungs. The resulting drop in blood volume reduces the work of the heart.

Other conditions for which diuretics are often prescribed include nephrotic syndrome (a kidney disorder that causes oedema), cirrhosis of the liver (in which fluid may accumulate in the abdominal cavity), and premenstrual syndrome (when hormonal activity can lead to fluid retention and bloating).

Less commonly, diuretics are used to treat glaucoma (see p.168) and Ménière's disease (see p.90).

How they work

The kidneys' normal filtration process takes water, salts (mainly potassium and sodium), and waste products out of the bloodstream. Most of the salts and water are returned to the bloodstream, but some are expelled from the body together with the waste products in the urine. Diuretics interfere with this filtration process by reducing the amounts of sodium and water taken back into the

ACTION OF DIURETICS

As blood passes through the kidney, water, sodium and potassium salts, and waste products are filtered out of the bloodstream. Most of the water and filtered salts are then reabsorbed by the bloodstream from the tubule; the remainder is excreted as urine.

By blocking the movement of sodium back into the blood-stream, diuretics prevent the reabsorption of water, so that more is expelled from the body as urine. Different diuretic drugs act on different parts of the tubule (see right).

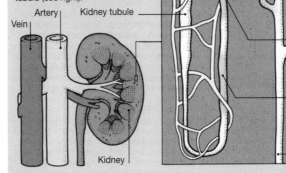

Diuretic action in the kidney tubule

Water, salts, and waste removed from blood in the glomerulus.

Sodium and water reabsorbed. Blocked by **osmotics.**

Sodium and water reabsorbed. Potassium lost. Blocked by **potassium-sparing diuretics.**

Water, sodium, and potassium reabsorbed. Blocked by **thiazides.**

Water, sodium, and potassium reabsorbed. Blocked by **loop diuretics.**

Urine to the bladder

Artery   Kidney tubule
Vein
Kidney

bloodstream, thus increasing the volume of urine produced. Modifying the filtration process in this way means that the water content of the blood is reduced; less water in the blood causes excess water present in the tissues to be drawn out and eliminated in urine.

How they affect you

All diuretics increase the frequency with which you need to pass urine. This is most noticeable at the start of treatment. People who have suffered from oedema may notice that swelling – particularly of the ankles – is reduced, and those with heart failure may find that breathlessness is relieved.

Risks and special precautions

Diuretics can cause blood chemical imbalances, of which a fall in potassium levels (hypokalaemia) is the most common. Hypokalaemia can cause confusion, weakness, and trigger abnormal heart rhythms (especially in people taking digitalis drugs). Potassium supplements or a potassium-sparing diuretic usually corrects the imbalance. A diet that is rich in potassium (containing plenty of fresh fruits and vegetables) may be helpful.

Some diuretics may raise blood levels of uric acid, increasing the risk of gout. They may also raise blood sugar levels, causing problems for diabetics.

TYPES OF DIURETIC

Thiazides The diuretics most commonly prescribed, thiazides may lead to potassium deficiency and they are, therefore, often given together with a potassium supplement or in conjunction with a potassium-sparing diuretic (see right).

Loop diuretics These fast-acting, powerful drugs increase the output of urine for a few hours, and are therefore sometimes used in emergencies. They may cause excessive loss of potassium, which may need to be countered as for thiazides. Large doses may disturb hearing.

Potassium-sparing diuretics These mild diuretics are usually used in conjunction with a thiazide or a loop diuretic to prevent excessive potassium loss.

Osmotic diuretics Prescribed only rarely, these drugs are used to maintain the flow of urine through the kidneys after surgery or injury, and to reduce pressure rapidly within fluid-filled cavities.

Acetazolamide This mild diuretic drug is used principally in the treatment of glaucoma (see p.168).

COMMON DRUGS

Loop diuretics
Bumetanide *
Ethacrynic acid
Frusemide *
Torasemide

Potassium-sparing diuretics
Amiloride *
Spironolactone *
Triamterene *

Thiazides
Bendroflumethiazide *
Chlortalidone
Chlorothiazide
Cyclopenthiazide *
Hydrochlorothiazide *
Hydroflumethiazide
Indapamide
Mefruside
Metolazone
Polythiazide
Xipamide

* See Part 4

ANTI-ARRHYTHMICS

The heart contains two upper and two lower chambers, which are known as the atria and ventricles (see p.95). The pumping actions of these two sets of chambers are normally coordinated by electrical impulses that originate in the pacemaker and then travel along conducting pathways so that the heart beats with a regular rhythm. If this coordination breaks down, the heart will beat abnormally, either irregularly or faster or slower than usual. The general term for abnormal heart rhythm is arrhythmia.

Arrhythmias may occur as a result of a birth defect, coronary heart disease, or other less common heart disorders. A variety of more general conditions, including overactivity of the thyroid gland, and certain drugs – such as caffeine and *anticholinergic* drugs – can also disturb heart rhythm.

SITES OF DRUG ACTION

Anti-arrhythmic drugs either slow the flow of electrical impulses to the heart muscle, or inhibit the muscle's ability to contract. Beta blockers reduce the ability of the pacemaker to pass electrical signals to the atria. Digitalis drugs reduce the passage of signals from the atrioventricular node. Calcium channel blockers interfere with the ability of the heart muscle to contract by impeding the flow of calcium into muscle cells. Other drugs such as quinidine and disopyramide reduce the sensitivity of muscle cells to electrical impulses.

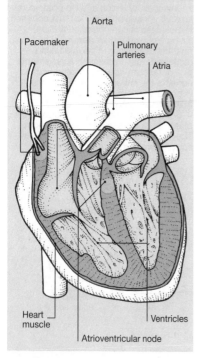

Aorta
Pacemaker
Pulmonary arteries
Atria
Heart muscle
Ventricles
Atrioventricular node

A broad selection of drugs is used to regulate heart rhythm, including beta blockers, digitalis drugs, and calcium channel blockers. Other drugs used are disopyramide, lignocaine, procainamide, and quinidine.

Why they are used

Minor disturbances of heart rhythm are common and do not usually require drug treatment. However, if the pumping action of the heart is seriously affected, the circulation of blood throughout the body may become inefficient, and drug treatment may be necessary.

Drugs may be taken to treat individual attacks of arrhythmia, or they may be taken on a regular basis to prevent or control abnormal heart rhythms. The particular drug prescribed depends on the type of arrhythmia to be treated, but because people differ in their response, it may be necessary to try several in order to find the most effective one. When the arrhythmia is sudden and severe, it may be necessary to inject a drug immediately to restore normal heart function.

How they work

The heart's pumping action is governed by electrical impulses under the control of the sympathetic nervous system (see Autonomic nervous system, p.79). These signals pass through the heart muscle, causing the two pairs of chambers – the atria and ventricles – to contract in turn (see Sites of drug action, left).

All anti-arrhythmic drugs alter the conduction of electrical signals in the heart. However, each drug or drug group has a different effect on the sequence of events controlling the pumping action. Some block the transmission of signals to the heart (beta blockers); some affect the way in which signals are conducted within the heart (digitalis drugs); others affect the response of the heart muscle to the signals received (calcium channel blockers, disopyramide, procainamide, and quinidine).

How they affect you

These drugs usually prevent symptoms of arrhythmia and may restore a regular heart rhythm. Although they do not prevent all arrhythmias, they usually reduce the frequency and severity of any symptoms.

Unfortunately, as well as suppressing arrhythmias, many of these drugs tend to depress normal heart function, and may produce dizziness on standing up, or increased breathlessness on exertion. Mild nausea and visual disturbances are also fairly frequent. Verapamil can cause constipation, especially when it is prescribed in high doses. Disopyramide may interfere with the parasympathetic nervous system (see p.79), resulting in a number of *anticholinergic* effects.

TYPES OF ARRHYTHMIA

Atrial fibrillation In this common type of arrhythmia, the atria contract irregularly at such a high rate that the ventricles cannot keep pace. It is treated with digoxin, sometimes in combination with quinidine.

Ventricular tachycardia This condition arises from abnormal electrical activity in the ventricles that causes the ventricles to contract rapidly. Regular treatment with quinidine, disopyramide, or procainamide is usually given. Amiodarone may be used if these are not effective.

Supraventricular tachycardia This condition occurs when extra electrical impulses arise in the pacemaker or atria. These extra impulses stimulate the ventricles to contract rapidly. Attacks may disappear on their own without treatment, but drugs such as adenosine, digoxin, verapamil, or propranolol may be given.

Heart block When impulses are not conducted from the atria to the ventricles, the ventricles start to beat at a slower rate. Some cases of heart block do not require treatment. For more severe heart block accompanied by dizziness and fainting, it is usually necessary to fit the patient with an artificial pacemaker.

Risks and special precautions

These drugs may further disrupt heart rhythm under certain circumstances and therefore they are used only when the likely benefit outweighs the risks.

Quinidine can be *toxic* if an overdose is taken, resulting in a syndrome called cinchonism, which includes disturbed hearing, giddiness, and impaired vision (even blindness). Because some people are particularly sensitive to this drug, a test dose is usually given before regular treatment is started.

Amiodarone may accumulate in the tissues over time, and may lead to light-sensitive rashes, changes in thyroid function, and lung problems.

COMMON DRUGS

Beta blockers (See p.97)	Other drugs
Calcium channel blockers	Adenosine
Verapamil *	Amiodarone *
	Bretylium
	Disopyramide
	Flecainide
Digitalis drugs	Lignocaine
Digitoxin	Mexiletine
Digoxin *	Moracizine
	Procainamide
	Propafenone
	Quinidine

* See Part 4

ANTI-ANGINA DRUGS

Angina is chest pain produced when insufficient oxygen reaches the heart muscle. This is usually caused by a narrowing of the blood vessels (coronary arteries) that carry blood and oxygen to the heart muscle. In the most common type of angina (classic angina), pain usually occurs during physical exertion or emotional stress. In variant angina, pain may also occur at rest. In classic angina, the narrowing of the coronary arteries results from deposits of fat – called atheroma – on the walls of the arteries. In the variant type, however, angina is caused by contraction (spasm) of the muscle fibres in the artery walls.

Atheroma deposits build up more rapidly in the arteries of smokers and people who eat a high-fat diet. This is why, as a basic component of angina treatment, doctors recommend that smoking should be given up and the diet changed. Overweight people are also advised to lose weight in order to reduce the demands placed on the heart. While such changes in lifestyle often produce an improvement in symptoms, drug treatment to relieve angina is also frequently necessary.

The drugs used to treat angina include beta blockers, nitrates, calcium channel blockers, and potassium channel openers.

Why they are used

Frequent episodes of angina can be disabling and, if left untreated, can lead to an increased risk of a heart attack. Drugs can be used both to relieve angina attacks and to reduce their frequency. People who suffer from only occasional episodes are usually prescribed a rapid-acting drug to take at the first signs of an attack, or before an activity that is known to bring on an attack. A rapid-acting nitrate – glyceryl trinitrate – is usually prescribed for this purpose.

If attacks become more frequent or more severe, regular preventative treatment may be advised. Beta blockers, long-acting nitrates, and calcium channel blockers are used as regular medication to prevent attacks. The introduction of adhesive patches to administer nitrates through the patient's skin has extended the duration of action of glyceryl trinitrate, making treatment easier.

Drugs can often control angina for many years, but they cannot cure the disorder. When severe angina cannot be controlled by drugs, then surgery to increase the blood flow to the heart may be recommended.

How they work

Nitrates and calcium channel blockers dilate blood vessels by relaxing the muscle layer in the blood vessel walls (see also Vasodilators, p.98). Blood is more easily pumped through the dilated vessels, reducing the strain on the heart.

Beta blockers reduce heart muscle stimulation during exercise or stress by interrupting signal transmission in the heart. Decreased heart muscle stimulation means less oxygen is required, reducing the risk of angina attacks. For further information on beta blockers, see p.97.

How they affect you

Treatment with one or more of these medicines usually effectively controls angina. Drugs to prevent attacks allow sufferers to undertake more strenuous activities without provoking pain, and if an attack does occur, nitrates usually provide effective relief.

ACTION OF ANTI-ANGINA DRUGS

Anginal pain occurs when the heart muscle runs short of oxygen as it pumps blood round the circulatory system. Nitrates, calcium channel blockers, and potassium channel openers reduce the heart's work by dilating blood vessels. Beta blockers impede the stimulation of heart muscle, reducing its oxygen requirement, thus relieving angina.

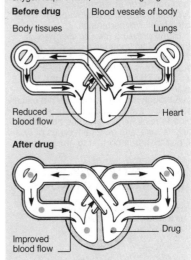

Before drug | Blood vessels of body

Body tissues | Lungs

Reduced blood flow | Heart

After drug

Improved blood flow | Drug

These drugs do not usually cause serious *adverse effects*, but they can produce a variety of minor symptoms. By dilating blood vessels throughout the body, the nitrates and calcium channel blockers can cause dizziness (especially when standing) and may cause fainting. Other possible side effects are headaches at the start of treatment, flushing of the skin (especially of the face), and ankle swelling. Beta blockers often cause cold hands and feet, and sometimes they may produce tiredness and a feeling of heaviness in the legs.

CALCIUM CHANNEL BLOCKERS

The passage of calcium through special channels into muscle cells is an essential part of the mechanism of muscle contraction (see right). These drugs prevent movement of calcium in the muscles of the blood vessels and so encourage them to dilate (see far right). The action helps to reduce blood pressure and relieves the strain on the heart muscle in angina by making it easier for the heart to pump blood throughout the body (see Action of anti-angina drugs, above right). Verapamil also slows the passage of nerve signals through the heart muscle. This can be helpful for correcting certain arrhythmias.

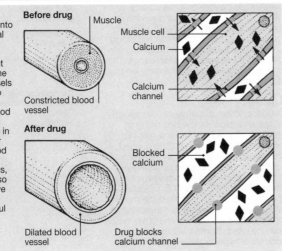

Before drug | Muscle

Muscle cell

Calcium

Calcium channel

Constricted blood vessel

After drug

Blocked calcium

Dilated blood vessel | Drug blocks calcium channel

COMMON DRUGS

Beta blockers
  see p.97)

Calcium channel blockers
Amlodipine ✳
Diltiazem ✳
Nicardipine
Nifedipine ✳

Nitrates
Glyceryl trinitrate ✳
Isosorbide dinitrate/
  mononitrate ✳

Potassium channel opener
Nicorandil ✳

Other drugs
Aspirin ✳
Simvastatin ✳
Heparin ✳

✳ See Part 4

ANTIHYPERTENSIVE DRUGS

Blood pressure is a measurement of the force exerted by the blood circulating in the arteries. Two readings are taken: one indicates force while the heart's ventricles are contracting (systolic pressure). This reading is a higher figure than the other one, which measures the blood pressure during ventricle relaxation (diastolic pressure). Blood pressure varies among individuals and normally increases with age. If a person's blood pressure is higher than normal on at least three separate occasions, a doctor may diagnose the condition as hypertension.

Blood pressure may be elevated as a result of an underlying disorder, which the doctor will try to identify. Usually, however, it is not possible to determine a cause. This condition is referred to as essential hypertension.

Although hypertension does not usually cause any symptoms, severely raised blood pressure may produce headaches, palpitations, and general feelings of ill-health. It is important to reduce high

blood pressure because it can have serious consequences, including stroke, heart attack, heart failure, and kidney damage. Certain groups are particularly at risk from high blood pressure. These risk groups include diabetics, smokers, people with pre-existing heart damage, and those whose blood contains a high level of fat. High blood pressure is more common among black people than among whites, and in countries, such as Japan, where the diet is high in salt.

A small reduction in blood pressure may be brought about by reducing weight, exercising regularly, and avoiding an excessive amount of salt in the diet. But for more severely raised blood pressure, one or more antihypertensive drugs may be prescribed. Several classes of drugs have antihypertensive properties, including the centrally acting antihypertensives, diuretics (p.99), beta blockers (p.97), calcium channel blockers (p.101), ACE (angiotensin-converting enzyme) inhibitors (p.98), and alpha blockers. See also Vasodilators, p.98.

Why they are used

Antihypertensive drugs are prescribed when diet, exercise, and other simple remedies have not brought about an adequate reduction in blood pressure, and your doctor sees a risk of serious consequences if the condition is not treated. These drugs do not cure hypertension and may have to be taken indefinitely. However, it is sometimes possible to taper off drug treatment when blood pressure has been reduced to a normal level for a year or more.

How they work

Blood pressure depends not only on the force with which the heart pumps blood, but also on the diameter of blood vessels and the volume of blood in circulation: blood pressure is increased either if the vessels are narrow or if the volume of blood is high. Antihypertensive drugs lower blood pressure either by dilating the blood vessels or by reducing blood volume. Antihypertensive drugs work in different ways and some have more than one action (see Action of antihypertensive drugs, left).

Choice of drug

Drug treatment depends on the severity of hypertension. At the beginning of treatment for mild or moderately high blood pressure, a single drug is used. A thiazide diuretic is often chosen for initial treatment, but it is also increasingly common to use a beta blocker, a calcium channel blocker, or an ACE inhibitor. If a single drug does not reduce the blood pressure sufficiently, a diuretic in combination with one of the other drugs may be used. Some people who have moderate hypertension require a third

drug, in which case a vasodilator, centrally acting antihypertensive, or alpha blocker, may also be prescribed.

Severe hypertension is usually controlled with a combination of several drugs, which may need to be given in high doses. Your doctor may need to try a number of drugs before finding a combination that controls blood pressure without unacceptable *side effects*.

How they affect you

Treatment with antihypertensive drugs relieves symptoms such as headache and palpitations. However, since most people with hypertension have few, if any, symptoms, side effects may be more noticeable than any immediate beneficial effect. Some antihypertensive drugs may cause dizziness and fainting at the start of treatment because they can sometimes cause an excessive fall in blood pressure. It may take a while for your doctor to determine a dosage that avoids such effects. For detailed information on the adverse effects of drugs used to treat hypertension, consult the individual drug profiles in Part 4.

Risks and special precautions

Since your doctor needs to know exactly how treatment with a particular drug affects your hypertension – the benefits as well as the side effects – it is important for you to keep using the antihypertensive medication as prescribed, even though you may feel the problem is under control. Sudden withdrawal of some of these drugs may cause a potentially dangerous rebound increase in blood pressure. To stop treatment, the dose needs to be reduced gradually under medical supervision.

ACTION OF ANTI-HYPERTENSIVE DRUGS

Each type of antihypertensive drug acts on a different part of the body to lower blood pressure.

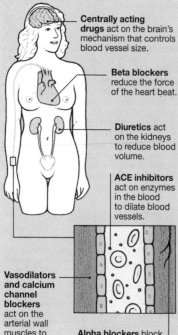

Centrally acting drugs act on the brain's mechanism that controls blood vessel size.

Beta blockers reduce the force of the heart beat.

Diuretics act on the kidneys to reduce blood volume.

ACE inhibitors act on enzymes in the blood to dilate blood vessels.

Vasodilators and calcium channel blockers act on the arterial wall muscles to prevent constriction.

Alpha blockers block nerve signals that trigger constriction of blood vessels.

COMMON DRUGS

ACE inhibitors (see p.98)	**Diuretics** (see p.99)
Beta blockers (see p.97)	**Alpha blockers** Doxazosin ✳ Prazosin Terazosin
Calcium channel blockers (see p.101)	
Centrally acting antihypertensives Clonidine Methyldopa ✳	**Vasodilators** (see p.98)

✳ See Part 4

LIPID-LOWERING DRUGS

The blood contains several types of fats, or lipids. They are necessary for normal body function but can be damaging if present in excess, particularly saturated fats such as cholesterol. The main risk is atherosclerosis, in which fatty deposits called atheroma build up in the arteries, restricting and disrupting the flow of blood. This can increase the likelihood of the formation of abnormal blood clots, leading to potentially fatal disorders such as stroke and heart attack.

For most people, cutting down the amount of fat in the diet is sufficient to reduce the risk of atherosclerosis. For those with an inherited tendency to high levels of fat in the blood (hyperlipidaemia), however, lipid-lowering drugs may also be recommended.

Why they are used

Lipid-lowering drugs are generally prescribed only when dietary measures have failed to control hyperlipidaemia. The drugs may be given at an earlier stage to individuals at increased risk of atherosclerosis – such as diabetics and people already suffering from circulatory disorders. The drugs may remove existing atheroma in the blood vessels and prevent accumulation of new deposits.

For maximum benefit, these drugs are used in conjunction with a low-fat diet and a reduction in other risk factors such as obesity and smoking. The choice of drug depends on the type of lipid causing problems, so a full medical history, examination, and laboratory analysis of blood samples are needed before drug treatment is prescribed.

How they work

Cholesterol and triglycerides are two of the major fats in the blood. One or both may be raised, influencing the choice of lipid-lowering drug. Bile salts contain a large amount of cholesterol and are normally released into the bowel to aid digestion before being reabsorbed into the blood. Drugs that bind to bile salts reduce cholesterol levels by blocking their reabsorption, allowing them to be lost from the body.

Other drugs act on the liver. Fibrates and nicotinic acid and its derivatives can reduce the level of both cholesterol and triglycerides in the blood. Statins and probucol lower blood cholesterol. Fish oil preparations reduce blood triglycerides, but they may raise cholesterol levels.

Lipid-lowering drugs do not correct the underlying cause of raised levels of fat in the blood, so it is usually necessary to continue with diet and drug treatment indefinitely. Stopping treatment usually leads to a return of high blood lipid levels.

How they affect you

Because hyperlipidaemia and athero-sclerosis are usually without symptoms,

ACTION OF LIPID-LOWERING DRUGS

Lipid-lowering drugs reduce the levels of fats in the blood by interfering with the absorption of bile salts in the bowel, or by altering the way in which the liver converts fatty acids in the blood into different types of lipids.

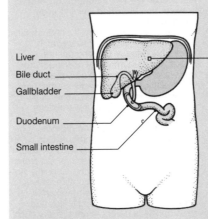

Liver
Bile duct
Gallbladder
Duodenum
Small intestine

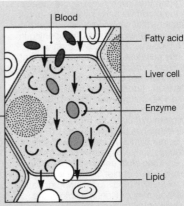

Blood
Fatty acid
Liver cell
Enzyme
Lipid

Drugs that act on the liver
Fatty acids in the blood are normally converted into lipids by enzyme activity in the liver (above). Several drugs alter the way fatty acids are taken into the liver cells and others alter the enzyme activity in the liver to prevent the manufacture of lipids.

Drugs that bind to bile salts
Bile is produced by the liver and released into the small intestine via the bile duct to aid digestion. Salts in the bile carry large amounts of cholesterol and are normally reabsorbed from the intestine into the bloodstream during digestion (right). Some drugs bind to bile salts in the intestine and prevent their reabsorption (far right). This action reduces the levels of bile salts in the blood, and triggers the liver to convert more cholesterol into bile salts, thus reducing blood cholesterol levels.

Before drug

After drug

Bile salts
Small intestine

Bile salt bound to drug
Blood vessel

you are unlikely to notice any short-term benefits from these drugs. Rather, the aim of treatment is to reduce long-term complications. There may be minor *side effects* from some of these drugs.

By increasing the amount of bile in the digestive tract, several drugs can cause gastrointestinal disturbances such as nausea and constipation or diarrhoea, especially at the start of treatment. The statin drugs appear to be well tolerated and are widely used to lower cholesterol levels when diet alone does not have sufficient effect.

Risks and special precautions

Drugs that bind to bile salts can limit absorption of some fat-soluble vitamins, so vitamin supplements may be needed. The fibrates can increase susceptibility to gallstones and occasionally upset the

balance of fats in the blood. Statins are used with caution in people with reduced kidney or liver function, and monitoring of blood samples is often advised.

COMMON DRUGS

Fibrates
Bezafibrate *
Ciprofibrate
Clofibrate
Fenofibrate
Gemfibrozil

Statins
Atorvastatin
Fluvastatin
Pravastatin
Simvastatin *

| * See Part 4 |

Drugs that bind to bile salts
Cholestyramine *
Colestipol
Ispaghula

Nicotinic acid and derivatives
Acipimox
Nicotinic acid

Other drugs acting on the liver
Omega-3 marine triglycerides

DRUGS THAT AFFECT BLOOD CLOTTING

When bleeding occurs from injury or surgery, the body normally acts swiftly to stem the flow by sealing the breaks in the blood vessels. This occurs in two stages – first when cells called platelets accumulate as a plug at the opening in the blood vessel wall, and then when these platelets produce chemicals that activate clotting factors in the blood to form a protein called fibrin. Vitamin K plays an important role in this process (see The clotting mechanism, below). An *enzyme* in the blood called plasmin ensures that clots are broken down when the injury has been repaired.

Some disorders interfere with this process, either preventing clot formation or creating clots uncontrollably. If the blood does not clot, there is a danger of excessive blood loss. Inappropriate development of clots may block the supply of blood to a vital organ.

Drugs used to promote blood clotting

Fibrin formation depends on the presence in the blood of several clotting-factor proteins. When Factor VIII is absent or at low levels, an inherited disease called haemophilia exists; the symptoms almost always appear only in males. Factor IX deficiency causes another bleeding condition called Christmas disease, named after the person in whom it was first identified. Lack of these clotting factors can lead to uncontrolled bleeding or excessive bruising following even minor injuries.

Regular drug treatment for haemophilia is not normally required. However, if severe bleeding or bruising occurs, a concentrated form of the missing factor, extracted from normal blood, may be injected in order to promote clotting and thereby halt bleeding. Injections may need to be repeated for several days after injury.

It is sometimes useful to promote blood clotting in non-haemophiliacs when bleeding is difficult to stop (for example, after surgery). In such cases, blood clots are sometimes stabilized by reducing the action of plasmin with an antifibrinolytic (or haemostatic) drug like tranexamic acid; this is also occasionally given to haemophiliacs before minor surgery such as tooth extraction.

A tendency to bleed may also occur as a consequence of vitamin K deficiency (see the box below).

Drugs used to prevent abnormal blood clotting

Blood clots normally form only as a response to injury. In some people, however, there is a tendency for clots to form in the blood vessels without apparent cause. Disturbed blood flow occurring as a result of the presence of fatty deposits – atheroma – inside the blood vessels increases the risk of the formation of this type of abnormal clot (or thrombus). In addition, a portion of a blood clot (known as an embolus) formed in response to injury or surgery may sometimes break off and be removed in the bloodstream. The likelihood of this happening is increased by long periods of little or no activity. When an abnormal clot forms, there is a risk that it may become lodged in a blood vessel, thereby blocking the blood supply to a vital organ such as the brain or heart.

THE CLOTTING MECHANISM

When a blood vessel wall is damaged, platelets accumulate at the site of damage and form a plug (1). Platelets clumped together release chemicals that activate blood clotting factors (2). These factors together with vitamin K act on a substance called fibrinogen and convert it to fibrin (3). Strands of fibrin become enmeshed in the platelet plug to form a blood clot (4).

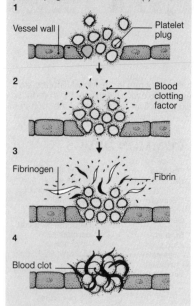

1

Vessel wall — Platelet plug

2

Blood clotting factor

3

Fibrinogen — Fibrin

4

Blood clot

VITAMIN K

Vitamin K is required for the production of several blood clotting factors. It is absorbed from the intestine in fats, but some diseases of the small intestine or pancreas cause fat to be poorly absorbed. As a result, the level of vitamin K in the circulation is low, causing impaired blood clotting. A similar problem sometimes occurs in newborn babies due to an absence of the vitamin. Injections of phytomenadione, a vitamin K preparation, are used to restore normal levels.

ACTION OF ANTIPLATELET DRUGS

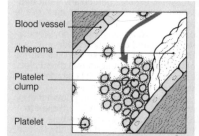

Blood vessel
Atheroma
Platelet clump
Platelet

Before drug
Where the blood flow is disrupted by an atheroma in the blood vessels, platelets tend to clump together.

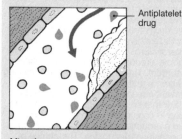

Antiplatelet drug

After drug
Antiplatelet drugs reduce the ability of platelets to stick together and so prevent clot formation.

Three main types of drugs are used to prevent and disperse clots: antiplatelet drugs, anticoagulants, and thrombolytics.

Antiplatelet drugs

Taken regularly by people with a tendency to form clots in the fast-flowing blood of the heart and arteries, these drugs are also given to prevent clots from forming after heart surgery. They reduce the tendency of platelets to stick together when blood flow is disrupted (see Action of antiplatelet drugs, above).

The most widely used antiplatelet drug is aspirin (see also Analgesics, p.80). This drug has an antiplatelet action even when given in much lower doses than would be necessary to reduce pain. In these low doses *adverse effects* that may occur when aspirin is given in pain-relieving doses are unlikely. Other antiplatelet drugs are clopidogrel and dipyridamole.

Anticoagulants

Anticoagulant drugs help to maintain normal blood flow in people who are at risk from clot formation. They can either prevent the formation of blood clots in the veins or stabilize an existing clot so that it does not break away and become a circulation-stopping embolism. All of the anticoagulant drugs reduce the activity of certain blood clotting factors, although the mode of action of each drug differs (see Action of anticoagulant drugs, right). However, these medicines do not dissolve the clots that have already formed: these clots are treated with thrombolytic drugs (below).

Anticoagulants fall into two groups: those that are given by intravenous injection and act immediately, and those that are given by mouth and take effect after a few days.

Intravenous anticoagulants

Heparin is the most widely used drug of this type and it is used mainly in hospital during or after surgery. In addition, it is also given during kidney dialysis to prevent clots from forming in the dialysis equipment. Because heparin cannot be taken by mouth, it is less suitable for long-term treatment in the home.

Heparin is sometimes given before starting regular treatment with one of the oral anticoagulants.

Versions of heparin, known as low molecular weight heparins (such as certoparin, dalteparin, enoxaparin, and tinzaparin), are as effective as ordinary heparin and their effects last longer.

Oral anticoagulants

Warfarin is the most widely used of the oral anticoagulants. These drugs are mainly prescribed to prevent the formation of clots in veins and in the chambers of the heart – they are less likely to prevent the formation of blood clots in arteries. Oral anticoagulants may be given following injury or surgery (in particular, heart valve replacement) when there is a high risk of embolism. They are also given long term as a preventative treatment to

ACTION OF ANTICOAGULANT DRUGS

Anticoagulant drugs block the action of certain blood clotting factors that convert fibrinogen into fibrin, the protein that binds platelets into blood clots.

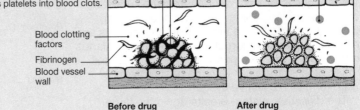

Before drug

After drug

people at risk from strokes. A common problem experienced with these drugs is that overdosage may lead to bleeding from the nose or gums, or in the urinary tract. For this reason, the dosage needs to be carefully calculated; regular blood tests are performed to ensure that the clotting mechanism is correctly adjusted.

The action of oral anticoagulant drugs may be affected by many other drugs and it may therefore be necessary to alter the dosage of anticoagulant when other drugs also need to be given. People who have been prescribed oral anticoagulants should carry a warning list of drugs that they should not be given. In particular, none of the anticoagulants should be taken together with aspirin except on the direction of a doctor.

Thrombolytics

Also known as fibrinolytics, these drugs are used to dissolve clots that have already formed. They are usually given in hospital intravenously to clear a blocked

blood vessel – for example, in coronary thrombosis. The sooner they are given after the start of symptoms, the more likely they are to reduce the size and severity of a heart attack. Thrombolytic drugs may be given either intravenously or directly into the blocked blood vessel. The main thrombolytics are streptokinase, anistreplase, and alteplase, all of which act by increasing the blood level of plasmin, the enzyme that breaks down fibrin (see Action of thrombolytic drugs, below). When given promptly, alteplase appears to be tolerated better than streptokinase and anistreplase.

The most common problems with use of these drugs are increased susceptibility to bleeding and bruising, and allergic reactions to streptokinase and anistreplase, often taking the form of rashes, breathing difficulty, or general discomfort. Once streptokinase has been administered, patients are given a card indicating this, because further treatment with the same drug is generally not advised.

ACTION OF THROMBOLYTIC DRUGS

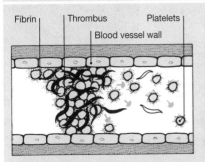

Before drug
When platelets accumulate in a blood vessel and are reinforced by strands of fibrin, the resultant blood clot, which is known as a thrombus, cannot be dissolved either by antiplatelet drugs or anticoagulant drugs.

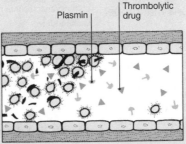

After drug
Thrombolytic drugs boost the action of plasmin, an enzyme in the blood that breaks up the strands of fibrin that bind the clot together. This allows the accumulated platelets to disperse and restores normal blood flow.

COMMON DRUGS

Blood clotting factors	**Heparin-like anticoagulants**
Clopidogrel *	Certoparin
Factor VIIa	Dalteparin
Factor VIII	Danaparoid
Factor IX	Enoxaparin *
	Heparin *
Antifibrinolytic or haemostatic drugs	Tinzaparin
Aprotinin	**Thrombolytic drugs**
Etamsylate	Alteplase
Tranexamic acid	Anistreplase
	Reteplase
Vitamin K	Streptokinase *
Phytomenadione	Urokinase
Antiplatelet drugs	**Oral anti-coagulants**
Aspirin *	Nicoumalone
Dipyridamole *	Warfarin *

* See Part 4

GASTROINTESTINAL TRACT

The gastrointestinal tract, also known as the digestive or alimentary tract, is the pathway through which food passes as it is processed to enable the nutrients it contains to be absorbed for use by the body. It consists of the mouth, oesophagus, stomach, duodenum, small intestine, large intestine (including the colon and rectum), and anus. In addition, a number of other organs are involved in the digestion of food: the salivary glands in the mouth, the liver, pancreas, and gallbladder. These organs, together with the gastrointestinal tract, form the digestive system.

The digestive system breaks down the large, complex chemicals – proteins, carbohydrates, and fats – present in the food we eat into simpler molecules that can be used by the body (see also Nutrition, p.148). Undigested or indigestible material, together with some of the body's waste products, pass to the large intestine, and, when a sufficient mass of such matter has accumulated, it is expelled from the body as faeces.

What can go wrong
Inflammation of the lining of the stomach or intestine (gastroenteritis) is usually the result of an infection or parasitic infestation. Damage may also be done by the inappropriate production of digestive juices, leading to minor complaints like acidity and major disorders like peptic ulcers. The lining of the intestine can be damaged by abnormal functioning of the immune system (inflammatory bowel disease). The rectum and anus can become painful and irritated by damage to the lining, tears in the skin at the opening of the anus (anal fissure), or enlarged veins (haemorrhoids).

The most frequently experienced gastrointestinal complaints – constipation, diarrhoea, and irritable bowel syndrome – usually occur when something disrupts the normal muscle contractions that propel food residue through the bowel.

Why drugs are used
Many drugs for gastrointestinal disorders are taken by mouth and act directly on the digestive tract without first entering the bloodstream. Such drugs include certain antibiotics and other drugs used to treat infestations. Some antacids for peptic ulcers and excess stomach acidity, and the bulk-forming agents for constipation and diarrhoea, also pass through the system unabsorbed.

However, for many disorders, drugs with a *systemic* effect are required, including anti-ulcer drugs, *opioid* antidiarrhoeal drugs, and some of the drugs for inflammatory bowel disease.

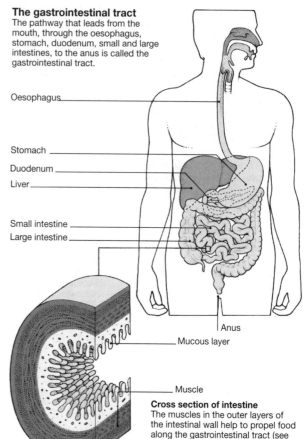

The gastrointestinal tract
The pathway that leads from the mouth, through the oesophagus, stomach, duodenum, small and large intestines, to the anus is called the gastrointestinal tract.

Oesophagus

Stomach

Duodenum

Liver

Small intestine

Large intestine

Anus

Mucous layer

Muscle

Cross section of intestine
The muscles in the outer layers of the intestinal wall help to propel food along the gastrointestinal tract (see facing page). The mucous lining of the intestine allows nutrients to be absorbed into the bloodstream.

Pancreas
The pancreas produces *enzymes* that digest fats, carbohydrates, and proteins into simpler substances. Pancreatic juices neutralize acidity of the stomach contents.

Gallbladder
Bile produced by the liver is stored in the gallbladder and released into the small intestine. Bile assists the digestion of fats by reducing them to smaller units that are more easily acted upon by digestive enzymes.

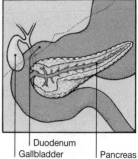

Duodenum

Gallbladder

Pancreas

MAJOR DRUG GROUPS

Antacids
Anti-ulcer drugs
Antidiarrhoeal drugs
Laxatives
Drugs for inflammatory
  bowel disease

Drugs for rectal and
  anal disorders
Drug treatment
  for gallstones

The lining of the gastrointestinal tract

The lining of the different sections of the gastrointestinal tract varies according to the function of that part, depending, for example, on whether its principal role is to secrete digestive juices or to absorb nutrients.

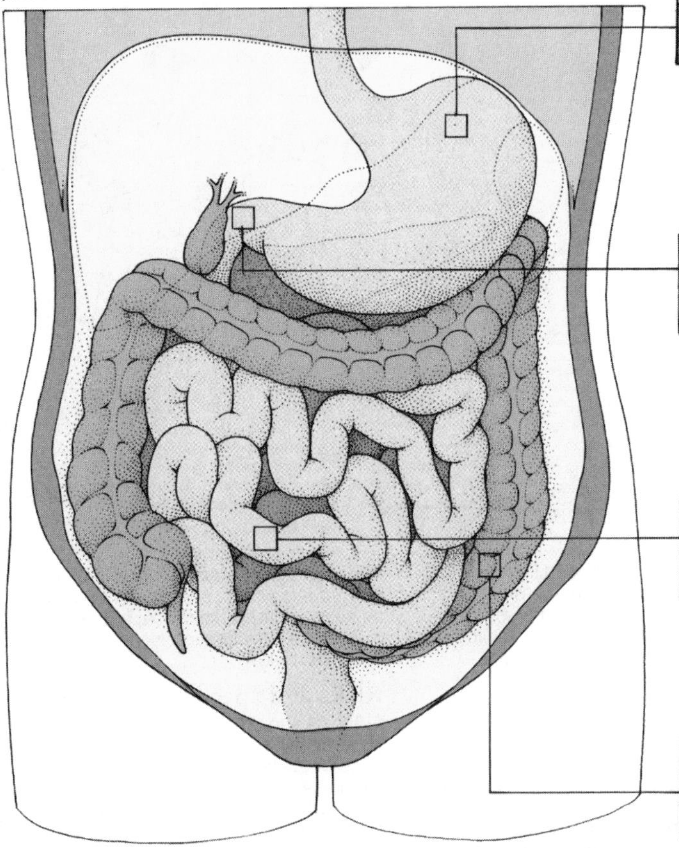

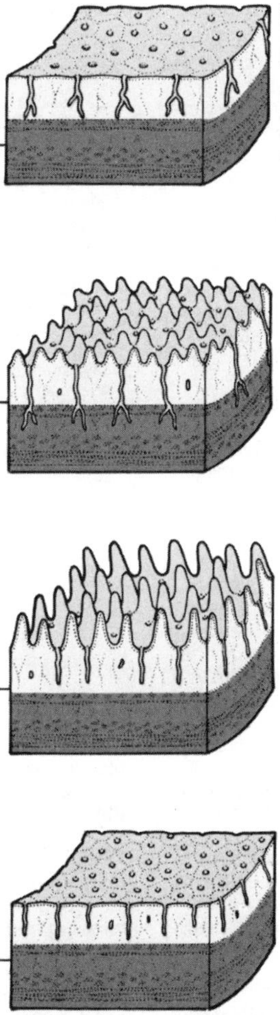

Stomach

The stomach stores food and passes it to the intestine. The lining of the stomach releases gastric juice that partly digests food. The stomach wall continuously produces thick mucus that forms a protective coating.

Duodenum

This is the tube that connects the stomach to the intestine. Its lining may be damaged by excess acid produced by the stomach.

Small intestine

The small intestine is a long tube in which food is broken down by digestive juices. The mucous lining is covered with tiny projections called villi that provide a large surface area through which the products of digestion are absorbed into the bloodstream.

Large intestine

The large intestine receives both undigested food and indigestible material from the small intestine. Water and mineral salts pass through the lining into the bloodstream.

MOVEMENT OF FOOD THROUGH THE GASTROINTESTINAL TRACT

Food is propelled through the gastrointestinal tract by rhythmic waves of muscular contraction called peristalsis. The illustration shows how peristaltic contractions of the bowel wall push food through the intestine.

Muscle contraction in the tract is controlled by the autonomic nervous system (p.79) and is therefore easily disrupted by drugs that either stimulate or inhibit the activity of the autonomic nervous system. Excessive peristaltic action may cause diarrhoea; slowed peristalsis may cause constipation.

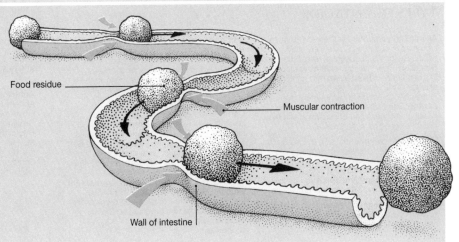

Food residue

Muscular contraction

Wall of intestine

ANTACIDS

Digestive juices in the stomach contain acid and *enzymes* that break down food before it passes into the intestine. The wall of the stomach is normally protected from the action of digestive acid by a layer of mucus that is constantly secreted by the stomach lining. Problems arise when the stomach lining is damaged or too much acid is produced and eats away at the mucous layer.

Excess acid that leads to discomfort, commonly referred to as indigestion, may result from anxiety, overeating or eating certain foods, coffee, alcohol, or smoking. Some drugs, notably aspirin and non-steroidal anti-inflammatory drugs, can irritate the stomach lining and even cause ulcers to develop.

Antacids are used to neutralize acid and thus relieve pain. They are simple chemical compounds that are mildly alkaline and some also act as chemical buffers. Their chalky taste is often disguised with flavourings.

Why they are used

Antacids may be needed when simple remedies (a change in diet or a glass of milk) fail to relieve indigestion. They are especially useful one to three hours after meals to neutralize after-meal acid surge.

Doctors prescribe these drugs in order to relieve dyspepsia (pain in the chest or upper abdomen caused by or aggravated by acid) in disorders such as inflammation or ulceration of the oesophagus, stomach lining, and duodenum. Antacids usually relieve pain resulting from ulcers in the oesophagus, stomach, or duodenum within a few minutes. Regular treatment with antacids reduces the acidity of the stomach, thereby encouraging the healing of any ulcers that may have formed.

How they work

By neutralizing stomach acid, antacids prevent inflammation, relieve pain, and

ACTION OF ANTACIDS

Excess acid in the stomach may eat away at the layer of mucus that protects the stomach. When this occurs, or when the mucous lining is damaged, for example, by an ulcer, stomach acid comes into contact with the underlying tissues, causing pain and inflammation (right). Antacids combine with stomach acid to reduce the acidity of the digestive juices. This helps to prevent pain and inflammation, and allows the mucous layer to repair itself (far right).

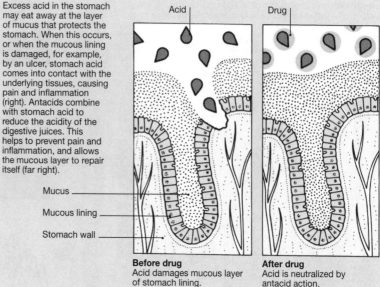

Mucus
Mucous lining
Stomach wall

Before drug
Acid damages mucous layer of stomach lining.

After drug
Acid is neutralized by antacid action.

allow the mucous layer and lining to mend. When used in the treatment of ulcers, they prevent acid from attacking damaged stomach lining and so allow the ulcer to heal.

How they affect you

If antacids are taken according to the instructions, they are usually effective in relieving abdominal discomfort caused by acid. The speed of action, dependent on the ability to neutralize acid, varies. Their duration of action also varies; the short-acting drugs may have to be taken quite frequently.

Although most antacids have few serious *side effects* when used only occasionally, some may cause diarrhoea, and others may cause constipation (see Types of antacids, below).

Risks and special precautions

Antacids should not be taken to prevent abdominal pain on a regular basis except under medical supervision, as they may suppress the symptoms of stomach cancer. Your doctor is likely to want to arrange tests such as endoscopy or barium X-rays before prescribing long-term treatment.

All antacids can interfere with the absorption of other drugs. For this reason, if you are taking a prescription medicine, you should check with your doctor before taking an antacid.

TYPES OF ANTACIDS

Aluminium compounds These drugs have a prolonged action and are widely used, especially for the treatment of indigestion and dyspepsia. They may cause constipation, but this is often countered by combining this type of antacid with one that contains magnesium. Aluminium compounds can interfere with the absorption of phosphate from the diet, causing weakness and bone damage if taken in high doses over a long period.

Magnesium compounds Like the aluminium compounds, these have a prolonged action. In large doses they can cause diarrhoea, and in people who have impaired kidney function, a high blood magnesium level may build up, causing weakness, lethargy, and drowsiness.

Sodium bicarbonate This antacid, the only sodium compound used as an antacid, acts quickly, but its effect soon passes. It reacts

with stomach acids to produce gas, which may cause bloating and belching. Sodium bicarbonate is not advised for people with heart or kidney disease, as it can lead to the accumulation of water (oedema) in the legs and lungs, or serious changes in the acid-base balance of the blood.

Combined preparations Antacids may be combined with other substances called alginates and antifoaming agents. Alginates are intended to float on the contents of the stomach and produce a neutralizing layer to subdue acid that can otherwise rise into the oesophagus, causing heartburn.

Antifoaming agents (usually dimeticone) are intended to relieve flatulence. In some preparations a local anaesthetic is combined with the antacid to relieve discomfort in oesophagitis. The value of these additives is dubious.

COMMON DRUGS

Antacids	Antifoaming
Aluminium	**agent**
hydroxide *	Dimeticone
Calcium carbonate	
Hydrotalcite	
Magnesium	
hydroxide *	
Sodium	
bicarbonate *	

* See Part 4

ANTI-ULCER DRUGS

Normally, the linings of the oesophagus, stomach, and duodenum are protected from the irritant action of stomach acids or bile by a thin covering layer of mucus. If this is damaged, or if large amounts of stomach acid are formed, the underlying tissue may become eroded, causing a peptic ulcer. An ulcer often leads to abdominal pain, vomiting, and changes in appetite. The most common type of ulcer occurs just beyond the stomach, in the duodenum. The exact cause of peptic ulcers is not understood, but a number of risk factors have been identified, including heavy smoking, the regular use of aspirin or similar drugs, and family history. An organism found in almost all patients who have peptic ulcers, *Helicobacter pylori*, is now believed to be the main causative agent.

The symptoms caused by ulcers may be relieved by an antacid (see facing page), but healing is slow. The usual treatment is with an anti-ulcer drug, such as an H_2 blocker, a proton pump inhibitor, bismuth, or sucralfate, often combined with antibiotics to eradicate the *Helicobacter pylori* infection which seems to cause many ulcers.

Why they are used

Anti-ulcer drugs are used to relieve symptoms and heal the ulcer. Untreated ulcers may erode blood vessel walls or perforate the stomach or duodenum.

Until recently, drugs could heal ulcers but not cure them. However, eradication of *Helicobacter pylori* by a proton pump inhibitor, or rantidine bismuth citrate combined with two antibiotics (triple therapy), may provide a cure in one to two weeks. Surgery is reserved for complications such as obstruction, perforation, haemorrhage, and when there is a possibility of cancer.

How they work

Drugs protect ulcers from the action of stomach acid, allowing the tissue to heal. H_2 blockers, misoprostol, and proton pump inhibitors reduce the amount of acid released; bismuth and sucralfate form a protective coating over the ulcer. Bismuth also has an antibacterial effects. It is combined with an H_2 blocker in ranitidine bismuth citrate.

How they affect you

These drugs begin to reduce pain in a few hours and usually allow the ulcer to heal in four to eight weeks. They produce few side effects, although H_2 blockers can cause confusion in the elderly. Bismuth and sucralfate may cause constipation; misoprostol, diarrhoea; and proton pump inhibitors, either constipation or diarrhoea. Triple therapy is given for one or two weeks. If *Helicobacter pylori* is eradicated, maintenance therapy should not be necessary. Sucralfate is usually prescribed for up to 12 weeks, and bismuth and misoprostol for four to six weeks. As they may mask symptoms of stomach cancer, H_2 blockers and proton pump inhibitors are normally prescribed only when tests have ruled out this disorder.

ACTION OF ANTI-ULCER DRUGS

Proton pump inhibitors

Acid secretion by the cells lining the stomach depends on an *enzyme* system (also known as the proton pump) that transports hydrogen ions across the cell walls. Omeprazole, lansoprazole, and similar drugs work by blocking the proton pump. They can stop stomach acid production until a new supply of the enzyme can be made by the body and, therefore, have a long duration of action.

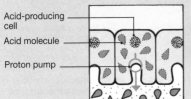

Acid-producing cell
Acid molecule
Proton pump

The proton pump
This enzyme system transports hydrogen ions across the cell wall into the stomach, thereby stimulating acid secretion.

Acid-producing cell
Acid molecule
Proton pump inhibitor

The action of proton pump inhibitors
Proton pump inhibitors block the enzyme system, stopping the transport of hydrogen ions and, thus, the secretion of acid.

H_2 blockers

Histamine is a chemical released by mast cells (see Allergies, p.123) that can produce a number of effects in different parts of the body. In the stomach, histamine stimulates H_2 receptors, causing acid production. To control stomach acid production, a class of antihistamine drugs was developed that acts by blocking the H_2 receptors. These drugs are known as H_2 blockers to distinguish them from antihistamines used for allergic disorders (see p.124), which are sometimes called H_1 blockers because they block H_1 receptors.

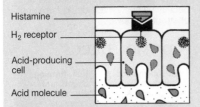

Histamine
H_2 receptor
Acid-producing cell
Acid molecule

The action of histamine on the stomach
Histamine binds to specialized H_2 receptors and stimulates acid-producing cells in the stomach wall to release acid.

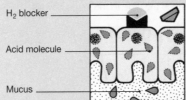

H_2 blocker
Acid molecule
Mucus

The action of H_2 blockers
H_2 blockers occupy H_2 receptors, preventing histamine from triggering the production of acid. This allows the mucous lining to heal.

Sucralfate and bismuth

Sucralfate forms a coating over the ulcer, protecting it from the action of stomach acid and allowing it to heal. Bismuth may stimulate production of *prostaglandins* or bicarbonate, and also kills the bacteria that are thought to cause most peptic ulcers. Bismuth is used in triple therapy with antibiotics to cure ulcers.

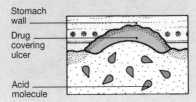

Stomach wall
Drug covering ulcer
Acid molecule

COMMON DRUGS

Proton pump inhibitors	Other drugs
Lansoprazole	Antacids (see p.108)
Omeprazole ✱	Antibiotics (see p. 128)
Pantoprazole	Bismuth
Rabeprazole	Carbenoxolone
	Misoprostol ✱
H_2 blockers	Ranitidine bismuth
Cimetidine ✱	citrate
Famotidine	Sucralfate ✱
Nizatidine	
Ranitidine ✱	

✱ See Part 4

ANTIDIARRHOEAL DRUGS

Diarrhoea is an increase in the fluidity and frequency of bowel movements. In some cases diarrhoea protects the body from harmful substances in the intestine by hastening their removal. The most common causes are viral infection, food poisoning, and parasites. But it also occurs as a symptom of other illnesses. It can be a *side effect* of some drugs and may follow radiation therapy for cancer. Diarrhoea may also be caused by anxiety.

An attack of diarrhoea usually clears up quickly without medical attention. The best treatment is to abstain from food and to drink plenty of clear fluids. Rehydration solutions containing sugar as well as potassium and sodium salts are widely recommended for preventing dehydration and chemical imbalances, particularly in children. You should consult your doctor if: the condition does not improve within 48 hours; the diarrhoea contains blood; severe abdominal pain and vomiting are present; you have just returned from a foreign country; or if the diarrhoea occurs in a small child or an elderly person.

Severe diarrhoea can impair absorption of drugs, and anyone taking a prescribed drug should seek advice from a doctor or pharmacist. A woman taking oral contraceptives may need additional contraceptive measures (see p.161).

The main types of drugs used to relieve non-specific diarrhoea are *opioids*, and bulk-forming and *adsorbent* agents. Antispasmodic drugs may also be used to relieve accompanying pain (see Drugs for irritable bowel syndrome, below).

Why they are used

An antidiarrhoeal drug may be prescribed to provide relief when simple remedies are not effective, and once it is certain the diarrhoea is neither infectious nor *toxic*.

Opioid drugs are the most effective antidiarrhoeals. They are used when the diarrhoea is severe and debilitating. The bulking and adsorbent agents have a

ACTION OF ANTIDIARRHOEAL DRUGS

Opioid antidiarrhoeals
These drugs reduce the transmission of nerve signals to the intestinal muscles, thus reducing muscle contraction. This allows more time for water to be absorbed from the food residue and therefore reduces the fluidity as well as the frequency of bowel movements.

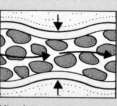

Bowel contents
Bowel wall

Before drug
Rapid bowel contraction prevents water from being absorbed.

After drug
Slowed bowel action allows more water to be absorbed.

Bulk-forming agents
These preparations contain particles that swell up as they absorb water from the large intestine. This makes the faeces firmer and less fluid. It is thought that bulk-forming agents may absorb irritants and harmful chemicals along with excess water.

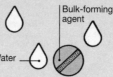

Bulk-forming agent

Water

Water is attracted by bulk-forming agent.

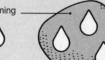

Bulk-forming agent swells as water is absorbed.

milder effect and are often used when it is necessary to regulate bowel action over a prolonged period – for example, in people with colostomies or ileostomies.

How they work

Opioids decrease the muscles' propulsive activity so that faecal matter passes more slowly through the bowel.

Bulk-forming agents and adsorbents absorb water and irritants present in the bowel, thereby producing larger and firmer stools at less frequent intervals.

How they affect you

Drugs that are used to treat diarrhoea reduce the urge to move the bowels.

Opioids and antispasmodics may relieve abdominal pain. All antidiarrhoeals may cause constipation if used in excess.

Risks and special precautions

Used in relatively low doses for a limited period of time, the opioid drugs are unlikely to produce adverse effects. However, these drugs should be used with caution when diarrhoea is caused by an infection, since they may slow the elimination of microorganisms from the intestine. All antidiarrhoeals should be taken with plenty of water. It is important not to take a bulk-forming agent together with an opioid or antispasmodic drug, because a bulky mass could form and obstruct the bowel.

DRUGS FOR IRRITABLE BOWEL SYNDROME

Irritable bowel syndrome is a common stress-related condition in which the normal coordinated waves of muscular contraction responsible for moving the bowel contents smoothly through the intestines become strong and irregular, often causing pain, and associated with diarrhoea or constipation.

Symptoms are often relieved by adjusting the amount of fibre in the diet, although medication may also be required. Bulk-forming agents may be given to regulate the consistency of the bowel contents. If pain is severe, an antispasmodic drug may be prescribed. These *anticholinergic* drugs reduce the transmission of nerve signals to the bowel wall, thus preventing spasm. Tricyclic antidepressants are sometimes used because their anticholinergic action has a calming effect on the bowel.

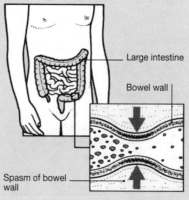

Large intestine

Bowel wall

Spasm of bowel wall

COMMON DRUGS

Antispasmodics	**Bulk-forming**
Atropine ✻	**agents and**
Dicyclomine ✻	**adsorbents**
Hyoscine ✻	Ispaghula
	Kaolin
Opioids	Methylcellulose ✻
Codeine ✻	
Diphenoxylate ✻	
Loperamide ✻	

✻ See Part 4

LAXATIVES

When your bowels do not move as frequently as usual and the faeces are hard and difficult to pass, you are suffering from constipation. The most common cause is lack of sufficient fibre in your diet; fibre supplies the bulk that makes the faeces soft and easy to pass. The simplest remedy is more fluid and a diet that contains plenty of foods that are high in fibre, but laxative drugs may also be used.

Ignoring the urge to defecate can also cause constipation, because the faeces become dry, hard to pass, and too small to stimulate the muscles that propel them through the intestine.

Certain drugs may be constipating: for example, *opioid* analgesics, tricyclic antidepressants, and antacids containing aluminium. Some diseases, such as hypo-thyroidism (underactive thyroid gland) and scleroderma (a rare disorder of connective tissue characterized by the hardening of the skin), can also lead to constipation.

The onset of constipation in a middle-aged or elderly person may be an early symptom of bowel cancer. Consult your doctor about any persistent change in bowel habit.

Why they are used

Since prolonged use is harmful, laxatives should be used for very short periods only. They may prevent pain and straining in people suffering from either hernias or haemorrhoids (p.113). Doctors may prescribe laxatives for the same reason after childbirth or abdominal surgery. Laxatives are also used to clear the bowel before investigative procedures such as colonoscopy. They may be prescribed for patients who are elderly or bedridden because lack of exercise can often lead to constipation.

How they work

Laxatives act on the large intestine – by increasing the speed with which faecal matter passes through the bowel, or increasing its bulk and/or water content.

ACTION OF LAXATIVES

Bulk-forming agents
Taken after a meal, these agents are not absorbed as they pass through the digestive tract. They contain particles that absorb many times their own volume of water. By doing so, they increase the bulk of the bowel movements and thus encourage bowel action.

Stimulant laxatives
These laxatives are thought to encourage bowel movements by acting on nerve endings in the wall of the intestines that trigger contraction of the intestinal muscles. This speeds the passage of faecal matter through the large intestine, allowing less time for water to be absorbed. Thus faeces become more liquid and are passed more frequently.

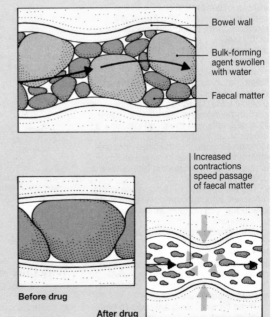

Bowel wall

Bulk-forming agent swollen with water

Faecal matter

Increased contractions speed passage of faecal matter

Before drug

After drug

Stimulants cause the bowel muscles to contract, increasing the speed at which faecal matter goes through the intestine. Bulk-forming laxatives absorb water in the bowel, thereby increasing the volume of faeces, making them softer and easier to pass. Lactulose also causes fluid to accumulate in the intestine. Osmotic laxatives act by keeping water in the bowel, and thereby make the bowel movements softer. This also increases the bulk of the faeces and enables them to be passed more easily. Lubricant liquid paraffin preparations make bowel movements softer and easier to pass

without increasing their bulk. Prolonged use can interfere with absorption of some essential vitamins.

Risks and special precautions

Laxatives can cause diarrhoea if taken in overdose, and constipation if overused. The most serious risk of prolonged use of most laxatives is developing dependence on the laxative for normal bowel action. Use of a laxative should therefore be discontinued as soon as normal bowel movements have been re-established. Children should not be given laxatives except in special circumstances on the advice of a doctor.

TYPES OF LAXATIVES

Bulk-forming agents These are relatively slow acting but are less likely than other laxatives to interfere with normal bowel action. Only after consultation with your doctor should they be taken for constipation accompanied by abdominal pain because of the risk of intestinal obstruction.

Stimulant (contact) laxatives These are for occasional use when other treatments have failed or when rapid onset of action is needed. Stimulant laxatives should not normally be used for longer than a week as they can cause abdominal cramps and diarrhoea.

Softening agents These are often used when hard bowel movements cause pain on defecation – for example, when haemorrhoids

are present, or after surgery when straining must be avoided. Liquid paraffin was once popular but can cause *side effects* and has generally been replaced by sodium docusate. and for the relief of faecal impaction (blockage of the bowel by faecal material).

Osmotic laxatives Salts such as Epsom salts (magnesium sulphate) may be used to evacuate the bowel before surgery or investigative procedures. They are not normally used for the long-term relief of constipation because they can cause chemical imbalances in the blood.

Lactulose is an alternative to bulk-forming laxatives for the long-term treatment of chronic constipation. It may cause stomach cramps and flatulence but is usually well tolerated.

COMMON DRUGS

Stimulant laxatives	Softening agents
Bisacodyl	Sodium docusate
Co-danthramer	Liquid paraffin
Co-danthrusate	
Docusate	**Osmotic laxatives**
Senna	Lactulose ✳
	Magnesium citrate
Bulk-forming agents	Magnesium hydroxide ✳
Ispaghula	Magnesium sulphate
Methylcellulose ✳	Sodium acid phosphate
Sodium alginate	

✳ See Part 4

DRUGS FOR INFLAMMATORY BOWEL DISEASE

Inflammatory bowel disease is the term used for disorders in which inflammation of the intestinal wall causes recurrent attacks of abdominal pain, general feelings of ill-health, and frequently diarrhoea, with blood and mucus present in the faeces. Loss of appetite and poor absorption of food may often result in weight loss.

There are two main types of inflammatory bowel disease: Crohn's disease and ulcerative colitis. In Crohn's disease (also called regional enteritis), any part of the digestive tract may become inflamed, although the small intestine is the most commonly affected site. In ulcerative colitis, it is the large intestine (colon) that becomes inflamed and ulcerated, often producing bloodstained diarrhoea (see right).

The exact cause of these disorders is unknown, although stress-related, dietary, infectious, and genetic factors may all be important.

Establishing a proper diet and a less stressful lifestyle may help to alleviate these conditions. Bed rest during attacks is also advisable. However, these simple measures alone do not usually relieve or prevent attacks, and drug treatment is often necessary.

Three types of drug are used to treat inflammatory bowel disease: corticosteroids (p.141), immunosuppressants (p.156), and aminosalicylate anti-inflammatory drugs such as sulfasalazine. Nutritional supplements (used especially for Crohn's disease) and antidiarrhoeal drugs (p.110) may also be used. Surgery to remove damaged areas of the intestine may be needed in severe cases.

SITES OF BOWEL INFLAMMATION

The two main types of bowel inflammation are ulcerative colitis and Crohn's disease. The former occurs in the large intestine. Crohn's disease can occur anywhere along the gastrointestinal tract, but it most often affects the small intestine.

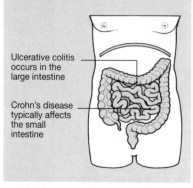

Ulcerative colitis occurs in the large intestine

Crohn's disease typically affects the small intestine

Why they are used

Drugs cannot cure inflammatory bowel disease, but treatment is needed, not only to control symptoms, but also to prevent complications, especially severe anaemia and perforation of the intestinal wall. Aminosalicylates are used to treat acute attacks of ulcerative colitis and Crohn's disease, and they may be continued as maintenance therapy. People who have severe bowel inflammation are usually prescribed a course of corticosteroids, particularly during a sudden flare-up.

Once the disease is under control, an immunosuppressant drug may be prescribed to prevent a relapse.

How they work

Corticosteroids and sulfasalazine damp down the inflammatory process, allowing the damaged tissue to recover. They act in different ways to prevent migration of white blood cells into the bowel wall, which may be responsible in part for the inflammation of the bowel.

How they affect you

Taken to treat attacks, these drugs relieve symptoms within a few days, and general health improves gradually over a period of a few weeks. Aminosalicylates usually provide long-term relief from the symptoms of inflammatory bowel disease.

Treatment with an immunosuppressant drug may take several months before the condition improves; and regular blood tests to monitor possible drug *side effects* are often required.

Risks and special precautions

Immunosuppressant and corticosteroid drugs can cause serious adverse effects and are only prescribed when potential benefits outweigh the risks involved.

The side effects of corticosteroids can be reduced by the use of budesonide in a new, topical preparation which releases the drug at the site of inflammation.

It is important to continue taking these drugs as instructed because stopping them abruptly may cause a sudden flare-up of the disorder. Doctors usually supervise a gradual reduction in dosage when such drugs are stopped, even when they are given as a short course for an attack. Antidiarrhoeal drugs should not be taken on a routine basis because they may mask signs of deterioration or cause sudden bowel dilation or rupture.

How they are administered

Antidiarrhoeal drugs are usually taken in the form of tablets, although mild ulcerative colitis in the last part of the large intestine may be treated with suppositories or an enema containing a corticosteroid or aminosalicylate.

ACTION OF DRUGS IN ULCERATIVE COLITIS

The most common form of inflammatory bowel disease is ulcerative colitis. It affects the large intestine, causing ulceration of the lining and producing pain and violent blood-stained diarrhoea. It is often treated with corticosteroids and aminosalicylates.

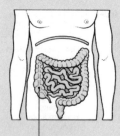

Large intestine

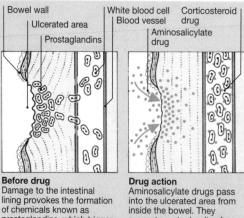

Bowel wall

Ulcerated area

Prostaglandins

White blood cell

Blood vessel

Corticosteroid drug

Aminosalicylate drug

Before drug
Damage to the intestinal lining provokes the formation of chemicals known as prostaglandins, which trigger the migration of white blood cells into the ulcerated area. The accumulation of white blood cells in the bowel wall causes inflammation.

Drug action
Aminosalicylate drugs pass into the ulcerated area from inside the bowel. They prevent prostaglandins from forming in the damaged tissue. Corticosteroids in the bloodstream reduce the ability of white blood cells to pass into the bowel wall.

COMMON DRUGS

Corticosteroids
Budesonide *
Hydrocortisone *
Prednisolone *

Immunosuppressants
Azathioprine *
Mercaptopurine *
Methotrexate *

Aminosalicylates
Balsalazide
Mesalazine *
Olsalazine
Sulfasalazine *

| * See Part 4 |

DRUGS FOR RECTAL AND ANAL DISORDERS

The most common disorder affecting the rectum (the last part of the large intestine) and anus (the opening from the rectum) is haemorrhoids, commonly known as piles. They occur when haemorrhoidal veins become swollen or irritated, often as a result of prolonged local pressure such as that caused by a pregnancy or a job requiring long hours of sitting. Haemorrhoids may cause irritation and pain, especially on defecation. The condition is aggravated by constipation and straining during defecation. In some cases haemorrhoids may bleed and occasionally clots form in the swollen veins, leading to severe pain, a condition called thrombosed haemorrhoids.

Other common disorders affecting the anus include anal fissure (painful cracks in the anus) and pruritus ani (itching around the anus). Anal disorders of all kinds occur less frequently in people who have soft, bulky stools.

A number of both over-the-counter and prescription-only preparations are available for the relief of such disorders.

Why they are used

Preparations for relief of haemorrhoids and anal discomfort fall into two main groups: creams or suppositories that act locally to relieve inflammation and irritation, and measures that relieve constipation, which contributes to the formation of, and the discomfort from, haemorrhoids and anal fissure.

Preparations from the first group often contain a soothing agent with *antiseptic*, *astringent*, or *vasoconstrictor* properties. Ingredients of this type include zinc oxide, bismuth, hamamelis (witch hazel), Peru balsam, and ephedrine. Some of these products also include a mild local anaesthetic (see p.80) such as lignocaine.

DISORDERS OF THE RECTUM AND ANUS

The rectum and anus form the last part of the digestive tract. Common conditions affecting the area include swelling of the veins around the anus (haemorrhoids), cracks in the anus (anal fissure), and inflammation or irritation of the anus and surrounding area (pruritus ani).

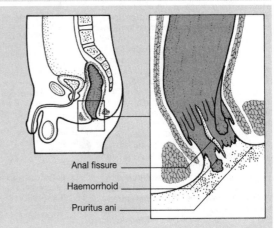

Anal fissure

Haemorrhoid

Pruritus ani

In some cases a doctor may prescribe an ointment containing a corticosteroid to relieve inflammation around the anus (see Topical corticosteroids, p.174).

People who suffer from haemorrhoids or anal fissure are generally advised to include in their diets plenty of fluids and fibre-rich foods, such as fresh fruits, vegetables, and whole grain products, both to prevent constipation and to ease defecation. A mild bulk-forming or softening laxative may also be prescribed (see p.111).

Neither of these treatments can shrink large haemorrhoids, although they may provide relief while anal fissures heal naturally. Severe, persistently painful haemorrhoids that continue to be troublesome in spite of these measures

may need to be removed surgically or, more commonly, by banding with specially applied small rubber bands (see below left).

How they affect you

The treatments described above usually relieve discomfort, especially during defecation. Most people experience no adverse effects, although preparations containing local anaesthetics may cause irritation or even a rash in the anal area. It is rare for ingredients in locally acting preparations to be absorbed into the body in sufficient quantities to cause generalized *side effects*.

The main risk is that self-treatment of haemorrhoids may delay diagnosis of bowel cancer. It is therefore always wise to consult your doctor if symptoms of haemorrhoids are present, especially if you have noticed bleeding from the rectum or a change in bowel habits.

SITES OF DRUG ACTION

The illustration below shows how and where drugs for the treatment of rectal disorders act to relieve symptoms.

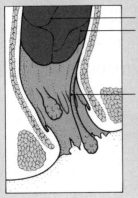

Faecal matter

Laxatives
These act in the large intestine to soften and ease the passage of faeces.

Creams and suppositories
Vasoconstrictors and astringents reduce the swelling and restrict blood supply, helping to relieve haemorrhoids. Local anaesthetics numb pain signals from the anus. Topical corticosteroids relieve inflammation.

Banding treatment
A small rubber band is applied tightly to a haemorrhoid, thereby blocking off its blood supply. The haemorrhoid will eventually wither away.

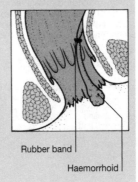

Rubber band

Haemorrhoid

COMMON DRUGS

Soothing and astringent agents Aluminium acetate Bismuth Peru balsam Zinc oxide	**Topical corticosteroids** Hydrocortisone ✳ **Local anaesthetics** (see p.80)
Vasoconstrictors Ephedrine ✳	**Laxatives** (see p.111)

✳ See Part 4

DRUG TREATMENT FOR GALLSTONES

The formation of gallstones is the most common disorder of the gallbladder, which is the storage and concentrating unit for bile, a digestive juice produced by the liver. During digestion, bile passes from the gallbladder via the bile duct into the small intestine, where it assists in the digestion of fats. Bile is composed of several ingredients, including bile acids, bile salts, and bile pigments. It also has a significant amount of cholesterol, which is dissolved in bile acid. If the amount of cholesterol in the bile increases, or if the amount of bile acid is reduced, a proportion of the cholesterol cannot remain dissolved, and under certain circumstances this excess accumulates in the gallbladder as gallstones.

Gallstones may be present in the gallbladder for years without causing symptoms. However, if they become lodged in the bile duct they cause pain and block the flow of bile. If the bile accumulates in the blood, it may cause an attack of jaundice, or the gallbladder may become infected and inflamed.

Drug treatment with chenodeoxycholic acid and ursodeoxycholic acid is only effective against stones made principally of cholesterol (some contain other substances), and even these take many months to dissolve. Therefore, surgery and ultrasound have become widely used, as techniques have improved. Surgery and ultrasound treatments are always used to remove stones blocking the bile duct.

Why they are used

Even if you have not experienced any symptoms, once gallstones have been diagnosed your doctor may advise treatment because of the risk of blockage of the bile duct. Drug treatment is usually preferred to surgery for small cholesterol stones when there is a possibility that surgery may be risky.

How they work

Chenodeoxycholic acid is a substance that is naturally present in bile. It acts on chemical processes in the liver to regulate the amount of cholesterol in the blood by controlling the amount that passes into the bile. Once the cholesterol level in the bile is reduced, the bile acids are able to start dissolving the stones in the gallbladder. To achieve maximum effect,

DIGESTION OF FATS

The digestion of fats (or lipids) in the small intestine is assisted by the action of bile, a digestive juice produced by the liver and stored in the gallbladder. A complex sequence of chemical processes enables fats to be absorbed through the intestinal wall, broken down in the liver, and converted for use in the body. Cholesterol, a lipid present in bile, plays an important part in this chain.

2 Bile salts act on fats to enable them to pass from the small intestine into the bloodstream, either directly or via the lymphatic system.

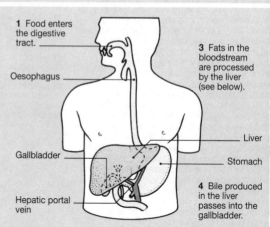

1 Food enters the digestive tract.

Oesophagus

3 Fats in the bloodstream are processed by the liver (see below).

Gallbladder

Liver

Stomach

Hepatic portal vein

4 Bile produced in the liver passes into the gallbladder.

How fats are processed in the liver

Fat molecules are broken down in the liver into fatty acids and glycerol. Glycerol, as well as some of the fatty acids, pass back into the bloodstream. Other fatty acids are used to form cholesterol, some of which in turn is used to make bile salts. Unchanged cholesterol is dissolved in the bile, which then passes into the gallbladder.

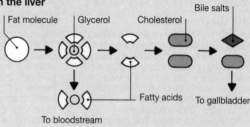

Fat molecule | Glycerol | Cholesterol | Bile salts

To bloodstream | Fatty acids | To gallbladder

chenodeoxycholic acid treatment usually needs to be accompanied by adherence to a low-cholesterol, high-fibre diet.

How they affect you

Drug treatment may often take years to dissolve gallstones completely. You will not, therefore, feel any immediate benefit from the drugs, but you may have some minor *side effects*, the most usual of which is diarrhoea. If this occurs, your doctor may adjust the dosage. The effect of drug treatment on the gallstones is usually monitored at regular intervals by means of ultrasound or X-ray examinations.

Even after successful treatment with drugs, gallstones often recur when the

drug is stopped. In some cases drug treatment and dietary restrictions may be continued even after the gallstones have dissolved, to prevent a recurrence.

Although these drugs reduce cholesterol in the gallbladder, they increase the level of cholesterol in the blood because they reduce its excretion in the bile. Doctors therefore prescribe them with caution to people who have atherosclerosis (fatty deposits in the blood vessels). These drugs are not usually given to people who have liver disorders because they can interfere with normal liver function. Surgical or ultrasound treatment is used for those with liver problems.

AGENTS USED IN DISORDERS OF THE PANCREAS

The pancreas releases certain *enzymes* into the small intestine that are necessary for digestion of a range of foods. If the release of pancreatic enzymes is impaired (caused by, for example, chronic pancreatitis or cystic fibrosis), enzyme replacement therapy may be necessary. Replacement of enzymes does not cure the underlying disorder, but it restores normal digestion. Pancreatic enzymes should

be taken just before or with meals, and usually take effect immediately. Your doctor will probably advise you to eat a diet that is high in protein and carbohydrates and low in fat.

Pancreatin, the generic name for those preparations containing pancreatic enzymes, is extracted from pig pancreas. Treatment must be continued indefinitely as long as the pancreatic disorder persists.

COMMON DRUGS

Drugs for gallstones	Pancreatic enzymes
Chenodeoxycholic acid	Amylase
Ursodeoxycholic acid	Lipase
	Pancreatin
	Protease

✳ See Part 4

MUSCLES, BONES, AND JOINTS

The basic architecture of the human body relies on 206 bones, over 600 muscles, and a complex assortment of other tissues – ligaments, tendons, and cartilage – that enable the body to move with remarkable efficiency.

What can go wrong

Although tough, these structures often suffer damage. Muscles, tendons, and ligaments can be strained or torn by violent movement, which may cause inflammation, making the affected tissue swollen and painful. Joints, especially those that bear the body's weight – hips, knees, ankles, and vertebrae – are prone to wear and tear. The cartilage covering the bone ends may tear, causing pain and inflammation. Joint damage also occurs in rheumatoid arthritis, which is thought to be a form of autoimmune disorder. Gout, in which uric acid crystals form in some joints, may also cause inflammation, a condition known as gouty arthritis.

Another problem affecting the muscles and joints includes nerve injury or degeneration, which alters nerve control over muscle contraction. Myasthenia gravis, in which transmission of signals between nerves and muscles is reduced, affects muscle control as a result. Bones may also be weakened by vitamin, mineral, or hormone deficiencies.

Why drugs are used

A simple analgesic drug or one that has an anti-inflammatory effect will provide pain relief in most of the above conditions. For severe inflammation, a doctor may inject a drug with a more powerful anti-inflammatory effect, such as a corticosteroid, into the affected site. In cases of severe progressive rheumatoid arthritis, antirheumatic drugs may halt the disease's progression and relieve symptoms.

Drugs that help to eliminate excess uric acid from the body are often prescribed to treat gout. Muscle relaxants that inhibit transmission of nerve signals to the muscles are used to treat muscle spasm. Drugs that increase nervous stimulation of the muscle are prescribed for myasthenia gravis. Bone disorders in which the mineral content of the bone is reduced are treated with supplements of minerals, vitamins, and hormones.

MAJOR DRUG GROUPS

Non-steroidal anti-inflammatory drugs
Antirheumatic drugs
Locally acting corticosteroids
Drugs for gout

Muscle-relaxant drugs
Drugs used for myasthenia gravis
Drugs for bone disorders

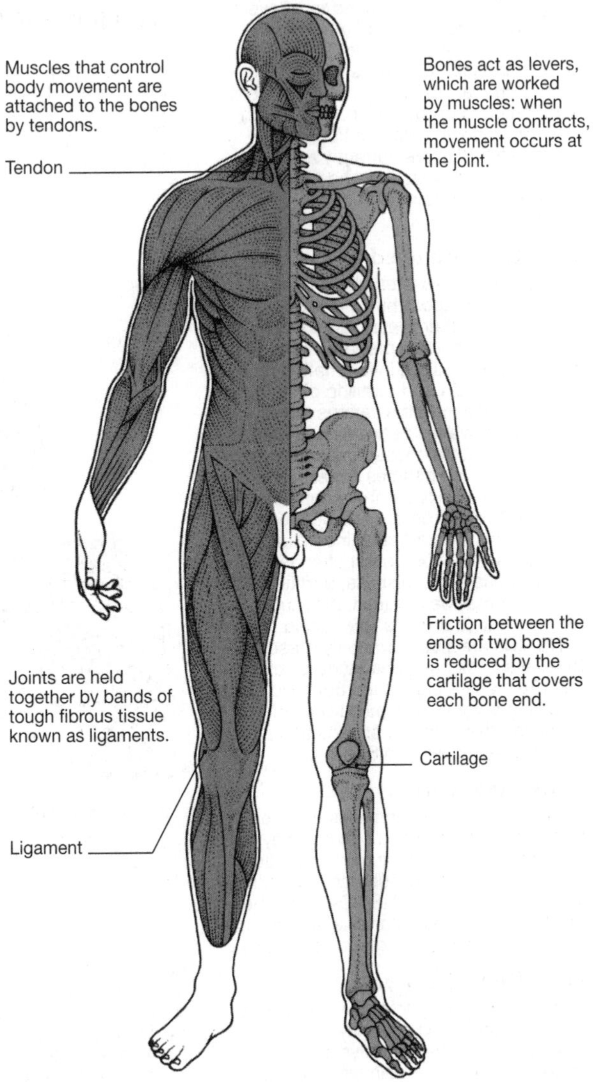

Muscles that control body movement are attached to the bones by tendons.

Tendon

Bones act as levers, which are worked by muscles: when the muscle contracts, movement occurs at the joint.

Friction between the ends of two bones is reduced by the cartilage that covers each bone end.

Joints are held together by bands of tough fibrous tissue known as ligaments.

Cartilage

Ligament

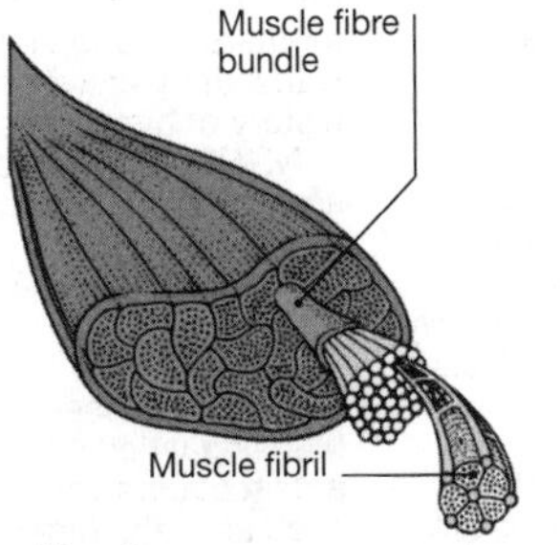

Muscle fibre bundle

Longitudinal canal

Transverse canal

Muscle fibril

Muscle
Each muscle is made of thick bundles of fibres: each bundle in turn is made of fibrils. Tiny nerves and blood vessels enable the muscle to function.

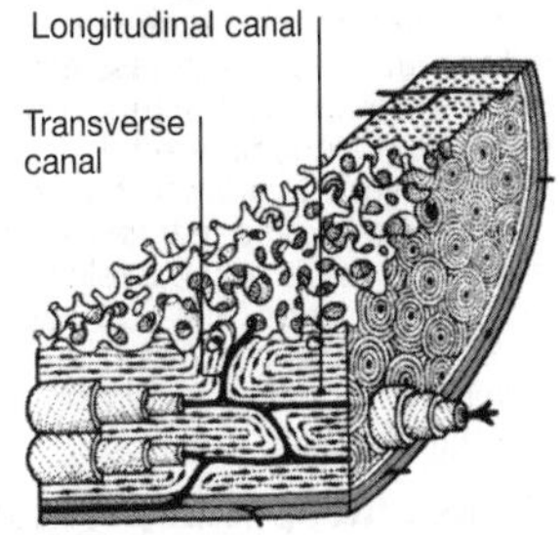

Bone
Long bones, such as the femur, contain a network of longitudinal and transverse canals to carry blood, nerves, and lymph vessels through the bone.

NON-STEROIDAL ANTI-INFLAMMATORY DRUGS

Drugs in this group are used to relieve the pain, stiffness, and inflammation of painful conditions affecting the muscles, bones, and joints. NSAIDs are called "non-steroidal" to distinguish them from corticosteroid drugs (see p.141), which also damp down inflammation.

Many NSAIDs are currently available, and others are being investigated in the hope of finding new compounds with fewer *side effects*.

Why they are used

NSAIDs are widely prescribed for the treatment of osteoarthritis, rheumatoid arthritis, and other rheumatic conditions. They do not alter the progress of these diseases, but reduce inflammation and thus relieve pain and swelling of joints.

The response to the various drugs in this group varies between individuals and the first drug chosen may not be effective. It is sometimes necessary for the doctor to prescribe a number of different NSAIDs before finding the one that best suits a particular individual.

Because NSAIDs do not change the progress of the disease, additional treatment may be required, particularly for rheumatoid arthritis (see facing page).

NSAIDs are also commonly prescribed to relieve back pain, headaches, gout (p.119), menstrual pain (p.160), mild pain following surgery, and pain from soft tissue injuries, such as sprains and strains (see also Analgesics, p.80).

How they work

Prostaglandins are chemicals released by the body at the site of injury. They are responsible for producing inflammation and pain following tissue damage and in immune reactions. NSAIDs block the production of prostaglandins and thus reduce pain and inflammation (see p.81).

How they affect you

NSAIDs are usually effective in reducing joint pain and swelling. They are rapidly absorbed from the digestive system and most start to relieve pain within an hour. When used regularly they reduce pain, inflammation, and stiffness and may restore or improve the function of a joint if this has been impaired.

Most NSAIDs are short acting and need to be taken a few times a day in order to provide optimal relief from pain. Some need to be taken only twice daily. Others, such as piroxicam, are very slowly eliminated from the body and are effective when taken once a day.

Risks and special precautions

With a few exceptions, most NSAIDs are free from serious *adverse effects* although nausea, indigestion, and altered bowel action are common. Aspirin has a higher potential to irritate the stomach than that of most other NSAIDs. However, the main

ACTION OF NSAIDs IN OSTEOARTHRITIS

Non-steroidal anti-inflammatory drugs (NSAIDs) are often prescribed to diminish the pain and stiffness associated with osteoarthritis, a disorder in which, typically, a weight-bearing joint such as the hip is damaged by wear and tear or other factors.

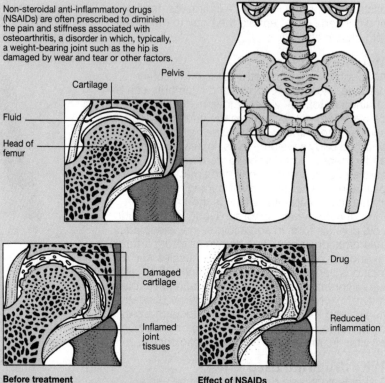

Before treatment
The protective layers of cartilage surrounding the joint are worn away and the joint becomes inflamed and painful.

Effect of NSAIDs
NSAIDs reduce inflammation and may thus relieve pain, but damage to the joint remains and symptoms are likely to worsen or recur if the drug is stopped.

risk from NSAIDs is that, occasionally, they can cause bleeding in the stomach or duodenum. They should therefore be avoided by people who have suffered from peptic ulcers.

Most NSAIDs are not recommended during pregnancy or for breast-feeding mothers. Caution is also advised for those with kidney or liver abnormalities or with a history of hypersensitivity to other drugs.

NSAIDs may impair blood clotting and are, therefore, prescribed with caution for people with bleeding disorders or who are taking drugs that reduce blood clotting.

Misoprostol

An NSAID causes the side effect of bleeding when its antiprostaglandin action occurs where it is not wanted, such as in the digestive tract. To protect against this side effect, a prostaglandin-like drug called misoprostol is sometimes prescribed with the NSAID. Preparations are now available that incorporate both misoprostol and an NSAID. Misoprostol

is also used to help heal peptic ulcers (see p.109). As an alternative to giving drugs such as misoprostol, NSAIDs are being developed that work selectively by preventing prostaglandin production in the joints but not in the digestive tract.

COMMON DRUGS

Aceclofenac	Flurbiprofen
Acemetacin	Ibuprofen *
Aspirin *	Indomethacin
Azapropazone	Ketoprofen *
Benorylate	Mefenamic acid *
Benzydamine	Meloxicam *
Diclofenac *	Nabumetone
Diflunisal	Naproxen *
Etodolac	Phenylbutazone
Felbinac *	Piroxicam *
Fenbufen	Sulindac
Fenoprofen	Tenoxicam
	Tiaprofenic acid

* See Part 4

ANTIRHEUMATIC DRUGS

These drugs are used in the treatment of various rheumatic disorders, the most crippling and deforming of which is rheumatoid arthritis, an autoimmune disease in which the body's mechanism for fighting infection contributes to the damage of its own joint tissue. The disease causes pain, stiffness, and swelling of the joints that, over many months, can lead to deformity. Flare-ups of rheumatoid arthritis also cause a general feeling of being unwell, fatigue, and loss of appetite.

Treatments for rheumatoid arthritis include drugs, rest, changes in diet, physiotherapy, and immobilization of joints. The disorder cannot yet be cured, although in many cases it does not progress far enough to cause permanent disability. It sometimes subsides spontaneously for prolonged periods.

Why they are used

The aim of drug treatment is to relieve the symptoms of pain and stiffness, maintain mobility, and prevent deformity. There are two main forms of drug treatment for rheumatoid arthritis: the first alleviates symptoms, and the second modifies, halts, or slows the underlying disease process. Drugs in the first category include aspirin (p.200) and the other non-steroidal anti-inflammatory drugs (NSAIDs, facing page). These drugs are usually prescribed as a first treatment.

However, if the rheumatoid arthritis is severe, or the initial drug treatment has proved to be ineffective, the second category of drugs may be given. These drugs may prevent any further joint damage and disability. They are not prescribed routinely because they have potentially severe adverse effects (see Types of Antirheumatic Drugs, below, for further information on individual drugs), and because the disease may stop spontaneously.

Corticosteroids (p.141) are sometimes used in the treatment of rheumatoid arthritis, but only for limited periods of time because these drugs depress the

THE EFFECTS OF ANTIRHEUMATIC DRUGS

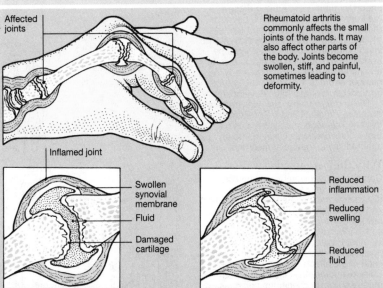

Rheumatoid arthritis commonly affects the small joints of the hands. It may also affect other parts of the body. Joints become swollen, stiff, and painful, sometimes leading to deformity.

Affected joints

Inflamed joint

Swollen synovial membrane

Fluid

Damaged cartilage

Reduced inflammation

Reduced swelling

Reduced fluid

Before treatment
The synovial membrane surrounding the joint is inflamed and thickened, producing increased fluid within the joint. The surrounding tissue is inflamed and joint cartilage damaged.

After treatment
Treatment with antirheumatic drugs relieves pain, swelling, and inflammation. Damage to cartilage and bone may be halted so that further deformity is minimized.

immune system, thereby increasing susceptibility to infection.

How they work

It is not known precisely how most antirheumatic drugs stop or slow the disease process. Some may reduce the body's immune response, which is thought to be partly responsible for the disease (see also Immunosuppressant drugs, p.156). When they are effective, antirheumatic drugs prevent damage to the cartilage and bone, thereby reducing progressive deformity and disability.

The effectiveness of each drug varies depending on the individual response.

How they affect you

These drugs are generally slow acting; it may be weeks or even months before benefit is noticed. So, aspirin or other NSAID treatment is usually continued until remission occurs. Prolonged treatment with antirheumatic drugs can cause a marked improvement in symptoms. Arthritic pain is relieved, joint mobility increased, and general symptoms of ill health fade. Side effects (which vary between individual drugs) may be noticed before any beneficial effect, so patience is required. Severe adverse effects may necessitate abandoning the treatment.

TYPES OF ANTIRHEUMATIC DRUGS

Chloroquine Originally developed to treat malaria (see p.137), chloroquine and related drugs are less effective than penicillamine or gold. Since prolonged use may cause eye damage, regular eye checks are needed.

Immunosuppressants These are prescribed if other drugs do not provide relief and if rheumatoid arthritis is severe and disabling. Regular observation and blood tests must be carried out because immunosuppressants can cause severe complications.

Sulfasalazine Used mainly for ulcerative colitis (p.112), sulfasalazine was originally introduced to treat rheumatoid arthritis and is effective in some cases.

Gold-based drugs These are believed to be the most effective and may be given orally or by injection for many years. Side effects can include a rash and digestive disturbances. Gold may sometimes damage the kidneys, which recover on stopping treatment; regular urine tests are usually carried out. It can also suppress blood cell production in bone marrow, so periodic blood tests are also carried out.

Penicillamine This drug may be used when rheumatoid arthritis is worsening, or when gold cannot be given. Improvement in symptoms may take 3 to 6 months. It has similar side effects to gold, and periodic blood and urine tests are usually performed.

COMMON DRUGS

Immunosuppressants	Gold-based drugs
Azathioprine *	Auranofin
Cyclophosphamide *	Sodium
Cyclosporin *	aurothiomalate
Methotrexate *	

NSAIDs
(see facing page)

Other drugs
Chloroquine *
Hydroxychloroquine *
Penicillamine
Sulfasalazine *

* See Part 4

LOCALLY ACTING CORTICOSTEROIDS

The adrenal glands, which lie on the top of the kidneys, produce a number of important hormones. Among these are the corticosteroids, so named because they are made in the outer part (cortex) of the glands. The corticosteroids play an important role, influencing the immune system and regulating the carbohydrate and mineral *metabolism* of the body. A number of drugs that mimic the natural corticosteroids have been developed.

These drugs have many uses and are discussed in detail under Corticosteroids (p.141). This section concentrates on those corticosteroids injected into an affected site to treat joint disorders.

Why they are used

Corticosteroids given by injection are particularly useful for treating joint disorders – notably rheumatoid arthritis and osteoarthritis – when one or only a few joints are involved, and when pain and inflammation have not been relieved by other drugs. In such cases, it is possible to relieve symptoms by injecting each of the affected joints individually. Corticosteroids may also be injected to relieve pain and inflammation caused by strained or contracted muscles, ligaments, and/or tendons – for example, in frozen shoulder or tennis elbow. They may also be given for bursitis, tendinitis, or swelling that is compressing a nerve. Corticosteroid injections are sometimes used in order to relieve pain and stiffness sufficiently to permit physiotherapy.

How they work

Corticosteroid drugs have two important actions that are believed to account for their effectiveness. They block the production of prostaglandins – chemicals responsible for triggering inflammation and pain – and depress the accumulation

COMMON INJECTION SITES

Corticosteroids are often injected into joints affected by osteo- and rheumatoid arthritis. Joints commonly treated in this way are knee, shoulder, and finger joints.

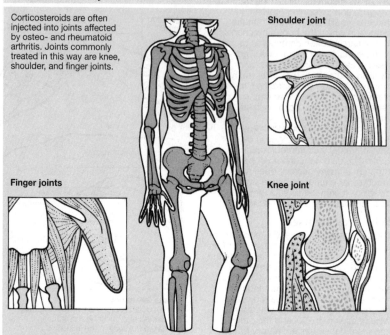

Shoulder joint

Finger joints

Knee joint

and activity of the white blood cells that cause the inflammation (below). Injection concentrates the corticosteroids, and their effects, at the site of the problem, thus giving the maximum benefit where it is most needed.

How they affect you

Corticosteroids usually produce dramatic relief from symptoms when the drug is injected into a joint. Often a single injection is sufficient to relieve pain and swelling, and to improve mobility. When used to treat muscle or tendon pain, they may not always be effective because it is difficult to position the needle so that the drug reaches the right spot. In some cases, repeated injections are necessary.

Because these drugs are concentrated in the affected area, rather than being dispersed in significant amounts in the body, the generalized *adverse effects* that sometimes occur when corticosteroids are taken by mouth are unlikely. Minor side effects, such as loss of skin pigment at the injection site, are uncommon. Occasionally, a temporary increase in pain (steroid flare) may occur. In such cases, rest, local application of ice, and analgesic medication may relieve the condition. Sterile injection technique is critically important.

ACTION OF CORTICOSTEROIDS ON INFLAMED JOINTS

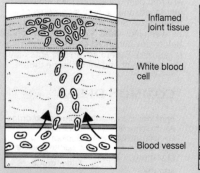

Inflamed joint tissue

White blood cell

Blood vessel

Inflamed tissue
Inflammation occurs when disease or injury causes large numbers of white blood cells to accumulate in the affected area. In joints this leads to swelling and stiffness.

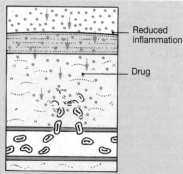

Reduced inflammation

Drug

Action of corticosteroids
Corticosteroids, when injected into the area, permeate the joint lining (synovial membrane), blocking prostaglandin production and preventing white blood cells accumulating.

COMMON DRUGS

Dexamethasone *   Prednisolone *
Hydrocortisone *   Triamcinolone
Methylprednisolone

* See Part 4

DRUGS FOR GOUT

Gout is a disorder that arises when the blood contains increased levels of uric acid, which is a by-product of normal body *metabolism*. When its concentration in the blood is excessive, uric acid crystals may form in various parts of the body, especially in the joints of the foot (most often the big toe), the knee, and the hand, causing intense pain and inflammation known as gouty arthritis. Crystals may form as white masses, known as tophi, in soft tissue, and in the kidneys as stones. Attacks of gouty arthritis can recur, and may lead to damaged joints and deformity. Kidney stones can cause kidney damage.

An excess of uric acid can be caused either by increased production or by decreased elimination by the kidneys, which remove it from the body. The disorder tends to run in families and is far more common in men than women. The risk of attack is increased by high alcohol intake, the consumption of certain foods

(red meat, sardines, anchovies, and offal such as liver, brains, and sweetbreads), and obesity. An attack may be triggered by drugs such as thiazide diuretics (see p.99) or anticancer drugs (see p.154), or excessive drinking. Changes in diet and a reduction in the consumption of alcohol may be an important part of treatment.

Drugs used to treat acute attacks of gouty arthritis include non-steroidal anti-inflammatory drugs (NSAIDs, see p.116), and colchicine. Other drugs, which lower the blood level of uric acid, are used for the long-term prevention of gout. These include the uricosuric drugs (probenecid and sulfinpyrazone), as well as allopurinol. Aspirin is not prescribed for pain relief because it slows the excretion of uric acid.

Why they are used

Drugs may be prescribed either to treat an attack of gout or to prevent recurrent attacks that could lead to deformity of affected joints and kidney damage. The

NSAIDs and colchicine are both used to treat an attack of gout and should be taken as soon as an attack begins. Because colchicine is relatively specific in relieving the pain and inflammation arising from gout, doctors sometimes administer it in order to confirm their diagnosis of the condition before prescribing an NSAID.

If symptoms recur, your doctor may advise long-term treatment with either allopurinol or a uricosuric drug. One of these drugs must usually be taken indefinitely. Since they can trigger attacks of gout at the beginning of treatment, colchicine is sometimes given with these drugs for a few months.

How they work

Allopurinol reduces the level of uric acid in the blood by interfering with the activity of xanthine oxidase, an *enzyme* that is involved in the production of uric acid in the body. Both sulfinpyrazone and probenecid increase the rate at which uric acid is excreted by the kidneys. The process by which colchicine reduces inflammation and relieves pain is not understood. The actions of NSAIDs are described on p.116.

How they affect you

Drugs used in the long-term treatment of gout are usually successful in preventing attacks and joint deformity. However, response may be slow.

Colchicine can disturb the digestive system, causing abdominal pain and diarrhoea, which your doctor can control by prescribing other drugs.

Risks and special precautions

Since they increase the output of uric acid through the kidneys, uricosuric drugs can cause uric acid crystals to form in the kidneys. They are not, therefore, usually prescribed for those people who already have kidney problems. In such cases, allopurinol may be preferred. It is always important to drink plenty of fluids while taking drugs for gout in order to prevent kidney crystals from forming. Regular blood tests to monitor levels of uric acid in the blood may be required.

ACTION OF URICOSURIC DRUGS

Uric acid is removed from the blood by the kidneys and excreted in the urine. Excess uric acid, caused by increased production or impaired kidney function, requires treatment with uricosuric drugs, which increase the rate at which uric acid is expelled.

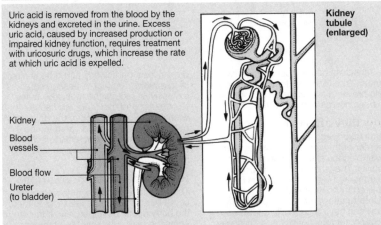

Kidney tubule (enlarged)

Kidney

Blood vessels

Blood flow

Ureter (to bladder)

Uric acid and gouty arthritis
Gouty arthritis occurs when uric acid crystals form in a joint, often a toe, knee, or hand, causing inflammation and pain. This is the result of excessively high levels of uric acid in the blood. In some cases this is caused by overproduction of uric acid, while in others it is the result of reduced excretion of uric acid by the kidneys.

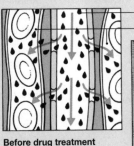

Uric acid

Blood vessels

Drug

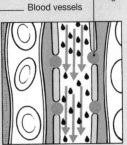

Before drug treatment
Excess uric acid from the kidney tubule is reabsorbed into the surrounding blood vessels. This leads to the formation of uric acid crystals, which can cause gouty arthritis.

After drug treatment
By blocking the reabsorption of uric acid into the blood vessels, the amount of uric acid excreted in the urine is increased.

COMMON DRUGS

Drugs to treat attacks
Colchicine ✳
NSAIDs (see p.116)
 (but not aspirin)

Drugs to prevent attacks
Allopurinol ✳
Probenecid
Sulfinpyrazone

✳ See Part 4

MUSCLE RELAXANTS

Several drugs are available to treat muscle spasm – the involuntary, painful contraction of a muscle or a group of muscles that can stiffen an arm or leg, or make it nearly impossible to straighten your back. There are various causes. It can follow an injury, or come on without warning. It may also be brought on by a disorder like osteoarthritis, the pain in the affected joint triggering abnormal tension in a nearby muscle.

Spasticity is another form of muscle tightness seen in some neurological disorders, such as multiple sclerosis, stroke, or cerebral palsy. Spasticity can sometimes be helped by physiotherapy but in severe cases drugs may be used to relieve symptoms.

Why they are used

Muscle spasm resulting from direct injury is usually treated with a non-steroidal anti-inflammatory drug (see p.80) or an analgesic. However, if the spasm is severe, a muscle relaxant may also be tried for a short period.

In spasticity, the sufferer's legs may become so stiff and uncontrollable that walking unaided is impossible. In such cases, a drug may be used to relax the muscles. Relaxation of the muscles often permits physiotherapy to be given for longer-term relief from spasms.

The muscle relaxant, botulinum toxin, may be injected locally to relieve muscle spasm in small groups of accessible muscles, such as those around the eye or in the neck.

How they work

Muscle-relaxant drugs work in one of several ways. The centrally acting drugs damp down the passage of the nerve signals from the brain and spinal cord that cause muscles to contract, thus reducing excessive stimulation of muscles as well as unwanted muscular contraction. Tizanidine stimulates the alpha receptors in the blood vessels. Dantrolene reduces

SITES OF ACTION OF MUSCLE RELAXANTS

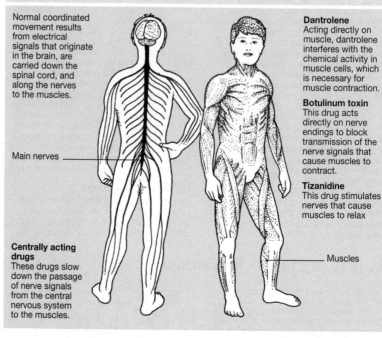

Normal coordinated movement results from electrical signals that originate in the brain, are carried down the spinal cord, and along the nerves to the muscles.

Main nerves

Centrally acting drugs
These drugs slow down the passage of nerve signals from the central nervous system to the muscles.

Dantrolene
Acting directly on muscle, dantrolene interferes with the chemical activity in muscle cells, which is necessary for muscle contraction.

Botulinum toxin
This drug acts directly on nerve endings to block transmission of the nerve signals that cause muscles to contract.

Tizanidine
This drug stimulates nerves that cause muscles to relax

Muscles

the sensitivity of the muscles to nerve signals. When injected locally, botulinum toxin prevents transmission of impulses between nerves and muscles.

How they affect you

Drugs taken regularly for a spastic disorder of the central nervous system usually reduce stiffness and improve mobility. They may restore the use of the arms and legs when this has been impaired by muscle spasm.

Unfortunately, most centrally acting drugs can have a generally depressant effect on nervous activity and produce

drowsiness, particularly at the beginning of treatment. Too high a dosage can excessively reduce the muscles' ability to contract and can therefore cause weakness. For this reason, the dosage needs to be carefully adjusted to find a level that controls symptoms but which, at the same time, maintains sufficient muscle strength.

Risks and special precautions

The main long-term risk associated with centrally acting muscle relaxants is that the body becomes dependent. If the drugs are withdrawn suddenly, the stiffness may become worse than before drug treatment.

Rarely, dantrolene can cause serious liver damage. Anyone who is taking this drug should have his or her blood tested regularly to assess liver function.

Unless used very cautiously, botulinum toxin can paralyse unaffected muscles, and might interfere with functions such as speech and swallowing.

ACTION OF CENTRALLY ACTING DRUGS

Centrally acting muscle relaxants restrict passage of nerve signals to the muscles by occupying a proportion of the *receptors* in the central nervous system that are normally used by *neurotransmitters* to transmit such impulses. Reduced nervous stimulation allows the muscles to relax; however, if the dose of the drug is too high, this action may give rise to excessive muscle weakness.

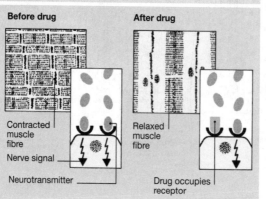

Before drug

After drug

Contracted muscle fibre

Nerve signal

Neurotransmitter

Relaxed muscle fibre

Drug occupies receptor

COMMON DRUGS

Centrally acting drugs
Baclofen *
Carisoprodol
Cyclobenzaprine
Diazepam *

Methocarbamol
Orphenadrine *

Other drugs
Botulinum toxin
Dantrolene
Quinine *
Tizanidine

| * See Part 4 |

DRUGS USED FOR MYASTHENIA GRAVIS

Myasthenia gravis is a disorder that occurs when the immune system (see p.152) becomes defective and produces antibodies that disrupt the signals being transmitted between the nervous system and muscles that are under voluntary control. As a result, the body's muscular response is progressively weakened. The first muscles to be affected are those controlling the eyes, eyelids, face, pharynx, and larynx, with muscles in the arms and legs becoming involved as the disease progresses. The disease is often linked to a disorder of the thymus gland, which is the source of the destructive antibodies concerned.

Various methods can be used in the treatment of myasthenia gravis, including the removal of the thymus gland (called a thymectomy) or temporarily clearing the blood of antibodies using a procedure known as plasmapheresis. Drugs that improve muscle function, principally neostigmine and pyridostigmine, may be prescribed. They may be used alone or together with other drugs that depress the immune system – usually azathioprine (see Immunosuppressant drugs, p.156) or corticosteroids (see p.141).

THE EFFECTS OF MYASTHENIA GRAVIS

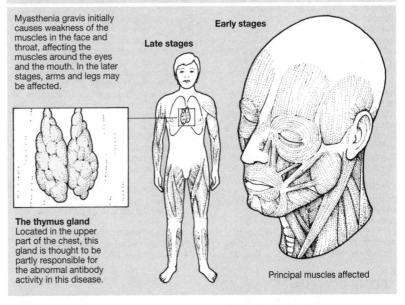

Myasthenia gravis initially causes weakness of the muscles in the face and throat, affecting the muscles around the eyes and the mouth. In the later stages, arms and legs may be affected.

Early stages

Late stages

The thymus gland
Located in the upper part of the chest, this gland is thought to be partly responsible for the abnormal antibody activity in this disease.

Principal muscles affected

Why they are used

Drugs that improve the muscle response to nerve impulses have several uses. One such drug, edrophonium, acts very quickly and, once administered, it brings about a dramatic improvement in the symptoms. This effect is used to confirm the diagnosis of myasthenia gravis. However, because of its short duration of action, edrophonium is not used for long-term treatment. Pyridostigmine and neostigmine are preferred for long-term treatment, especially when surgery to remove the thymus gland is not feasible or does not provide adequate relief.

These drugs may be given following surgery to counteract the effects of a muscle-relaxant drug given prior to certain surgical procedures.

How they work

Normal muscle action occurs when a nerve impulse triggers a nerve ending to release a *neurotransmitter*, which combines with a specialized *receptor* on the muscle cells and causes the muscles to contract. In myasthenia gravis, the body's immune system destroys many of these receptors, so that the muscle is less responsive to nervous stimulation. Drugs used to treat the disorder increase the amount of neurotransmitter at the nerve ending by blocking the action of an *enzyme* that normally breaks it down. Increased levels of the neurotransmitter permit the remaining receptors to function more efficiently (see Action of drugs used for myasthenia gravis, below).

How they affect you

These drugs usually restore the muscle function to a normal or near-normal level, particularly when the disease takes a mild form. Unfortunately, the drugs can produce unwanted muscular activity by enhancing the transmission of nerve impulses elsewhere in the body.

Common side effects include vomiting, nausea, diarrhoea, and muscle cramps in the arms, legs, and abdomen.

Risks and special precautions

Muscle weakness can suddenly worsen even when it is being treated with drugs. Should this occur, it is important not to take larger doses of the drug in an attempt to relieve the symptoms, since excessive levels can interfere with the transmission of nerve impulses to muscles, causing further weakness. The administration of other drugs, including some antibiotics, can also markedly increase the symptoms of myasthenia gravis. If your symptoms suddenly become worse, consult your doctor.

ACTION OF DRUGS USED FOR MYASTHENIA GRAVIS

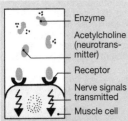

Enzyme

Acetylcholine (neurotransmitter)

Receptor

Nerve signals transmitted

Muscle cell

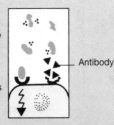

Antibody

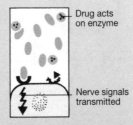

Drug acts on enzyme

Nerve signals transmitted

Normal nerve transmission
Muscles contract when a neurotransmitter (acetylcholine) binds to receptors on muscle cells. An enzyme breaks down acetylcholine.

In myasthenia gravis
Abnormal antibody activity destroys many receptors, reducing stimulation of the muscle cells and weakening the muscle action.

Drug action
Anticholinesterase drugs block enzyme action, increasing acetylcholine and prolonging the muscle cell response to nervous stimulation.

COMMON DRUGS

Neostigmine
Pyridostigmine *
Distigmine
Edrophonium

Azathioprine *
Corticosteroids (see p.141)

* See Part 4

DRUGS FOR BONE DISORDERS

Bone is a living structure. Its hard, mineral quality is created by the action of the bone cells. These cells continuously deposit and remove phosphorus and calcium, stored in a honeycombed protein framework called the matrix. Because the rates of deposit and removal (the bone metabolism) are about equal in adults, the bone mass remains fairly constant.

Removal and renewal is regulated by hormones and influenced by a number of factors, notably the level of calcium in the blood, which depends on the intake of calcium and vitamin D from the diet, the actions of various hormones, plus everyday movement and weight-bearing stress. When normal bone metabolism is altered, various bone disorders result.

Osteoporosis

In osteoporosis, the strength and density of bone are reduced. Such wasting occurs when the rate of removal of mineralized bone exceeds the rate of deposit. In most people, bone density decreases very gradually from the age

of 30. But bone loss can dramatically increase when a person is immobilized for a period, and this is an important cause of osteoporosis in elderly people. Hormone deficiency is another important cause, commonly occurring in women with lowered oestrogen levels after the menopause or removal of the ovaries. Osteoporosis also occurs in disorders in which there is excess production of adrenal or thyroid hormones. Osteoporosis can result from long-term treatment with corticosteroid drugs.

People with osteoporosis often have no symptoms, but, if the vertebrae become so weakened that they are unable to bear the body's weight, they may collapse spontaneously or after a minor accident. Subsequently, the individual suffers from back pain, reduced height, and a round-shouldered appearance. Osteoporosis also makes a fracture of an arm, leg, or hip more likely.

Most doctors emphasize the need to prevent the disorder by an adequate intake of protein and calcium and by

regular exercise throughout adult life. Oestrogen supplements during and after the menopause may be used to prevent osteoporosis in older women. (See Hormone replacement therapy, p.147.)

The condition of bones damaged by osteoporosis cannot usually be improved, although drug treatment can help prevent further deterioration and help fractures to heal. For people whose diet is deficient in calcium or vitamin D, supplements may be prescribed. However, these are of limited value and are often less useful than drugs that inhibit removal of calcium from the bones. In the past, the hormone calcitonin was used, but it has now been largely superseded by drugs such as etidronate and alendronate. These drugs, known as bisphosphonates, bind very tightly to bone matrix, preventing its removal by bone cells.

Osteomalacia and rickets

In osteomalacia – called rickets when it affects children – lack of vitamin D leads to loss of calcium, resulting in softening of the bones. Sufferers experience pain and tenderness and there is a risk of fracture and bone deformity. In children, growth is retarded.

Osteomalacia is most commonly caused by a lack of vitamin D. This can result from an inadequate diet, inability to absorb the vitamin, or insufficient exposure of the skin to sunlight (the action of the sun on the skin produces vitamin D inside the body). People who are at special risk include those whose absorption of vitamin D is impaired by an intestinal disorder, like Crohn's disease or coeliac disease. People with dark skins living in Northern Europe are also susceptible. Chronic kidney disease is an important cause of rickets in children and of osteomalacia in adults, since healthy kidneys play an essential role in the body's metabolism of vitamin D.

Long-term relief depends on treating the underlying disorder where possible. In rare cases, treatment may be lifelong.

Vitamin D

A number of substances that are related to vitamin D may be used in the treatment of bone disorders. These drugs include alfacalcidol, calcitriol, and ergocalciferol. The one prescribed depends on the underlying problem (see also page 448).

BONE WASTING

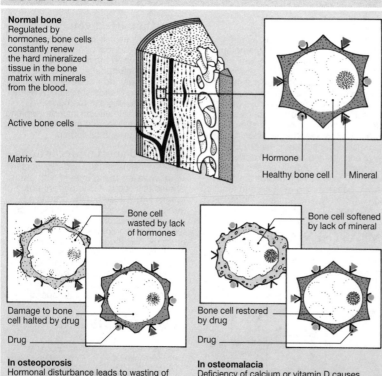

Normal bone
Regulated by hormones, bone cells constantly renew the hard mineralized tissue in the bone matrix with minerals from the blood.

Active bone cells

Matrix

Hormone
Healthy bone cell | Mineral

Bone cell wasted by lack of hormones

Bone cell softened by lack of mineral

Damage to bone cell halted by drug

Drug

Bone cell restored by drug

Drug

In osteoporosis
Hormonal disturbance leads to wasting of active bone cells. The bones become less dense and more fragile. Drug treatment with hormone and mineral supplements usually only prevents further bone loss.

In osteomalacia
Deficiency of calcium or vitamin D causes softening of the bone tissue. The bones become weaker and sometimes deformed. Drug treatment with vitamin D and minerals usually restores bone strength.

COMMON DRUGS

Alendronate	Conjugated
Alfacalcidol	oestrogens ✳
Calcitonin	Ergocalciferol
Calcitriol	Etidronate ✳
Calcium carbonate	Fluoride
	Salcatonin
	(calcitonin (salmon))
✳ See Part 4	Vitamin D ✳

ALLERGY

Allergy, which is a hypersensitivity to certain substances, is a extreme reaction of the body's immune system. Through a variety of mechanisms (see Malignant and immune disease, p.152), the immune system protects the body by eliminating foreign substances that it does not recognize, such as microorganisms (bacteria or viruses).

One way in which the immune system acts is through the production of *antibodies*. When the body encounters a particular foreign substance (or allergen) for the first time, one type of white blood cell, the lymphocytes, produces antibodies that attach themselves to another type of white blood cell, the mast cells. If the same substance is encountered again, the allergen binds to the antibodies on the mast cells, causing the release of chemicals known as mediators.

The most important mediator is histamine. This can produce a rash, swelling, narrowing of the airways, and a drop in blood pressure. Although these effects are important in protecting the body against infection, they may also be triggered inappropriately in an allergic reaction.

What can go wrong

One of the most common allergic disorders, hay fever, is caused by an allergic reaction to inhaled grass pollen leading to allergic rhinitis – swelling and irritation of the nasal passages and watering of the nose and eyes. Other substances, such as house-dust mites, animal fur, and feathers, may cause a similar reaction in susceptible people.

Asthma, another allergic disorder, may result from the action of leukotrienes rather than histamine. Other allergic conditions include urticaria (hives) or other rashes (sometimes in response to a drug), some forms of eczema and dermatitis, and allergic alveolitis (farmer's lung). Anaphylaxis is a serious systemic allergic reaction (p.496) that occurs when an allergen reaches the bloodstream.

Why drugs are used

Antihistamines and drugs that inhibit mast cell activity are used to prevent and treat allergic reactions. Other drugs minimize allergic symptoms, such as decongestants (p.93) to clear the nose in allergic rhinitis, bronchodilators (p.92) to widen the airways of those with asthma, and corticosteroids applied to skin affected by eczema (p.179).

MAJOR DRUG GROUPS

Antihistamines	Corticosteroids (see p.141)

Allergic response

Lymphocytes produce antibodies to allergens and these attach to mast cells. If the allergen enters the body again, it binds to the antibodies, and the mast cells release histamine.

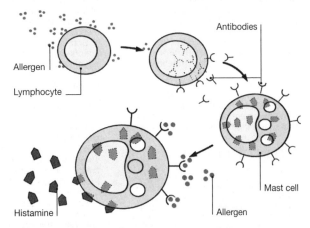

Histamine and histamine receptors

Histamine, released in response to injury or the presence of allergens, acts on H_1 *receptors* in the skin, blood vessels, nasal passages, and airways, and on H_2 receptors in the stomach lining, salivary glands, and lacrimal (tear) glands. It provokes dilation of blood vessels, inflammation and swelling of tissues, and narrowing of the airways. In some cases a reaction called anaphylactic shock may occur, caused by a dramatic fall in blood pressure, which may lead to collapse. Antihistamine drugs block the H_1 receptors, and H_2 blockers block the H_2 receptors (see also Antihistamines, p.124, and Anti-ulcer drugs, p.109).

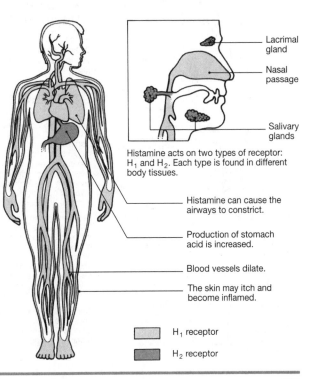

Histamine acts on two types of receptor: H_1 and H_2. Each type is found in different body tissues.

Histamine can cause the airways to constrict.

Production of stomach acid is increased.

Blood vessels dilate.

The skin may itch and become inflamed.

H_1 receptor

H_2 receptor

ANTIHISTAMINES

Antihistamines are the most widely used drugs in the treatment of allergic reactions of all kinds. They can be subdivided according to their chemical structure, each subgroup having slightly different actions and characteristics (see table on facing page). Their main action is to counter the effects of histamine, one of the chemicals released in the body when there is an allergic reaction. (For a full explanation of the allergy mechanism, see p.123.)

Histamine is also involved in other body functions, including blood vessel dilation and constriction, contraction of muscles in the respiratory and gastrointestinal tracts, and the release of digestive juices in the stomach. The antihistamine drugs described here are also known as H_1 blockers because they only block the action of histamine on certain *receptors*, known as H_1 receptors. Another group of antihistamines, known as H_2 blockers, is used in the treatment of peptic ulcers (see Anti-ulcer drugs, p.109).

Some antihistamines have a significant *anticholinergic* action. This is used to advantage in a variety of conditions, but it also accounts for certain undesired side effects.

Why they are used

Antihistamines relieve allergy-related symptoms when it is not possible or practical to prevent exposure to the substance that has provoked the reaction. They are most commonly used in the prevention of allergic rhinitis (hay fever), the inflammation of the nose and upper airways that results from an allergic reaction to a substance such as pollen, house dust, or animal fur. Antihistamines are more effective when taken before the start of an attack. If they are taken only after an attack has begun, beneficial effects may be delayed.

Antihistamines are not usually effective in asthma caused by similar allergens because the symptoms of this allergic disorder are not solely caused by the action of histamine, but are likely to be the result of more complex mechanisms. Antihistamines are usually the first drugs to be tried in the treatment of allergic disorders but there are alternatives that can be prescribed (see below).

Antihistamines are also prescribed to relieve the itching, swelling, and redness that are characteristic of allergic reactions involving the skin – for example, urticaria (hives), infantile eczema, and other forms of dermatitis. Irritation from chickenpox may be reduced by these drugs. Allergic reactions to insect stings may also be reduced by antihistamines. In such cases the drug may be taken by mouth or applied *topically*. Applied as drops, antihistamines can reduce inflammation and irritation of the eyes and eyelids in allergic conjunctivitis.

An antihistamine is often included as an ingredient in cough and cold preparations (see p.94), when the anticholinergic effect of drying mucus secretions and their sedative effect on the coughing mechanism may be helpful.

Because most antihistamines have a depressant effect on the brain, they are sometimes used to promote sleep, especially when discomfort from itching is disturbing sleep (see also Sleeping drugs, p.82). The depressant effect of antihistamines on the brain also extends to the centres that control nausea and vomiting. Antihistamines are therefore often effective for preventing and controlling these symptoms (see Anti-emetics, p.90).

Occasionally, antihistamines are used to treat fever, rash, and breathing difficulties that may occur in adverse reactions to blood transfusions and allergic reactions to drugs. Promethazine and trimeprazine are also used as *premedication* to provide sedation and to dry secretions during surgery, particularly in children.

How they work

Antihistamines block the action of histamine on H_1 receptors. These are found in various body tissues, particularly the small blood vessels in the skin, nose, and eyes. This helps prevent the dilation of the vessels, thus reducing the redness,

SITES OF ACTION

Antihistamines act on a variety of sites and systems throughout the body. Their main action is on the muscles surrounding the small blood vessels that supply the skin and mucous membranes. They also act on the airways in the lungs and on the brain.

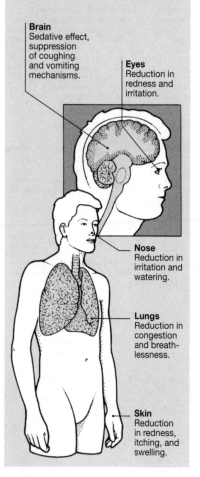

Brain
Sedative effect, suppression of coughing and vomiting mechanisms.

Eyes
Reduction in redness and irritation.

Nose
Reduction in irritation and watering.

Lungs
Reduction in congestion and breath-lessness.

Skin
Reduction in redness, itching, and swelling.

OTHER ALLERGY TREATMENTS

Sodium cromoglicate
This drug (p.404) prevents the release of histamine from mast cells (see p.123) in response to exposure to an allergen, thus preventing the physical symptoms of allergies. It is commonly given by inhaler for the prevention of allergy-induced rhinitis (hay fever) or asthma attacks and by drops for the treatment of allergic eye disorders.

Leukotriene antagonists
Like histamines, leukotrienes are substances that occur naturally in the body and seem to play an important part in asthma. Drugs such as zileuton, montelukast (p.352), and zafirlukast, known as leukotriene antagonists, have been developed to prevent an asthma attack. They are not bronchodilators and will not relieve an existing attack.

Corticosteroids
These are used to treat allergic rhinitis and asthma. They are given by inhaler, which use much lower doses than tablets.

Desensitization
This may be tried in conditions such as allergic rhinitis due to pollen sensitivity and insect venom hypersensitivity, when avoidance, antihistamines, and other treatments have not been effective and tests have shown one or two specific allergens to be responsible. Desensitization often provides incomplete relief and can be time consuming.

Treatment involves giving a series of injections containing gradually increasing doses of an extract of the allergen. The way in which this prevents allergic reactions is not understood. Perhaps controlled exposure triggers the immune system into producing increasing levels of antibodies so that the body no longer responds dramatically when the allergen is encountered naturally.

Desensitization must be carried out under medical supervision because it can provoke a severe allergic response. It is important to remain near emergency medical facilities for at least one hour after each injection.

COMPARISON OF ANTIHISTAMINES

Although antihistamines have broadly similar effects and uses, differences in their strength of anticholinergic action and the amount of drowsiness they produce, as well as in their duration of action, affect the uses for which each drug is commonly selected. The table indicates the main uses of some of the common antihistamines and gives an indication of the relative strengths of their anticholinergic and sedative effects and of their duration of action.

- ● Drug used
- ■ Strong
- ◪ Medium
- □ Minimal
- ▲ Long (over 12 hours)
- ◮ Medium (6–12 hours)
- △ Short (4–6 hours)

Drugs	Common uses — Allergic rhinitis	Skin allergy	Sedation	Premedication	Nausea/vomiting	Cough/cold remedies	Actions and effects — Drowsiness	Anticholinergic action	Duration of action
Alimemazine	●	●	●				■	□	◮
Azatadine	●	●					◪	□	▲
Brompheniramine	●	●				●		□	△
Cetirizine	●	●					□	□	▲
Chlorphenamine	●	●	●				◪	◪	△
Dimenhydrinate					●			◪	△
Diphenhydramine			●		●	●	■	◪	△
Diphenylpyraline	●	●					◪	■	
Hydroxyzine		●	●					◪	△
Loratadine	●	●					□	□	▲
Promethazine	●	●	●	●	●		■	◪	◮
Terfenadine	●	●					◪	□	◮
Triprolidine	●	●				●		□	◮

watering, and swelling. In addition, the anticholinergic action of these drugs contributes to this effect by reducing the secretions from tear glands and nasal passages.

Antihistamine drugs pass from the blood into the brain. In the brain, the blocking action of the antihistamines on histamine activity may produce general sedation and depression of various brain functions, including the vomiting and coughing mechanisms.

How they affect you

Antihistamines frequently cause a degree of drowsiness and may adversely affect coordination, leading to clumsiness. Some of the newer drugs have little or no sedative effect (see table above).

Anticholinergic side effects, including dry mouth, blurred vision, and difficulty passing urine, are common. Most side effects diminish with continued use and can often be helped by an adjustment in dosage or a change to a different drug.

Risks and special precautions

It may be advisable to avoid driving or operating machinery while taking antihistamines, particularly those that are more likely to cause drowsiness (see table above). The sedative effects of alcohol, sleeping drugs, opioid analgesics, and anti-anxiety drugs can also be increased by antihistamines.

In high doses, or in children, some antihistamines can cause excitement, agitation, and even, in extreme cases, hallucinations and convulsions. Abnormal heart rhythms have occurred after high doses with some antihistamines or when drugs that interact with them, such as antifungals and antibiotics, have been taken at the same time. Heart rhythm problems may also affect people with liver disease, electrolyte disturbances, or abnormal heart activity. A person who has these conditions, or who has glaucoma or prostate trouble, should seek medical advice before taking antihistamines because their various drug actions may make such conditions worse.

ANTIHISTAMINES AND ALLERGIC RHINITIS

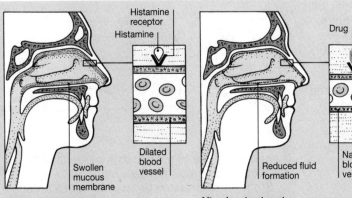

Before drug treatment
In allergic rhinitis, histamine released in response to an allergen acts on histamine receptors and produces dilation of the blood vessels supplying the lining of the nose, leading to swelling and increased mucus production. There is also irritation that causes sneezing, and often redness and watering of the eyes.

After drug treatment
Antihistamine drugs prevent histamine from attaching to histamine receptors, thereby preventing the body from responding to allergens. Over a period of time, the swelling, irritation, sneezing, and watery discharge are reduced, and further contact with the allergen responsible usually produces only minor allergic symptoms.

COMMON DRUGS

Non-sedating
Acrivastine
Cetirizine ✱
Fexofenadine
Loratadine ✱
Mizolastine
Terfenadine ✱

Sedating
Azatadine
Brompheniramine
Chlorphenamine
Clemastine
Dimenhydrinate
Diphenhydramine
Diphenylpyraline
Doxylamine
Promethazine ✱
Trimeprazine
Triprolidine

✱ See Part 4

INFECTIONS AND INFESTATIONS

The human body provides a suitable environment for the growth of many types of microorganisms, including bacteria, viruses, fungi, yeasts, and protozoa. It may also become the host for animal parasites such as insects, worms, and flukes.

Microorganisms (microbes) exist all around us and can be transmitted from person to person in many ways: direct contact, inhalation of infected air, and consumption of contaminated food or water (see Transmission of infection, facing page). Not all microorganisms cause disease; many types of bacteria exist on the skin surface or in the bowel without causing ill effects, while others cannot live either in or on the body.

Normally the immune system protects the body from infection. Invading microbes are killed before they can multiply in sufficient numbers to cause serious disease. (See also Malignant and immune disease, p.152.)

What can go wrong

Infectious diseases occur when the body is invaded by microbes. This may be caused by the body having little or no natural immunity to the invading organism, or the number of invading microbes being too great for the body's immune system to overcome. Serious infections can occur when the immune system does not function properly or when a disease weakens or destroys the immune system, as occurs in AIDS (acquired immune deficiency syndrome).

Infections (such as childhood infectious diseases or those with flu-like symptoms) can cause generalized illness or they may affect a specific part of the body (as in wound infections). Some parts are more susceptible to infection than others – respiratory tract infections are relatively common, whereas bone and muscle infections are rare.

Some symptoms are the result of damage to body tissues by the infection, or by *toxins* released by the microbes. In other cases, the symptoms result from the body's defence mechanisms.

Most bacterial and viral infections cause fever. Bacterial infections may also cause inflammation and pus formation in the affected area.

Why drugs are used

Treatment of an infection is necessary only when the type or severity of symptoms shows that the immune system has not overcome the infection.

Bacterial infection can be treated with antibiotic or antibacterial drugs. Some of these drugs actually kill the infecting bacteria, whereas others merely prevent them from multiplying.

Types of infecting organisms
Bacteria
A typical bacterium (right) consists of a single cell that has a protective wall. Some bacteria are aerobic – that is, they require oxygen – and therefore are more likely to infect surface areas such as the skin or respiratory tract. Others are anaerobic and multiply in oxygen-free surroundings such as the bowel or deep puncture wounds.

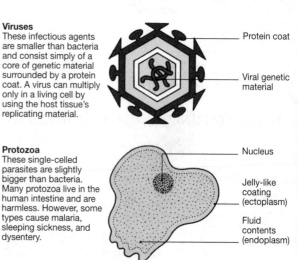

Nucleus

Cell wall

Cocci (spherical)
Streptococcus (above) can cause sore throats and pneumonia.

Bacilli (rod-shaped)
Mycobacterium tuberculosis (above) causes tuberculosis.

Spirochaete (spiral-shaped) This group includes bacteria that cause syphilis and gum infections.

Viruses
These infectious agents are smaller than bacteria and consist simply of a core of genetic material surrounded by a protein coat. A virus can multiply only in a living cell by using the host tissue's replicating material.

Protein coat

Viral genetic material

Protozoa
These single-celled parasites are slightly bigger than bacteria. Many protozoa live in the human intestine and are harmless. However, some types cause malaria, sleeping sickness, and dysentery.

Nucleus

Jelly-like coating (ectoplasm)

Fluid contents (endoplasm)

Unnecessary use of antibiotics may result in the development of resistant bacteria.

Some antibiotics can be used to treat a broad range of infections, while others are effective against a particular type of bacterium or in a certain part of the body. Antibiotics are most commonly given by mouth, or by injection in severe infections, but they may be applied topically for a local action.

Antiviral drugs are used for severe viral infections that threaten body organs or survival. Antivirals may

How bacteria affect the body

Bacteria can cause symptoms of disease in two principal ways: first, by releasing toxins that harm body cells; second, by provoking an inflammatory response in the infected tissues.

Effects of toxins

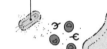

The invading bacterium gives off poisons (toxins) that attack the body cell.

The toxins emanating from the bacterium break through the cell structure and destroy the cell.

Inflammatory response

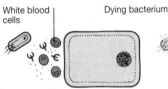
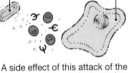

White blood cells of the immune system attack the bacterium directly by releasing inflammatory substances and, later, antibodies.

A side effect of this attack of the immune system on the bacterium is damage to, and inflammation of, the body's own cells.

Transmission of infection

Infecting organisms can enter the human body through a variety of routes, including direct contact between an infected person and someone else, and eating or inhaling infected material.

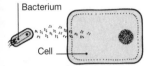

Droplet infection
Coughing and sneezing spread infected secretions.

Insects
Insect bites may transmit infection.

Physical contact
Everyday contact may spread infection.

Sexual contact
Certain infections and infestations may be spread by genital contact.

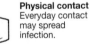

Food
Many infecting organisms can be ingested in food.

Water
Infections can be spread in polluted water.

be used in topical preparations, given by mouth, or administered in hospital by injection.

Other drugs used in the fight against infection include antiprotozoal drugs for protozoal infections such as malaria; antifungal drugs for infection by fungi and yeasts, including *Candida* (thrush); and anthelmintics to eradicate worm and fluke infestations. Cases of infestation by skin parasites are usually treated with the topical application of insecticides (see p.176.)

INFESTATIONS

Invasion by parasites that live on the body (such as lice) or in the body (such as tapeworms) is known as infestation. Since the body lacks strong natural defences against infestation, antiparasitic treatment is necessary. Infestations are often associated with tropical climates and poor standards of hygiene.

Tapeworms and roundworms live in the intestines and may cause diarrhoea and anaemia. Roundworm eggs may be passed in faeces. Hookworm larvae in infected soil usually enter the body through the skin. Tapeworms may grow to 9m (30 feet) and infection occurs through undercooked meat containing larvae.

Flukes are of various types. The liver fluke (acquired from infected vegetation) lives near the bile duct in the liver and can cause jaundice. A more serious type (which lives in small blood vessels supplying the bladder or intestines) causes schistosomiasis and is acquired from contact with infected water.

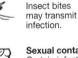

Lice and scabies spread by direct contact. Head, clothing, and pubic lice need human blood to survive and die away from the body. Dried faeces of clothing lice spread typhus by infecting wounds or being inhaled. Scabies (caused by a tiny mite that does not carry disease) makes small, itchy tunnels in the skin.

Life cycle of a worm

Many worms have a complex life cycle. The life cycle of the worm that causes the group of diseases known as filariasis is illustrated below.

A mosquito ingests the filarial larvae and bites a human, thereby transmitting the larvae.

The mature larvae enter the lymph glands and vessels and reproduce there, often causing no ill effects.

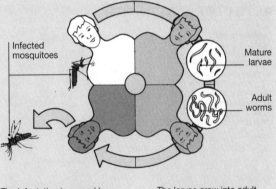

Infected mosquitoes

Mature larvae

Adult worms

The infestation is spread by mosquitoes biting infected people and restarting the cycle.

The larvae grow into adult worms, which release larvae into the bloodstream.

MAJOR DRUG GROUPS

Antibiotics and antibacterial drugs (including antituberculosis drugs)
Antiviral drugs
Vaccines and immunizations

Antiprotozoal drugs (including antimalarial drugs)
Antifungal drugs
Anthelmintic drugs

ANTIBIOTICS

One out of every six prescriptions that British doctors write every year is for antibiotics. These drugs are usually safe and effective in the treatment of bacterial disorders ranging from minor infections, like conjunctivitis, to life-threatening diseases like pneumonia, meningitis, and septicaemia. They are similar in function to the antibacterial drugs (see p.131), but the early antibiotics all had a natural origin in moulds and fungi, although most are now synthesized.

Since 1941, when the first antibiotic, penicillin, was introduced, many different classes have been developed. Each one has a different chemical composition and is effective against a particular range of bacteria. None is effective against viral infections (see Antiviral drugs, p.133).

Some of the antibiotics have a broad spectrum of activity against a wide variety of bacteria. Others are used in the treatment of infection by only a few specific organisms. For a description of each common class of antibiotic, see Classes of antibiotics p.130.

Why they are used

We are surrounded by bacteria – in the air we breathe, on the mucous membranes of our mouth and nose, on our skin, and in our intestines – but we are protected, most of the time, by our immunological defences. When these break down, or when bacteria already present migrate to a vulnerable new site, or when harmful

ANTIBIOTIC RESISTANCE

The increasing use of antibiotics in the treatment of infection has led to resistance in certain types of bacteria to the effects of particular antibiotics. This resistance to the drug usually occurs when bacteria develop mechanisms of growth and reproduction that are not disrupted by the effects of the antibiotics. In other cases, bacteria produce *enzymes* that neutralize the antibiotics.

Antibiotic resistance may develop in a person during prolonged treatment when a drug has failed to eliminate the infection quickly. The resistant strain of bacteria is able to multiply, thereby prolonging the illness. It

may also infect other people, and result in the spread of resistant infection. One particularly important example is methicillin-resistant staphylococcus aureus, which resists most antibiotics but can be treated with other drugs such as teicoplanin and vancomycin.

Doctors try to prevent the development of antibiotic resistance by selecting the drug most likely to eliminate the bacteria present in each individual case as quickly and as thoroughly as possible. Failure to complete a course of antibiotics that has been prescribed by your doctor increases the likelihood that the infection will recur in a resistant form.

bacteria not usually present invade the body, infectious disease sets in.

The bacteria multiply uncontrollably, destroying tissue, releasing toxins, and, in some cases, threatening to spread via the bloodstream to such vital organs as the heart, brain, lungs, and kidneys. The symptoms of infectious disease vary widely, depending on the site of the infection and the type of bacteria.

Confronted with a sick person and suspecting a bacterial infection, the doctor should identify the organism causing the disease before prescribing any drug. However, tests to analyse blood, sputum, urine, stool, or pus usually take 24 hours or more. In the meantime, especially if the person is in discomfort

or pain, the doctor usually makes a preliminary drug choice, something of an educated guess as to the causative organism. In starting this "empirical treatment", as it is called, the doctor is guided by the site of the infection, the nature and severity of the symptoms, the likely source of infection, and the prevalence of any similar illnesses in the community at that time.

In such circumstances, pending laboratory identification of the trouble-making bacteria, the doctor may initially prescribe a broad-spectrum antibiotic, which is effective against a wide variety of bacteria. As soon as tests provide more exact information, the doctor may switch the person to the recommended antibiotic treatment for the identified bacteria. In some cases, more than one antibiotic is prescribed, to be sure of eliminating all strains of bacteria.

In most cases, antibiotics can be given by mouth. However, in serious infections when high blood levels of the drug are needed rapidly, or when a type of antibiotic is needed that cannot be given by mouth, the drug may be given by injection. Antibiotics are also included in *topical* preparations for localized skin, eye, and ear infections (see also Anti-infective skin preparations, p.175, and Drugs for ear disorders, p.171).

How they work

Depending on the type of drug and the dosage, antibiotics are either bactericidal, killing organisms directly, or bacteriostatic, halting the multiplication of bacteria and enabling the body's natural defences to overcome the remaining infection.

Penicillins and cephalosporins are bactericidal, destroying bacteria by preventing them from making normal cell walls; most other antibiotics act inside the bacteria by interfering with the chemical activities essential to their life cycle.

How they affect you

Antibiotics stop most common types of infection within days. Because they do not relieve symptoms directly, your doctor

ACTION OF ANTIBIOTICS

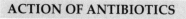

Penicillins and cephalosporins
Drugs from these groups are bactericidal – that is, they kill bacteria. They interfere with the chemicals needed by bacteria to form normal cell walls (right). The cell's outer lining disintegrates and the bacterium dies (far right).

Other antibiotics
These drugs alter chemical activity inside the bacteria, thereby preventing the production of proteins that the bacteria need to multiply and survive (right). This may have a bactericidal effect in itself, or it may prevent reproduction (bacteriostatic action) (far right).

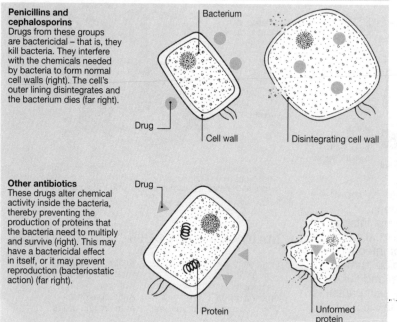

Bacterium

Drug

Cell wall

Disintegrating cell wall

Drug

Protein

Unformed protein

USES OF ANTIBIOTICS

The table below shows which common drugs in each class of antibiotic are used for the treatment of infections in different parts of the body. For the purposes of comparison, this table also includes (in the Other drugs category) some antibacterial drugs that are discussed on page 131. This table is not intended to be used as a guide to prescribing but indicates the possible applications of each drug. Some drugs have a wide range of possible uses; this table concentrates on the most common ones.

Antibiotic	Ear, nose, throat, and mouth	Respiratory tract	Skin and soft tissue	Gastrointestinal tract	Eye	Kidney and urinary tract	Brain and nervous system	Heart	Bones and joints	Genital tract
Penicillins										
Amoxycillin	●	●	●			●		●	●	●
Ampicillin	●	●	●			●	●		●	●
Benzylpenicillin	●	●	●				●	●	●	●
Co-amoxiclav	●	●	●			●			●	
Flucloxacillin	●		●					●	●	
Phenoxymethylpenicillin	●	●	●							
Cephalosporins										
Cefaclor	●	●				●				
Cefotaxime		●					●			
Cefoxitin		●	●			●				●
Cefalexin		●	●			●				
Macrolides										
Azithromycin	●	●	●							●
Erythromycin	●	●	●	●	●				●	●
Tetracyclines										
Doxycycline	●	●				●				●
Oxytetracycline	●	●								
Tetracycline	●	●			●	●				●
Aminoglycosides										
Amikacin		●	●	●		●	●		●	
Gentamicin		●	●	●	●	●	●	●	●	
Neomycin			●	●						
Netilmicin		●	●			●	●		●	
Streptomycin		●						●		
Tobramycin		●	●	●		●	●		●	
Sulphonamides										
Co-trimoxazole						●				
Sulphafurazole	●	●				●				
Other drugs										
Chloramphenicol	●	●		●	●		●			
Ciprofloxacin		●		●		●				
Clindamycin		●	●	●					●	
Colistin		●				●				
Dapsone			●							
Fusidic acid			●						●	
Metronidazole	●		●	●			●	●	●	●
Nalidixic acid						●				
Nitrofurantoin						●				
Teicoplanin				●				●	●	
Trimethoprim		●				●				
Vancomycin				●				●		

ANTIBIOTICS continued

may advise additional medication, such as analgesics (see p.80), to relieve pain and fever until the antibiotics take effect.

It is important to complete the course of medication as it has been prescribed by your doctor, even if all your symptoms have disappeared. Failure to do this can lead to a resurgence of the infection in an antibiotic-resistant form (see Antibiotic resistance, p.128).

Most antibiotics used in the home do not cause any adverse effects if taken in the recommended dosage. In people who do experience adverse effects, nausea and diarrhoea are among the more common ones (see also individual drug profiles in Part 4). Some people may be sensitive to certain types of

DRUG TREATMENT FOR MENINGITIS

Meningitis is inflammation of the meninges (the membranes surrounding the brain and spinal cord) and is caused by both bacteria and viruses. Bacterial meningitis can kill previously well individuals within hours.

If bacterial meningitis is suspected, intravenous antibiotics are needed immediately and admission to hospital is arranged.

In cases of bacterial meningitis caused by *Haemophilus influenzae* or *Neisseria meningitidis*, close contacts of these patients are advised to have a preventative course of antibiotics, usually rifampicin.

antibiotics, which can result in a variety of serious adverse effects.

Risks and special precautions

Most antibiotics used for short periods outside a hospital setting are safe for most people. The most common risk, particularly with cephalosporins and penicillins, is a severe allergic reaction to the drug that can cause rashes and sometimes swelling of the face and throat. If this happens, the drug should be stopped and immediate medical advice sought. If you have had a previous allergic reaction to an antibiotic, all other drugs in that class and related classes should be avoided. It is therefore important to inform your doctor if you have previously suffered an adverse reaction to treatment with an antibiotic (with the exception of minor bowel disturbances).

Another risk of antibiotic treatment, especially if it is prolonged, is that the balance among microorganisms normally inhabiting the body may be disturbed. In particular, antibiotics may destroy the bacteria that normally limit the growth of *Candida*, a yeast that is often present in the body in small amounts. This can lead to overgrowth of *Candida* (thrush) in the mouth, vagina, or bowel, and an antifungal drug (p.138) may be needed.

A rarer, but more serious, result of disruption of normal bacterial activity in the body is a disorder known as pseudomembranous colitis, in which

bacteria that are resistant to the antibiotic multiply in the bowel, causing violent, bloody diarrhoea. This potentially fatal disorder can occur with any antibiotic, but is most common with the lincosamides.

COMMON DRUGS

Aminoglycosides	Penicillins
Amikacin	Amoxicillin *
Gentamicin *	Ampicillin
Neomycin	Azlocillin
Netilmicin	Aztreonam
Streptomycin	Benzylpenicillin
Tobramycin	Co-amoxiclav
	Co-fluampicil
Cephalosporins	Flucloxacillin
Cefaclor *	Imipenem
Cefalexin *	Phenoxymethyl-
Cefamandole	penicillin *
Cefazolin	
Cefixime	**Tetracyclines**
Cefodizime	Doxycycline *
Cefoxitin	Oxytetracycline
Cefpodoxime	Tetracycline *
Cefradine	
Ceftazidime	**Other drugs**
Cafadroxil	Chloramphenicol *
	Colistin
Lincosamides	Fusidic acid
Clindamycin	Metronidazole *
	Rifampicin *
Macrolides	Spectinomycin
Azithromycin	Teicoplanin
Clarithromycin	Trimethoprim *
Erythromycin *	Vancomycin

| * See Part 4 |

CLASSES OF ANTIBIOTICS

Penicillins
The first antibiotic drugs to be developed, penicillins are still widely used to treat many common infections. Some penicillins are not effective when they are taken by mouth and therefore have to be given by injection in hospital. Unfortunately, certain strains of bacteria are resistant to penicillin treatment, and other drugs may have to be substituted. Penicillins often cause allergic reactions.

Cephalosporins
These are broad-spectrum antibiotics similar to the penicillins. They are often used when penicillin treatment has proved ineffective. Some cephalosporins can be given by mouth, but others are only given by injection. About 10 per cent of people who are allergic to penicillins may be allergic to cephalosporins. Some cephalosporins can occasionally damage the kidneys, particularly if used with aminoglycosides. Another serious, although rare, adverse effect of a few cephalosporins is that they occasionally interfere with normal blood clotting, leading to abnormally heavy bleeding, especially in the elderly.

Macrolides
Erythromycin is the most common drug in this group. It is a broad-spectrum antibiotic that is often prescribed as an alternative to penicillins or cephalosporins. Erythromycin is also effective against certain diseases, such as Legionnaires' disease (a rare type of

pneumonia), that cannot be treated with other antibiotics. The main risk with erythromycin is that it can occasionally impair liver function.

Tetracyclines
These have a broader spectrum of activity than other classes of antibiotic. However, increasing bacterial resistance (see Antibiotic resistance, p.128) has limited their use, although they are still widely prescribed. As well as being used for the treatment of infections, tetracyclines are also used in the long-term treatment of acne, although this application is probably not related to their antibacterial action. A major drawback to the use of tetracycline antibiotics in young children and in pregnant women is that they are deposited in developing bones and teeth.

With the exception of doxycycline, drugs from this group are poorly absorbed through the intestines, and when given by mouth they have to be administered in high doses in order to reach effective levels in the blood. Such high doses increase the likelihood of diarrhoea as a side effect. The absorption of tetracyclines can be further reduced by interaction with calcium and other minerals. Drugs from this group should not therefore be taken with iron tablets or milk products. Tetracyclines deteriorate and may become poisonous with time, so leftover tablets or capsules should always be discarded.

Aminoglycosides
These potent drugs are effective against a broad range of bacteria. However, they are not

as widely used as some other antibiotics since they have to be given by injection and they have potentially serious side effects. Their use is therefore limited to hospital treatment of serious infections. They are often given with other antibiotics. Possible adverse effects include damage to the kidneys and the nerves in the ear, and severe skin rashes.

Lincosamides
The lincosamide clindamycin is not commonly used as it is more likely to cause serious disruption of bacterial activity in the bowel than other antibiotics. It is mainly reserved for the treatment of bone, joint, abdominal, and pelvic infections that do not respond well to the safer antibiotics. Clindamycin is also used topically for acne and vaginal infections.

Quinolones
These drugs are often called antibacterials because they are derived from chemicals rather than living organisms. Quinolones have a broad spectrum of activity. They are used in the treatment of urinary infections and are widely effective in acute diarrhoeal diseases, including that caused by salmonella, as well as in the treatment of enteric fever.

The absorption of quinolones is reduced by antacids containing magnesium and aluminium. They are well tolerated but should be avoided by epileptics, as they may rarely cause convulsions, and by children, as studies have shown that they may cause arthritis.

ANTIBACTERIAL DRUGS

This broad classification of drugs comprises agents that are similar to the antibiotics (p.128) in function but dissimilar in origin. The original antibiotics were derived from living organisms, for example, moulds and fungi. Antibacterials were developed from chemicals. The sulphonamides were the first drugs to be given for the treatment of bacterial infections and provided the mainstay of the treatment of infection before penicillin (the first antibiotic) became generally available. Increasing bacterial resistance and the development of antibiotics that are more effective and less *toxic* have reduced the use of sulphonamides.

Why they are used

Sulphonamides have a number of uses. Because certain strains of bacteria have developed a resistance to their actions (see Antibiotic resistance, p.128), the sulphonamides have in many cases been superseded by antibiotics that are more effective and safer. Yet there are still many circumstances in which doctors prescribe the sulphonamides.

Because sulphonamides reach high concentrations in the urine, they are especially useful for treating many urinary tract infections. They are often used for chlamydial pneumonia and some middle ear infections. Trimethoprim is used for chest and urinary tract infections. The drug used to be combined with sulfamethoxazole as co-trimoxazole, but because of the side effects of sulfamethoxazole, trimethoprim on its own is usually preferred now.

Not all antibacterials are sulphonamides. Antibacterials used for tuberculosis are discussed on p.132. Others, sometimes classified as antimicrobials, include metronidazole, prescribed for a variety of genital infections and for some serious

ACTION OF SULPHONAMIDES

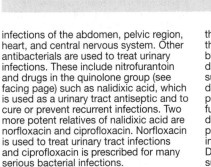

Before drug treatment
Folic acid, a chemical that is necessary for the growth of bacteria, is produced within bacterial cells by an *enzyme* that acts on a chemical called para-aminobenzoic acid.

Bacterium

Enzyme

Para-aminobenzoic acid

Folic acid

After drug treatment
Sulphonamides interfere with the release of the enzyme. This prevents folic acid from being formed. The bacterium is therefore unable to function properly and dies.

Drug

Dying bacterium

infections of the abdomen, pelvic region, heart, and central nervous system. Other antibacterials are used to treat urinary infections. These include nitrofurantoin and drugs in the quinolone group (see facing page) such as nalidixic acid, which is used as a urinary tract antiseptic and to cure or prevent recurrent infections. Two more potent relatives of nalidixic acid are norfloxacin and ciprofloxacin. Norfloxacin is used to treat urinary tract infections and ciprofloxacin is prescribed for many serious bacterial infections.

How they work

Most antibacterials function by preventing growth and multiplication of bacteria (see also Action of antibiotics, p.128, and Action of sulphonamides, above).

How they affect you

Antibacterials usually take several days to eliminate bacteria. During this time your doctor may recommend additional medication to alleviate pain and fever. Possible side effects of sulphonamides include loss of appetite, nausea, a rash, and drowsiness.

Risks and special precautions

Like antibiotics, most antibacterials can cause allergic reactions in susceptible people. Possible symptoms that should always be brought to your doctor's attention include rashes and fever. If such symptoms occur, a change to another drug is likely to be necessary. Treatment with sulphonamides carries a number of serious, but rare risks. Some drugs in

this group can cause crystals to form in the kidneys, a risk that can be reduced by drinking adequate amounts of fluid during prolonged treatment. Because sulphonamides may also occasionally damage the liver, they are not usually prescribed for people with impaired liver function. There is also a slight risk of damage to bone marrow, lowering the production of white blood cells and increasing the chances of infection. Doctors therefore try to avoid prescribing sulphonamides for prolonged periods. Liver function and blood composition are often monitored during unavoidable long-term treatment.

DRUG TREATMENT FOR HANSEN'S DISEASE

Hansen's disease, better known as leprosy, is a bacterial infection caused by *Mycobacterium leprae*. It is rare in the United Kingdom, but relatively common in parts of Africa, Asia, and Latin America.

The disease progresses slowly, first affecting the peripheral nerves and causing loss of sensation in the hands and feet. This leads to frequent unnoticed injuries and consequent scarring. Later, the nerves of the face may also be affected.

Treatment uses three drugs together to prevent the development of resistance. Usually, dapsone, rifampicin, and clofazimine will be given for at least 2 years. If one of these cannot be used, then a second line drug (ofloxacin, minocycline, or clarithromycin) might be substituted. Complications during treatment may require use of prednisolone, aspirin, chloroquine, or even thalidomide.

COMMON DRUGS

Quinolones
Cinoxacin
Ciprofloxacin ✳
Grepafloxacin
Levofloxacin ✳
Nalidixic acid
Norfloxacin
Ofloxacin

Sulphonamides
Co-trimoxazole ✳
Sulfadiazine
Sulfadimidine

Urinary antiseptic
Nitrofurantoin ✳

Other drugs
Clofazimine
Dapsone
Metronidazole ✳
Tinidazole
Trimethoprim ✳

✳ See Part 4

ANTITUBERCULOUS DRUGS

Tuberculosis is a contagious bacterial disease acquired, often in childhood, by inhaling the tuberculosis bacilli present in the spray caused by a sneeze or cough from someone who is actively infected. It may also be acquired from infected cow's milk. The disease usually starts in a lung and takes one of two forms: either primary infection or reactivated infection.

In 90 to 95 per cent of those with a primary infection, the body's immune system suppresses the infection but does not kill the bacilli. They remain alive but dormant and may cause the reactivated form of the disease. After they are reactivated, the tuberculosis bacilli may spread via the lymphatic system and bloodstream throughout the body (see Sites of infection, below).

The first symptoms of the primary infection may include a cough, fever, tiredness, night sweats, and weight loss. Tuberculosis is confirmed through clinical investigations, which may include a chest X-ray, isolation of the bacilli from the person's sputum, and a positive reaction – localized inflammation – to the Mantoux test, an injection of tuberculin (a protein extracted from tuberculosis bacilli) into the skin.

The gradual emergence in adults of the destructive and progressive form of tuberculosis is caused by the reactivated infection. It occurs in 5 to 10 per cent of those who have had a previous primary infection. Another form, reinfection tuberculosis, occurs when someone with the dormant, primary form is reinfected. This type of tuberculosis is clinically identical to the reactivated form. Reactivation is more likely in those people whose immune system is suppressed, such as the elderly, those on corticosteroids or other immunosuppressant drugs, and those who have AIDS. Reactivation tuberculosis may be difficult to identify because the symptoms may start in any part of the body seeded with the bacilli. It is most often first seen in the upper lobes of the lung, and is frequently diagnosed after a chest X-ray. The early symptoms may be identical to those of primary infection: a cough, tiredness, night sweats, fever, and weight loss.

If left untreated, tuberculosis continues to destroy tissue, spreading throughout the body and eventually causing death. It was one of the most common causes of death in the United Kingdom until the 1940s and the disease is on the increase again. Vulnerable groups are people with suppressed immune systems and the homeless.

Why they are used

A person who has been diagnosed as having tuberculosis is likely to be treated with three or four antituberculous drugs. This helps to overcome the risk of drug-resistant strains of the bacilli emerging (see Antibiotic resistance, p.128).

The standard drug combination for the treatment of tuberculosis consists of rifampicin, isoniazid, and pyrazinamide. In areas where there is a high prevalence of drug-resistant tuberculosis ethambutol may be added. However, other drugs may be substituted if the initial treatment fails or if drug sensitivity tests indicate that the bacilli are resistant to these drugs.

The standard duration of treatment for a newly diagnosed tuberculosis infection is a six-month regimen as follows: isoniazid, rifampicin, and pyrazinamide (perhaps with ethambutol) daily for two months, followed by isoniazid and rifampicin for four months. The duration of treatment can be extended from nine months to up to two years in people at particular risk, such as those with a suppressed immune system.

Corticosteroids may be added to the treatment, if the patient does not have a suppressed immune system, to reduce the amount of tissue damage.

Both the number of drugs required and the long duration of treatment may make treatment difficult, particularly for those who are homeless. To help with this problem, supervised administration of treatment is available when required, both in the community and in hospital.

Tuberculosis infection in patients with HIV infection or AIDS is treated with the standard antituberculous drug regimen; but lifelong preventative treatment with isoniazid may be necessary.

SITES OF INFECTION

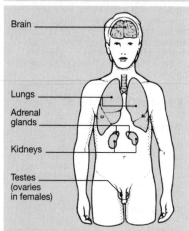

Brain

Lungs

Adrenal glands

Kidneys

Testes (ovaries in females)

Tuberculosis usually affects only part of one lung at first. However, later outbreaks usually spread to both lungs and may also affect the kidneys, leading to pyelonephritis; the adrenal glands, causing Addison's disease; and the membranes surrounding the brain, which may lead to meningitis. The testes (in men) and the ovaries (in women) may also be affected.

TUBERCULOSIS PREVENTION

A vaccine prepared from an artificially weakened strain of cattle tuberculosis bacteria can provide immunity from tuberculosis by provoking the development of natural resistance to the disease (see Vaccines and immunization, p.134). The BCG (Bacille Calmette-Guérin) vaccine is a form of tuberculosis bacillus that provokes the body's immune response but does not cause the illness because it is not infectious. The vaccine is usually given to children between the ages of 10 and 14 years who are shown to have no natural immunity when given a skin test. BCG vaccination may be given to newborn babies if, for example, someone in the family has tuberculosis.

How it is done
The vaccine is usually injected into the upper arm. A small pustule usually appears 6–12 weeks later, by which time the person can be considered immune.

How they work

Antituberculous drugs act in the same way as antibiotics, either by killing bacilli or preventing them from multiplying (see Action of antibiotics, p.128).

How they affect you

Although the drugs start to combat the disease within days, benefits of drug treatment are not usually noticeable for a few weeks. As the infection is eradicated, the body repairs the damage caused by the disease. Symptoms such as fever and coughing gradually subside, and appetite and general health improve.

Risks and special precautions

Antituberculous drugs may cause adverse effects (nausea, vomiting, and abdominal pain), and they occasionally lead to serious allergic reactions. When this happens, another drug is substituted.

Rifampicin and isoniazid may affect liver function; isoniazid may adversely affect the nerves as well. Ethambutol can cause changes in colour vision. Dosage is carefully monitored, especially in children, the elderly, and those with reduced kidney function.

COMMON DRUGS

Capreomycin	Pyrazinamide
Cycloserine	Rifampicin *
Ethambutol *	Rifabutin
Isoniazid *	Streptomycin

* See Part 4

ANTIVIRAL DRUGS

Viruses are simpler and smaller organisms than bacteria and are less able to sustain themselves. These organisms can survive and multiply only by penetrating body cells (see Action of antiviral drugs, right). Because viruses perform few functions independently, medicines that disrupt or halt their life cycle without harming human cells have been difficult to develop.

There are many different types of virus, and viral infections cause illnesses with various symptoms and degrees of severity. Common viral illnesses include the cold, influenza and flu-like illnesses, cold sores, and the usual childhood diseases such as chickenpox and mumps. Throat infections, pneumonia, acute bronchitis, gastroenteritis, and meningitis are often, but not always, caused by a virus.

Fortunately, the natural defences of the body are usually strong enough to overcome infections such as these, with drugs given to ease pain and lower fever. However, the more serious viral diseases, such as pneumonia and meningitis, need close medical supervision.

Another difficulty with viral infections is the speed with which the virus multiplies. By the time symptoms appear, the viruses are so numerous that antiviral drugs have little effect. Antiviral agents must be given early in the course of a viral infection or they may be used prophylactically (as a preventative). Some viral infections can be prevented by vaccination (see p.134).

Why they are used

The main area where antiviral drugs are helpful is in the treatment of various conditions caused by the herpes virus: cold sores, encephalitis, genital herpes, chickenpox, and shingles.

Some drugs are applied *topically* to treat outbreaks of cold sores, herpes eye infections, and genital herpes. They can reduce the severity and duration of an outbreak, but they do not eliminate the infection permanently. Other antiviral drugs are given by mouth or, under exceptional circumstances by injection, to prevent chickenpox or severe, recurrent attacks of the herpes virus infections in those who are already weakened by other conditions.

Antiviral agents are also given to prevent influenza A, as is amantadine, a drug for parkinsonism that also has antiviral properties.

The interferons are proteins produced by the body and involved in the immune response and cell function. Interferon alpha and beta have recently been shown to be effective in reducing disease activity in people infected with hepatitis B and hepatitis C. Further research into the antiviral activity of these agents is under way, including their use in the treatment of central nervous system conditions, such as multiple sclerosis.

ACTION OF ANTIVIRAL DRUGS

In order to reproduce, a virus requires a living cell. The invaded cell eventually dies and the new viruses are released, spreading and infecting other cells. Most antiviral drugs act to prevent the virus from using the host cell's genetic material, DNA, to multiply. Unable to divide, the virus dies and the spread of infection is halted.

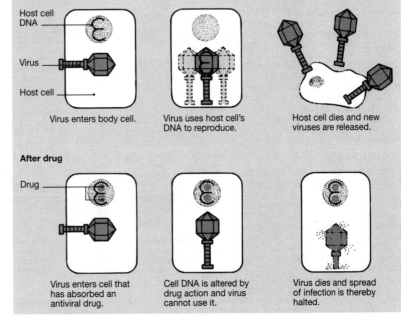

Before drug

Host cell DNA
Virus
Host cell

Virus enters body cell.

Virus uses host cell's DNA to reproduce.

Host cell dies and new viruses are released.

After drug

Drug

Virus enters cell that has absorbed an antiviral drug.

Cell DNA is altered by drug action and virus cannot use it.

Virus dies and spread of infection is thereby halted.

AIDS (acquired immune deficiency syndrome) is caused by a viral infection, HIV, that reduces the body's resistance to infection by other viruses, bacteria, and protozoa, as well as to some types of cancer. Drug treatment for AIDS is discussed more fully on p.157.

How they work

Some antiviral drugs, such as idoxuridine, act by altering the cell's genetic material (DNA) so that the virus cannot use it to multiply. Other drugs stop multiplication of viruses by blocking enzyme activity within the host cell. Halting multiplication prevents the virus from spreading to uninfected cells and improves symptoms rapidly. However, in herpes infections, it does not eradicate the virus from the body. Infection may therefore flare up on another occasion.

Amantadine has a different action: it prevents the virus from entering the cells. It is therefore most effective when it is given as a *prophylactic*, before the infection has spread widely.

How they affect you

Topical antiviral drugs usually start to act at once. Providing that the treatment is applied early enough, an outbreak of herpes can be cut short. Symptoms usually clear up within two to four days. Antiviral ointments may cause irritation and redness. Antiviral drugs given by mouth or injection can occasionally cause nausea and dizziness.

Risks and special precautions

Because some of these drugs may affect the kidneys adversely, they are prescribed with caution for people with reduced kidney function. Some antiviral drugs can adversely affect the activity of normal body cells, particularly those in the bone marrow. Idoxuridine is, for this reason, available only for topical application.

COMMON DRUGS

Aciclovir ✳	Inosine pranobex
Amantadine ✳	Interferon ✳
Cidofovir	Penciclovir
Famciclovir	Tribavirin
Foscarnet	Valaciclovir
Ganciclovir	Zanamivir ✳
Idoxuridine	

✳ See Part 4	See also Drugs for HIV, p.157

VACCINES AND IMMUNIZATION

Many infectious diseases, including most of the common viral infections, occur only once during a person's lifetime. The reason is that the antibodies produced in response to the disease remain afterwards, prepared to repel any future invasion as soon as the first infectious germs appear. The duration of such immunity varies, but it can last a lifetime.

Protection against many infections can now be provided artificially by the use of vaccines derived from altered forms of the infecting organism. These vaccines stimulate the immune system in the same way as a genuine infection, and provide lasting, active immunity. Because each type of microbe stimulates the production of a specific antibody, a different vaccine must be given for each disease.

Another type of immunization, called passive immunization, relies on giving antibodies (see Immune globulins, below).

Why they are used

Some infectious diseases cannot be treated effectively or are potentially so serious that prevention is the best treatment. Routine immunization not only protects the individual but may gradually eradicate the disease completely, as has been achieved with smallpox.

Newborn babies receive antibodies for many diseases from their mothers, but this protection lasts only for about three months. Most children between the ages of 2 months and 15 years are routinely vaccinated against common childhood infectious diseases. In addition, travellers to many underdeveloped countries, especially those in the tropics, are often advised to be vaccinated against the diseases common in those regions.

Effective lifelong immunization can sometimes be achieved by a single dose of the vaccine. However, in many cases reinforcing doses, commonly called booster shots, are needed later in order to maintain reliable immunity.

Vaccines do not provide immediate protection against infection and it may be

ACTIVE AND PASSIVE IMMUNIZATION

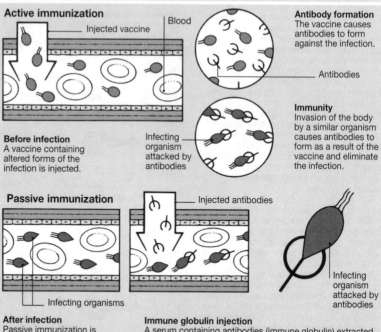

Active immunization

Injected vaccine — Blood

Before infection
A vaccine containing altered forms of the infection is injected.

Infecting organism attacked by antibodies

Antibody formation
The vaccine causes antibodies to form against the infection.

Antibodies

Immunity
Invasion of the body by a similar organism causes antibodies to form as a result of the vaccine and eliminate the infection.

Passive immunization

Injected antibodies

After infection
Passive immunization is needed when the infection has entered the blood.

Infecting organisms

Infecting organism attacked by antibodies

Immune globulin injection
A serum containing antibodies (immune globulin) extracted from donated blood is injected. This helps the body to fight the infection.

up to four weeks before full immunity is able to develop. When immediate protection from infectious disease is needed – for example, following exposure to infection – it may be necessary to establish passive immunity with immune globulins (see below).

How they work

Vaccines provoke the immune system into creating antibodies that help the body to resist specific infectious diseases. Many vaccines (known as live vaccines) are made from artificially

weakened forms of the disease-causing germ. But even these weakened germs are effective in stimulating sufficient growth of antibodies. Other vaccines rely either on inactive (or killed) disease-causing germs, or inactive derivatives of these germs, but their effect on the immune system remains the same. Effective antibodies are created, thereby establishing active immunity.

How they affect you

The degree of protection varies among different vaccines. Some provide reliable lifelong immunity; others may not give full protection against a disease, or the effects may last for as little as six months. Influenza vaccines usually protect only against the variety of virus causing the latest outbreak of flu. New varieties appear during most years.

Any vaccine may cause side effects but they are usually mild and soon disappear. The most common reactions are a red, slightly raised, tender area at the site of injection, and a slight fever or a flu-like illness lasting for one or two days.

Risks and special precautions

Serious reactions are rare and, for most children, the risk is far outweighed by the protection given. Children who have had fits may be advised against vaccinations

IMMUNE GLOBULINS

Antibodies, which can result from exposure to snake and insect venom as well as infectious disease, permeate the serum of the blood (the part remaining after the red cells and clotting agents are removed). The concentrated serum of people who have survived diseases or poisonous bites is called immune globulin, and, given by injection, it creates passive immunity. Immune globulin from blood donated by a wide cross-section of donors is likely to contain antibodies to most common diseases. Specific immune globulins against rare diseases or toxins are derived from the blood of selected donors likely to have high levels of antibodies to that disease. These are called hyperimmune globulins. Some

immune globulins are extracted from horse blood following repeated doses of the toxin.

Because immune globulins do not stimulate the body to produce its own antibodies, their effect is not long-lasting and diminishes progressively over three or four weeks. Continued protection requires repeated injections of immune globulins.

Adverse effects from immune globulins are uncommon. Some people are sensitive to horse globulins, and about a week after the injection they may experience a reaction known as serum sickness, with fever, a rash, joint swelling, and pain. This usually ends in a few days but should be reported to your doctor before any further immunization.

for pertussis (whooping cough) or measles. Children who have any infection more severe than a common cold will not be given any routine vaccination until they have recovered.

Live vaccines should not be given during pregnancy because they can affect the developing baby, nor should they be given to people whose immune systems are weakened by disease or drug treatment. It is also advisable for those taking high doses of corticosteroids (p.141) to delay their vaccinations until the end of drug treatment.

The risk of high fever following the DPT (combined diphtheria, pertussis, and tetanus) vaccine can be reduced by giving paracetamol at the time of vaccination. The pertussis vaccine may rarely cause a mild fit, which is brief, usually associated with fever, and stops without treatment. Children who have experienced such fits recover completely without neurological or developmental problems.

COMMON VACCINATIONS

Disease	Age at which vaccination is given	How given	General information
Diphtheria	2 months, 3 months, 4 months, 3–5 years. Booster on leaving school.	Injection	Given in infancy with tetanus and pertussis vaccines. Immunity may diminish in later life.
Tetanus	2 months, 3 months, 4 months, 3–5 years. Boosters on leaving school and every 10 years thereafter.	Injection	Given in infancy with diphtheria and pertussis, this gives protection for 5 to 10 years. Injury likely to result in tetanus infection is treated with a booster shot.
Pertussis (whooping cough)	2 months, 3 months, 4 months.	Injection	Given in infancy with diphtheria and tetanus, pertussis vaccine may not give complete protection, but reduces the severity of the illness. The vaccine may cause mild fever, irritability, and fits.
Polio	2 months, 3 months, 4 months, 3–5 years. Boosters on leaving school.	By mouth	Many doctors recommend a booster every 10 years, especially for people who are travelling to countries where polio is still prevalent.
Haemophilus influenzae type b (Hib)	2 months, 3 months, 4 months.	Injection	Routinely given in infancy to prevent serious disease up to the age of 4 years.
Rubella (German measles)	12–15 months and 3–5 years	Injection	This is given in infancy with measles and mumps vaccines (MMR. Rubella is important because it can damage the fetus if it affects a woman in early pregnancy. Women of childbearing age who have had the vaccine should avoid becoming pregnant for at least 3 months afterwards.
Measles	12–15 months and 3–5 years.	Injection	Given with mumps and rubella vaccines (MMR) in infancy. It may cause a brief fever, rash, and fits. Measles vaccine does not always provide complete protection, but it reduces the severity of illness.
Mumps	12–15 months and 3–5 years.	Injection	Given together with measles and rubella vaccines (MMR) in infancy.
Tuberculosis (BCG)	6 weeks or 10–14 years.	Injection	Usually given at 10–14 years. See p.132.
Influenza	People of any age who are at risk of serious illness or death if they develop influenza.	Injection	Long-term immunity against all forms of influenza is impossible, but protection against the latest strains may be given to people at risk. Annual vaccinations are needed to protect against the latest strains.
Hepatitis A	Single dose for people of any age who are at risk. Booster 6–12 months after initial shot. Boosters every 10 years if needed.	Injection	Given to people travelling to areas of poor hygiene or where hepatitis infection is likely and to those exposed at school or work.
Hepatitis B	3 inoculations at any age, with the second and third shots 1 and 6 months after the first. Booster after 5 years if needed.	Injection	Efficacy is checked by a blood test. Recommended for "at risk" groups, such as health-care providers, travellers to tropical countries, and intravenous drug users.
Pneumococcal pneumonia	Single dose for people at any age who are at risk.	Injection	Given to persons at risk of contracting pneumococcal pneumonia. This includes people who have had their spleen removed, immunodeficient persons, or those with chronic liver or lung disease or diabetes mellitus.
Meningococcal meningitis	Single dose for people at any age who are at risk.	Injection	Given to persons at risk of contracting meningitis; for example to travellers to the "Meningitis belt" of tropical and subtropical countries where there is a high risk of meningitis infection, also contacts of cases in UK.

ANTIPROTOZOAL DRUGS

Protozoa are single-celled organisms that are present in soil and water. They may be transmitted to or between humans through contaminated food or water, sexual contact, or insect bites. There are many types of protozoal infection, each of which causes a different disease depending on the organism involved. Trichomoniasis, toxoplasmosis, cryptosporidium, giardiasis, and pneumocystis pneumonia are probably the most common protozoal infections seen in the United Kingdom. The rarer infections are usually contracted as a result of exposure to infection in another part of the world.

Many types of protozoa infect the bowel, causing diarrhoea and generalized symptoms of ill-health. Others may infect the genital tract or skin. Some protozoa may penetrate vital organs such as the lungs, brain, and liver. Prompt diagnosis and treatment are important in order to limit the spread of the infection within the body and, in some cases, prevent it from spreading to other people. Increased attention to hygiene is an important factor in controlling the spread of the disease.

A variety of medicines is used in the treatment of these diseases. Some, such as metronidazole and tetracycline, are also commonly used for their antibacterial action. Others, such as pentamidine, are rarely used except in treating specific protozoal infections.

How they affect you

Protozoa are often difficult to eradicate from the body. Drug treatment may therefore need to be continued for several months in order to eliminate the infecting organisms completely and thus prevent recurrence of the disease. In addition, unpleasant side effects such as nausea, diarrhoea, and abdominal cramps are often unavoidable because of the limited choice of drugs and the need to maintain dosage levels that will effectively cure the disease. For detailed information on the risks and adverse effects of individual antiprotozoal drugs, consult the appropriate drug profile in Part 4.

The table below describes the principal protozoal infections and some of the drugs used in their treatment. Malaria, probably the most common protozoal disease in the world today, is discussed on the facing page.

SUMMARY OF PROTOZOAL DISEASES

Disease	Protozoan	Description	Drugs
Amoebiasis (amoebic dysentery)	*Entamoeba histolytica*	Infection of the bowel and sometimes of the liver and other organs. Usually transmitted in contaminated food or water. Major symptom is violent, sometimes bloody diarrhoea.	Diloxanide Metronidazole Tinidazole
Balantidiasis	*Balantidium coli*	Infection of the bowel, specifically the colon. Usually transmitted through contact with infected pigs. Possible symptoms include diarrhoea and abdominal pain.	Tetracycline Metronidazole Di-odohydroxyquinoline
Cryptosporidiosis	*Cryptosporidium*	Infection of the bowel, also occasionally of the respiratory tract and bile ducts. Symptoms include diarrhoea and abdominal pain	No specific drugs but Paromomycin, azithromycin, eflornithine may be effective.
Giardiasis (lambliasis)	*Giardia lamblia*	Infection of the bowel. Usually transmitted in contaminated food or water but may also be spread by some types of sexual contact. Major symptoms are general ill health, diarrhoea, flatulence, and abdominal pain.	Mepacrine Metronidazole Tinidazole
Leishmaniasis	*Leishmania*	A mainly tropical and subtropical disease caused by organisms spread through sandfly bites. It affects the mucous membranes of the mouth, nose, and throat, and may in its severe form invade organs such as the liver.	Paromomycin Sodium stibogluconate Pentamidine Amphotericin
Pneumocystis pneumonia	*Pneumocystis carinii*	Potentially fatal lung infection that usually affects only those with reduced resistance to infection, such as AIDS sufferers. The symptoms include cough, breathlessness, fever, and chest pain.	Atovaquone Co-trimoxazole Pentamidine Trimetrexate
Toxoplasmosis	*Toxoplasma gondii*	Infection is usually spread via cat faeces or by eating undercooked meat. Although usually symptomless, infection may cause generalized ill-health, mild fever, and eye inflammation. Treatment is necessary only if the eyes are involved or if the patient is immunosuppressed (such as in AIDS). It may also pass from mother to baby during pregnancy, leading to severe disease in the fetus.	Pyrimethamine with sulfadiazine or with azithromycin, clarithromycin, or clindamycin Spiramycin (during pregnancy)
Trichomoniasis	*Trichomonas vaginalis*	Infection most often affects the vagina, causing irritation and an offensive discharge. In men, infection may occur in the urethra. The disease is usually sexually transmitted.	Metronidazole Tinidazole
Trypanosomiasis	*Trypanosoma*	African trypanosomiasis (sleeping sickness) is spread by the tsetse fly and causes fever, swollen glands, and drowsiness. South American trypanosomiasis (Chagas' disease) is spread by assassin bugs and causes inflammation, enlargement of internal organs, and infection of the brain.	Pentamidine (sleeping sickness) Suramin eflornithine melarsoprol (sleeping sickness) Primaquine (Chagas' disease) Nifurtimox, (Chagas' disease)

ANTIMALARIAL DRUGS

Malaria is one of the main killing diseases in the tropics (see map below). It is most likely to affect people who live in or travel to such places.

The disease is caused by protozoa (see also facing page) whose life cycle is far from simple. The malaria parasite, which is called *Plasmodium*, lives in and depends on the female *Anopheles* mosquito during one part of its life cycle. It lives in and depends on human beings during other parts of its life cycle.

Transferred to humans in the saliva of the female mosquito as she penetrates ("bites") the skin, the malaria parasite enters the bloodstream and settles in the liver, where it multiplies asexually.

Following its stay in the liver, the parasite (or plasmodium) enters another phase of its life cycle, circulating in the bloodstream, penetrating and destroying red blood cells, and reproducing again. If the plasmodia then transfer back to a female *Anopheles* mosquito via another "bite", they breed sexually, and are again ready to start a human infection.

Following the emergence of plasmodia from the liver, the symptoms of malaria occur: episodes of high fever and profuse sweating alternate with equally agonizing episodes of shivering and chills. One of the four strains of malaria (*Plasmodium falciparum*) can produce a single severe attack that can be fatal unless treated.

The others cause recurrent attacks, sometimes extending over many years.

A number of drugs are available for preventing malaria, the choice depending on the region in which the disease can be contracted and the resistance to the commonly used drugs. In most malarial areas, *Plasmodium falciparum* is resistant to chloroquine (see Choice of drugs, below). In all regions, three drugs are commonly used for treating malaria: quinine, mefloquine, and Malarone.

Why they are used

The medical response to malaria takes three forms: prevention, treatment of attacks, and the complete eradication of the plasmodia (radical cure).

For someone planning a trip to an area where malaria is prevalent, drugs are given that destroy the parasites in the liver. Dosing begins one week (2–3 weeks for mefloquine) before the traveller arrives in the malarial area and should continue for four to six weeks after return from the area.

Drugs such as mefloquine and Fansidar can produce a radical cure but chloroquine does not. So after chloroquine treatment of non-falciparum malaria, a 14- to 21-day course of primaquine is administered. Although it is highly effective in destroying plasmodia in the liver, the drug is weak against the plasmodia circulating in the bloodstream.

Primaquine is recommended only after a person leaves the malarial area because of the high risk of reinfection.

How they work

Taken to prevent the disease, the drugs kill the plasmodia in the liver, preventing them from multiplying. Once plasmodia have multiplied in the liver, the same drugs may be used in higher doses to kill plasmodia that re-enter the bloodstream. If these drugs are not effective, primaquine may be used to destroy any plasmodia that is still present in the liver.

How they affect you

The low doses of antimalarial drugs taken to prevent the disease rarely produce noticeable effects. Drugs taken for an attack usually begin to relieve symptoms within a few hours. Most of them can cause nausea, vomiting, and diarrhoea. Quinine can cause disturbances in vision and hearing. Mefloquine can cause sleep disturbance, dizziness, and difficulties in coordination.

Risks and special precautions

When drugs are given to prevent or cure malaria, the full course of treatment must be taken. No drugs give long-term protection; a new course of treatment is needed for each journey.

Most of these drugs do not produce severe adverse effects, but primaquine can cause the blood disorder haemolytic anaemia, particularly in people with glucose-6-phosphate dehydrogenase (G6PD) deficiency. Blood tests are taken before treatment to identify susceptible individuals. Halofantrine can have an adverse effect on heart rhythm. Mefloquine is not prescribed for those who have had psychological disorders or convulsions.

Other protective measures

Because *Plasmodium* strains continually develop resistance to the available drugs, prevention using drugs is not absolutely reliable. Protection from mosquito bites is of the highest priority. Such protection includes the use of insect repellents and mosquito nets impregnated with permethrin insecticide, as well as covering any exposed skin after dark.

CHOICE OF DRUGS

The parts of the world in which malaria is prevalent (illustrated on the map, right), and travel to which may make antimalarial drug treatment advisable, can be divided into six zones. The table below indicates the drug(s) currently used for the prevention of malaria in each zone. As prevalent strains of malaria change very rapidly, you must always seek specific medical advice before travelling to these areas.

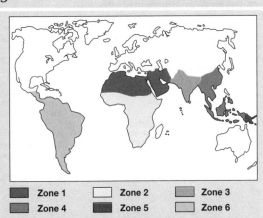

	Zone 1		Zone 2		Zone 3
	Zone 4		Zone 5		Zone 6

Zone	Countries	Recommended antimalarial drugs for prevention
1	North Africa and the Middle East	Chloroquine, plus proguanil in areas of chloroquine resistance
2	Sub-Saharan Africa	Mefloquine, or chloroquine with proguanil
3	South Asia	Mefloquine or chloroquine with proguanil
4	Southeast Asia	Mefloquine in high-risk areas, or chloroquine with proguanil; doxycycline in mefloquine-resistant areas
5	Oceania	Mefloquine, or doxycycline
6	Latin America	Central America: chloroquine or proguanil. South America: mefloquine in high-risk areas, or chloroquine with proguanil

COMMON DRUGS

Artemether
Chloroquine *
Doxycycline *
Halofantrine
Mefloquine *
Primaquine
Proguanil *

Proguanil/
atovaquone
("Malarone") *
Pyrimethamine/
dapsone
("Malaprim") * or
Pyrimethamine/
sulphadoxine
("Fansidar")
Quinine *

* See Part 4

ANTIFUNGAL DRUGS

We are continually exposed to fungi – in the air we breathe, the food we eat, and the water we drink. Fortunately, most of them cannot live in the body, and few are harmful. But some can grow in the mouth, skin, hair, or nails, causing irritating or unsightly changes, and a few can cause serious and possibly fatal disease. The most common fungal infections are caused by the tinea group. These include tinea pedis (athlete's foot), tinea cruris (jock itch), tinea corporis (ringworm), and tinea capitis (scalp ringworm). Caused by a variety of organisms, they are spread by direct or indirect contact with infected humans or animals. Infection is encouraged by warm, moist conditions.

Problems may also result from the proliferation of a fungus normally present in the body; the most common example is excessive growth of *Candida*, a yeast that causes thrush infection of the mouth, vagina, and bowel. It can also infect other organs if it spreads through the body via the bloodstream. Overgrowth of *Candida* may occur in people taking antibiotics (p.128) or oral contraceptives (p.161), in pregnant women, or in those with diabetes or immune system disorders such as AIDS.

Superficial fungal infections – those that attack only the outer layer of the skin and mucous membranes – are relatively common and, although irritating, do not usually present a threat to general health. Internal fungal infections – for example, of the lungs, heart, or other organs – are rare, but may be serious and prolonged.

As antibiotics and other antibacterial drugs have no effect on fungi and yeasts, a different type of drug is needed. Drugs for fungal infections are either applied *topically* to treat minor infections of the skin, nails, and mucous membranes, or they are given by mouth or injection to eliminate serious fungal infections of the internal organs and nails.

Why they are used

Drug treatment is necessary for most fungal infections since they rarely improve alone. Measures such as careful washing and drying of affected areas may help but are not a substitute for antifungal drugs. The use of over-the-counter preparations to increase the acidity of the vagina is not usually effective except when accompanied by drug treatment.

Fungal infections of the skin and scalp are usually treated with a cream or shampoo. Drugs for vaginal thrush are most commonly applied in the form of vaginal pessaries or cream applied with a special applicator. For very severe or persistent vaginal infections, fluconazole or itraconazole may be given as a short course by mouth. Mouth infections are usually eliminated by lozenges dissolved in the mouth or an antifungal solution or gel applied to the affected areas. When *Candida* infects the bowel, an antifungal drug that is not absorbed into the bloodstream, such as nystatin, is given in tablet form. For severe or persistent infections of the nails, either griseofulvin or terbinafine are given by mouth until the infected nails have grown out.

In the rare cases of fungal infections affecting internal organs, such as the blood, the heart, or the brain, potent drugs such as fluconazole and itraconazole are given by mouth, or amphotericin and flucytosine are given by injection. These drugs pass into the bloodstream to fight the fungi.

ACTIONS OF ANTIFUNGAL DRUGS

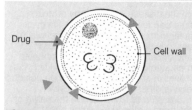

Drug — Cell wall

Stage one
The drug acts on the wall of the fungal cell.

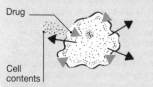

Drug

Cell contents

Stage two
The drug damages the cell wall and the cell contents leak out. The cell dies.

How they work

Most antifungals alter the permeability of the fungal cell's walls. Chemicals needed for cell life leak out and the fungal cell dies.

How they affect you

The speed with which antifungal drugs provide benefit varies with the type of infection. Most fungal or yeast infections of the skin, mouth, and vagina improve within a week. The condition of nails affected by fungal infections improves only when new nail growth occurs, which takes months. *Systemic* infections of the internal organs can take weeks to cure.

Antifungal drugs applied topically rarely cause side effects, although they may irritate the skin. However, treatment by mouth or injection for systemic and nail infections may produce more serious side effects. Amphotericin, injected in cases of life-threatening, systemic infections, can cause potentially dangerous effects, including kidney damage.

CHOICE OF ANTIFUNGAL DRUG

The table below shows the range of uses for some antifungal drugs. The particular drug chosen in each case depends on the precise nature and site of the infection. The usual route of administration for each drug is also indicated.

Drug	Infection									Administration		
	Oesophageal thrush	Cryptococcal meningitis	Skin ringworm	Scalp ringworm	Nail infection	Mouth thrush	Vaginal thrush	Candida of the skin	Systemic candida	Topical	Injection	Oral
Amphotericin	●	●				●		●	●		●	●
Clotrimazole			●	●		●	●	●		●		
Fluconazole	●	●						●	●		●	●
Flucytosine	●	●							●		●	●
Griseofulvin			●	●	●							●
Ketoconazole			●	●		●	●	●				●
Miconazole			●	●		●	●	●		●		
Nystatin						●	●	●		●		
Terbinafine			●	●	●							●

COMMON DRUGS

Amorolfine
Amphotericin ✳
Benzoyl
  peroxide ✳
Co-trimazole ✳
Econazole
Fenticonazole
Fluconazole ✳

Flucytosine
Griseofulvin
Isoconazole
Itraconazole
Ketoconazole ✳
Miconazole ✳
Nystatin ✳
Sulconazole
Terbinafine ✳
Tioconazole

✳ See Part 4

ANTHELMINTIC DRUGS

Anthelmintics are drugs that are used to eliminate the many types of worm (helminths) that can enter the body and live there as parasites, producing a general weakness in some cases and serious harm in others. The body may be host to many different worms (see Choice of drug, below). Most species spend part of their life cycle in another animal, and the infestation is often passed on to humans in food contaminated with the eggs or larvae. In some cases, such as hookworm, larvae enter the body through the skin. Larvae or adults may attach themselves to the intestinal wall and feed on the bowel contents; others feed off the intestinal blood supply, causing *anaemia*. Worms can also infest the bloodstream or lodge in the muscles or internal organs.

Many people have worms at some time during their life, especially during childhood; most can be effectively eliminated with anthelmintic drugs.

Why they are used

Most worms common in the United Kingdom cause only mild symptoms and usually do not pose a serious threat to general health. Anthelmintic drugs are usually necessary, however, because the body's natural defences against infection are not effective against most worm infestations. Certain types of infestation must always be treated since they can cause serious complications. In some cases, such as threadworm infestation, doctors may recommend anthelmintic treatment for the whole family to prevent reinfection. If worms have invaded tissues and formed cysts, they may have to be removed surgically. Laxatives are given with some anthelmintics to hasten expulsion of worms from the bowel. Other drugs may be prescribed to ease symptoms or to compensate for any blood loss or nutritional deficiency.

How they work

The anthelmintic drugs act in several ways. Many of them kill or paralyse the worms, which pass out of the body in the faeces. Others, which act *systemically*, are used to treat infection in the tissues.

Many anthelmintics are specific for particular worms, and the doctor must identify the worm before selecting the most appropriate treatment (see Choice of drug, below). Most of the common intestinal infestations are easily treated, often with only one or two doses of the drug. However, tissue infections may require more prolonged treatment.

How they affect you

Once the drug has eliminated the worms, symptoms caused by infestation rapidly disappear. Taken as a single dose or a short course, anthelmintics do not usually produce side effects. However, treatment can disturb the digestive system, causing abdominal pain, nausea, and vomiting.

COMMON DRUGS

Albendazole
Diethylcarbamazine
Ivermectin
Levamisole
Mebendazole
Niclosamide
Piperazine
Praziquantel
Thiabendazole

✳ See Part 4

CHOICE OF DRUG

Threadworm (enterobiasis)
The most common worm infection in the United Kingdom, particularly among young children. The worm lives in the intestine, but it travels to the anus at night to lay eggs. This causes itching; scratching leaves eggs on the fingers, usually under the fingernails. These eggs are transferred to the mouth, often by sucking the fingers or eating food with unwashed hands. Keeping nails short and good hygiene, including washing the hands after using the toilet and before each meal, and an early morning bath to remove the eggs, are all important elements in the eradication of infection.
Drugs Mebendazole, piperazine. All members of the family should be treated simultaneously.

Common roundworm (ascariasis)
The most common worm infection worldwide. Transmitted to humans in contaminated raw food or in soil. Infects the intestine. The worms are large and dense clusters of them can block the intestine.
Drugs Levamisole, mebendazole, piperazine

Tropical threadworm (strongyloidiasis)
Occurs in the tropics and southern Europe. Larvae from contaminated soil penetrate skin, pass into the lungs, and are swallowed into the gut.
Drugs Albendazole, thiabendazole, ivermectin

Whipworm (trichuriasis)
Mainly occurs in tropical areas as a result of eating contaminated raw vegetables. Worms infest the intestines.
Drugs Mebendazole

Hookworm (uncinariasis)
Mainly found in tropical areas. Worm larvae penetrate skin and pass via the lymphatic system and bloodstream to the lungs. They then travel up the airways, are swallowed, and attach themselves to the intestinal wall, where they feed off the intestinal blood supply.
Drugs Mebendazole

Pork roundworm (trichinosis)
Transmitted in infected undercooked pork. Initially worms lodge in the intestines, but larvae may invade muscle to form cysts that are often resistant to drug treatment and may require surgery.
Drugs Mebendazole, thiabendazole

Toxocariasis (visceral larva migrans)
Usually occurs as a result of eating soil or eating with fingers contaminated with dog or cat faeces. Eggs hatch in the intestine and may travel to the lungs, liver, kidney, brain, and eyes. Treatment is not always effective.
Drugs Mebendazole, thiabendazole, diethylcarbamazine

Creeping eruption (cutaneous larva migrans)
Mainly occurs in tropical areas and coastal areas of southeastern United States as a result of skin contact with larvae from cat and dog faeces. Infestation is usually confined to the skin.
Drugs Thiabendazole, ivermectin, albendazole

Filariasis (including onchocerciasis and loiasis)
Tropical areas only. Infection by this group of worms is spread by bites of insects that are carriers of worm larvae or eggs. May affect the lymphatic system, blood, eyes, and skin.
Drugs Diethylcarbamazine, ivermectin

Flukes
Sheep liver fluke (fascioliasis) is indigenous to the United Kingdom. Infestation usually results from eating watercress grown in contaminated water. Mainly affects the liver and biliary tract. Other flukes only found abroad may infect the lungs, intestines, or blood.
Drugs Praziquantel

Tapeworms (including beef, pork, fish, and dwarf tapeworms)
Depending on the type may be carried by cattle, pigs, or fish and transmitted to humans in undercooked meat. Most types affect the intestines. Larvae of the pork tapeworm may form cysts in muscle and other tissues.
Drugs Niclosamide, praziquantel

Hydatid disease (echinococciasis)
Eggs are transmitted in dog faeces. Larvae may form cysts over many years, commonly in the liver. Surgery is the usual treatment for cysts.
Drugs Albendazole

Bilharzia (schistosomiasis)
Occurs in polluted water in tropical areas. Larvae may be swallowed or penetrate the skin; they migrate to the liver: adult worms live in the bladder.
Drugs Praziquantel

HORMONES AND ENDOCRINE SYSTEM

The endocrine system is a collection of glands located throughout the body that produce *hormones* and release them into the bloodstream. Each endocrine gland produces one or more hormones, each of which governs a particular body function, including growth and repair of tissues, sexual development and reproductive function, and the body's response to stress.

Most hormones are released continuously from birth, but the amount produced fluctuates with the body's needs. Others are produced mainly at certain times – for example, growth hormone is released mainly during childhood and adolescence. Sex hormones are produced by the testes and ovaries from puberty onwards (see p.158).

Many endocrine glands release their hormones in response to triggering hormones produced by the pituitary gland. The pituitary releases a variety of pituitary hormones, each of which, in turn, stimulates the appropriate endocrine gland to produce its hormone.

A "feedback" system usually regulates blood hormone levels: if the blood level rises too high, the pituitary responds by reducing the amount of stimulating hormone produced, thereby allowing the blood hormone level to return to normal.

What can go wrong

Endocrine disorders, usually resulting in too much or too little of a particular hormone, have a variety of causes. Some are congenital in origin; others may be caused by autoimmune disease (including some forms of diabetes mellitus), malignant or benign tumours, injury, or certain drugs.

Why drugs are used

Natural hormone preparations or their synthetic versions are often prescribed to treat deficiency. Sometimes drugs are given to stimulate increased hormone production in the endocrine gland, such as oral antidiabetic drugs, which act on the insulin-producing cells of the pancreas. When too much hormone is produced, drug treatment may reduce the activity of the gland.

Hormones or related drugs are also used to treat certain other conditions. Corticosteroids related to adrenal hormones are prescribed to relieve inflammation and to suppress immune system activity (see p.156). Several types of cancer are treated with sex hormones (see p.154). Female sex hormones are used as contraceptives (see p.161) and to treat menstrual disorders (see p.160).

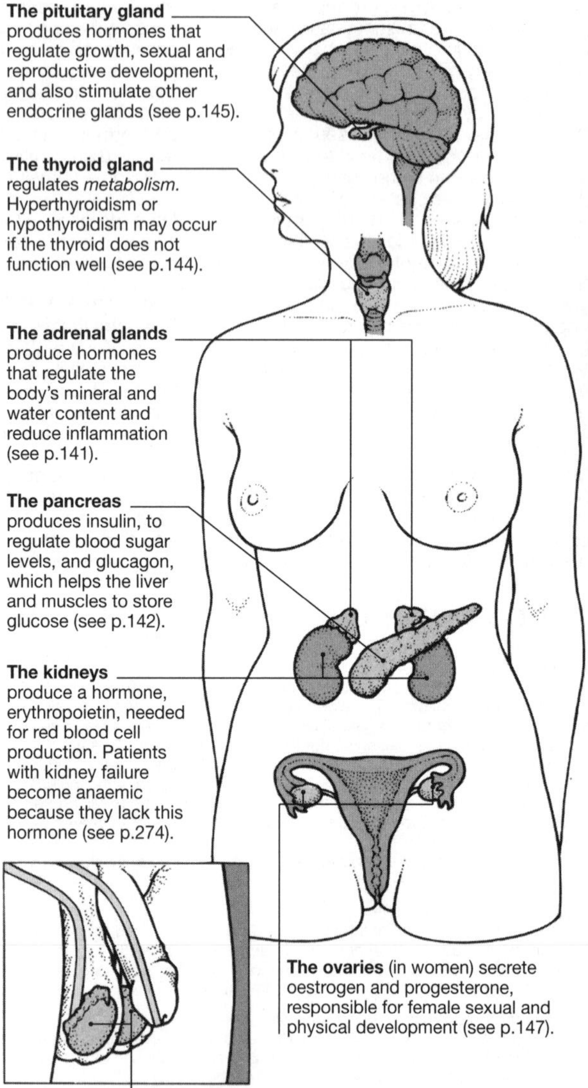

The pituitary gland produces hormones that regulate growth, sexual and reproductive development, and also stimulate other endocrine glands (see p.145).

The thyroid gland regulates *metabolism*. Hyperthyroidism or hypothyroidism may occur if the thyroid does not function well (see p.144).

The adrenal glands produce hormones that regulate the body's mineral and water content and reduce inflammation (see p.141).

The pancreas produces insulin, to regulate blood sugar levels, and glucagon, which helps the liver and muscles to store glucose (see p.142).

The kidneys produce a hormone, erythropoietin, needed for red blood cell production. Patients with kidney failure become anaemic because they lack this hormone (see p.274).

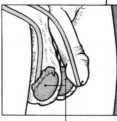

The ovaries (in women) secrete oestrogen and progesterone, responsible for female sexual and physical development (see p.147).

The testes (in men) produce testosterone, which controls the development of male sexual and physical characteristics (see p.146).

MAJOR DRUG GROUPS

Corticosteroids
Drugs used in diabetes
Drugs for thyroid disorders
Drugs for pituitary disorders
Male sex hormones
Female sex hormones

CORTICOSTEROIDS

Corticosteroid drugs – often referred to simply as steroids – are derived from, or are synthetic variants of, the natural corticosteroid *hormones* formed in the outer part (cortex) of the adrenal glands, situated on top of each kidney. Release of these hormones is governed by the pituitary gland (see p.145).

Corticosteroids may have either mainly glucocorticoid or mainly mineralocorticoid effects. Glucocorticoid effects include the maintenance of normal levels of sugar in the blood and the promotion of recovery from injury and stress. The main mineralocorticoid effects are the regulation of the balance of mineral salts and the water content of the body. When present in large amounts, corticosteroids act to reduce inflammation and suppress allergic reactions and immune system activity. They are distinct from another group of steroid hormones, the anabolic steroids (see p.146).

Although corticosteroids have broadly similar actions to each other, they vary in their relative strength and duration of action. The mineralocorticoid effects of these drugs also vary in strength.

Why they are used

Corticosteroid drugs are used primarily for their effect in controlling inflammation, whatever its cause. *Topical* preparations containing corticosteroids are often used for the treatment of many inflammatory skin disorders (see p.174). These drugs may also be injected directly into a joint or around a tendon to relieve inflammation caused by injury or disease (see p.118). However, when local administration of the drug is either not possible or not effective, corticosteroids may be given *systemically*, either by mouth or by intravenous injection.

Corticosteroids are commonly part of the treatment of many disorders in which inflammation is thought to be caused by excessive or inappropriate activity of the immune system. These disorders include inflammatory bowel disease (p.112), rheumatoid arthritis (p.117), glomerulonephritis (a kidney disease), and some rare connective tissue disorders, such as systemic lupus erythematosus. In these conditions corticosteroids relieve symptoms and may also temporarily halt the disease.

Corticosteroids may be given regularly by mouth or inhaler to treat asthma, although they are not effective for the relief of asthma attacks in progress (see Bronchodilators, p.92).

An important use of oral corticosteroids is to replace the natural hormones that are deficient when adrenal gland function is reduced, as in Addison's disease. In these cases, the drugs most closely resembling the actions of the natural hormones are selected and a combination of these may be used.

Some cancers of the lymphatic system (lymphomas) and the blood (leukaemias) may also respond to corticosteroid treatment. These drugs are also widely used to prevent or treat rejection of organ transplants, usually in conjunction with other drugs, such azathioprine (see Immunosuppressants, p.156).

How they work

Given in high doses, corticosteroid drugs reduce inflammation by blocking the action of chemicals called prostaglandins that are responsible for triggering the inflammatory response. These drugs also temporarily depress the immune system by reducing the activity of certain types of white blood cell.

How they affect you

Corticosteroid drugs often produce a dramatic improvement in symptoms. Given systemically, corticosteroids may also act on the brain to produce a heightened sense of well-being and, in some people, a sense of euphoria.

Troublesome day-to-day side effects are rare. Long-term corticosteroid treatment, however, carries a number of serious risks for the patient.

Risks and special precautions

In the treatment of Addison's disease, corticosteroids can be considered as "hormone replacement therapy", with drugs replacing the natural hormone hydrocortisone. Because replacement doses are given, the adverse effects of high-dose corticosteroids do not occur.

Drugs with strong mineralocorticoid effects, such as fludrocortisone, may cause water retention, swelling (especially of the ankles), and an increase in blood pressure. Because corticosteroids reduce the effect of insulin, they may create problems in diabetics, and may even give rise to diabetes in susceptible individuals. They can also cause peptic ulcers.

Because corticosteroids suppress the immune system, they increase susceptibility to infection. They also suppress symptoms of infectious disease. People who are taking corticosteroids should avoid exposure to chickenpox or shingles, but if they catch either disease, aciclovir tablets may be prescribed. With long-term use, corticosteroids may cause a variety of adverse effects as described at left. Doctors try to avoid long-term prescription of corticosteroids drugs to children because prolonged use may retard growth.

Long-term use of corticosteroids suppresses the production of the body's own corticosteroid hormones. For this reason, treatment that lasts for more than a few weeks should be withdrawn gradually to give the body time to adjust. If the drug is stopped abruptly, the lack of corticosteroid hormones may lead to sudden collapse.

People taking corticosteroids by mouth for longer than one month are advised to carry a warning card. If someone who is taking steroids long-term has an accident or serious illness, his or her defences against shock may need to be quickly strengthened with extra hydrocortisone, administered intravenously.

ADVERSE EFFECTS OF CORTICOSTEROIDS

Corticosteroids are effective and useful drugs that often provide benefit in cases where other drugs are ineffective. However, long-term use of high doses can lead to a variety of unwanted effects on the body, as shown below.

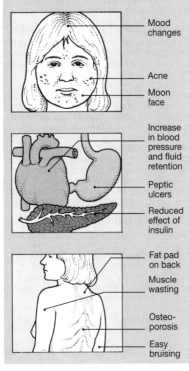

- Mood changes
- Acne
- Moon face
- Increase in blood pressure and fluid retention
- Peptic ulcers
- Reduced effect of insulin
- Fat pad on back
- Muscle wasting
- Osteoporosis
- Easy bruising

COMMON DRUGS

Alclometasone	Fluocinonide
Beclometasone *	Fluocinolone
Betamethasone *	Fluocortolone
Budesonide *	Fluticasone *
Clobetasol *	Flurandrenolone
Clobetasone	Halcinonide
Desoximetasone	Hydrocortisone *
Dexamethasone *	Methylprednisolone
Diflucortolone	Mometasone *
Fludrocortisone	Prednisolone *
Flunisolide	Triamcinolone
Flumetasone	

* See Part 4

DRUGS USED IN DIABETES

The body obtains most of its energy from glucose, a simple form of sugar made in the intestine from the breakdown of starch and other sugars. Insulin, one of the hormones produced in the pancreas, enables body tissues to take up glucose from the blood, either to use it for energy or to store it. In diabetes mellitus (or sugar diabetes), insulin production is defective. This results in reduced uptake of glucose by the tissues and therefore the glucose level in the blood rises abnormally. A high blood glucose level is medically known as hyperglycaemia.

There are two main types of diabetes mellitus. Insulin-dependent (Type 1) diabetes usually appears in young people, 50 per cent of cases occurring around the time of puberty. The insulin-secreting cells in the pancreas are gradually destroyed. An autoimmune condition (where the body recognizes its pancreas as "foreign" and tries to eliminate it) or a childhood viral infection is the most likely cause. Although the decline in insulin production is slow, the condition often appears suddenly, brought on by periods of stress (for example, infection or puberty) when the body's insulin requirements are high. Symptoms of Type 1 diabetes include extreme thirst, increased urination, lethargy, and weight loss. This type of diabetes is fatal if it is left untreated.

In Type 1 diabetes, insulin treatment is the only treatment option. It has to be continued for the rest of the patient's life. Several types of insulin are available, which are broadly classified by their duration of action (short-, medium-, and long-acting).

Non-insulin-dependent diabetes mellitus (NIDDM), also known as Type 2 or maturity-onset diabetes, appears at an older age (usually over 40) and tends to come on much more gradually – there may be a delay in its diagnosis for several years because of the gradual onset of symptoms. In this type of diabetes, the levels of insulin in the blood are usually high. However, the cells of the body are resistant to the effects of insulin and have a reduced glucose uptake despite the

ADMINISTRATION OF INSULIN

The non-diabetic body produces a background level of insulin, with additional insulin being produced as required during meals. The insulin delivery systems that are currently available cannot mimic this precisely. In young people with Type 1 diabetes, short-acting insulin is usually given before meals, and a medium-acting insulin is given either before the evening meal or at bedtime. Insulin pen injectors are particularly useful for administration during the day because

they are discreet and easy to carry and use. In patients with Type 2 diabetes who require insulin, a mixture of short- and medium-acting insulin may be given twice a day. Special pumps that deliver continuous subcutaneous insulin appear to have no advantage over multiple subcutaneous injections. Some new types of insulins called "insulin analogues" (e.g. Insulin lispro) may be better at mimicking the insulin-producing behaviour of the normal pancreas.

Duration of action of types of insulin

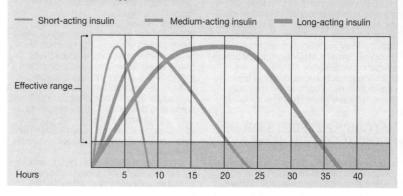

high insulin levels. This results in hyperglycaemia. Obesity is the most common cause of Type 2 diabetes.

In both types of diabetes, an alteration in diet is vital. A healthy diet consisting of a low-fat, high-fibre, low simple sugar (cakes, sweets) and high complex sugar (pasta, rice, potatoes) intake is advised. In Type 2 diabetes, a reduction in weight alone may be sufficient to lower the body's energy requirements and restore blood glucose to normal levels. If an alteration in diet fails, oral antidiabetic drugs, such as metformin, acarbose, or sulphonylureas, are prescribed. Insulin may need to be given to people with Type 2 diabetes if the above treatments

fail, or in pregnancy, during severe illness, and before the patient undergoes any surgery requiring a general anaesthetic.

Importance of treating diabetes
If diabetes is left untreated, the continuous high blood glucose levels damage various parts of the body. The major problems are caused by the build-up of atherosclerosis in arteries, which narrows the vessels, reducing the flow of blood. This can result in heart attacks, blindness, kidney failure, reduced circulation in the legs, and even gangrene. The risk of these conditions is greatly reduced with treatment. Careful control of diabetes in young people, during puberty and afterwards, is of great importance in reducing possible long-term complications. Good diabetic control before conception reduces the chance of miscarriage or abnormalities in the baby.

How antidiabetic drugs work
All drugs for diabetes promote the uptake of glucose into body tissues and help to prevent an excessive rise in the level of glucose in the blood. Insulin treatment directly replaces the natural hormone that is deficient in diabetes mellitus. Human and pork insulins are the most widely available. When transferring between animal and human insulin, alteration of the dose may be required.

Unfortunately, insulin cannot be given by mouth because it is broken down in the

ACTION OF SULPHONYLUREA DRUGS

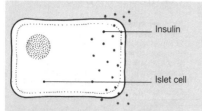

Before drug treatment
In Type 2 diabetes, the islet cells of the pancreas secrete insufficient insulin to meet the body's needs.

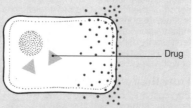

After drug treatment
The drug stimulates the islet cells to release increased amounts of insulin.

digestive tract before it reaches the blood-stream. Regular injections are therefore necessary (see Administration of insulin, facing page).

Sulphonylurea oral antidiabetic drugs encourage the pancreas to produce insulin. They are therefore effective only when some insulin-secreting cells remain active, and this is why they are ineffective in the treatment of Type 1 diabetes. Metformin alters the way in which the body *metabolizes* sugar. Acarbose slows digestion of starch and sugar and thereby slows the increase in blood sugar that occurs after a meal.

Insulin treatment and you

The insulin requirements in diabetes vary greatly between individuals and also depend on physical activity and calorie intake. Hence, insulin regimens are tailored to each person's particular needs, and the diabetic is encouraged to take an active role in his or her own management.

A regular record of home blood glucose monitoring should be kept. This is the basis on which insulin doses are adjusted, preferably by diabetics themselves.

A person with diabetes should learn to recognize the warning signs of hypoglycaemia. A hypoglycaemic event may be induced by giving insulin under medical supervision. The symptoms of sweating, faintness, or palpitations are produced but disappear with the administration of glucose, so a diabetic should always carry glucose tablets or sweets. Recurrent "hypos" at specific

times of the day or night may require a reduction of insulin dose. Rarely, undetected low glucose levels may lead to coma. The injection of glucagon (a substance that raises blood glucose) rapidly reverses this. A relative may be instructed how to perform this procedure.

Other complications may arise from insulin injection. Repeated injection at the same site may disturb the fat layer beneath the skin, producing either swelling or dimpling. This alters the rate of insulin absorption and can be avoided by regularly rotating injection sites.

Insulin requirements are increased during illness and pregnancy. During an illness, the urine should be checked for ketones, which are produced when there is insufficient insulin to permit the normal uptake of glucose by the tissues. If high ketone levels occur in a diabetic's urine during an illness, urgent medical advice should be sought. The combination of high blood sugars, high urinary ketones, and vomiting is a diabetic emergency and the person should attend an Accident and Emergency department immediately.

Exercise increases the body's need for glucose, and therefore extra calories should be taken prior to exertion. The effects of vigorous exercise on blood sugar levels may last up to 18 hours, and the subsequent (post-exercise) doses of insulin may need to be reduced by 10–25 per cent to avoid hypoglycaemia.

It is advisable for diabetics to carry a card or bracelet detailing their treatment. This may be useful in an emergency.

SITES OF INJECTION

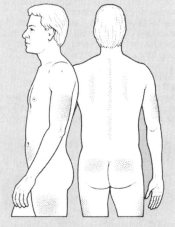

The shaded areas indicate suitable sites for the injection of insulin.

Antidiabetic drugs and you

Oral antidiabetic drugs relieve symptoms of diabetes by returning the blood glucose to normal. A normal, healthy, active lifestyle should be encouraged. However, the sulphonylureas may lower the blood glucose too much, a condition called hypoglycaemia. This condition can be avoided by starting treatment with low doses and ensuring a regular food intake. Rarely, these drugs cause a decrease in the blood cell count, a rash, or intestinal or liver disturbances. Interactions may occur with other drugs, so your doctor should be informed of your treatment before prescribing any medicines for you.

Unlike the sulphonylureas, metformin does not cause hypoglycaemia. Its most common side effects are nausea, weight loss, abdominal distension, and diarrhoea. It should not be used in people with liver, kidney, or heart problems. Acarbose does not cause hypoglycaemia if used on its own. The tablets must either be chewed with the first mouthful of food at mealtimes or swallowed whole with a little liquid immediately before food.

MONITORING BLOOD GLUCOSE

Diabetics need to check either their blood or urine glucose level at home. Blood tests give the most accurate results. The kit illustrated (right) consists of a programmable meter that reads the glucose levels of blood samples applied to a special card testing strip.

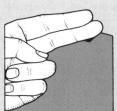

1 Prick your finger to give a large drop of blood.

2 Touch the blood on to the test pads of the testing strip.

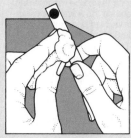

3 Press the time button on the meter. After 60 seconds wipe the blood from the test pads with a clean, dry cotton ball.

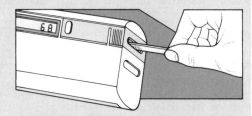

4 Within 120 seconds insert the test strip into the meter as shown. Your reading will appear after 120 seconds.

COMMON DRUGS

Sulphonylurea drugs	Other drugs
Chlorpropamide	Acarbose
Glibenclamide ✳	Glucagon
Gliclazide ✳	Guar gum
Glimepiride	Insulin ✳
Gliquidone	Insulin lispro
Glipizide	Metformin ✳
Tolbutamide ✳	Repaglinide ✳
Tolazamide	

✳ See Part 4

143

DRUGS FOR THYROID DISORDERS

The thyroid gland produces the *hormone* thyroxine, which regulates the body's *metabolism*. During childhood, thyroxine is essential for normal physical and mental development. Calcitonin, also produced by the thyroid, regulates calcium metabolism and is used as a drug for certain bone disorders (p.122).

Hyperthyroidism

In this condition (often called thyrotoxicosis), the thyroid is overactive and produces too much thyroxine. Women are more commonly affected than men.

ACTION OF DRUGS FOR THYROID DISORDERS

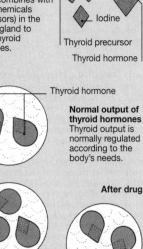

Thyroid hormone production
Iodine combines with other chemicals (precursors) in the thyroid gland to make thyroid hormones.

Iodine

Thyroid precursor

Thyroid hormone

Thyroid hormone

Normal output of thyroid hormones
Thyroid output is normally regulated according to the body's needs.

After drug

Drug

Before drug

Action of antithyroid drugs
In hyperthyroidism, antithyroid drugs partly reduce the production of thyroid hormones by preventing iodine from combining with thyroid precursors in the thyroid gland.

Before drug

After drug

Synthetic thyroid hormone

Action of thyroid hormones
In hypothyroidism, when the thyroid gland is underactive, supplements of synthetic or (rarely) natural thyroid hormones restore hormone levels to normal.

Symptoms include anxiety, palpitations, weight loss, increased appetite, heat intolerance, diarrhoea, and menstrual disturbances. Graves' disease is the most common form of hyperthyroidism. It is an autoimmune disease in which the body produces antibodies that stimulate the thyroid to produce excess thyroxine. Patients with Graves' disease may develop abnormally protuberant eyes (exophthalmos) or a swelling involving the skin over the shins (pretibial myxoedema). Hyperthyroidism can be caused by a benign single tumour of the thyroid or a pre-existing multinodular goitre. Rarely, an overactive thyroid may follow a viral infection, a condition called thyroiditis. Inflammation of the gland leads to the release of stored thyroxine.

Management of hyperthyroidism

There are three possible treatments: antithyroid drugs, radio-iodine, and surgery. The most commonly used antithyroid drug is carbimazole. This drug inhibits the formation of thyroid hormones and reduces their levels to normal over a period of about 4–8 weeks. In the early stage of treatment a beta blocker (p.97) may be prescribed to control symptoms. This should be stopped once thyroid function returns to normal. Long-term carbimazole is usually given for 18 months to prevent relapse. A "block and replace" regimen may also be used. In this treatment, the thyroid gland is blocked by high doses of carbimazole and thyroxine is added when the level of thyroid hormone in the blood falls below normal.

Carbimazole may produce minor side effects such as nausea, vomiting, skin rashes, or headaches. Rarely, the drug may reduce the white blood cell count. Propylthiouracil may be used as an alternative antithyroid drug.

Radio-iodine (radioactive iodine) is frequently chosen as a first-line therapy, especially in the elderly, and is the second choice if hyperthyroidism recurs following use of carbimazole. It acts by destroying thyroid tissue. Hypothyroidism occurs in up to 80 per cent of people within 20 years after treatment. Long-term studies show radio-iodine to be safe, but its use should be avoided during pregnancy.

Surgery is a third-line therapy. Its use may be favoured for patients with a large goitre, particularly if it causes difficulty in swallowing or breathing. Exophthalmos may require corticosteroids (p.141) as it does not respond to other treatments.

Hypothyroidism

This is a condition resulting from too little thyroxine. Sometimes it may be caused by an autoimmune disorder, in which the body's immune system attacks the thyroid gland. Other cases may follow

TREATMENT FOR GOITRE

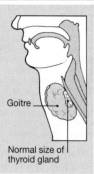

A goitre is a swelling of the thyroid gland. It may occur only temporarily, during puberty or pregnancy, or it may be due to an abnormal growth of thyroid tissue that requires surgical removal. It may rarely be brought about by iodine deficiency. This last cause is treated with iodine supplements (see also p.441).

Goitre

Normal size of thyroid gland

treatment for hyperthyroidism. In newborn babies, hypothyroidism may be the result of an inborn *enzyme* disorder. In the past, it also arose from a deficiency of iodine in the diet.

The symptoms of adult hypothyroidism develop slowly and include weight gain, mental slowness, dry skin, hair loss, increased sensitivity to cold, and heavy menstrual periods. In babies, low levels of thyroxine cause permanent mental and physical retardation and, for this reason, babies are tested for hypothyroidism within a week of birth.

Management of hypothyroidism

Lifelong oral treatment with synthetic thyroid hormones (thyroxine (levothyroxine), or liothyronine) is the only option. Blood tests are performed regularly to monitor the treatment and permit dosage adjustments. In the elderly, as well as people with heart disease, gradual introduction of thyroxine is used to prevent heart strain.

In severely ill patients, thyroid hormone may be given by injection. This method of administration may also be used to treat newborn infants with low levels of thyroxine.

Symptoms of thyrotoxicosis may appear if excess thyroxine replacement is given. Otherwise, no adverse events occur since treatment is adjusted to replace the natural hormone that the body should produce itself.

COMMON DRUGS

Drugs for hypothyroidism	**Drugs for hyperthyroidism**
Liothyronine	Carbimazole ✳
Thyroxine (levothyroxine) ✳	Iodine
	Nadolol
	Propranolol ✳
	Propylthiouracil ✳
	Radio-iodine

✳ See Part 4

DRUGS FOR PITUITARY DISORDERS

The pituitary gland, which lies at the base of the brain, produces a number of *hormones* that regulate physical growth, *metabolism*, sexual development, and reproductive function. Many of these hormones act indirectly by stimulating other glands, such as the thyroid, adrenal glands, ovaries, and testes, to release their own hormones. A summary of the actions and effects of each pituitary hormone is given below.

An excess or a lack of one of the pituitary hormones may produce serious effects, the nature of which depends on the hormone involved. Abnormal levels of a particular hormone may be caused by a pituitary tumour, which may be treated surgically, with radiotherapy, or with drugs. In other cases, drugs may be used to correct the hormonal imbalance.

The more common pituitary disorders that can be treated with drugs are those involving growth hormone, antidiuretic hormone, prolactin, adrenal hormones, and the gonadotrophins. The first three are discussed below. For information on the use of drugs to treat infertility arising from inadequate levels of gonadotrophins, see p.164. Lack of corticotrophin, leading to inadequate production of adrenal hormones, is usually treated with corticosteroids (see p.141).

Drugs for growth hormone disorders

Growth hormone (somatotropin) is the principal hormone required for normal growth in childhood and adolescence.

Lack of growth hormone impairs normal physical growth. Doctors administer hormone treatment only after tests have proven that a lack of this hormone is the cause of the disorder. If treatment is started at an early age, regular injections of somatropin, a synthetic form of natural growth hormone, administered until the end of adolescence usually allow normal growth and development to take place.

Less often, the pituitary produces an excess of growth hormone. In children this can result in pituitary gigantism; in adults, it can produce a disorder known as acromegaly. This disorder, which is usually the result of a pituitary tumour, is characterized by thickening of the skull, face, hands, and feet, and enlargement of some internal organs.

The pituitary tumour may either be surgically removed or destroyed by radiotherapy. In the frail or elderly, drugs such as bromocriptine and octreotide are used to reduce growth hormone levels. Octreotide is also used as an adjunctive treatment before surgery and in those with increased growth hormone levels occurring after surgery. People who have undergone surgery and/or radiotherapy may require long-term replacement with other hormones (such as sex hormones, thyroid hormone, or corticosteroids).

Drugs for diabetes insipidus

Antidiuretic hormone (also known as ADH or vasopressin) acts on the kidneys, controlling the amount of water retained in the body and returned to the blood.

A lack of ADH is usually caused by damage to the pituitary, and this in turn causes diabetes insipidus. In this rare condition, the kidneys cannot retain water and large quantities pass into the urine. The chief symptoms of diabetes insipidus are constant thirst and the production of large volumes of urine.

Diabetes insipidus is treated with ADH or a related synthetic drug, desmopressin. These replace naturally produced ADH and may be given by injection or in the form of a nasal spray. Chlorpropamide may be used to treat mild cases; it works by increasing ADH release from the pituitary and by sensitizing the kidneys to the effect of ADH.

Alternatively, a thiazide diuretic (such as chlortalidone) may be prescribed for mild cases (see Diuretics, p.99). The usual effect of such drugs is to increase urine production, but in diabetes insipidus they have the opposite effect, reducing water loss from the body.

Drugs used to reduce prolactin levels

Prolactin, also called lactogenic hormone, is produced in both men and women. In women, prolactin controls the secretion of breast milk following childbirth. The function of this hormone in men is not understood, although it appears to be necessary for normal sperm production.

The disorders associated with prolactin are all concerned with overproduction. High levels of prolactin in women can cause lactation that is unassociated with pregnancy and birth (galactorrhoea), lack of menstruation (amenorrhoea), and infertility. If excessive amounts are produced in men, the result may be galactorrhoea, impotence, or infertility.

Some drugs, notably methyldopa, oestrogen, and the phenothiazine antipsychotics, can raise the prolactin level in the blood. More often, however, the increased prolactin results from a pituitary tumour and is usually treated with bromocriptine or cabergoline. These drugs inhibit prolactin production.

THE EFFECTS OF PITUITARY HORMONES

The pituitary gland produces a large number of hormones, many of which control the activities of other glands. The illustration shows the principal sites of action of the major pituitary hormones.

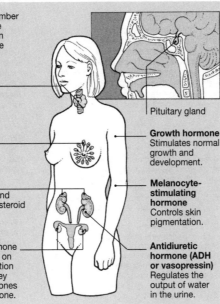

Thyroid-stimulating hormone
Stimulates production and release of thyroid hormones.

Prolactin
Stimulates glands in the breast to produce milk in women.
Helps sperm production in men.

Corticotrophin (ACTH)
Controls the production and release of adrenal corticosteroid hormones.

Gonadotrophins
Two hormones, follicle-stimulating hormone (FSH) and luteinizing hormone (LH), act on the sex glands to stimulate egg production and release, and sperm production. They also control the output of the sex hormones oestrogen, progesterone, and testosterone.

Pituitary gland

Growth hormone
Stimulates normal growth and development.

Melanocyte-stimulating hormone
Controls skin pigmentation.

Antidiuretic hormone (ADH or vasopressin)
Regulates the output of water in the urine.

COMMON DRUGS

Drugs for growth hormone disorders
Bromocriptine ✳
Lanreotide
Octreotide
Somatropin

Drugs for diabetes insipidus
Carbamazepine ✳
Chlorpropamide
Chlortalidone
Desmopressin ✳
Vasopressin (ADH)

Drugs to reduce prolactin levels
Bromocriptine ✳
Cabergoline
Quinagolide

✳ See Part 4

MALE SEX HORMONES

Male sex hormones – androgens – are responsible for the development of male sexual characteristics. The principal androgen is testosterone, which in men is produced by the testes from puberty onwards. Women produce testosterone in small amounts in the adrenal glands, but its exact function in the female body is not known.

Testosterone has two major effects: an androgenic effect and an anabolic effect. Its androgenic effect is to stimulate the appearance of the secondary sexual characteristics at puberty, such as the growth of body hair, deepening of the voice, and an increase in genital size. Its anabolic effects are to increase muscle bulk and accelerate growth rate.

There are a number of synthetically produced derivatives of testosterone that produce varying degrees of the androgenic and anabolic effects mentioned above. Derivatives that have a mainly anabolic effect are known as anabolic steroids (see box below).

Testosterone and its derivatives have been used under medical supervision in both men and women to treat a number of conditions.

Why they are used

Male sex hormones are mainly given to men to promote the development of male sexual characteristics when hormone production is deficient. This may be the result of an abnormality of the testes or of inadequate production of the pituitary hormones that stimulate the testes to release testosterone.

A course of treatment with male sex hormones is sometimes prescribed for adolescent boys in whom the onset of puberty is delayed by pituitary problems. The treatment may also help to stimulate development of secondary male sexual characteristics and to increase sex drive (libido) in adult men who are producing inadequate testosterone levels. However, this type of hormone treatment has been found to reduce the production of sperm. (For information on the drug treatment of male infertility, see p.164.)

EFFECTS OF MALE SEX HORMONES

Anabolic effects
These are the tissue-building effects of male sex hormones.

Increase in muscle size

Increased muscle bulk
Anabolic hormones promote development of muscles, especially of the upper body.

Pelvis

Growing end of femur

Bone growth
Anabolic hormones increase bone density. They also halt growth of the bone ends.

Androgenic effects
These are the effects of male sex hormones on the development of secondary male sexual characteristics.

Voice changes
Androgenic hormones cause enlargement of the larynx and, thus, deepen the voice.

Facial hair

Larynx

Facial and body hair
Androgenic hormones stimulate hair growth on face and body areas.

Penis

Testis

Genital development
Androgenic hormones stimulate enlargement of the testes and penis.

Androgens may also be prescribed for women to treat certain types of cancer of the breast and uterus (see Anticancer drugs, p.154). Testosterone can be given by injection, capsules, patches, or pellets that are surgically inserted.

How they work

Taken in low doses as part of replacement therapy when natural production is low, male sex hormones act in the same way as the natural hormones. In adolescents suffering from delayed puberty, hormone treatment produces both androgenic and anabolic effects (above), initiating the development of secondary sexual

characteristics over a few months; full sexual development usually takes place over three to four years. When sex hormones are given to adult men, the effects on physical appearance and libido may begin to be felt within a few weeks.

Risks and special precautions

The main risks with these drugs occur when they are given to boys with delayed puberty and to women with breast cancer. Given to initiate the onset of puberty, they may stunt growth by prematurely sealing the growing ends of the long bones. Doctors normally try to avoid prescribing hormones in these circumstances until growth is complete. High doses given to women have various masculinizing effects, including increased facial and body hair, and a deeper voice. The drugs may also produce enlargement of the clitoris, changes in libido, and acne.

ANABOLIC STEROIDS

Anabolic steroids are synthetically produced variants that mimic the anabolic effects of the natural hormones. They increase muscle bulk and body growth.

Doctors occasionally prescribe anabolic steroids and a high-protein diet to promote recovery after serious illness or major surgery. The steroids may also help to increase the production of blood cells in some forms of anaemia and to reduce itching in chronic obstructive jaundice.

Anabolic steroids have been widely abused by athletes because these drugs speed up

the recovery of muscles after a session of intense exercise. This enables the athlete to go through a more demanding daily exercise programme, which results in a significant improvement in muscle power. The use of anabolic steroids by athletes to improve their performance is condemned by doctors and athletic organizations because of the risks to health, particularly for women. The side effects range from acne and baldness to fluid retention, reduced fertility in men and women, hardening of the arteries, a long-term risk of liver disease, and certain forms of cancer.

COMMON DRUGS

Primarily androgenic
Mesterolone
Testosterone ✳

Primarily anabolic
Nandrolone
Oxymetholone
Stanozolol

Anti-androgens
Cyproterone
Finasteride ✳

✳ See Part 4

FEMALE SEX HORMONES

There are two types of female sex hormones: oestrogen and progesterone. In women, these hormones are secreted by the ovaries from puberty until the menopause. Each month, the levels of oestrogen and progesterone fluctuate, producing the menstrual cycle (see p.159). During pregnancy, oestrogen and progesterone are produced by the placenta. The adrenal gland also makes small amounts of oestrogen. Production of oestrogen and progesterone is regulated by the two gonadotrophin hormones (FSH and LH) produced by the pituitary gland (see p.145).

Oestrogen is responsible for the development of female sexual characteristics, including breast development, growth of pubic hair, and widening of the pelvis. Progesterone prepares the lining of the uterus for implantation of a fertilized egg. This hormone is also important for the maintenance of pregnancy.

Synthetic forms of these hormones are used medically to treat a number of conditions and are known as oestrogens and progestogens.

Why they are used

The best-known use of oestrogens and progestogens is in oral contraceptives These drugs are discussed on p.161. Other uses include the treatment of menstrual disorders (p.160) and certain hormone-sensitive cancers (p.154). This page discusses the drug treatments that are used for natural hormone deficiency.

Hormone deficiency

Deficiency of female sex hormones may occur as a result of deficiency of gonadotrophins caused by a pituitary disorder or by abnormal development of the ovaries (ovarian failure). This may lead to the absence of menstruation and lack of sexual development. If tests show a deficiency of gonadotrophins, preparations of these hormones may be prescribed (see p.164). These trigger the release of oestrogen and progesterone from the ovaries. If pituitary function is normal and ovarian failure is diagnosed as the cause of hormone deficiency, oestrogens and progestogens may be given as supplements. In this situation, these supplements ensure development of normal female sexual characteristics but cannot stimulate ovulation.

Menopause

A decline in levels of oestrogen and progesterone occurs naturally after the menopause, when the menstrual cycle ceases. The sudden reduction in levels of oestrogen often causes distressing symptoms and many doctors suggest that hormone supplements be used following the menopause (see below) Such hormone replacement therapy (HRT) helps to reduce the symptoms of the menopause and to delay some of the long-term consequences of reduced oestrogen levels in old age, including osteoporosis (p.122) and atherosclerosis (the deposition of fat in the arteries). A

balance between the benefits and risk for individual women must be considered, however, because there can be a slight increase in risk of breast cancer. When dryness of the vagina is a particular problem, a cream containing an oestrogen drug may be prescribed. It is used together with a progestogen unless the woman has had a hysterectomy, in which case the oestrogen alone is used. Some women with very severe symptoms respond poorly to oral drugs and may be helped by oestrogen implants. Hormone replacement therapy may also be prescribed for women who have undergone a premature menopause as a result of surgical removal of the ovaries or radiotherapy for ovarian cancer.

How they affect you

Hormones given to treat ovarian failure or delayed puberty take three to six months to produce a noticeable effect on sexual development. Taken for menopausal symptoms, they can dramatically reduce the number of hot flushes within a week.

Both oestrogens and progestogens can cause fluid retention, and oestrogens may cause nausea, vomiting, breast tenderness, headache, dizziness, and depression. Progestogens may cause "breakthrough" bleeding between menstrual periods. In the comparatively low doses used to treat these disorders, side effects are unlikely.

Risks and special precautions

The use of oestrogens and progestogens for the treatment of ovarian failure carries few risks for otherwise healthy young women. Because oestrogens increase the risk of hypertension (raised blood pressure) and thrombosis (abnormal blood clotting), however, there are risks associated with long-term treatment in older women. For this reason, treatment is prescribed with caution for women who have heart or circulatory disorders, or those who are overweight or smoke. Oestrogens may also trigger the onset of diabetes mellitus in susceptible people or aggravate blood sugar control in diabetic women. Tibolone has both oestrogen and progestogen properties and can therefore be used on its own.

EFFECTS OF HORMONE REPLACEMENT THERAPY (HRT)

Besides alleviating the symptoms of the menopause, such as hot flushes and vaginal dryness, HRT has a beneficial effect on many parts of the body, including the cardiovascular system and the brain and is important in preventing osteoporosis (p.122). Benefits must, however, be weighed against a slightly increased risk of breast cancer.

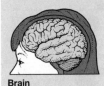

Brain
The risk of stroke is reduced, and HRT may play a part in preventing Alzheimer's disease and Parkinsonism.

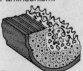

Bones
HRT reduces the thinning of bone that occurs in osteoporosis and thus protects against fractures.

Heart
HRT prevents accumulation of fat deposits in the artery walls, reducing the risk of coronary artery disease.

Breasts
There is a slightly increased risk of breast cancer with long-term use of HRT, especially in older women.

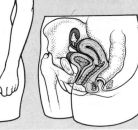

Reproductive organs
Thinning of the vaginal tissues leading to painful intercourse can be prevented by HRT.

COMMON DRUGS

Oestrogens	Progestogens
Conjugated oestrogens *	Dydrogesterone *
Estradiol *	Hydroxyprogesterone
Estriol	Levonorgestrel *
Estrone	Medroxyprogesterone *
Estropipate	Norethisterone *
Mestranol	Norgestrel
Tibolone *	Progesterone
	Raloxifene *

* See Part 4

NUTRITION

Food provides energy (as calories) and materials called nutrients needed for growth and renewal of tissues. Protein, carbohydrate, and fat are the three major nutrient components of food. Vitamins and minerals are found only in small amounts in food, but are just as important for normal function of the body. Fibre, found only in foods from plants, is needed for a healthy digestive system.

During digestion, large molecules of food are broken down into smaller molecules, releasing nutrients that are absorbed into the bloodstream. Carbohydrate and fat are then *metabolized* by body cells to produce energy. They may also be incorporated with protein into the cell structure. Each metabolic process is promoted by a specific *enzyme* and often requires the presence of a particular vitamin or mineral.

Why drugs are used

Dietary deficiency of essential nutrients can lead to illness. In poorer countries where there is a shortage of food, marasmus (resulting from lack of food energy) and kwashiorkor (from lack of protein) are common. In the developed world, however, excessive food intake leading to obesity is more common. Nutritional deficiencies in developed countries result from poor food choices and usually stem from a lack of a specific vitamin or mineral, such as in iron-deficiency anaemia.

Some nutritional deficiencies may be caused by an inability of the body to absorb nutrients from food (malabsorption) or to utilize them once they have been absorbed. Malabsorption may be caused by lack of an enzyme or an abnormality of the digestive tract. Errors of metabolism are often inborn and are not yet fully understood. They may be caused by failure of the body to produce the chemicals required to process nutrients for use.

Why supplements are used

Deficiencies such as kwashiorkor or marasmus are usually treated by dietary improvement and, in some cases, food supplements, rather than drugs. Vitamin and mineral deficiencies are usually treated with appropriate supplements. Malabsorption disorders may require changes in diet or long-term use of supplements. Metabolic errors are not easily treated with supplements or drugs, and a special diet may be the main treatment.

Obesity was formerly treated with appetite-suppressants related to amphetamines (p.452), the use of which is now discouraged. The preferred treatment includes reduction of food intake, altered eating patterns, and increased exercise.

Major food components

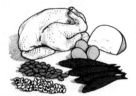

Proteins
Vital for tissue growth and repair. In meat and dairy products, cereals, and pulses. Moderate amounts required.

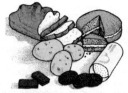

Carbohydrates
A major energy source, stored as fat when taken in excess. In cereals, sugar, and vegetables. Starchy foods preferable to sugar.

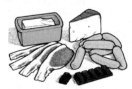

Fats
A concentrated energy form that is needed only in small quantities. In animal products such as butter and in plant oils.

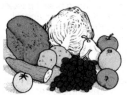

Fibre (non-starch polysaccharides)
The indigestible part of any plant product that, although it contains no nutrients, adds bulk to faeces.

Absorption of nutrients

Food passes through the mouth, oesophagus, and stomach to the small intestine. The lining of the small intestine secretes many enzymes and is covered by tiny projections (villi) that enable nutrients to pass into the blood.

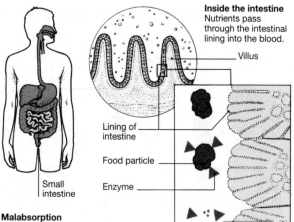

Inside the intestine
Nutrients pass through the intestinal lining into the blood.

Villus

Lining of intestine

Food particle

Enzyme

Small intestine

Food molecule absorbed

Malabsorption
Enzyme action breaks food down into molecules that can be absorbed. Lack of certain enzymes may cause malabsorption of nutrients. Other causes include flattened villi and scars on the intestine.

MAJOR DRUG GROUPS

Vitamins

VITAMINS

Vitamins are complex chemicals that are essential for a variety of body functions. With the exception of vitamin D, the body cannot manufacture these substances itself and therefore we need to include them in our diet. There are 13 major vitamins: A, C, D, E, K, and the B complex vitamins – thiamine (B_1), riboflavin (B_2), niacin (B_3), pantothenic acid (B_5), pyridoxine (B_6), and cobalamin (B_{12}) folic acid and biotin. Most vitamins are required in very small amounts and each vitamin is present in one or more foods (see Main food sources of vitamins, p.150). Vitamin D is also produced in the body when the skin is exposed to sunlight. Vitamins fall into two groups, depending on whether they dissolve in fat or water (see Fat-soluble and water-soluble vitamins, p.151).

A number of vitamins (such as vitamins A, C, and E) have now been recognized as having strong antioxidant properties. Antioxidants neutralize the effect of free radicals, substances produced during the body's normal processes that may be potentially harmful if they are not neutralized. Free radicals are believed to play a role in cardiovascular disease, ageing, and cancer.

A balanced diet that includes a variety of different types of food is likely to contain adequate amounts of all the vitamins. Inadequate intake of any vitamin over an extended period can lead to symptoms of deficiency. The nature of these symptoms depends on the vitamin concerned.

A doctor may recommend taking supplements of one or more vitamins in a variety of circumstances: to prevent vitamin deficiency occurring in people who are considered at special risk, to treat symptoms of deficiency, and in the treatment of certain medical conditions.

Why they are used

Preventing deficiency

Most people in the United Kingdom obtain sufficient quantities of vitamins in their diet, and it is therefore not usually necessary to take additional vitamins in the form of supplements. People who are unsure if their present diet is adequate are advised to look at the table on p.150 to check that foods that are rich in vitamins are eaten regularly. Vitamin intake can often be boosted simply by increasing the quantities of fresh foods and raw fruit and vegetables in the diet. Certain groups in the population are, however, at increased

risk of vitamin deficiency. These include people who have an increased need for certain vitamins that may not be met from dietary sources – in particular, women who are pregnant or breast-feeding, and infants and young children. The elderly, who may not be eating a varied diet, may also be at risk. Strict vegetarians, vegans, and others on restricted diets may not receive adequate amounts of all vitamins.

In addition, people who suffer from disorders in which absorption of nutrients from the bowel is impaired, or who need to take drugs that reduce the absorption of vitamins (for example, some types of lipid-lowering drugs), are usually given additional vitamins.

In these cases, the doctor is likely to advise supplements of one or more vitamins. Although most preparations are available without a prescription, it is important to seek specialist advice before starting a course of vitamin supplements, so that a proper assessment is made of your individual requirements.

Vitamin supplements should not be used as a general tonic to improve well-being – they are not effective for this purpose – nor should they ever be used as a substitute for a balanced diet.

PRIMARY FUNCTIONS OF VITAMINS

The role of vitamins in the body is not yet fully understood; much of our knowledge is based on the evidence that is provided by symptoms occurring as a result of deficiency of a particular vitamin. Most vitamins have been found to have a number of important actions on one or more body systems or functions. Many are involved in the activity of *enzymes* (substances that promote or enable biochemical reactions in the body). The illustration below indicates the organs and body systems on which each vitamin has its principal effect.

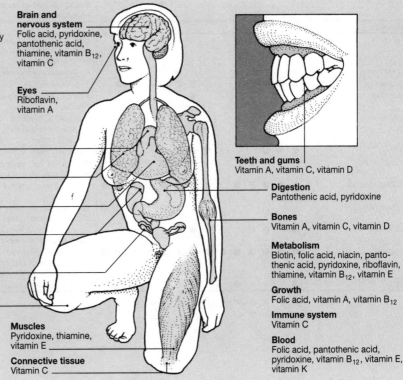

Brain and nervous system
Folic acid, pyridoxine, pantothenic acid, thiamine, vitamin B_{12}, vitamin C

Eyes
Riboflavin, vitamin A

Blood vessels
Vitamin E

Lungs
Vitamin A, vitamin E

Heart
Thiamine, vitamin E

Adrenal hormones
Pantothenic acid, riboflavin, vitamin C

Fertility
Folic acid, vitamin A

Skin
Niacin, pyridoxine, riboflavin, vitamin A, vitamin E

Muscles
Pyridoxine, thiamine, vitamin E

Connective tissue
Vitamin C

Teeth and gums
Vitamin A, vitamin C, vitamin D

Digestion
Pantothenic acid, pyridoxine

Bones
Vitamin A, vitamin C, vitamin D

Metabolism
Biotin, folic acid, niacin, pantothenic acid, pyridoxine, riboflavin, thiamine, vitamin B_{12}, vitamin E

Growth
Folic acid, vitamin A, vitamin B_{12}

Immune system
Vitamin C

Blood
Folic acid, pantothenic acid, pyridoxine, vitamin B_{12}, vitamin E, vitamin K

VITAMINS continued

MAIN FOOD SOURCES OF VITAMINS AND MINERALS

The table below indicates which foods are especially good sources of particular vitamins and minerals. Ensuring that you regularly select foods from a variety of categories helps to maintain adequate intake for most people, without a need for supplements. It is important to remember that processed and overcooked foods are likely to contain fewer vitamins than fresh, raw, or lightly cooked foods.

Vitamins	Red meat	Poultry	Liver	Milk	Cheese	Butter/margarine	Eggs	Fish	Cereals and bread	Green vegetables	Root vegetables	Pulses/legumes	Nuts	Fruit	Other	
Biotin		●					●			●	●					Especially peanuts. Cauliflower and mushrooms are good sources.
Folic acid		●					●			●					●	Wheat germ and mushrooms are rich sources.
Niacin as nicotinic acid	●	●	●				●	●		●	●					Protein-rich foods such as milk and eggs contain tryptophan, which can be converted to niacin in the body.
Pantothenic acid			●				●	●								Each food group contributes some pantothenic acid.
Pyridoxine	●	●	●				●	●	●							Especially white meat (poultry), fish, and wholemeal cereals.
Riboflavin		●	●	●	●		●		●	●	●	●				Found in most foods.
Thiamine	●		●					●		●	●					Brewer's yeast, wheat germ, and bran are also good sources.
Vitamin A		●	●	●	●	●	●			●					●	Fish liver oil, dark green leafy vegetables such as spinach, and orange or yellow-orange vegetables and fruits such as carrots, apricots, and peaches, are especially good sources of vitamin A.
Vitamin B$_{12}$	●		●	●	●		●	●								Obtained only from animal products, especially liver and red meat.
Vitamin C										●				●		Especially citrus fruits, tomatoes, potatoes, broccoli, strawberries, and melon.
Vitamin D				●			●									Dietary products are the best source, but the vitamin is also obtained by the body when the skin is exposed to sunlight.
Vitamin E						●	●		●	●		●	●			Vegetable oils, wholemeal cereals, and wheat germ are the best sources.
Vitamin K								●								Found in small amounts in fruits, seeds, root vegetables, dairy and meat products.
Minerals																
Calcium				●	●					●		●	●			Dark green leafy vegetables, soya bean products, and nuts are good non-dairy alternatives. Also present in hard, or alkaline, water supplies.
Chromium	●			●					●	●						Especially unrefined wholemeal cereals.
Copper	●	●	●					●	●	●		●	●			Especially shellfish, wholemeal cereals, and mushrooms.
Fluoride								●								Primarily obtained from fluoridated water supplies. Also in seafood and tea.
Iodine				●	●			●	●							Provided by "iodized" table salt, but adequate amounts can be obtained without using table salt from dairy products, saltwater fish, and bread.
Iron	●	●	●				●	●	●	●						Especially liver, red meat, and enriched or whole grains.
Magnesium				●				●	●	●		●	●			Dark green leafy vegetables such as spinach are rich sources. Also present in alkaline water supplies.
Phosphorus	●	●	●	●	●		●	●	●	●	●	●	●		●	Common food additive. Large amounts found in some carbonated beverages.
Potassium								●	●		●			●		Best sources are fruits and vegetables, especially oranges, bananas, and potatoes.
Selenium	●			●	●		●	●								Seafood is the richest source. Amounts in most foods are variable, depending on soil where plants were grown and animals grazed.
Sodium	●	●	●	●	●	●	●	●	●	●	●	●	●		●	Sodium is present in all foods, especially table salt, processed foods, potato crisps, crackers, and pickled, cured, or smoked meats, seafood, and vegetables. Also present in "softened" water.
Zinc	●			●			●	●				●				Highest amounts in wholemeal breads and cereals.

Vitamin deficiency

It is rare for a diet to be completely lacking in a particular vitamin. But if intake of a particular vitamin is regularly lower than the body's requirements, over a period of time the body's stores of vitamins may become depleted and symptoms of deficiency may begin to appear. In Britain, vitamin deficiency disorders are most common among vagrants and alcoholics and those on low incomes who fail to eat an adequate diet. Deficiencies of water-soluble vitamins are more likely since most of these are not stored in large quantities in the body. For descriptions of individual deficiency disorders, see the appropriate vitamin profile in Part 4.

Dosages of vitamins prescribed to treat vitamin deficiency are likely to be larger than those used to prevent deficiency. Medical supervision is required when correcting vitamin deficiency.

Other medical uses of vitamins

Various claims have been made for the value of vitamins in the treatment of medical disorders other than vitamin deficiency. High doses of vitamin C have been said to be effective in the prevention and treatment of the common cold, but such claims are not yet proved; zinc, however, may be helpful for this purpose. Vitamin and mineral supplements do not improve IQ in well-nourished children, but quite small dietary deficiencies can cause poor academic performance.

Certain vitamins have recognized medical uses apart from their nutritional role. Vitamin D has long been used to treat bone-wasting disorders (p.122). Niacin is sometimes used (in the form of nicotinic acid) as a lipid-lowering drug (p.103). Derivatives of vitamin A (retinoids) are an established part of the treatment

MINERALS

Minerals are elements – the simplest form of substances – many of which are essential in trace amounts for normal metabolic processes. A balanced diet usually contains all of the minerals that the body requires; mineral deficiency diseases, except iron-deficiency anaemia, are uncommon.

Dietary supplements are necessary only when a doctor has diagnosed a specific deficiency or as part of the prevention or treatment of a medical disorder. Doctors often prescribe minerals for people with intestinal diseases that reduce the absorption of minerals from the diet. Iron supplements are often advised for pregnant or breast-feeding women, and iron-rich foods are recommended for infants over six months.

Much of the general advice given for vitamins also applies to minerals: taking supplements unless under medical direction is not advisable, exceeding the body's daily requirements is not beneficial, and large doses may be harmful.

CALCULATING DAILY VITAMIN REQUIREMENTS

Everyone needs a minimum amount of each vitamin for maintenance of health. The amount may vary with age, sex, and whether a woman is pregnant or breast-feeding. Guidelines for assessing the nutritional value of diets are called Reference Nutrient Intakes (RNI), and are based on the amount of a nutrient that is enough, or more than enough, for 97 per cent of people. Those consuming much less than the RNI on a daily basis may not be consuming less than their needs but the risk of doing so is increased.

The current RNI (see table below) were set by the UK Department of Health Committee on Medical Aspects of Food Policy (COMA) in 1991, and replace the Recommended Dietary Allowances (RDA). Where no RNI exists, the 1989 US RDA is given.

Daily reference nutrient intakes of vitamins for adults (aged 19–50)

Vitamin (unit)	Reference Nutrient Intake		
	Men	Women	Pregnancy and breast-feeding
Biotin (mcg)	10–200*	10–200*	Not established
Folic acid as folate (mcg)	200	200	260–300
Niacin as nicotinic acid (mg)	17	13	13–15
Pantothenic acid (mg)	3–7*	3–7*	3–7*
Pyridoxine (mg)	1.4	1.2	1.2
Riboflavin (mg)	1.3	1.1	1.4–1.6
Thiamine (mg)	1.0	0.8	0.9–1.0
Vitamin A (mcg)	700	600	700–950
Vitamin B_{12} (mcg)	1.5	1.5	1.5–2.0
Vitamin C (mg)	40	40	50–70
Vitamin D (mcg)	Ø	Ø	10
Vitamin E (mg)	4–10†	3–8†	10–12†

*Estimated requirement; Ø See Vitamin D, p.448; † US figure

for severe acne (p.177). Many women who suffer from pre-menstrual syndrome take pyridoxine (vitamin B_6) supplements to relieve their symptoms. See also Drugs for menstrual disorders, p.160.

Risks and special precautions

Vitamins are natural substances, and supplements can be taken without risk by most people. It is important, however, not to exceed the recommended dosage, particularly in the case of fat-soluble vitamins, which may accumulate in the body. Dosage needs to be carefully calculated, taking into account the degree of deficiency, the dietary intake, and the duration of treatment. Overdosage has at best no therapeutic value and at worst it may incur the risk of serious harmful effects. Multivitamin preparations containing a large number of different vitamins are widely available. Fortunately, the amounts of each vitamin contained in each tablet are not usually large and are not likely to be harmful unless the dose is greatly exceeded. Single vitamin supplements can be harmful because an excess of one vitamin may increase requirements for others; hence, they should be used only on medical advice. For specific information on each vitamin, see Part 4, pp.437–449.

FAT-SOLUBLE AND WATER-SOLUBLE VITAMINS

Fat-soluble vitamins
Vitamins A, D, E, and K are absorbed from the intestine into the bloodstream together with fat (see also How drugs pass through the body, p.17). Deficiency of these vitamins may occur as a result of any disorder that affects the absorption of fat (for example, coeliac disease). These vitamins are stored in the liver and reserves of some of them may last for several years. Taking an excess of a fat-soluble vitamin for a long period may cause it to build up to a harmful level in the body. Ensuring that foods rich in these vitamins are regularly included in the diet usually provides a sufficient supply without the risk of overdosage.

Water-soluble vitamins
Vitamin C and the B vitamins dissolve in water. Most are stored in the body for only a short period and are rapidly excreted by the kidneys if taken in higher amounts than the body requires. Vitamin B_{12} is the exception; it is stored in the liver, which may hold up to six years' supply. For these reasons, foods containing water-soluble vitamins need to be eaten daily. They are easily lost in cooking, so uncooked foods containing these vitamins should be eaten regularly. An overdose of water-soluble vitamins does not usually cause toxic effects, but adverse reactions to large dosages of vitamin C and pyridoxine (vitamin B_6) have been reported.

MALIGNANT AND IMMUNE DISEASE

New cells are continuously needed by the body to replace those that wear out and die naturally and to repair injured tissue. In normal circumstances the rate at which cells are created is carefully regulated. However, sometimes abnormal cells are formed that multiply uncontrollably. They may form lumps, warts, or nodules of abnormal tissue. These tumours are usually confined to one place and cause few problems; these are benign growths. In other types of tumour the cells may invade or destroy the structures around the tumour, and abnormal cells may spread to other parts of the body, forming satellite or metastatic tumours. These malignant growths are also called cancers.

Opposing the development of tumours is the body's immune system. This can recognize as foreign not only invading bacteria and viruses but also transplanted tissue and cells that have become cancerous. The immune system relies on different types of white blood cells produced in the lymph glands and the bone marrow. They respond to foreign cells in a variety of ways, which are described on the facing page.

Overactivity of the immune system also causes allergic reactions (see Allergy, p.123).

What can go wrong

A single cause for cancer has not been identified, and an individual's risk of developing cancer may depend both upon genetic predisposition (some families seem particularly prone to cancers of one or more types) and upon exposure to external risk factors, known as carcinogens. These include tobacco smoke, which increases the risk of lung cancer, and ultraviolet light, which makes skin cancer more likely in those who spend long periods in the sun. Long-term suppression of the immune system by disease (as in AIDS) or by drugs – for example, those given to prevent rejection of transplanted organs – also increases the risk of developing not only infections but also certain cancers. This fact demonstrates the importance of the immune system in removing abnormal cells with the potential to cause a tumour.

Excessive activity of the immune system may also cause problems. It may respond excessively to an innocuous stimulus, as in hay fever, or may mount a reaction against normal tissues, leading to a variety of disorders known as autoimmune diseases. These include rheumatoid arthritis, certain inflammatory skin disorders (for example, systemic lupus erythematosus), pernicious anaemia, and some forms of hypothyroidism. Immune system activity can also be troublesome

Types of cancer

Uncontrolled multiplication of cells leads to the formation of tumours that may be benign or malignant. Benign tumours do not spread to other tissues; however, malignant (cancerous) tumours do. Some of the main types of cancer are defined below.

Type of cancer	Tissues affected
Carcinoma	Skin and glandular tissue lining cells of internal organs
Sarcoma	Muscles, bones, and fibrous tissues and lining cells of blood vessels
Leukaemia	White blood cells
Lymphoma	Lymph glands

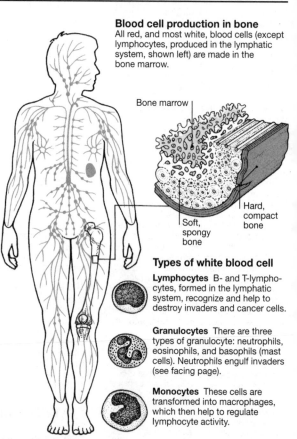

Blood cell production in bone
All red, and most white, blood cells (except lymphocytes, produced in the lymphatic system, shown left) are made in the bone marrow.

Bone marrow

Hard, compact bone

Soft, spongy bone

Types of white blood cell

Lymphocytes B- and T-lymphocytes, formed in the lymphatic system, recognize and help to destroy invaders and cancer cells.

Granulocytes There are three types of granulocyte: neutrophils, eosinophils, and basophils (mast cells). Neutrophils engulf invaders (see facing page).

Monocytes These cells are transformed into macrophages, which then help to regulate lymphocyte activity.

following an organ or tissue transplant, when it may lead to rejection of the foreign tissue. This shows the need for medication that can dampen the immune system and enable the body to accept the foreign tissue.

Why drugs are used

In cancer treatment, cytotoxic (cell-killing) drugs are used to eliminate abnormally dividing cells. This has the effect of slowing the growth rate of tumours and sometimes leading to their complete

Types of immune response

A specific response occurs when the immune system recognizes an invader. Two types of specific response, humoral and cellular, are described below. Phagocytosis, a non-specific response that does not depend on recognition of the invader, is also described.

Humoral response

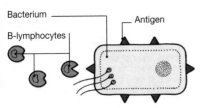

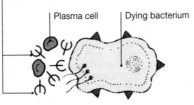

B-lymphocytes are activated by unfamiliar proteins (antigens) on the surface of the invading bacterium.

The activated B-lymphocytes form plasma cells, which release antibodies that bind to the invader and kill it.

Cellular response

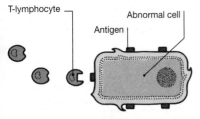

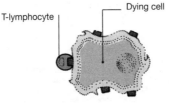

T-lymphocytes recognize the antigens on abnormal or invading cells.

The T-lymphocytes bind to the abnormal cell and destroy it by altering chemical activity within the cell.

Engulfing invaders (phagocytosis)

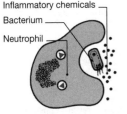

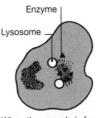

Certain cells, such as neutrophils, are attracted by inflammatory chemicals to an area of bacterial infection.

The neutrophil flows around the bacterium, enclosing it within a fluid-filled space called a vacuole.

When the vacuole is formed, enzymes from areas called lysosomes in the neutrophil destroy the bacterium.

INTERFERONS

Interferons are natural proteins that limit viral infection by inhibiting viral replication within body cells. These substances also assist in the destruction of cancer cells.

Effect on viral infection

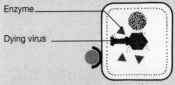

Interferon binds to receptors on a virus-infected cell.

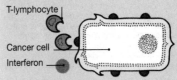

The presence of interferon triggers the release of enzymes that block viral replication. The virus is thus destroyed.

Effect on cancer cells

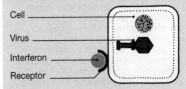

Interferon produced in response to a cancer cell activates T-lymphocytes.

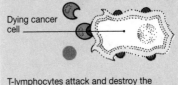

T-lymphocytes attack and destroy the cancer cell.

---

disappearance. Because these drugs act against all rapidly dividing cells, they also reduce the number of normal cells, including blood cells, being produced from the bone marrow. This can produce serious adverse effects, like *anaemia* and neutropenia in cancer patients, but it can be useful in limiting white cell activity in autoimmune disorders.

Other drugs that have immunosuppressant effects include corticosteroids and cyclosporin, which are used following transplant surgery. No drugs are yet available that directly stimulate the entire immune system. However, growth factors may be used to increase the number and activity of some white blood cells, and antibody infusions may help those with deficient production or be used against specific targets in organ transplantation and cancer.

MAJOR DRUG GROUPS

Anticancer drugs
Immunosuppressant drugs
Drugs for AIDS and immune deficiency

ANTICANCER DRUGS

Cancer is a general term that covers a wide range of disorders, ranging from the leukaemias (blood cancers) to solid tumours of the lung, breast, and other organs. In all cancers, a group of cells escape from the normal controls on cell growth and multiplication. As a result, the malignant (cancerous) cells begin to crowd out the normal cells and a tumour develops. Cancerous cells are frequently unable to perform their usual functions, and this may lead to progressively impaired function of the organ or area concerned. Cancers may develop from cells of the blood, skin, muscle, or any other tissue.

Malignant tumours spread into nearby structures, blocking blood vessels and compressing nerves and other structures. Fragments of the tumour may become detached and carried in the bloodstream to other parts of the body, where they form secondary growths (metastases).

Many different factors, or a combination of them, can provoke cancerous changes in cells. These include an individual's

genetic background, immune system failure, and exposure to cancer-causing agents (carcinogens). Known carcinogens include strong sunlight, tobacco smoke, radiation, certain chemicals, viruses, and dietary factors.

Treating cancer is a complicated process that depends on the type of cancer, its stage of development, and the patient's condition and wishes. Any of the following treatments may be used alone or in combination with the others: surgical removal of the cancer, radiation treatment, and chemotherapy (that is, the use of anticancer drugs).

Anticancer drugs that kill cancer cells are sometimes referred to as cytotoxic drugs. They fall into several classes, depending on their chemical composition and principal mode of action. Alkylating agents, antimetabolites, and cytotoxic antibiotics are among the most widely used classes. In addition to these drugs, sex hormones and related substances are also used to treat some types of cancer.

Increasingly, attempts are being made to stimulate the body's own immune defences using drugs like interferon or interleukin and antibodies which recognise specific tumour types.

Why they are used

Cytotoxic drugs can cure rapidly growing cancers and are the treatment of choice for leukaemias, lymphomas, and certain cancers of the testis. They are less effective against slow-growing solid tumours, such as those of the breast and bowel, but they can relieve symptoms and prolong life (see below). *Adjuvant* chemotherapy is increasingly being used after surgery, especially for breast and bowel tumours, to prevent regrowth of the cancer from cells left behind after surgery. Hormone treatment is offered in cases of hormone-sensitive cancer, including many breast, uterine, and prostatic cancers.

Since all anticancer drugs may produce severe adverse effects (see facing page), they are used only in cases where there

SUCCESSFUL CHEMOTHERAPY

Not all cancers respond to treatment with anticancer drugs. Some cancers can be cured by drug treatment. In others, drug treatment can slow or temporarily halt the progress of the disease. In certain cases, drug treatment has no beneficial effect, but in some of these cases other treatments, such as surgery, often produce significant benefits. The table (right) summarizes the main cancers that fall into each of the three groups described.

Successful drug treatment of cancer usually requires repeated courses of anticancer drugs

because the treatment needs to be halted periodically to allow the blood-producing cells in the bone marrow to recover. The diagram below shows the number of cancer cells and normal blood cells before and after each course of treatment with cytotoxic anticancer drugs during successful chemotherapy. Both cancer cells and blood cells are reduced, but the blood cells recover quickly between courses of drug treatment. When treatment is effective, the number of cancer cells is reduced, so they no longer cause symptoms.

Response to chemotherapy

Cancers that can be cured by drugs
Some cancers of the lymphatic system (including Hodgkin's disease)
Acute leukaemias (forms of blood cancer)
Choriocarcinoma (cancer of the placenta)
Germ cell tumours (cancers affecting sperm and egg cells)
Wilms' tumour (a rare form of kidney cancer that affects children)
Cancer of the testis

Cancers in which drugs produce worthwhile benefits
Breast cancer
Ovarian cancer
Some leukaemias
Multiple myeloma (a bone marrow cancer)
Many types of lung cancer
Head and neck cancers
Cancer of the stomach
Cancer of the prostate
Some cancers of the lymphatic system
Bladder cancer
Cancer of the islet cells of the pancreas
Endometrial cancer (cancer affecting the lining of the uterus)
Cancer of the large intestine
Cancer of the oesophagus

Cancers in which drugs are unlikely to be of benefit
Thyroid cancer
Brain cancer in adults
Malignant melanoma (a form of skin cancer)
Liver cancer
Cancer of the pancreas
Cancer of the cervix
Kidney cell cancer

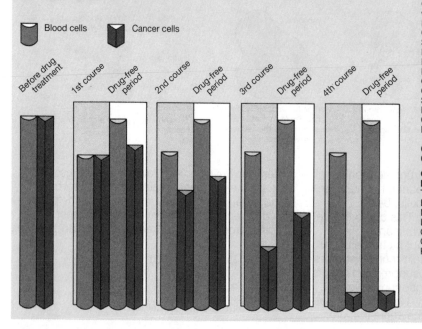

Blood cells   Cancer cells

Before drug treatment | 1st course | Drug-free period | 2nd course | Drug-free period | 3rd course | Drug-free period | 4th course | Drug-free period

is a reasonable chance of achieving a complete cure, significantly prolonging life, or relieving distressing symptoms. Their effectiveness varies a great deal, depending primarily on the type of cancer and the extent of its spread.

The choice of anticancer drug depends on the type of cancer and the condition of the person who is being treated. Often a combination of several drugs is used, either simultaneously or successively. Special regimes of different drugs used together and in succession have been devised to maximize their activity and minimize side effects.

Certain anticancer drugs are also used for their effect in suppressing immune system activity (see p.156).

How they work

All cytotoxic anticancer drugs kill cancer cells by preventing them from growing or dividing. Cells grow and divide in several stages. Most anticancer drugs act at one specific stage of cell growth or division. During treatment, several drugs may be given in sequence to eliminate abnormal cells at all stages of development.

Hormone treatments act by opposing the effects of the hormone that is encouraging growth of the cancer. For example, some breast cancers are stimulated by the female sex hormone oestrogen, whose action is opposed by the drug tamoxifen. Other cancers are damaged by high doses of a particular sex hormone. For example, medroxy-progesterone, a progesterone, often halts the spread of endometrial cancer.

Monoclonal antibodies, such as rituximab, bind to certain cells, marking them out for destruction. Interferon alfa and interleukin 2 are cytokines which stimulate the immune system to attack certain cancers by mechanisms that are not entirely understood.

How they affect you

At the start of treatment, adverse effects of cytotoxic anticancer drugs are likely to be more noticeable than benefits. The most common side effect is nausea and vomiting, for which an anti-emetic drug (see p.90) will usually be prescribed. Effects on the blood are also common. Many anticancer drugs cause hair loss because of the effect of their activity on the hair follicle cells, but the hair usually starts to grow back after chemotherapy has been completed. Individual drugs may produce other side effects.

Anticancer drugs are, in most cases, administered in the highest doses that can be tolerated in order to kill as many cancer cells as quickly as possible.

The unpleasant side effects of intensive chemotherapy, combined with a delay of several weeks before any beneficial effects are seen, and the seriousness of the underlying disease often lead to

ACTION OF CYTOTOXIC ANTICANCER DRUGS

Each type of cytotoxic drug affects a separate stage of the cancer cell's development, and each type of drug kills the cell by a different mechanism of action. The action of some of the principal classes of cytotoxic drugs is described below.

Alkylating agents and cytotoxic antibiotics
These act within the cell's nucleus to damage the cell's genetic material, DNA. This prevents the cell from growing and dividing.

Antimetabolites
These drugs prevent the cell from *metabolizing* (processing) nutrients and other substances that are necessary for normal activity in the cell.

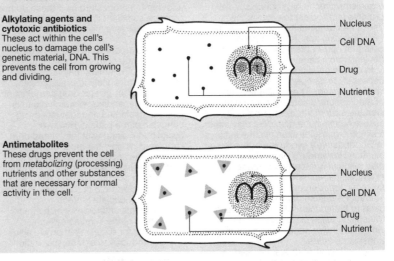

Nucleus
Cell DNA
Drug
Nutrients

Nucleus
Cell DNA
Drug
Nutrient

depression in those who are receiving anticancer drugs. Specialist counselling, support from family and friends, and, in some cases, treatment with antidepressant drugs, may be helpful.

Risks and special precautions

All cytotoxic anticancer drugs interfere with the activity of noncancerous cells and, for this reason, they often produce serious adverse effects during long-term treatment. In particular, these drugs often adversely affect rapidly dividing cells such as the blood-producing cells in the bone marrow. The numbers of red and white cells and the number of platelets (particles in the blood responsible for clotting) may all be reduced. In some cases, symptoms of *anaemia* (weakness and fatigue) and an increased risk of abnormal or excessive bleeding may develop as a result of treatment with anticancer drugs. Reduction in the number of white blood cells may result in an increased susceptibility to infection. A simple infection such as a sore throat may be a sign of depressed white cell production in a patient taking anticancer drugs, and it must be reported to the doctor without delay. In addition, wounds may take longer to heal, and susceptible people can develop gout as a result of increased uric acid production due to cells being broken down.

Because of these problems, anticancer chemotherapy is often given in hospital, where the adverse effects can be closely monitored. Several short courses of drug treatment are usually given, thus allowing the bone marrow time to recover in the

period between courses (see Successful chemotherapy, facing page). Blood tests are performed regularly. When necessary, blood transfusions, antibiotics, or other forms of treatment are used to overcome the adverse effects. When relevant, contraceptive advice is given early in treatment because most anticancer drugs can damage a developing baby.

In addition to these general effects, individual drugs may have adverse effects on particular organs. These are described under individual drug profiles in Part 4.

COMMON DRUGS

Alkylating agents
Chlorambucil
Cyclophosphamide *
Melphalan

Antimetabolites
Azathioprine *
Cytarabine
Fluorouracil
Mercaptopurine *
Methotrexate *

Cytotoxic antibiotics
Doxorubicin *
Epirubicin

Hormone treatments
Anastrozole
Bicalutamide
Cyproterone acetate

Flutamide
Formestane
Goserelin *
Letrozole
Leuprorelin
Medroxy-progesterone *
Megestrol *
Tamoxifen *

Cytokines
Interferon alfa *
Interleukin 2

Taxanes
Docetaxel
Paclitaxel

Other drugs
Carboplatin
Cisplatin *
Etoposide
Irinotecan
Rituximab

| * See Part 4 |

IMMUNOSUPPRESSANT DRUGS

The body is protected against attack from bacteria, fungi, and viruses by the specialized cells and proteins in the blood and tissues that make up the immune system (see p.152). White blood cells known as lymphocytes either kill invading organisms directly or produce special proteins (*antibodies*) to destroy them. These mechanisms are also responsible for eliminating abnormal or unhealthy cells that could otherwise multiply and develop into a cancer.

In certain conditions it is medically necessary to dampen the activity of the immune system. These include a number of autoimmune disorders in which the immune system attacks normal body tissue. Autoimmune disorders may affect a single organ – for example, the kidneys in Goodpasture's syndrome or the thyroid gland in Hashimoto's disease – or they may result in widespread damage, for example, in rheumatoid arthritis or systemic lupus erythematosus.

Immune system activity may also need to be reduced following an organ transplant, when the body's defences would otherwise attack and reject the transplanted tissue.

Several types of drugs are used as immunosuppressants: anticancer drugs (p.154), corticosteroids (p.141), and cyclosporin (p.249).

Why they are used

Immunosuppressant drugs are given to treat autoimmune disorders, such as rheumatoid arthritis, when symptoms are severe and other treatments have not provided adequate relief. Corticosteroids are usually prescribed initially. The pronounced anti-inflammatory effect of these drugs, as well as their immuno-suppressant action, helps to promote healing of tissue damaged by abnormal immune system activity. Anticancer drugs such as methotrexate may be used in addition to corticosteroids if these do not produce sufficient improvement or if their effect wanes (see also Antirheumatic drugs, p.117).

Immunosuppressant drugs are given before and after organ and other tissue transplants. Treatment may have to be continued indefinitely to prevent rejection. A number of drugs and drug combinations are used, depending on which organ is being transplanted and the underlying condition of the patient. However, cyclosporin, along with the related drug tacrolimus, is now the most widely used drug for preventing organ rejection. It is also increasingly used to treat autoimmune disorders. It is often used in combination with a corticosteroid or the more specific drug mycophenolate mofetil.

Monoclonal antibodies which attack those parts of the immune system responsible for organ rejection are also being introduced to aid transplantation.

How they work

Immunosuppressant drugs reduce the effectiveness of the immune system, either by depressing the production of lymphocytes or by altering their activity.

How they affect you

When immunosuppressants are given to treat an autoimmune disorder, they reduce the severity of the symptoms and may temporarily halt the progress of the disease. However, they cannot restore major tissue damage.

Immunosuppressant drugs can produce a variety of unwanted side effects. The side effects caused by corticosteroids are described in more detail on p.141. Anticancer drugs, when prescribed as immunosuppressants, are given in low doses that produce only mild side effects. They may cause nausea and vomiting, for which an anti-emetic drug (p.90) may be prescribed. Hair loss is rare and regrowth usually occurs when the drug treatment is discontinued. Cyclosporin may cause increased growth of facial hair, swelling of the gums, and tingling in the hands.

Risks and special precautions

All of these drugs may produce potentially serious adverse effects. By reducing the activity of the patient's immune system, immunosuppressant drugs can affect the body's ability to fight invading micro-organisms, thereby increasing the risk of serious infections. Because lymphocyte activity is also important for preventing the multiplication of abnormal cells, there is an increased risk of certain types of cancer. A major drawback of anticancer drugs is that, in addition to their effect on the production of lymphocytes, they interfere with the growth and division of other blood cells in the bone marrow. Reduced production of red blood cells can cause *anaemia*; when the production of blood platelets is suppressed, blood clotting may be less efficient.

Although cyclosporin is more specific in its action than either corticosteroids or anticancer drugs, it can cause kidney damage and, in too high a dose, may affect the brain, causing hallucinations or fits. Cyclosporin also tends to raise blood pressure, and another drug may be required to counteract this effect (see Antihypertensive drugs, p.102).

ACTION OF IMMUNOSUPPRESSANTS

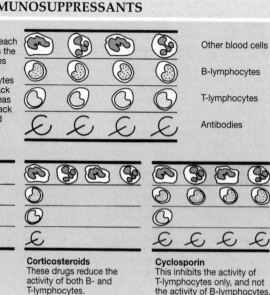

Before treatment
Many types of blood cell, each with a distinct role, form in the bone marrow. Lymphocytes respond to infection and foreign tissue. B-lymphocytes produce antibodies to attack invading organisms, whereas T-lymphocytes directly attack invading cells. Other blood cells help the action of the B- and T-cells.

Other blood cells

B-lymphocytes

T-lymphocytes

Antibodies

Anticancer drugs
These drugs slow the production of all cells in the bone marrow.

Corticosteroids
These drugs reduce the activity of both B- and T-lymphocytes.

Cyclosporin
This inhibits the activity of T-lymphocytes only, and not the activity of B-lymphocytes.

COMMON DRUGS

Anticancer drugs
Azathioprine ✳
Chlorambucil
Cyclophosphamide ✳
Methotrexate
Mycophlenolate mofetil

Other drugs
Cyclosporin ✳
Tacrolimus

Corticosteroids
(see p.141)

Antibodies
Anti-lymphocyte globulin
Basiliximab
Daclizumab

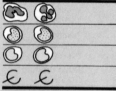

✳ See Part 4

DRUGS FOR HIV AND AIDS

The disease AIDS (acquired immune deficiency syndrome) is caused by infection with the human immunodeficiency virus (HIV). This virus invades certain cells of the immune system, particularly the white blood cells called T-helper lymphocytes, which normally activate other cells in the immune system to fight infection. Since HIV kills T-helper lymphocytes, the body cannot fight the virus or subsequent infections. Currently, it is not known whether all individuals who become infected with HIV will develop full-blown AIDS, which is defined by the occurrence of certain infections and/or cancers.

Why they are used

Drug treatments for HIV infection can be divided into the treatment of the initial infection with HIV, and the treatment of diseases that are associated with AIDS.

There are two groups of drugs which act directly against HIV. Both work by interfering with enzymes vital for virus replication. The first group, which inhibit an enzyme known as the reverse transcriptase enzyme, are divided according to their chemical structure into nucleoside and non-nucleoside inhibitors. The second group interfere with an enzyme called protease.

These drugs are much more effective when used in combination. Treatment is now usually started with a combination of two nucleoside transcriptase inhibitors plus a non-nucleoside drug or a protease inhibitor. If this so-called "triple therapy" is started before damage to the immune system is too great, it can dramatically reduce the levels of HIV virus in the body and improve the outlook for HIV-infected patients, though it is not a cure for the disease and patients remain infectious.

The mainstay of drug treatment for AIDS-related diseases are the antimicrobial drugs for the bacterial, viral, fungal, and protozoal infections to which people with AIDS are susceptible. These drugs include the antituberculous drugs (p.132), co-trimoxazole for the treatment of pneumocystis carinii pneumonia (PCP), and ganciclovir for the treatment of CMV (cytomegalovirus) infection.

COMMON DRUGS

Nucleoside reverse transcriptase inhibitors	Non-nucleoside transcriptase inhibitors
Didanosine ✱	Efavirenz
Lamivudine ✱	Nevirapine
Stavudine	
Zalcitabine ✱	**Protease inhibitors**
Zidovudine (AZT) ✱	Indinavir
	Nelfinavir
	Ritonavir
	Saquinavir

✱ See Part 4

HIV INFECTION AND POSSIBLE TREATMENTS

The illustrations below show how the human immunodeficiency virus (HIV) enters body cells and, once inside, replicates itself to produce new viruses. The action of already existing drugs, along with the possible action of future drugs is also shown.

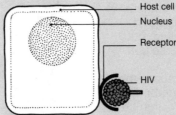
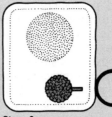

Stage 1
The virus binds to a specialized site (receptor) on a body cell.

Possible drug intervention
Binding could be blocked by giving specific antibodies that themselves bind to the virus or cell receptor.

Stage 2
The virus enters the cell.

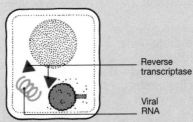
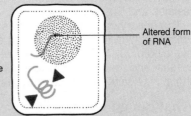

Stage 3
The virus loses its protective coat and releases RNA, its genetic material, and an enzyme known as reverse transcriptase.

Possible drug intervention
Drugs may be developed to prevent the virus losing its protective coat. Amantadine has this effect on the influenza A virus but not on HIV.

Stage 4
The enzyme reverse transcriptase converts viral RNA into a form that can enter the host cell's nucleus and may become integrated with the cell's genetic material.

Drug intervention
Zidovudine and other related drugs, such as didanosine and zalcitabine, inhibit the action of reverse transcriptase.

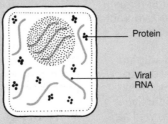
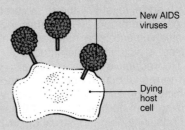

Stage 5
The host cell starts to produce new viral RNA and protein from the viral material that has been incorporated into its nucleus.

Drug intervention
Protease inhibitor drugs such as nelfinavir, ritonavir, and saquinavir act by preventing the production of viral proteins.

Stage 6
The new viral RNA and proteins assemble to produce new viruses. These leave the host cell (which then dies) and are free to attack other cells in the body.

Drug intervention
The new protease inhibitors prevent formation of viral proteins and viral assembly. Alpha interferon inhibits virus release from the cell.

REPRODUCTIVE & URINARY TRACTS

The reproductive systems of men and women consist of those organs that produce and release sperm (male), or store and release eggs, and then nurture a fertilized egg until it develops into a baby (female).

The urinary system filters wastes and water from the blood, producing urine, which is then expelled from the body. The reproductive and urinary systems of men are partially linked, but those of women form two physically close but functionally separate systems.

The female reproductive organs comprise the ovaries, fallopian tubes, and uterus (womb). The uterus opens via the cervix (neck of the uterus) into the vagina. The principal male reproductive organs are the two sperm-producing glands, the testes (testicles), which lie within the scrotum, and the penis. Other structures of the male reproductive tract include the prostate gland and several tubular structures – the tightly coiled epididymides, the vas deferens, the seminal vesicles and the urethra (see right).

The urinary organs in both sexes comprise the kidneys, which filter the blood and excrete urine (see also p.99), the ureters down which urine passes, and the bladder, where urine is stored until it is released from the body via the urethra.

What can go wrong
The reproductive and urinary tracts are both subject to infection. Such infections (apart from those transmitted by sexual activity) are relatively uncommon in men because the long male urethra prevents bacteria and other organisms passing easily to the bladder and upper urinary tract, and to the male sex organs. The shorter female urethra allows urinary tract infections, especially of the bladder (cystitis) and of the urethra (urethritis), to occur commonly. The female reproductive tract is also vulnerable to infection, which, in some cases, is sexually transmitted.

Reproductive function may also be disrupted by hormonal disturbances that lead to reduced fertility. Women may be troubled by symptoms arising from normal activity of the reproductive organs, including menstrual disorders as well as problems associated with childbirth.

The most common urinary problems apart from infection are those related to bladder function. Urine may be released involuntarily (incontinence) or it may be retained in the bladder. Such disorders are usually the result of abnormal nerve signals to the bladder or sphincter muscle. The filtering action of the kidneys may be affected by alteration

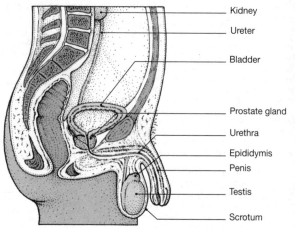

Male reproductive system
Sperm produced in each testis pass into the epididymis, a tightly coiled tube in which the sperm mature before passing along the vas deferens to the seminal vesicle. Sperm are stored in the seminal vesicle until they are ejaculated from the penis via the urethra, together with seminal fluid and secretions from the prostate gland.

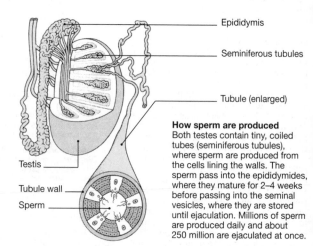

How sperm are produced
Both testes contain tiny, coiled tubes (seminiferous tubules), where sperm are produced from the cells lining the walls. The sperm pass into the epididymides, where they mature for 2–4 weeks before passing into the seminal vesicles, where they are stored until ejaculation. Millions of sperm are produced daily and about 250 million are ejaculated at once.

of the composition of the blood or the hormones that regulate urine production, or by damage (from infection or inflammation) to the filtering units themselves.

Why drugs are used
Antibiotic drugs (p.128) are used to eliminate both urinary and reproductive tract infections (including sexually transmitted infections). Certain infections of the vagina are caused by fungi or yeasts and require antifungal drugs (p.138).

Hormone drugs are used both to reduce fertility deliberately (oral contraceptives) and to increase fertility in certain conditions in which it has not been

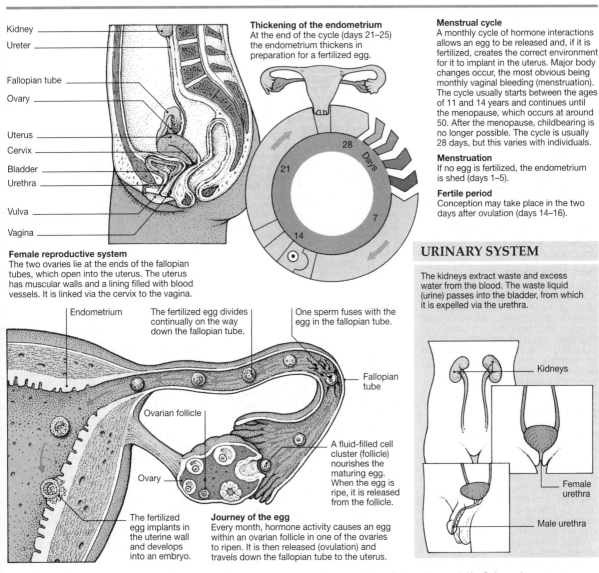

Female reproductive system
The two ovaries lie at the ends of the fallopian tubes, which open into the uterus. The uterus has muscular walls and a lining filled with blood vessels. It is linked via the cervix to the vagina.

Kidney
Ureter
Fallopian tube
Ovary
Uterus
Cervix
Bladder
Urethra
Vulva
Vagina

Thickening of the endometrium
At the end of the cycle (days 21–25) the endometrium thickens in preparation for a fertilized egg.

Menstrual cycle
A monthly cycle of hormone interactions allows an egg to be released and, if it is fertilized, creates the correct environment for it to implant in the uterus. Major body changes occur, the most obvious being monthly vaginal bleeding (menstruation). The cycle usually starts between the ages of 11 and 14 years and continues until the menopause, which occurs at around 50. After the menopause, childbearing is no longer possible. The cycle is usually 28 days, but this varies with individuals.

Menstruation
If no egg is fertilized, the endometrium is shed (days 1–5).

Fertile period
Conception may take place in the two days after ovulation (days 14–16).

Endometrium
The fertilized egg divides continually on the way down the fallopian tube.
One sperm fuses with the egg in the fallopian tube.
Fallopian tube
Ovarian follicle
A fluid-filled cell cluster (follicle) nourishes the maturing egg. When the egg is ripe, it is released from the follicle.
Ovary
The fertilized egg implants in the uterine wall and develops into an embryo.

Journey of the egg
Every month, hormone activity causes an egg within an ovarian follicle in one of the ovaries to ripen. It is then released (ovulation) and travels down the fallopian tube to the uterus.

URINARY SYSTEM

The kidneys extract waste and excess water from the blood. The waste liquid (urine) passes into the bladder, from which it is expelled via the urethra.

Kidneys
Female urethra
Male urethra

possible for a couple to conceive. Hormones may also be used to regulate menstruation when it is irregular or excessively painful or heavy. Analgesic drugs (p.80) are used to treat menstrual period pain and are also widely used for pain relief in labour. Other drugs used in labour include those that increase contraction of the muscles of the uterus and those that limit blood loss after the birth. Drugs may also be employed to halt premature labour.

Drugs that alter the transmission of nerve signals to the bladder muscles have an important role in the treatment of urinary incontinence and retention. Drugs that increase the kidneys' filtering action are commonly used to reduce blood pressure and fluid

retention (see Diuretics, p.99). Other drugs may alter the composition of the urine – for example, the uricosuric drugs that are used in the treatment of gout (p.119) increase the amount of uric acid.

MAJOR DRUG GROUPS

Drugs used to treat menstrual disorders
Oral contraceptives
Drugs for infertility
Drugs used in labour
Drugs used for urinary disorders

DRUGS USED TO TREAT MENSTRUAL DISORDERS

The menstrual cycle results from the actions of female sex hormones that cause ovulation (the release of an egg) and thickening of the endometrium (the lining of the uterus) each month in preparation for pregnancy. Unless the egg is fertilized, the endometrium will be shed about two weeks later during menstruation (see also p.158).

The main problems associated with menstruation that may require medical treatment are excessive blood loss (menorrhagia), pain during menstruation (dysmenorrhoea), and distressing physical and psychological symptoms occurring prior to menstruation (premenstrual syndrome). The absence of periods (amenorrhoea) is discussed under female sex hormones (p.147).

The drugs most commonly used to treat the menstrual disorders described above include oestrogens, progestogens, danazol, and analgesics.

Why they are used

Drug treatment for menstrual disorders is undertaken only when the doctor has ruled out the possibility of an underlying gynaecological disorder, such as a pelvic infection or fibroids. In some cases, especially in women over the age of 35, a D and C (dilatation and curettage) may be recommended. When no underlying reason for the problem is found, drug treatment aimed primarily at the relief of symptoms is usually prescribed.

Dysmenorrhoea

Painful menstrual periods are usually treated initially with a simple analgesic (see p.80). Non-steroidal anti-inflammatory drugs (NSAIDs; see p.116), are often most effective because they counter the effects of prostaglandins, chemicals that are partly responsible for transmission of pain to the brain. Diclofenac and mefenamic acid are also used to reduce the excessive blood loss of menorrhagia (see below).

When these drugs are not sufficient to provide adequate pain relief, hormonal drug treatment may be recommended. If contraception is also required, treatment may involve an oral contraceptive pill containing both an oestrogen and a progestogen, or a progestogen alone. However, non-contraceptive progestogen preparations may also be prescribed. These are usually taken for only a few days during each month. The treatment of dysmenorrhoea caused by endometriosis is described in the box above right.

Menorrhagia

Excessive blood loss during menstruation can sometimes be reduced by some NSAIDs. Tranexamic acid, an antifibrinolytic drug, is an effective treatment for menorrhagia. Alternatively, danazol, a drug that reduces production

ENDOMETRIOSIS

Endometriosis is a condition in which fragments of endometrial tissue (uterine lining) occur outside the uterus in the pelvic cavity. This disorder causes severe pain during menstruation, often causes pain during intercourse, and may sometimes lead to infertility.

Drugs used for this disorder are similar to those prescribed for heavy periods (menorrhagia). However, in this case the intention is to suppress endometrial development for an extended period so that the abnormal tissue eventually withers away. Progesterone supplements that suppress endometrial thickening may be prescribed throughout the menstrual cycle. Alternatively, danazol, which suppresses endometrial development by reducing oestrogen production, may be prescribed. Any drug treatment usually needs to be continued for a minimum of six months.

When drug treatment is unsuccessful, surgical removal of the abnormal tissue is usually necessary.

Sites of endometriosis

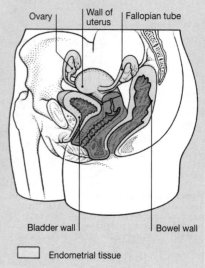

Ovary | Wall of uterus | Fallopian tube

Bladder wall | Bowel wall

☐ Endometrial tissue

of the female sex hormone oestrogen, may be prescribed to reduce blood loss.

Premenstrual syndrome

This is a collection of psychological and physical symptoms that affect many women to some degree in the days before menstruation. Psychological symptoms include mood changes such as increased irritability, depression, and anxiety. Principal physical symptoms are bloating, headache, and breast tenderness. Because some doctors believe that premenstrual syndrome is the result of a drop in progesterone levels in the last half of the menstrual cycle, non-contraceptive supplements of this hormone may be given in the week or so before menstruation. Oral contraceptives may be considered as an alternative. Other drugs sometimes used include pyridoxine (vitamin B$_6$), diuretics (p.99) if bloating due to fluid retention is a problem, and bromocriptine when breast tenderness is the major symptom. Anti-anxiety drugs (p.83) may be prescribed in rare cases where severe premenstrual psychological disturbance is experienced.

How they work

Drugs used in menstrual disorders act in a variety of ways. Hormonal treatments are aimed at suppressing the pattern of hormonal changes that is causing troublesome symptoms. Contraceptive preparations override the woman's normal menstrual cycle. Ovulation does not occur, and the endometrium does not

thicken normally. Bleeding that occurs at the end of a cycle is less likely to be abnormally heavy, to be accompanied by severe discomfort, or to be preceded by distressing symptoms. For further information on oral contraceptives, see facing page.

Non-contraceptive progestogen preparations taken in the days before menstruation do not suppress ovulation. Increased progesterone during this time reduces premenstrual symptoms and prevents excessive thickening of the endometrium.

Danazol, a potent drug, prevents the thickening of the endometrium, thereby correcting excessively heavy periods. Blood loss is reduced, and in some cases menstruation ceases altogether during treatment.

COMMON DRUGS

Oestrogens and progestogens (see p.147)	**Diuretics** (see p.99)
NSAID analgesics	**Other drugs**
Aspirin ✳	Bromocriptine ✳
Diclofenac ✳	Buserelin
Diflunisal	Danazol ✳
Flurbiprofen	Gestrinone
Ibuprofen ✳	Goserelin ✳
Ketoprofen ✳	Leuprorelin
Mefenamic acid ✳	Nafarelin
Naproxen ✳	Pyridoxine ✳
	Tranexamic Acid

✳ See Part 4

ORAL CONTRACEPTIVES

There are many different methods of ensuring that conception and pregnancy do not follow sexual intercourse, but for most women the oral contraceptive is the most effective method (see Comparison of reliability of different methods of contraception, right). It has the added advantage of being convenient and unobtrusive during lovemaking. About 25 per cent of the women who seek contraceptive protection in Britain choose a form of oral contraceptive.

There are three main types of oral contraceptive: the combined pill, the progestogen-only pill, and the phased pill. All three types contain a progestogen (a synthetic form of the female sex hormone, progesterone). Both the combined and phased pills also contain a natural or synthetic oestrogen (see also Female sex hormones, p.147).

COMPARISON OF RELIABILITY OF DIFFERENT METHODS OF CONTRACEPTION

The table indicates the number of pregnancies that occur with each method of contraception among 100 women using that method in a year. The wide variation that occurs with some methods takes into account pregnancies that occur as a result of incorrect use of the method.

Method	Pregnancies*
Combined and phased pills	2–3
Progestogen-only pill	2.5–10
IUD (Intrauterine device)	4–9
Condom	3–4
Diaphragm	10–20
Rhythm	25–30
Contraceptive sponge	9–27
Vaginal spermicide alone	2–30
Norethisterone implant	Less than 1
No contraception	80–85
"Morning after" pill	20–25

* Per 100 users per year.

Why they are used

The combined pill

The combined pill is the most widely prescribed form of oral contraceptive and has the lowest failure rate in terms of unwanted pregnancies. It is referred to as the "pill" and is the type thought most suitable for young women who want to use a hormonal form of contraception. The combined pill is particularly suitable for those women who regularly experience exceptionally painful, heavy, or prolonged periods (see Drugs used to treat menstrual disorders, facing page).

There are many different products available containing a fixed dose of an oestrogen and a progestogen drug. They are generally divided into three groups according to their oestrogen content (see Hormone content of common oral contraceptives, below). Low-dose products are chosen when possible to minimize the risk of adverse effects.

Progestogen-only pill

The progestogen-only pill is often recommended for those women who react adversely to the oestrogen in the combined pill or for whom the combined pill is not considered suitable because of their age or medical history (see Risks and special precautions, p.163). It is also prescribed for women who are breast-feeding since it does not reduce milk production. The progestogen pill has a higher failure rate than the combined pill and must be taken at precisely the same time each day for maximum contraceptive effect.

Phased pills

The newest form of oral contraceptive is a pack of pills divided into two or three groups or phases. Each phase contains a different proportion of an oestrogen and a progestogen. The aim is to provide a hormonal balance that closely resembles the fluctuations of a normal menstrual cycle. Phased pills provide effective protection for many women who suffer side effects from other available forms of oral contraceptive.

How they work

In a normal menstrual cycle, the ripening and release of an egg and the preparation of the uterus for implantation of the fertilized egg are the result of a complex interplay between the natural female sex hormones, oestrogen and progesterone, and the pituitary hormones, follicle-stimulating hormone (FSH) and luteinizing hormone (LH) (see also p.147). The oestrogen and progestogens contained in oral contraceptives disrupt the normal menstrual cycle in such a way that conception is less likely.

With combined and phased pills, the increased levels of oestrogen and progesterone produce similar effects to the hormonal changes of pregnancy. The actions of the hormones inhibit the production of FSH and LH, thereby preventing the egg from ripening in the ovary and from being released.

The progestogen-only pill has a slightly different effect. It does not always prevent release of an egg; its main contraceptive action may be on the mucus that lines the cervix, which thickens so sperm cannot cross it. This effect occurs to some extent with combined pills and phased pills.

How they affect you

Each course of combined and phased pills lasts for 21 days, followed by a pill-free seven days, during which time

HORMONE CONTENT OF COMMON ORAL CONTRACEPTIVES

The oestrogen-containing forms are classified according to oestrogen content as follows: Low: 20 micrograms; standard: 30–35 micrograms; high: 50 micrograms; phased pills: 30–40 micrograms; morning after: 100 micrograms dose.

Type of pill (oestrogen content)	Brand names
Combined (20mcg)	Loestrin 20, Mercilon
(30–35mcg)	Binovum, Brevinor, Cilest, Eugynon 30, Femodene, Femodene ED, Loestrin 30, Norimin, Marvelon, Microgynon 30, Microgynon 30 ED Minulet, Ovran 30, Ovranette, Ovysmen,
(50mcg)	Norinyl-1, Ovran.
Phased (30–40mcg)	Logynon, Logynon ED, Synphase, Triadene, Tri-Minulet, Trinordiol, TriNovum.
Progestogen-only (no oestrogen)	Femulen, Micronor, Microval, Neogest, Norgeston, Noriday.
Post-coital (morning after) (50mcg x 2)	Schering PC4

ORAL CONTRACEPTIVES continued

BALANCING THE RISKS AND BENEFITS OF ORAL CONTRACEPTIVES

Oral contraceptives are safe for the vast majority of young women. However, every woman who is considering oral contraception should discuss with her doctor the risks and possible adverse effects of the drugs before deciding that a hormonal method is the most suitable in her case. A variety of factors must be taken into account, including the woman's age, her own medical history and that of her close relatives, and factors such as whether she is a smoker. The importance of such factors varies depending on the type of contraceptive. The table below gives the main advantages and disadvantages of oestrogen-containing and progestogen-only pills.

Type of oral contraceptive	Oestrogen-containing combined and phased	Progestogen-only

Advantages	● Very reliable
	● Convenient/unobtrusive
	● Regularizes menstruation
	● Reduced menstrual pain and blood loss
	● Reduced risk of:
	  ▼ benign breast disease
	  ▼ endometriosis
	  ▼ ectopic pregnancy
	  ▼ ovarian cysts
	  ▼ pelvic infection
	  ▼ ovarian and endometrial cancer
		● Reasonably reliable
		● Convenient/unobtrusive
		● Suitable during breast-feeding
		● Avoids oestrogen-related side effects and risks
		● Allows rapid return to fertility

Side effects	● Weight gain ● Depression ● Breast swelling ● Reduced sex drive ● Headaches ● Increased vaginal discharge ● Nausea	● Irregular menstruation
Risks	● Thrombosis/embolism ● Heart disease ● High blood pressure ● Jaundice ● Cancer of the liver (rare) ● Gallstones	● Ectopic pregnancy ● Ovarian cysts
Factors that may prohibit use	● Previous thrombosis* ● Heart disease ● High levels of lipid in blood ● Liver disease ● Blood disorders ● High blood pressure ● Unexplained vaginal bleeding ● Migraine ● Otosclerosis ● Presence of several risk factors (below)	● Previous ectopic pregnancy ● Heart or circulatory disease ● Unexplained vaginal bleeding
Factors that increase risks	● Smoking* ● Obesity* ● Increasing age ● Diabetes mellitus ● Family history of heart or circulatory disease* ● Current treatment with other drugs	● As for oestrogen-containing pills, but to a lesser degree

*Products containing desogestrel or gestodene have a higher excess risk with these factors than other progestogens.

How to minimize your health risks while taking the pill

▼ Give up smoking.
▼ Maintain a healthy weight and diet.
▼ Have regular blood pressure and blood lipid checks.
▼ Have regular cervical smear tests.

▼ Remind your doctor that you are taking oral contraceptives before taking other prescription drugs.
▼ Stop taking oestrogen-containing oral contraceptives four weeks before planned major surgery (use alternative contraception).

menstruation occurs. Some brands contain seven additional inactive pills. With these, the new course directly follows the last so that the habit of taking the pill daily is not broken. Progestogen-only pills are taken for 28 days each month. Menstruation usually occurs during the last few days of the menstrual cycle.

Women taking oral contraceptives, especially drugs that contain oestrogen, usually find that their menstrual periods are lighter and relatively pain-free. Some women cease to menstruate altogether. This is not a cause for concern in itself, provided no pills have been missed, but it may make it difficult to determine if pregnancy has occurred. An apparently missed period probably indicates a light one, rather than pregnancy. However, if you have missed two consecutive periods and you feel that you may be pregnant, it is advisable to have a pregnancy test.

All forms of oral contraceptive may cause spotting of blood in mid-cycle ("breakthrough bleeding"), especially at first, but this can be a particular problem of the progestogen-only pill.

Oral contraceptives that contain oestrogen may produce any of a large number of mild side effects depending on the dose. Symptoms similar to those experienced early in pregnancy may occur, particularly in the first few months of pill use: some women complain of nausea and vomiting, weight gain, depression, altered libido, increased appetite, and cramps in the legs and abdomen. The pill may also affect the circulation, producing minor headaches

and dizziness. All these effects usually disappear within a few months, but if they persist, it may be advisable to change to a brand containing a lower dose of oestrogen or to some other contraceptive method.

Risks and special precautions

All oral contraceptives need to be taken regularly for maximum protection against pregnancy. Contraceptive protection can be reduced by missing a pill (see What to do if you miss a pill, below). It may also be reduced by vomiting or diarrhoea. If you suffer from either of these symptoms, it is advisable to act as if you had missed your last pill. Many drugs may also affect the action of oral contraceptives and it is essential to tell your doctor that you are taking oral contraceptives, before taking additional prescribed medications.

Oral contraceptives, particularly those containing an oestrogen, have been found to carry a number of risks. These are summarized in the box on the facing page. One of the most serious potential adverse effects of oestrogen-containing pills is development of a thrombus (blood clot) in a vein or artery. The thrombus may travel to the lungs or cause a stroke or heart attack. The risk of thrombus-formation increases with age and other factors, notably obesity, high blood pressure, and smoking. Doctors assess these risk factors for each person when prescribing oral contraceptives. A woman who is over 35 may be advised against taking a combined pill, especially if she

POSTCOITAL CONTRACEPTION

Pregnancy following intercourse without contraception may be avoided by taking a short course of postcoital ("morning after") pills. The preparations used for this purpose usually contain an oestrogen and a progestogen and are usually taken in two doses 12 hours apart, within 72 hours following intercourse. These drugs postpone ovulation and act on the lining of the uterus to prevent implantation of the egg. However, the high doses required make them unsuitable for regular use. This method has a higher failure rate than the usual oral contraceptives.

smokes or has an underlying medical condition such as diabetes mellitus. Concerns have been expressed about contraceptive pills containing the progestogens gestodene or desogestrel because several studies have found that these preparations carry a higher risk of thrombus formation than those containing other progestogens. The Committee on the Safety of Medicines has advised that these preparations should be used only by those women who are intolerant of other contraceptive pills and are aware of the higher risk. The drugs that contain desogestrel include Marvelon and Mercilon, while those that contain gestodene include Femodene, Femodene ED, Minulet, Triadene, and Tri-Minulet.

High blood pressure is a possible complication of oral contraceptives for some women. Measurement of blood pressure before the pill is prescribed and every six months after the woman starts taking oral contraceptives is advised for all women taking oral contraceptives.

Some very rare liver cancers have occurred in pill-users, and breast cancer may be slightly more common, but cancers of the ovaries and uterus are less common.

Although there is no evidence that oral contraceptives reduce a woman's fertility or that they damage the babies conceived after they are discontinued, doctors recommend that you wait for at least one normal menstrual period before you attempt to become pregnant.

WHAT TO DO IF YOU MISS A PILL

Contraceptive protection may be reduced if blood levels of the hormones in the body fall as a result of missing a pill. It is particularly important to ensure that the progestogen-only pills are taken punctually. If you miss a pill, the action you should take depends on the degree of lateness and the type of pill being used (see below).

	Combined and phased pills	Progestogen-only pills
3–12 hours late	Take the missed pill now. No additional precautions necessary.	Take the missed pill now. Take additional precautions for the next 7 days.
Over 12 hours late	Take the missed pill now and take the next pill on time (even if on the same day). If more than one pill has been missed, take the latest missed pill now and the next on time. Take additional precautions for the next 7 days. If the 7 days extends into the pill-free (or inactive pill) period, start the next packet without a break (or without taking inactive pills).	Take the missed pill now, and take the next on time. Take additional precautions for the next 7 days.

COMMON DRUGS

Progestogens	Oestrogens
Desogestrel	Ethinyloestradiol *
Gestodene	Mestranol
Levonorgestrel *	
Norethisterone *	
Norgestimate	

* See Part 4

DRUGS FOR INFERTILITY

Conception and the establishment of pregnancy require a healthy reproductive system in both partners. The man must be able to produce sufficient numbers of healthy sperm; the woman must be able to produce a healthy egg that is able to pass freely down the fallopian tube to the uterus. The lining of the uterus must be in a condition that allows the implantation of the fertilized egg.

The cause of infertility may sometimes remain undiscovered, but in the majority of cases it is due to one of the following factors: intercourse taking place at the wrong time during the menstrual cycle; the man producing too few or unhealthy sperm; the woman either failing to ovulate (release an egg) or having blocked fallopian tubes perhaps as a result of previous pelvic infection. Alternatively, production of gonadotrophin hormones – follicle-stimulating hormone (FSH) and luteinizing hormone (LH) – needed for ovulation and implantation of the egg may be affected by illness or psychological stress.

If no simple explanation can be found, the man's semen will be analyzed. If these tests show that abnormally low numbers of sperm are being produced, or if a large proportion of the sperm produced are unhealthy, drug treatment may be tried.

If no abnormality of sperm production is discovered, the woman will be given a thorough medical examination. Ovulation is monitored and blood tests may be performed to assess hormone levels. If ovulation does not occur, the woman may be offered drug treatment.

Why they are used

In men, low sperm production may be treated with gonadotrophins (FSH or HCG) or a pituitary-stimulating drug (for example, clomifene) and unhealthy sperm may be controlled with corticosteroids.

In women, drugs are useful in helping to achieve pregnancy only when a hormone defect inhibiting ovulation has been diagnosed. Treatment may continue for months and does not always produce a pregnancy. Women in whom the pituitary gland produces some FSH and

ACTION OF FERTILITY DRUGS

Ovulation (release of an egg) and implantation are governed by hormones that are produced by the pituitary gland. FSH stimulates ripening of the egg follicle. LH triggers ovulation and ensures that progesterone is produced to prepare the uterus for the implantation of the egg. Drugs for female infertility boost the actions of these hormones.

FSH and HCG FSH adds to the action of the natural FSH early in the menstrual cycle. HCG mimics the action of natural LH at mid-cycle.

Clomifene Normally, oestrogen suppresses the output of FSH and LH by the pituitary gland. Clomifene opposes the action of oestrogen so that FSH and LH continue to be produced.

Comparison of normal hormone fluctuation and timing of drug treatment

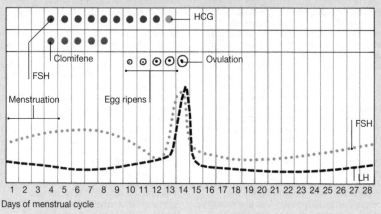

Days of menstrual cycle

LH may be given courses of clomifene for several days during each month. Usually, up to three courses may be tried. An effective dose produces ovulation five to ten days after the last tablet is taken.

Clomifene may thicken the cervical mucus, impeding the passage of sperm but the advantage of achieving ovulation outweighs the risk of this side effect. If treatment with clomifene fails to produce ovulation, or if a disorder of the pituitary gland prevents the production of FSH and LH, treatment with FSH and human chorionic gonadotrophin (HCG) may be given. FSH is given during the second week of the menstrual cycle, followed by an injection of HCG.

How they work

Fertility drugs raise the chance of ovulation by boosting levels of LH and FSH. Clomifene stimulates the pituitary gland to increase its output of these hormones. Artificially produced FSH and HCG mimic the action of naturally produced FSH and LH respectively. Both treatments, when successful, stimulate ovulation and implantation of the fertilized egg.

How they affect you

Clomifene may produce hot flushes, nausea, headaches, and, rarely, ovarian cysts and visual disturbance, while HCG can cause tiredness, headaches, and mood changes. FSH can cause the ovaries to enlarge, producing abdominal discomfort. These drugs increase the likelihood of multiple births, usually twins.

DRUGS FOR IMPOTENCE

Impotence is a common male disorder and is defined as the inability to achieve or maintain an erection. The penis contains three cylinders of erectile tissue, the corpora cavernosa and the corpus spongiosum. Normally, when a man is sexually aroused, the arteries in the penis relax and widen, allowing more blood than usual to flow into the organ, filling the corpora cavernosa and the corpus spongiosum. As these tissues expand and harden, the veins that carry blood out of the penis become compressed, reducing outflow and resulting in an erection. In some forms of

impotence, this does not happen. Drugs can then be used that will increase the blood flow into the penis to produce an erection.

Sildenafil (p.401) not only increases the blood flow into the penis but also prevents the muscle wall from relaxing, so the blood does not drain out of the blood vessels and the penis remains erect.

Alprostadil (p.190) is a prostaglandin drug that helps men achieve an erection by widening the blood vessels, but it must be injected directly into the penis, or applied into the urethra using a special syringe.

COMMON DRUGS

Chorionic
    gonadotrophin
    (HCG) *
Clomifene *
Follicle-stimulating
    hormone (FSH)
Follitropin
Goserelin

Luteinizing
    hormone (LH)
Menotrophin
Menopausal
    gonadotrophins
Tamoxifen *
Urofollitropin

**Drugs for
impotence**
Alprostadil *
Sildenafil *

* See Part 4

DRUGS USED IN LABOUR

Normal labour has three stages. In the first stage, the uterus begins to contract, initially irregularly and then gradually more regularly and powerfully, while the cervix dilates until it is fully stretched. During the second stage, powerful contractions of the uterus push the baby down the mother's birth canal and out of her body. The third stage involves the delivery of the placenta.

Drugs may be required during one or more stages of labour for any of the following reasons: to induce or augment labour; to delay premature labour (see Uterine muscle relaxants, below right); and to relieve pain. The administration of some drugs may be viewed as part of normal obstetric care; for example, the uterine stimulant ergometrine may be injected routinely before the third stage of labour. Other drugs are administered only when the condition of the mother or baby requires intervention. The possible adverse effects of the drug on both mother and baby are always carefully balanced against the benefits.

Drugs to induce or augment labour

Induction of labour may be advised when a doctor considers it risky for the health of the mother or baby for the pregnancy to continue – for example, if natural labour does not occur within two weeks of the due date or when a woman has pre-eclampsia. Other common reasons for inducing labour include premature rupture of the membrane surrounding the baby (breaking of the waters), slow growth of the baby due to poor nourishment by the placenta, or death of the fetus in the uterus.

When labour needs to be induced, oxytocin, a uterine stimulant, may be administered intravenously. Alternatively, a prostaglandin pessary may be given to soften and dilate the cervix. If these methods are ineffective or cannot be used because of potential adverse effects (see Risks and special precautions, above right), a caesarean delivery may have to be performed.

DRUGS USED TO TERMINATE PREGNANCY

Drugs may be used in a hospital or clinic to terminate pregnancy up to 20 weeks, or to empty the uterus after the death of the baby. Before the 14th week of pregnancy, a prostaglandin may be given as a vaginal pessary to dilate the cervix before removing the fetus under general anaesthetic.

After the 14th week, labour is induced by a prostaglandin drug in a vaginal pessary, injected into the uterus, or via a catheter placed through the cervix. These methods may be supplemented by oxytocin given by intravenous drip (see Drugs to induce or augment labour, above).

Oxytocin may also be used to strengthen the force of contractions in labour that has started spontaneously but has not continued normally.

A combination of oxytocin and another uterine stimulant, ergometrine, is given to most women as the baby is being born or immediately following birth to prevent excessive bleeding after the delivery of the placenta. This combination encourages the uterus to contract after delivery, which restricts the flow of blood.

Risks and special precautions
When oxytocin is used to induce labour, the dosage is carefully monitored throughout to prevent the possibility of excessively violent contractions. It is administered to women who have had surgery of the uterus only with careful monitoring. The drug is not known to affect the baby adversely. Ergometrine is not given to women who have suffered from high blood pressure during the course of pregnancy.

Drugs used for pain relief
Opioid analgesics
Pethidine, morphine, or other opioids may be given once active labour has been established (see Analgesics, p.80). Possible side effects for the mother include drowsiness, nausea, and vomiting. Opioid drugs may cause breathing difficulties for the new baby, but these problems may be reversed by the antidote naloxone.

Epidural anaesthesia
This provides pain relief during labour and birth by numbing the nerves leading to the uterus and pelvic area. It is often used during a planned caesarean delivery, thus enabling the mother to be fully conscious for the birth.

An epidural involves the injection of a local anaesthetic drug (see p.80) into the epidural space between the spinal cord and the vertebrae. An epidural may block the mother's urge to push during the second stage, and a forceps delivery may be necessary. Headaches may occasionally occur following epidural anaesthesia.

Oxygen and nitrous oxide
These gases are combined to produce a mixture that reduces the pain caused by contractions. During the first and second stages of labour, gas is self-administered by inhalation through a mouthpiece or mask. If it is used over too long a period, it may produce nausea, confusion, and dehydration in the mother.

Local anaesthetics
These drugs are injected inside the vagina or near the vaginal opening and are used to numb sensation during forceps delivery, before an episiotomy (an incision

WHEN DRUGS ARE USED IN LABOUR

The drugs used in each stage of labour are described below.

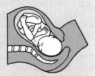

Before labour
Oxytocin
Prostaglandins

First stage
Epidural anaesthetics
Morphine
Oxytocin
Pethidine

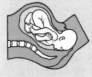

Second stage
Local anaesthetics
Nitrous oxide
Oxytocin

Third stage
Ergometrine
Oxytocin

made to enlarge the vaginal opening), and when stitches are necessary. Side effects are rare.

Uterine muscle relaxants
When contractions of the uterus start before the 34th week of pregnancy, doctors usually advise bed rest and may also administer a drug that relaxes the muscles of the uterus and thus halts labour. Initially, the drug is given in hospital by injection, but it may be continued orally at home. These drugs work by stimulating the sympathetic nervous system (see Autonomic nervous system, p.79) and may cause palpitations and anxiety in the mother. They have not been shown to have adverse effects on the baby.

COMMON DRUGS

Prostaglandins
Carboprost
Dinoprostone
Gemeprost

Pain relief
Entonox® (oxygen and nitrous oxide)

Opioids
Fentanyl
Morphine *
Pethidine

Uterine muscle relaxants
Ritodrine
Salbutamol *
Terbutaline *

Uterine stimulants
Ergometrine
Oxytocin

Local anaesthetics
Bupivacaine
Lignocaine

Sex hormones
Mifepristone

| * See Part 4 |

DRUGS USED FOR URINARY DISORDERS

Urine is produced by the kidneys and stored in the bladder. As the urine accumulates, the bladder walls stretch and pressure within the bladder increases. Eventually, the stretching stimulates nerve endings that produce the urge to urinate. The ring of muscle (sphincter) around the bladder neck normally keeps the bladder closed until it is consciously relaxed, allowing urine to pass via the urethra out of the body.

A number of disorders can affect the urinary tract. The most common of these disorders are infection in the bladder (cystitis) or the urethra (urethritis), and loss of reliable control over urination (urinary incontinence). A less common problem is inability to expel urine (urinary retention). Drugs used to treat these problems include antibiotics and antibacterial drugs, analgesics, drugs to increase the acidity of the urine, and drugs that act on nerve control over the muscles of the bladder and sphincter.

Drugs for urinary infection

Nearly all infections of the bladder are caused by bacteria. Symptoms include a continual urge to urinate, although often nothing is passed; pain on urinating; and lower abdominal pain.

Many antibiotic and antibacterial drugs are used to treat urinary tract infections. Among the most widely used – because of their effectiveness – are trimethoprim and amoxycillin (see Antibiotics, p.128, and Antibacterial drugs, p.131).

Measures are also sometimes taken to increase the acidity of the urine, thereby making it hostile to bacteria. Ascorbic acid (vitamin C) and acid fruit juices have this effect, although making the urine less

acidic with potassium or sodium citrate during an attack of cystitis helps to relieve the discomfort. Symptoms are commonly relieved within a few hours of the start of treatment.

For maximum effect, all drug treatments prescribed for urinary tract infections need to be accompanied by increased fluid intake.

Drugs for urinary incontinence

Urinary incontinence can occur for a several reasons. A weak sphincter muscle allows the involuntary passage of urine when abdominal pressure is raised by coughing or physical exertion. This is known as stress incontinence and commonly affects women who have had children. Urgency – the sudden need to urinate – stems from oversensitivity of the bladder muscle; small quantities of urine stimulate the urge to urinate frequently.

Incontinence can also occur due to loss of nerve control in neurological disorders such as multiple sclerosis. In children, inability to control urination at night (nocturnal enuresis) is also a form of urinary incontinence.

Drug treatment is not necessary or appropriate for all forms of incontinence. In stress incontinence, exercises to strengthen the pelvic floor muscles or surgery to tighten stretched ligaments may be effective. In urgency, regular emptying of the bladder can often avoid the need for medical intervention. Incontinence caused by loss of nerve control is unlikely to be helped by drug treatment. Frequency of urination in urgency may be reduced by *anticholinergic* and *antispasmodic* drugs. These reduce nerve signals from the

muscles in the bladder, allowing greater volumes of urine to accumulate without stimulating the urge to pass urine. Tricyclic antidepressants, such as imipramine, have a strong anticholinergic action, and have been prescribed for nocturnal enuresis in children, but many doctors believe the risk of overdosage is unacceptable. Desmopressin, a synthetic derivative of antidiuretic hormone (see p.145), is also used for nocturnal enuresis.

Drugs for urinary retention

Urinary retention is the inability to empty the bladder. This usually results from the failure of the bladder muscle to contract sufficiently to expel accumulated urine. Possible causes include an enlarged prostate gland or tumour, or a long-standing neurological disorder. Some drugs can cause urinary retention.

Most cases of urinary retention need to be relieved by inserting a tube (catheter) into the urethra. Surgery may be needed to prevent a recurrence of the problem. Drugs that relax the sphincter or stimulate bladder contraction are now rarely used in the treatment of urinary retention, but two types of drug are used in the long-term management of prostatic enlargement. Finasteride prevents production of male hormones that stimulate prostatic growth and alpha blockers, such as prazosin, indoramine, and terazosin, relax prostatic and urethral smooth muscle, thereby improving urine outflow. Long-term drug treatment can relieve symptoms and delay the need for surgery.

ACTION OF DRUGS ON URINATION

Normal bladder action

Urination occurs when the sphincter keeping the exit from the bladder into the urethra closed is consciously relaxed in response to signals from the bladder indicating that it is full. As the sphincter opens, the bladder wall contracts and urine is expelled.

Ureter

Openings of the ureters into bladder

Bladder wall

Urethra

Bladder

Sphincter muscle

How drugs act to improve bladder control

Anticholinergic drugs relax the bladder muscle by interfering with the passage of nerve impulses to the muscle.

Sympathomimetics act directly on the sphincter muscle, causing it to contract.

How drugs act to relieve urinary retention

Parasympathomimetics (cholinergics) stimulate contraction of the bladder wall.

Alpha blockers relax the muscle of the sphincter.

COMMON DRUGS

Antibiotics and antibacterials (see pp.128–131)

Anticholinergics
Flavoxate
Imipramine *
Oxybutynin *
Propiverine
Tolterodine *

Parasympatho-mimetic
Distigmine

Alpha blockers
Alfuzosin
Doxazosin *
Indoramin *
Prazosin
Tamsulosin *
Terazosin

Other drugs
Desmopressin *
Finasteride *
Potassium citrate
Vitamin C *
Dimethyl sulphoxide

* See Part 4

EYES AND EARS

The eyes and ears are the two sense organs that provide us with the most information about the world around us. The eye is the organ of vision that converts light images into nerve signals, which are transmitted to the brain for interpretation. The ear not only provides the means by which sound is detected and communicated to the brain, but it also contains the organ of balance that tells the brain about the position and movement of the body. It is divided into three parts – outer, middle, and inner ear.

What can go wrong

The most common eye and ear disorders are infection and inflammation (sometimes caused by allergy). Many parts of the eye may be affected, notably the conjunctiva (the membrane that covers the front of the eye and lines the eyelids) and the iris. The middle and outer ear are more commonly affected by infection than the inner ear.

The eye may also be damaged by glaucoma, a disorder in which pressure of fluid within the eye builds up and may eventually threaten vision. Eye problems such as retinopathy (disease of the retina) or cataracts (clouding of the lens) may occur as a result of diabetes or for other reasons, but both are now treatable. Disorders for which no drug treatment is appropriate are beyond the scope of this book.

Other disorders affecting the ear include build-up of wax (cerumen) in the outer ear canal and disturbances to the balance mechanism (see Vertigo and Ménière's disease, p.90).

Why drugs are used

Doctors usually prescribe antibiotics (see p.128) to clear ear and eye infections. These may be given by mouth or *topically*. Topical eye and ear preparations may contain a corticosteroid (p.141) to reduce inflammation. When inflammation has been caused by allergy, antihistamines (p.124) may also be taken. Decongestant drugs (p.93) are often prescribed to help clear the eustachian tube in middle ear infections.

Various drugs are used to reduce fluid pressure in glaucoma. These include diuretics (p.99), beta blockers (p.97), and *miotics* to narrow the pupil. In other cases, the pupil may need to be widened by *mydriatic* drugs.

MAJOR DRUG GROUPS

Drugs for glaucoma
Drugs affecting the pupil

Drugs for ear disorders

How the eye works

Light enters the eye through the cornea. The muscles of the iris control pupil size and thus the amount of light passing into the eye. In the eye, light hits the retina, which converts it to nerve signals that are carried by the optic nerve to the brain.

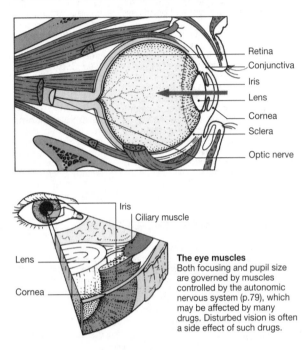

Retina
Conjunctiva
Iris
Lens
Cornea
Sclera
Optic nerve

Iris
Ciliary muscle

Lens

Cornea

The eye muscles
Both focusing and pupil size are governed by muscles controlled by the autonomic nervous system (p.79), which may be affected by many drugs. Disturbed vision is often a side effect of such drugs.

The ear

The outer ear canal is separated from the middle ear by the eardrum. Three bones in the middle ear connect it to the inner ear. This contains the cochlea (organ of hearing) and the labyrinth (organ of balance).

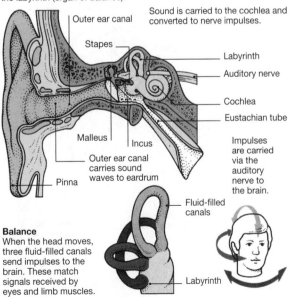

Outer ear canal

Sound is carried to the cochlea and converted to nerve impulses.

Stapes

Labyrinth
Auditory nerve

Cochlea
Eustachian tube

Malleus
Incus

Outer ear canal carries sound waves to eardrum

Pinna

Impulses are carried via the auditory nerve to the brain.

Fluid-filled canals

Balance
When the head moves, three fluid-filled canals send impulses to the brain. These match signals received by eyes and limb muscles.

Labyrinth

DRUGS FOR GLAUCOMA

Glaucoma is the name given to a group of conditions in which the pressure in the eye builds up to an abnormally high level. This compresses the blood vessels that supply the nerve connecting the eye to the brain (optic nerve) and may result in irreversible nerve damage and permanent loss of vision.

In the most common type of glaucoma, called chronic (or open-angle) glaucoma, reduced drainage of fluid from the eye causes pressure inside the eye to build up slowly. Progressive reduction in the peripheral field of vision may take months or years to be noticed. Acute (or closed-angle) glaucoma occurs when drainage of fluid is suddenly blocked by the iris. Fluid pressure usually builds up quite suddenly, blurring vision in the affected eye (see below). The eye becomes red and painful, accompanied by a headache and sometimes vomiting. The main attack is often preceded by milder warning attacks, such as seeing haloes around

lights in the previous weeks or months. Elderly, far-sighted people are particularly at risk of developing acute glaucoma. The angle may also narrow suddenly following injury or after taking certain drugs, for example, *anticholinergic* drugs. Closed-angle glaucoma may develop more slowly (chronic closed-angle glaucoma).

Drugs are used in the treatment of both types of glaucoma. These include miotics (see Drugs affecting the pupil, p.170) and beta blockers (p.97), as well as certain diuretics (carbonic anhydrase inhibitors and osmotics, p.99).

Why they are used

Chronic glaucoma
In this form of glaucoma, drugs are used to reduce pressure inside the eye. These drugs will prevent further deterioration of vision but cannot restore damage that has already been sustained, and therefore these drugs may be required lifelong. In most patients, treatment is begun with

eyedrops containing a beta blocker to reduce the production of fluid inside the eye. Miotic eyedrops to constrict the pupil and improve fluid drainage may be given. The prostaglandin, latanoprost, is also used to increase fluid outflow. If none of these drugs are effective, epinephrine, dipivefrine, or brimonidine may be tried to reduce secretion and help outflow. Sometimes a carbonic anhydrase inhibitor such as acetazolamide may be given by mouth to reduce fluid production. Laser treatment and surgery may also be used to improve fluid drainage from the eye.

Acute glaucoma
In acute glaucoma immediate medical treatment is required in order to prevent total loss of vision. Drugs are used initially to bring down the pressure within the eye. Laser treatment or surgery is then carried out to prevent a recurrence of the problem so that long-term drug treatment is seldom required.

WHAT HAPPENS IN GLAUCOMA

Normal eye
The ciliary body, situated at the root of the iris, continuously produces aqueous humour – a watery fluid that helps to maintain the normal shape of the eyeball. Aqueous humour drains via the angle between the cornea and iris through a mesh of fibres (the trabecular meshwork) into a channel in the sclera (white of the eye).

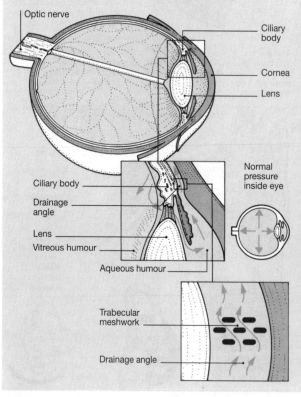

Optic nerve
Ciliary body
Cornea
Lens

Ciliary body
Drainage angle
Lens
Vitreous humour
Aqueous humour
Trabecular meshwork
Drainage angle

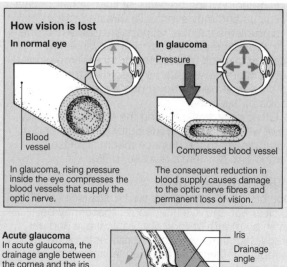

How vision is lost

In normal eye

In glaucoma
Pressure

Blood vessel

Compressed blood vessel

In glaucoma, rising pressure inside the eye compresses the blood vessels that supply the optic nerve.

The consequent reduction in blood supply causes damage to the optic nerve fibres and permanent loss of vision.

Normal pressure inside eye

Acute glaucoma
In acute glaucoma, the drainage angle between the cornea and the iris becomes completely closed, so the pressure inside the eye rises rapidly. This may cause permanent damage to the nerve fibres.

Iris
Drainage angle

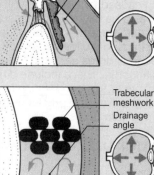

Chronic glaucoma
In chronic glaucoma, the trabecular meshwork through which the aqueous humour normally drains slowly closes off, so that fluid pressure builds up gradually and damages the optic nerve.

Trabecular meshwork
Drainage angle

Acetazolamide is often the first drug administered when the condition is diagnosed. This drug may be injected for rapid effect and thereafter administered by mouth. Frequent applications of eye drops containing pilocarpine or another miotic drug are given. An osmotic diuretic such as mannitol may be administered. This draws fluid out of all body tissues, including the eye, and reduces pressure within the eye.

How they work

The drugs used to treat glaucoma act in various ways to reduce the pressure of fluid in the eye. Miotics improve the drainage of the fluid out of the eye. In chronic glaucoma, this is achieved by increasing the outflow of aqueous humour through the drainage channel called the trabecular meshwork. In acute glaucoma, the pupil-constricting effect of miotics pulls the iris away from the drainage channel, allowing the aqueous humour to flow out normally. Latanoprost acts by improving drainage from the eye but has no miotic action. Beta blockers and carbonic anhydrase inhibitors act on the fluidproducing cells inside the eye to reduce the output of aqueous humour. Sympathomimetic drugs such as epinephrine, brimonidine, and apraclonidine are also thought to act partly in this way and partly by improving fluid drainage.

How they affect you

Drugs for acute glaucoma relieve pain and other symptoms within a few hours of their being used. The benefits of treatment in chronic glaucoma, however, may not be immediately apparent since treatment is only able to halt a further deterioration of vision.

People receiving miotic eye drops are likely to notice darkening of vision and difficulty seeing in the dark. Increased shortsightedness may be noticeable. Some miotics also cause irritation and redness of the eyes.

Beta blocker eye drops have few day-to-day side effects but carry risks for a few people (see right). Acetazolamide usually causes an increase in frequency of urination and thirst. Nausea and general malaise are also common.

ACTION OF DRUGS FOR GLAUCOMA

Miotics
These act on the circular muscle in the iris to reduce the size of the pupil. In acute glaucoma, this relieves any obstruction to the flow of aqueous humour by pulling the iris away from the cornea (right). In chronic glaucoma, miotic drugs act directly to increase the outflow of aqueous humour.

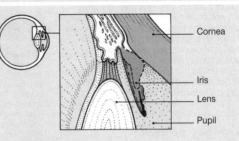

- Cornea
- Iris
- Lens
- Pupil

Beta blockers
The fluid-producing cells in the ciliary body are stimulated by signals passed through beta receptors. Beta blocking drugs prevent the transmission of signals through these receptors, thereby reducing the stimulus to produce fluid.

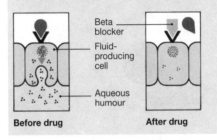

- Beta blocker
- Fluid-producing cell
- Aqueous humour

Before drug **After drug**

- Fluid-producing cell
- Carbonic anhydrase
- Drug

Carbonic anhydrase inhibitors
These block carbonic anhydrase, an *enzyme* involved in the production of aqueous humour in the ciliary body.

Risks and special precautions

Miotics can cause alteration in vision. Beta blockers are absorbed into the body and can affect the lungs, heart, and circulation. As a result, a cardioselective beta blocker, such as betaxolol, may be prescribed with caution to people with asthma or certain circulatory disorders and, in some cases, such drugs are withheld altogether. The amount of the drug absorbed into the body can be reduced by applying the eye drops carefully, as described (left). Acetazolamide may cause troublesome adverse effects, including painful tingling of the hands and feet, the formation of kidney stones, and, rarely, kidney damage. People with existing kidney problems are not usually given this drug.

APPLYING EYE DROPS IN GLAUCOMA

To reduce the amount of drug absorbed into the blood via the lacrimal (tear) duct, apply eye drops as described. This also improves the effectiveness of the drug.

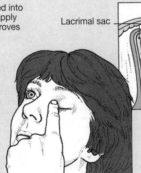

Lacrimal sac

Lacrimal duct

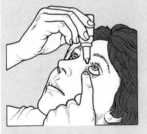

1 Press firmly on the lacrimal sac in the corner of the eye and apply the number of drops prescribed by your doctor.

2 Maintain pressure on the lacrimal sac for a few moments after applying the drops.

COMMON DRUGS

Miotics
Carbachol
Physostigmine
Pilocarpine *

Carbonic anhydrase inhibitors
Acetazolamide
Dorzolamide *

Other drugs
Latanoprost

Beta blockers
Betaxolol
Carteolol
Levobunolol
Metipranolol
Timolol *

Sympathomimetics
Apraclonidine
Brimonidine
Dipivefrine
Epinephrine *
Guanethidine

* See Part 4

DRUGS AFFECTING THE PUPIL

The pupil of the eye is the circular opening in the centre of the iris (the coloured part of the eye) through which light enters. It continually changes in size to adjust to variations in the intensity of light; in bright light it becomes quite small (constricts), but in dim light the pupil enlarges (dilates).

Eye drops containing drugs that act on the pupil are widely used by specialists. They are grouped into two categories: *mydriatics*, which dilate the pupil, and *miotics*, which constrict it.

Why they are used

Mydriatics are most often used to allow the doctor to view the inside of the eye – particularly the retina, the optic nerve head, and the blood vessels that supply the retina. Many of these drugs cause a temporary paralysis of the eye's focusing mechanism, a state called cycloplegia. Cycloplegia is sometimes induced to help determine the presence of any focusing errors, especially in babies and young children. By producing cycloplegia, it is possible to determine the precise optical prescription required for a small child, especially in the case of a squint.

Dilation of the pupil is part of the treatment for uveitis, an inflammatory disease of the iris and focusing muscle. In uveitis, the inflamed iris may stick to the lens, and thus cause severe damage to the eye. This complication can be prevented by early dilation of the pupil so that the iris is no longer in contact with the lens.

Constriction of the pupil with miotic drugs is often required in the treatment of glaucoma (see p.168). Miotics can also be used to restore the pupil to a normal size after dilation is induced by drugs.

How they work

The size of the pupil is controlled by two separate sets of muscles in the iris, the circular muscle and the radial muscle. The two sets of muscles are governed by separate branches of the autonomic nervous system (see p.79): the radial muscle is controlled by the sympathetic nervous system, and the circular muscle is controlled by the parasympathetic nervous system.

Individual mydriatic and miotic drugs affect different branches of the autonomic nervous system, and cause the pupil to dilate or to contract, depending on the type of drug used (see above).

How they affect you

Mydriatic drugs – especially the long-acting types – impair the ability to focus

ACTION OF DRUGS AFFECTING THE PUPIL

The muscles of the iris
Pupil size is controlled by the coordinated action of the circular and radial muscles in the iris. The circular muscle forms a ring around the pupil; when this muscle contracts, the pupil becomes smaller. The radial muscle is composed of fibres that run from the pupil to the base of the iris like the spokes of a wheel. Contraction of these fibres causes the pupil to become larger.

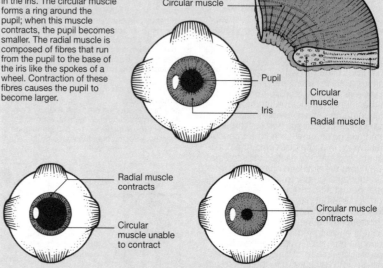

Section of iris
Circular muscle
Pupil
Iris
Circular muscle
Radial muscle

Radial muscle contracts
Circular muscle unable to contract

Circular muscle contracts

Mydriatics
Mydriatics enlarge the pupil in one of two ways. The *sympathomimetics* stimulate the radial muscle to contract. The *anticholinergics* prevent the circular muscle from contracting.

Miotics
Most miotics reduce the size of the pupil by stimulating the activity of the parasympathetic nervous system, which causes the circular muscle to contract.

the eye(s) for several hours after use. This interferes particularly with close activities such as reading. Bright light may cause discomfort. Miotics often interfere with night vision and may cause temporary short sight.

Normally, these eye drops produce few serious adverse effects. *Sympathomimetic* mydriatics may raise blood pressure and are used with caution in people with hypertension or heart disease. Miotics may irritate the eyes, but rarely cause generalized effects.

ARTIFICIAL TEAR PREPARATIONS

Tears are continually produced to keep the front of the eye covered with a thin moist film. This is essential for clear vision and for keeping the front of the eye free from dirt and other irritants. In some conditions, known collectively as dry eye syndromes (for example, Sjögren's syndrome), inadequate tear production may make the eyes feel dry and sore. Sore eyes can also occur in disorders where the eyelids do not close properly, causing the eye to become dry.

Why they are used
Since prolonged deficiency of natural tears can damage the cornea, regular application

of artificial tears in the form of eye drops is recommended for all of the conditions described above. Artificial tears may also be used to provide temporary relief from any feeling of discomfort and dryness in the eye caused by irritants, exposure to wind or sun, or following the initial wearing of contact lenses.

Although artificial tears are non-irritating, they often contain a preservative (for example, thimerosal or benzalkonium chloride) that may cause irritation. This risk of irritation is increased for wearers of soft contact lenses, who should ask their optician for advice before using any type of eye drops.

COMMON DRUGS

Sympathomimetic mydriatics
Epinephrine ✳
Phenylephrine

Miotics
Carbachol
Pilocarpine ✳
Tropicamide

Anticholinergic mydriatics
Atropine ✳
Cyclopentolate
Homatropine
Physostigmine

✳ See Part 4

DRUGS FOR EAR DISORDERS

Inflammation and infection of the outer and middle ear are the most common ear disorders that are treated with drugs. Drug treatment for Ménière's disease, a condition that affects the inner ear, is described under Vertigo and Ménière's disease, p.90.

The type of drug treatment given for ear inflammation depends on the cause of the trouble and the site affected.

Inflammation of the outer ear

Inflammation of the external ear canal (otitis externa) can be caused by eczema or by a bacterial or fungal infection. The risk of inflammation is increased by swimming in dirty water, accumulation of wax in the ear, or scratching or poking too frequently at the ear.

Symptoms vary, but in many cases there is itching, pain (which may be severe if there is a boil in the ear canal), tenderness, and possibly some loss of hearing. If the ear is infected there will probably be a discharge.

Drug treatment
A corticosteroid (see p.141) in the form of ear drops may be used to treat inflammation of the outer ear when there is no infection. Aluminium acetate solution, as drops or applied on a piece of gauze, may also be used. Relief is usually obtained within a day or two. Prolonged use of corticosteroids is not advisable because they may reduce the ear's resistance to infection.

If there is both inflammation and infection, your doctor may prescribe ear drops containing an antibiotic (see p.128) combined with a corticosteroid to relieve the inflammation. Usually, a combination of antibiotics is prescribed to make the treatment effective against a wide range of bacteria. Commonly used antibiotics include framycetin, neomycin, and polymyxin B. These antibiotics are not used if the eardrum is perforated. They

EAR WAX REMOVAL

Ear wax (cerumen) is a natural secretion from the outer ear canal that keeps it free from dust and skin debris. Occasionally, wax may build up in the outer ear canal and become hard, leading to irritation and/or hearing loss.

A number of over-the-counter remedies are available to soften ear wax and hasten its expulsion. Such products may contain irritating substances that can cause inflammation. Doctors advise instead application of olive or almond oil. A cotton plug should be inserted to retain the oil in the outer ear. When ear wax is not dislodged by such home treatment, a doctor may syringe the ear with warm water. Do not use a stick or cotton bud.

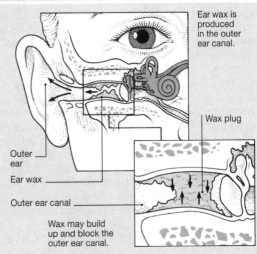

Ear wax is produced in the outer ear canal.

Wax plug

Outer ear

Ear wax

Outer ear canal

Wax may build up and block the outer ear canal.

are not usually applied for long periods because prolonged application can irritate the skin that lines the ear canal.

Sometimes an antibiotic given in the form of drops is not effective, and another type of antibiotic may also have to be taken by mouth.

Infection of the middle ear
Infection of the middle ear (otitis media) often causes severe pain and hearing loss. It is particularly common in young children in whom infecting organisms are able to spread easily into the middle ear from the nose or throat via the eustachian tube.

Viral infections of the middle ear usually cure themselves and are less serious than those caused by bacteria, which are treated with antibiotics given by mouth or injection. Bacterial infections often cause the eustachian tube to swell and become blocked. When a blockage occurs, pus builds up in the middle ear and puts pressure on the eardrum, which may perforate as a result.

Drug treatment
Doctors usually prescribe a decongestant (see p.93) or antihistamine (see p.124) to reduce swelling in the eustachian tube, thus allowing the pus to drain out of the middle ear. Usually, an antibiotic is also given by mouth to clear the infection.

Although antibiotics are not effective against viral infections, it is often difficult to distinguish between a viral and a bacterial infection of the middle ear, so your doctor may prescribe an antibiotic as a precautionary measure. Paracetamol, an analgesic (see p.80), may be given to relieve pain.

HOW TO USE EAR DROPS

Ear drops for outer ear disorders are more easily and efficiently administered if you have someone to help you. Lie on your side while the other person drops the medication into the ear cavity, ensuring that the dropper does not touch the ear. If possible, it is advisable to remain lying in that position for a few minutes in order to allow the drops to bathe the ear canal. Ear drops should be discarded when the course of treatment has been completed.

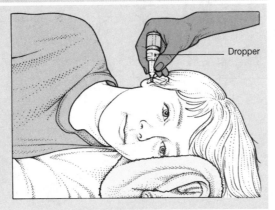

Dropper

COMMON DRUGS

Antibiotic and antibacterial ear drops
Chloramphenicol *
Clioquinol
Clotrimazole *
Framycetin
Gentamicin *
Neomycin

Decongestants
Ephedrine *
Oxymetazoline
Xylometazoline

Corticosteroids
Betamethasone *
Dexamethasone *
Flumethasone
Hydrocortisone *
Prednisolone *
Triamcinolone

Other drugs
Aluminium acetate
Antihistamines
(see p.124)

* See Part 4

SKIN

The skin waterproofs, cushions, and protects the rest of the body and is, in fact, its largest organ. It provides a barrier against innumerable infections and infestations, it helps the body to retain its vital fluids; it plays a major role in temperature control, and it houses the sensory nerves of touch.

The skin consists of two main layers: a thin, tough top layer, the epidermis, and below it a thicker layer, the dermis. The epidermis also has two layers: the skin surface, or stratum corneum (horny layer) consisting of dead cells, and below, a layer of active cells. The cells in the active layer divide and eventually die, maintaining the horny layer. Living cells produce keratin, which toughens the epidermis and is the basic substance of hair and nails. Some living cells in the epidermis produce melanin, a pigment released in increased amounts following exposure to sunlight.

The dermis contains different types of nerve ending for sensing pain, pressure, and temperature; sweat glands to cool the body; sebaceous glands that release an oil (sebum) that lubricates and waterproofs the skin; and white blood cells that help to keep the skin clear of infection.

What can go wrong
Most skin complaints are not serious, but they may be distressing if visible. They include infection, inflammation and irritation, infestation by skin parasites, and changes in skin structure and texture (for example, psoriasis, eczema, and acne).

Why drugs are used
Skin problems often resolve themselves without drug treatment. Over-the-counter preparations containing active ingredients are available, but doctors generally advise against their use without medical supervision because they could aggravate some skin conditions if used inappropriately. The drugs prescribed by doctors, however, are often highly effective, including antibiotics (p.128) for bacterial infections, antifungal drugs (p.138) for fungal infections, anti-infestation agents for skin parasites (p.176) and topical corticosteroids (p.174) for inflammatory conditions. Specialized drugs are available for conditions like psoriasis and acne.

Although many drugs are *topical* medications, they must be used carefully because, like drugs taken orally, they can also cause adverse effects.

Structure of the skin
The epidermis contains keratin and melanin, while the dermis contains sweat glands, sebaceous glands, and nerve endings that sense pain, temperature, and pressure.

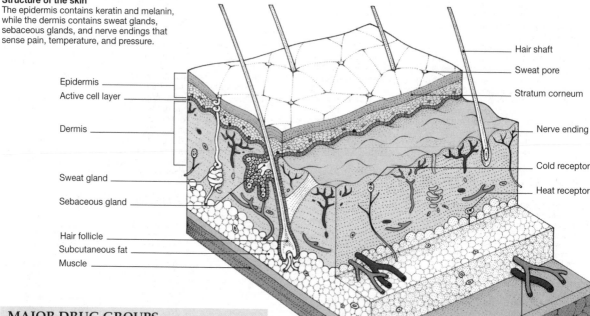

Epidermis
Active cell layer
Dermis
Sweat gland
Sebaceous gland
Hair follicle
Subcutaneous fat
Muscle

Hair shaft
Sweat pore
Stratum corneum
Nerve ending
Cold receptor
Heat receptor
Blood vessel

MAJOR DRUG GROUPS

Antipruritics
Topical corticosteroids
Anti-infective skin preparations
Drugs to treat skin parasites
Drugs used to treat acne

Drugs for psoriasis
Drugs for eczema
Drugs for dandruff
Drugs for hair loss
Sunscreens

ANTIPRURITICS

Itching (irritation of the skin that creates the urge to scratch), also known as pruritus, most often occurs as a result of minor physical irritation or chemical changes in the skin caused by disease, allergy, inflammation, or exposure to irritant substances. People differ in their tolerance to itching, and an individual's threshold can be altered by stress and other psychological factors.

Itching is a common symptom of many skin disorders, including eczema and psoriasis and allergic conditions such as urticaria (hives). It is also sometimes caused by a localized fungal infection or parasitic infestation. Diseases such as chickenpox may also cause itching. Less commonly, itching may also occur as a symptom of diabetes mellitus, jaundice, and kidney failure.

In many cases, generalized itching is caused by dry skin. Itching in particular parts of the body is often caused by a specific problem. For example, itching around the anus (pruritus ani) may result from haemorrhoids or worm infestation, while genital itching in women (pruritus vulvae) may be caused either by vaginal infection or, in older women, may be the result of a hormone deficiency.

Although scratching frequently provides temporary relief, it can often increase skin inflammation and make the condition worse. Continued scratching of an area of irritated skin may occasionally lead to a vicious circle of scratching and itching that continues long after the original cause of the trouble has been removed.

There are a number of different types of medicines used to relieve skin irritation. These products include soothing *topical* preparations applied to the affected skin and drugs that are taken by mouth. The main drugs used in antipruritic products include corticosteroids (see Topical corticosteroids, p.174), antihistamines (p.124), and local anaesthetics (p.80). Simple *emollient* or cooling creams or ointments, which do not contain active ingredients, are often recommended.

Why they are used
For mild itching arising from sunburn, urticaria, or insect bites, a cooling lotion such as calamine, perhaps containing menthol, phenol, or camphor, may be the most appropriate treatment. Local anaesthetic creams are sometimes helpful for small areas of irritation, such as insect bites, but are unsuitable for widespread itching. The itching caused by dry skin is often soothed by a simple emollient. Avoiding excessive bathing and using moisturizing bath oils may also help.

Severe itching from eczema or other inflammatory skin conditions may be treated with a topical corticosteroid preparation. When the irritation prevents sleep, a doctor may prescribe an antihistamine drug to be taken at night to promote sleep as well as to relieve itching (see also sleeping drugs, p.82). Antihistamines are also often included in topical preparations for the relief of skin irritation, but their effectiveness when administered in this way is doubtful. For the treatment of pruritus ani, see drugs for rectal and anal disorders (p.113). Post-menopausal pruritus vulvae may be helped by vaginal creams containing oestrogen; for further information, see female sex hormones (p.147). Itching that is caused by an underlying illness cannot be helped by skin creams and requires treatment for the principal disorder.

Risks and special precautions
The main risk from any antipruritic, with the exception of simple emollient and soothing preparations, is skin irritation, and therefore aggravated itching, that is caused by prolonged or heavy use. Antihistamine and local anaesthetic creams are especially likely to cause a reaction, and must be stopped if they do so. Antihistamines taken by mouth to relieve itching are likely to cause drowsiness. The special risks of topical corticosteroids are discussed on p.174.

Because itching can be a symptom of many underlying conditions, self-treatment should be continued for no longer than a week before seeking medical advice.

ACTION OF ANTIPRURITICS

Irritation of the skin causes the release of substances, such as histamine, that cause blood vessels to dilate and fluid to accumulate under the skin, which results in itching and inflammation. Antipruritic drugs act either by reducing inflammation, and therefore irritation, or by numbing the nerve impulses that transmit sensation to the brain.

Corticosteroids applied to the skin surface reduce itching caused by allergy within a few days, although the soothing effect of the cream may produce an immediate improvement. They pass into the underlying tissues and blood vessels and reduce the release of histamine, the chemical that causes itching and inflammation.

Antihistamines act within a few hours to reduce allergy-related skin inflammation. Applied to the skin, they pass into the underlying tissue and block the effects of histamine on the blood vessels beneath the skin. Taken by mouth, they also act on the brain to reduce the perception of irritation.

Local anaesthetics absorbed through the skin numb the transmission of signals from the nerves in the skin to the brain.

Soothing and emollient creams Calamine lotion and similar preparations applied to the skin surface reduce inflammation and itching by cooling the skin. Emollient creams lubricate the skin surface and prevent dryness.

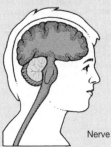

Antihistamines by mouth
The action of these drugs on histamine in the brain reduces the response to signals from irritated skin.

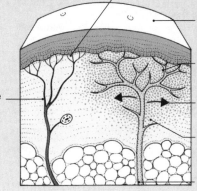

Nerve

Topical antipruritics
These antipruritics act locally to reduce itching.

Local anaesthetics numb nerve endings.

Soothing creams act on the skin surface.

Corticosteroids reduce histamine release.

Histamine released into the tissues.

Antihistamines block the effects of histamine in the tissues.

Blood vessel

COMMON DRUGS

Antihistamines
(see also p.124)
Antazoline
Diphenhydramine
Mepyramine
Trimeprazine

Corticosteroids
(see also p.141)
Hydrocortisone *

Local anaesthetics
Amethocaine
Benzocaine
Lignocaine

Emollient and cooling preparations
Aqueous cream
Calamine lotion
Cold cream
Emulsifying ointment

Other drugs
Colestyramine *
Crotamiton
Doxepin

* See Part 4

TOPICAL CORTICOSTEROIDS

Corticosteroid drugs (often simply called steroids) are related to the hormones produced by the adrenal glands. For a full description of these drugs, see p.141. *Topical* preparations containing a corticosteroid drug are often used to treat skin conditions in which inflammation is a prominent symptom.

Why they are used

Corticosteroid creams and ointments are most commonly given to relieve itching and inflammation associated with skin diseases such as eczema and dermatitis. These preparations may also be prescribed for psoriasis (see p.178). Corticosteroids do not affect the underlying cause of skin irritation, and the condition is therefore likely to recur unless the substance (allergen or irritant) that has provoked the irritation is removed, or the underlying condition is treated.

A doctor might not prescribe a corticosteroid as the initial treatment, preferring to try a topical medicine that has fewer adverse effects (see Antipruritics, p.173).

In most cases, treatment is started with a preparation containing a low concentration of a mild corticosteroid drug. A stronger preparation may be prescribed subsequently if the first product is ineffective.

How they affect you

Corticosteroids prevent the release of chemicals that trigger inflammation (see Action of corticosteroids on the skin, above right). Conditions treated with these drugs improve within a few days of starting the drug. Applied topically, corticosteroids rarely cause side effects, but the stronger drugs used in high concentrations have certain risks.

Risks and special precautions

Prolonged use of potent corticosteroids in high concentrations usually leads to

permanent changes in the skin. The most common effect is thinning of the skin, sometimes resulting in permanent stretch marks. Fine blood vessels under the skin surface may become prominent (this condition is known as telangiectasia). Because the skin on the face is especially vulnerable to such damage, only weak corticosteroids may be prescribed for use on the face. Dark-skinned people sometimes suffer a temporary reduction in pigmentation at the site of application.

When corticosteroids have been used on the skin for a prolonged period, abrupt discontinuation can cause a reddening of the skin called rebound erythroderma. This effect may be avoided by a gradual reduction in dosage. Corticosteroids suppress the body's immune system (see p.156), thereby increasing the risk of infection. For this reason, they are never used alone to treat skin inflammation caused by bacterial or fungal infection. However, they are sometimes included in a topical preparation that also contains an antibiotic or antifungal agent (see Anti-infective skin preparations, facing page).

ACTION OF CORTICOSTEROIDS ON THE SKIN

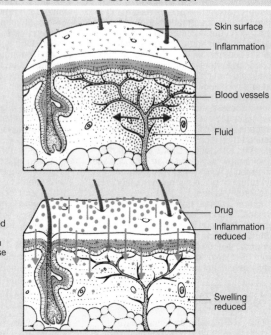

Skin inflammation
Irritation of the skin, caused by allergens or irritant factors, provokes white blood cells to release substances that dilate the blood vessels. This makes the skin hot, red, and swollen.

Skin surface
Inflammation
Blood vessels
Fluid

Drug action
Applied to the skin surface, corticosteroids are absorbed into the underlying tissue. There they inhibit the action of the substances that cause inflammation, allowing the blood vessels to return to normal and reducing the swelling.

Drug
Inflammation reduced
Swelling reduced

LONG-TERM EFFECTS OF TOPICAL CORTICOSTEROIDS

Prolonged use of topical corticosteroids causes drying and thinning of the epidermis, so that tiny blood vessels close to the skin surface become visible. In addition, long-term use of these drugs weakens the underlying connective tissue of the dermis, leading to an increased susceptibility to stretch marks.

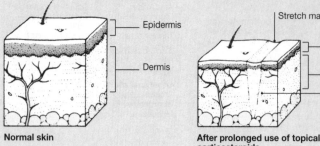

Epidermis
Dermis

Normal skin

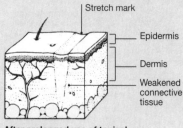

Stretch mark
Epidermis
Dermis
Weakened connective tissue

After prolonged use of topical corticosteroids

COMMON DRUGS

Very potent
Clobetasol ✱
Halcinonide

Potent
Beclomethasone ✱
Betamethasone ✱
Desoxymethasone
Diflucortolone
Fluocinolone
Fluocinonide
Fluticasone ✱
Mometasone ✱
Triamcinolone

Moderate
Alclometasone
Clobetasone
Fluocortolone
Flurandrenolone

Mild
Hydrocortisone ✱

✱ See Part 4

ANTI-INFECTIVE SKIN PREPARATIONS

The skin is the body's first line of defence against infection. Yet the skin can also become infected itself, especially if the outer layer (epidermis) is damaged by a burn, cut, scrape, insect bite, or an inflammatory skin condition – for example, eczema or dermatitis.

Several different types of organism may infect the skin, including bacteria, viruses, fungi, and yeasts. This page concentrates on drugs applied *topically* to treat bacterial skin infections. These drugs include antiseptics, antibiotics, and other antibacterial agents. Infection by other organisms is covered elsewhere (see Antiviral drugs, p.133, Antifungal drugs, p.138, and Drugs used to treat skin parasites, p.176).

Why they are used

Bacterial infection of a skin wound can usually be prevented by thorough cleansing of the damaged area and the application of antiseptic creams or lotions as described in the box (right). If infection does occur, the wound usually becomes inflamed and swollen, and pus may form. If you develop these signs, you should see your doctor. The usual treatment for a wound infection is an antibiotic taken orally, although often an antibiotic cream is also prescribed.

An antibiotic or antibacterial skin cream may also be used to prevent infection when your doctor considers this to be a particular risk – for example, in the case of severe burns.

Other skin disorders in which topical antibiotic treatment may be prescribed include impetigo and infected eczema, skin ulcers, bedsores, and nappy rash.

Often, a preparation containing two or more antibiotics is used in order to ensure that all bacteria are eradicated. The antibiotics selected for inclusion in topical preparations are usually drugs

ANTISEPTICS

Antiseptics (sometimes called germicides or skin disinfectants) are chemicals that kill or prevent the growth of microorganisms. They are weaker than household disinfectants, which are irritating to the skin.

Antiseptic lotions, creams, and solutions may be effective for preventing infection following wounds to the surface of the skin. Solutions can be added to water to clean wounds (if they are used undiluted, they may

Soaps, shampoos, throat lozenges and mouthwashes, skin lotions, creams, and ointments may contain antiseptic ingredients.

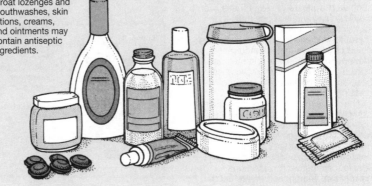

cause inflammation and increase the risk of infection). Creams may be applied to wounds after cleansing.

Antiseptics are also included in some soaps and shampoos for the prevention of acne and dandruff, but their benefit in these disorders is doubtful. They are also included in some throat lozenges, but their effectiveness in curing throat infections is unproven.

that are poorly absorbed through the skin (for example, the aminoglycosides). Thus the drug remains concentrated on the surface and in the skin's upper layers where it is intended to have its effect. However, if the infection is deep under the skin, or is causing fever and malaise, antibiotics may need to be given by mouth or injection.

Risks and special precautions

Any topical antibiotic product can irritate the skin or cause an allergic reaction.

Irritation is sometimes provoked by another ingredient of the preparation rather than the active drug, for example, a preservative contained in the product. An allergic reaction causing swelling and reddening of the skin is more likely to be caused by the antibiotic drug itself. Any adverse reaction of this kind should be reported to your doctor, who may substitute another drug, or prescribe a different preparation.

Always follow your doctor's instructions on how long the treatment with antibiotics should be continued. Stopping too soon may cause the infection to flare up again.

Never use a skin preparation that has been prescribed for someone else since it may aggravate your condition. Always throw away any unused medication.

BASES FOR SKIN PREPARATIONS

Drugs that are applied to the skin are usually in a preparation known as a base (or vehicle), such as a cream, lotion, ointment, or paste. Many bases are beneficial on their own.

Creams These have an *emollient* effect. They are usually composed of an oil-in-water emulsion and are used in the treatment of dry skin disorders, such as psoriasis and dry eczema. They may contain other ingredients, such as camphor or menthol.

Barrier preparations These may be creams or ointments. They protect the skin against water and irritating substances. They may be used in the treatment of nappy rash and to protect the skin around an open sore. They may contain powders and water-repellent substances, such as silicones.

Lotions These thin, semi-liquid preparations are often used to cool and soothe inflamed skin. They are most suitable for use on large,

hairy areas. Preparations known as shake lotions contain fine powder that remains on the surface of the skin when the liquid has evaporated. They are used to encourage scabs to form.

Ointments These are usually greasy and are suitable for treating wet (weeping) eczema.

Pastes These are ointments containing large amounts of finely powdered solids such as starch or zinc oxide. Pastes protect the skin and absorb unwanted moisture. They are used for skin conditions that affect clearly defined areas, such as psoriasis.

Collodions These are preparations that, when applied to damaged areas of the skin such as ulcers and minor wounds, dry to form a protective film. They are sometimes used to keep a dissolved drug in contact with the skin.

COMMON DRUGS

Antibiotics	Antiseptics and other antibacterials
Bacitracin	
Chlortetracycline	Cetrimide
Colistin	Chlorhexidine
Framycetin	Hexachlorophene
Fusidic acid	Metronidazole ✳
Gramicidin	Povidone iodine
Mupirocin	Silver sulfadiazine
Neomycin	Triclosan
Polymyxin B	
Tetracycline ✳	

✳ See Part 4

DRUGS TO TREAT SKIN PARASITES

Mites and lice are the most common parasites that live on the skin. One common mite causes the skin disease scabies. The mite burrows into the skin and lays eggs, causing intense itching. Scratching the affected area results in bleeding and scab formation, as well as increasing the risk of infection.

There are three types of lice, each of which infests a different part of the human body: the head louse, the body (or clothes) louse, and the crab louse, which often infests the pubic areas but is also sometimes found on other hairy areas such as the eyebrows. All of these lice cause itching and lay eggs (nits) that look like white grains attached to hairs.

Both mites and lice are passed on by direct contact with an infected person (during sexual intercourse in the case of pubic lice) or, particularly in the case of body lice, by contact with infected bedding or clothing.

The drugs most often used to eliminate skin parasites are insecticides that kill both the adult insects and their eggs. The most effective drugs for scabies are malathion and permethrin; benzyl benzoate is occasionally used. For lice infestations, carbaryl, malathion, permethrin, and phenothrin are used.

Why they are used

Skin parasites do not represent a serious threat to health, but they require prompt treatment since they can cause severe irritation and spread rapidly if untreated. Drugs are used to eradicate the parasites from the body, but bedding and clothing may need to be disinfected to avoid the possibility of reinfestation.

How they are used

Lotions for the treatment of scabies are applied to the whole body – with the exception of the head and neck – after a bath or shower. Many people find these lotions messy to use, but they should not be washed off for 12 hours (malathion) or

SITES AFFECTED BY SKIN PARASITES

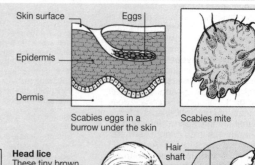

Scabies
The female scabies mite burrows into the skin and lays its eggs under the skin surface. After hatching, larvae travel to the skin surface, where they mature for 10–17 days before starting the cycle again.

Skin surface · Eggs · Epidermis · Dermis

Scabies eggs in a burrow under the skin

Scabies mite

Head lice
These tiny brown insects are transmitted from person to person (commonly among children). Their bites often cause itching.

Head louse

Hair shaft · Nit

Nits
Head lice lay and attach their eggs near the base of the hair shaft, especially around the ears.

48 hours (benzyl benzoate), otherwise they will not be effective. It is probably most convenient to apply malathion before going to bed. The lotion may then be washed off the following morning.

One or two treatments are normally sufficient to remove the scabies mites. However, the itch associated with scabies may persist after the mite has been removed, so it may be necessary to use a soothing cream or medication containing an antipruritic drug (see p.173) to ease this. People who have direct skin-to-skin contact with a sufferer from scabies, such as family members and sexual partners, should also be treated with antiparasitic preparations at the same time.

Head and pubic lice infestations are usually treated by applying a preparation of one of the products and washing it off with water when and as instructed by the leaflet given with the preparation. If the skin has become infected as a result of scratching, a *topical* antibiotic (see Anti-infective skin preparations, p.175) may also be prescribed.

Risks and special precautions

Lotions prescribed to control parasites can cause irritation and stinging that may be intense if the medication is allowed to come into contact with the eyes, mouth, or other moist membranes. Therefore, lotions and shampoos should be applied carefully, following the instructions of your doctor or the manufacturer.

Because they are applied topically, antiparasitic drugs do not usually have generalized effects. Nevertheless, it is important not to apply these preparations more often than directed.

ELIMINATING PARASITES FROM BEDDING AND CLOTHING

Most skin parasites may also infest bedding and clothing that has been next to an infected person's skin. Therefore, to avoid reinfestation following removal of the parasites from the body, any insects and eggs lodged in the bedding or clothing must be eradicated.

Washing
Since all skin parasites are killed by heat, washing affected items of clothing and bedding in hot water and drying them in a hot dryer is an effective and convenient method of dealing with the problem.

Non-washable items
Items that cannot be washed should be isolated in plastic bags. The insects and their eggs cannot survive long without their human

hosts and die within days. The length of time they can survive, and therefore the period of isolation, varies depending on the type of parasite (see the table below).

Parasite	Maximum survival time away from host Insects	Eggs	Isolation period
Scabies	2 days	0 days	2 days
Head lice	2 days	10 days	10 days
Crab lice	1 day	10 days	10 days
Body lice	10 days	30 days	30 days

COMMON DRUGS

Benzyl benzoate	Malathion *
Carbaryl *	Permethrin *
Crotamiton	Phenothrin

* See Part 4

DRUGS USED TO TREAT ACNE

Acne, known medically as acne vulgaris, is a common condition caused by excess production of the skin's natural oil (sebum), leading to blockage of hair follicles (see What happens in acne, right). It chiefly affects adolescents but it may occur at any age, due to taking certain drugs, exposure to industrial chemicals, oily cosmetics, or hot, humid conditions.

Acne primarily affects the the face, neck, back, and chest. The primary symptoms are blackheads, papules (inflamed spots), and pustules (raised pus-filled spots with a white centre). Mild acne may produce only blackheads and an occasional papule or pustule. Moderate cases are characterized by larger numbers of pustules and papules. In severe cases of acne, painful, inflamed cysts also develop. These can cause permanent pitting and scarring.

Medication for acne can be divided into two groups: *topical* preparations applied directly to the skin and *systemic* treatments taken by mouth.

Why they are used

Mild acne usually does not need medical treatment. It can be controlled by regular washing and by moderate exposure to sunlight or ultraviolet light. Over-the-counter antibacterial soaps and lotions are limited in use and may cause irritation.

When a doctor or dermatologist thinks acne is severe enough to need medical treatment, he or she usually recommends

CLEARING BLOCKED HAIR FOLLICLES

The most common treatment for acne is the application of keratolytic skin ointments. These encourage the layer of dead and hardened skin cells that form the skin surface to peel off. At the same time, this clears blackheads that block hair follicles and give rise to the formation of acne spots.

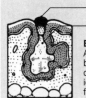

Blackhead

Trapped sebum

Blocked hair follicle
A hair follicle blocked by a plug of skin debris and sebum is ideal for acne spot formation.

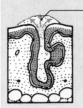

Freed sebum

Cleared hair follicle
Once the follicle is unblocked, sebum can escape and air can enter, thereby limiting bacterial activity.

WHAT HAPPENS IN ACNE

In normal, healthy skin, sebum produced by a sebaceous gland attached to a hair follicle is able to flow out of the follicle along the hair. An acne spot forms when the flow of the sebum from the sebaceous gland is blocked by a plug of skin debris and hardened sebum, leading to an accumulation of sebum.

Acne papules and pustules
Bacterial activity leads to the formation of pustules and papules. Irritant substances may leak into the surrounding skin, causing inflammation.

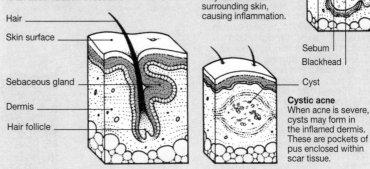

Hair

Skin surface

Sebaceous gland

Dermis

Hair follicle

Sebum

Blackhead

Cyst

Cystic acne
When acne is severe, cysts may form in the inflamed dermis. These are pockets of pus enclosed within scar tissue.

a topical preparation containing benzoyl peroxide or salicylic acid. If this does not produce an improvement, an ointment containing tretinoin, a drug related to vitamin A; azelaic acid, or tetracycline, an antibiotic, may be prescribed.

If acne is severe or does not respond to topical treatments, a doctor may prescribe a course of antibiotics by mouth (usually tetracycline or minocycline). If these measures are unsuccessful, the more powerful vitamin A-like drug isotretinoin, taken by mouth, may be prescribed.

Oestrogen drugs may have a beneficial effect on acne. A woman suffering from acne who also needs contraception may be given an oestrogen-containing oral contraceptive (p.161). Alternatively, a preparation containing an oestrogen and cyproterone (a drug that opposes male sex hormones) may be prescribed.

How they work

Drugs used to treat acne act in different ways. Some have a keratolytic effect – that is, they loosen the dead cells on the skin surface (see Clearing blocked hair follicles, left). Other drugs work by countering bacterial activity in the skin or reducing sebum production.

Topical preparations, such as benzoyl peroxide, salicylic acid, and tretinoin, have a keratolytic effect. Benzoyl peroxide also has an antibacterial effect. Topical or systemic tetracyclines reduce bacteria but may also have a direct anti-inflammatory effect on the skin. Isotretinoin reduces sebum production, soothes inflammation, and helps to unblock hair follicles.

How they affect you

Keratolytic preparations often cause soreness of the skin, especially at the

start of treatment. If this persists, a change to a milder preparation may be recommended. Day-to-day side effects are rare with antibiotics.

Treatment with isotretinoin often causes dry and scaly skin, particularly on the lips. The skin may become itchy and some hair loss may occur.

Risks and special precautions

Antibiotics in skin ointments may, in rare cases, provoke an allergic reaction requiring discontinuation of treatment. The tetracyclines, which are some of the most commonly used antibiotics for acne, have the advantage of being effective both topically and systemically. However, they are not suitable for use by mouth in pregnancy since they can affect the bones and teeth of the developing baby.

Isotretinoin sometimes increases levels of lipids in the blood. More seriously, the drug is known to damage the developing baby if taken during pregnancy. Women taking this drug need to make sure that they avoid conception during treatment.

COMMON DRUGS

Topical treatments	Oral and topical antibiotics
Adapalene	Clindamycin
Azelaic acid	Erythromycin ✳
Benzoyl peroxide ✳	Minocycline ✳
Isotretinoin ✳	Tetracycline ✳
Nicotinamide (Niacin) ✳	
Salicylic acid	**Other oral drugs**
Tretinoin	Cyproterone acetate
	Isotretinoin ✳

✳ See Part 4

DRUGS FOR PSORIASIS

The skin is constantly being renewed; as fast as dead cells in the outermost layer (epidermis) are shed, they are replaced by cells from the base of the epidermis. Psoriasis occurs when the production of new cells increases while the shedding of old cells remains normal. As a result of increased cell production, the live skin cells accumulate and produce patches of inflamed, thickened skin covered by silvery scales. In some cases, the area of skin affected is extensive and causes severe embarrassment and physical discomfort. Psoriasis may occasionally be accompanied by arthritis, in which the joints become swollen and painful.

The underlying cause of psoriasis is not known. The disorder usually first occurs between the ages of 10 and 30, and it recurs throughout life. Outbreaks may be triggered by emotional stress, skin damage, and physical illness. Psoriasis can also occur as a consequence of the withdrawal of corticosteroid drugs.

There is no complete cure for psoriasis. Simple measures, including careful sunbathing or using an ultraviolet lamp, may help to clear mild psoriasis. An *emollient* cream (see Antipruritics, p.173) often soothes the irritation. When such measures fail to provide adequate relief, additional drug therapy is needed.

Why they are used

Drugs are used to decrease the size of affected skin areas and to reduce inflammation and scaling. Mild and moderate psoriasis are usually treated with a *topical* preparation. Coal tar preparations, available in the form of creams, pastes, or bath additives, are often helpful, although some people dislike the smell. Dithranol is also widely used. Applied to the affected areas, the preparation is left for a few minutes or overnight (depending on which product is used), after which it is washed off. Both dithranol and coal tar can stain clothes and bed linen.

If these agents alone do not produce adequate benefit, ultraviolet light therapy in the form of regulated exposure to natural sunlight or to ultraviolet lamps (UVB) may be advised. Salicylic acid may be applied to help remove thick scale and crusts, especially from the scalp.

Topical corticosteroids (see p.174) may be used in difficult cases that do not respond to those treatments. They are particularly useful for the skinfold areas and may be given to counter irritation caused by dithranol.

If psoriasis is very severe and other treatments have not been effective, specialist treatment may include the use of more powerful drugs. These drugs include vitamin A derivatives (acitretin) taken by mouth in courses lasting approximately six months, and metho-trexate, which is an anticancer drug.

PUVA

PUVA is the combined use of a psoralen drug (methoxsalen) and ultraviolet A light (UVA). The drug is applied *topically* or taken by mouth some hours before exposure to UVA, which enhances the effect of the drug on skin cells.

This therapy is given two to three times a week and produces an improvement in skin condition within about four to six weeks.

Possible adverse effects include nausea, itching, and painful reddening of the normal areas of skin. More seriously, there is a risk of the skin ageing prematurely and a long-term risk of skin cancer, particularly in fair-skinned people. For these reasons, PUVA therapy is generally recommended only for severe psoriasis, when other treatments have failed.

In psoriasis
Skin cells form at the base of the epidermis faster than they can be shed from the skin surface. This causes the formation of patches of thickened, inflamed skin covered by a layer of flaking dead skin.

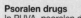

Normal skin / Skin in psoriasis — Epidermis, Rapidly dividing skin cells, Dermis

Psoralen drugs
In PUVA, psoralen drugs administered by mouth or as ointment penetrate the skin cells.
— Skin cell, DNA, Drug

Ultraviolet light
The drug is activated by exposure of the skin to ultraviolet light. It acts on the cell's genetic material (DNA) to regulate its rate of division.
— UVA rays, Drug, DNA restricted

Another form of specialist treatment, PUVA, is described in the box above.

How they work

Dithranol and methotrexate slow down the rapid rate of cell division that causes skin thickening. Acitretin also reduces production of keratin, the hard protein that forms in the outer layer of skin. Salicylic acid and coal tar remove the layers of dead skin cells. Corticosteroids reduce inflammation of underlying skin.

How they affect you

Appropriate treatment of psoriasis usually improves the appearance of the skin. However, since drugs cannot cure the underlying cause of the disorder, psoriasis tends to recur, even following successful treatment of an outbreak.

Individual drugs may cause side effects. Topical preparations can cause stinging and inflammation, especially if applied to normal skin. Coal tar and methoxsalen increase the skin's sensitivity to sunlight; excessive sunbathing or overexposure to artificial ultraviolet light may damage skin and worsen the condition.

Acitretin and methotrexate can have several serious side effects, including gastrointestinal upsets, liver damage (acitretin) and bone marrow damage (methotrexate). Both are contraindicated in pregnancy, and women are advised not to become pregnant for two years after completing treatment with acitretin. Topical corticosteroids may cause rebound worsening of psoriasis when these drugs are stopped.

COMMON DRUGS

Acitretin	Methotrexate ✳
Calcipotriol ✳	Methoxsalen
Coal tar	Salicylic acid
Cyclosporin ✳	Tacalcitol
Dithranol	Tazarotene
	Topical cortico-
	steroids (see p.174)

✳ See Part 4

DRUGS AND OTHER TREATMENTS FOR ECZEMA

Eczema is a skin condition causing a dry, itchy rash that may be inflamed and blistered. There are several types, some of which are called dermatitis. Eczema can be triggered by allergy but often occurs for no known reason. In the long term, it can thicken the skin as a result of persistent scratching.

The most common type, atopic eczema, may appear in infancy, but many children grow out of it. There is often a family history of eczema, asthma, or allergic rhinitis. Atopic eczema commonly appears on the hands, due to their exposure to detergents, and the feet, due to the warm, moist conditions of enclosed footwear.

Contact dermatitis, another common form of eczema, is caused by chemicals, detergents, or soap. It may only appear after repeated exposure to the substance, but strong acids or alkalis can cause a reaction within minutes. It can also result from irritation of the skin by traces of detergent on clothes and bedding.

Allergic contact dermatitis can appear days or even years after initial contact has been made with triggers such as nickel, rubber, elastic, or drugs (e.g., antibiotics, antihistamines, antiseptics, or local anaesthetics). Sunlight can also trigger contact dermatitis following use of aftershave or perfume.

Nummular eczema causes circular dry, scaly, itchy, patches to develop anywhere on the body, and bacteria are often found in these areas. The cause of nummular eczema is unknown.

Seborrhoeic dermatitis mainly affects the scalp and face (see Dandruff and hair loss p.180).

Why they are used
Emollients are used to soften and moisten the skin. Oral antihistamines (p.124) may be prescribed for a particularly itchy rash (*topical* antihistamines make the skin

COMMON SUBSTANCES THAT CAN CAUSE ECZEMA

Some substances produce an allergic reaction and some irritate the skin, causing eczema. The most common are listed below.

Allergens	Irritants
● Nickel, chromium	● Detergents
● Perfumes	● Soaps
● Plants	● Disinfectants
● Drugs	● Household cleaning products
● Rubber, elastic	
● Sticking plasters (especially zinc oxide ones)	● Paints
	● Glues and resins
● Cats and dogs	● Vegetable and fruit juices
● Tanning agents and dyes in leather and clothing	● Extremes of weather

PATCH TESTING

Low concentrations of the suspected substances are applied as spots to the skin of the back and held in place with non-absorbent adhesive tape. This method allows a number of potential allergens (substances that can cause an allergic reaction) to be tested at the same time.

After 48 hours, the adhesive tape is removed and the skin inspected for any redness, swelling, or blistering that has developed, which would indicate a positive reaction. The skin will be checked after a further 24 and 48 hours, in case the reaction has taken longer to develop.

Patches being applied

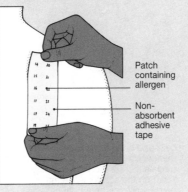

Patch containing allergen

Non-absorbent adhesive tape

Results of patch test

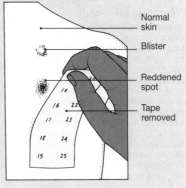

Normal skin

Blister

Reddened spot

Tape removed

more sensitive and should not be used). Coal tar or ichthammol may be used for chronic atopic eczema, but topical corticosteroids (p.174) may be needed to help control a flare up. Rarely, severe cases that are resistant to other treatments may need to be treated with the immuno-suppressant drug cyclosporin (p.249). Oral corticosteroids may be used to treat contact dermatitis. Nummular eczema usually requires corticosteroid treatment. If it is resistant, antibiotics (p.128) may be prescribed because infection is likely.

How they work
Emollients make the skin less dry and itchy. They are available as ointments, creams, lotions, soap substitutes, or bath oils. The effect is not long-lasting, so they need to be applied frequently. Emollients do not usually contain an active drug.

Antihistamines block the action of histamine (a chemical present in all cells). Histamine dilates the blood vessels in the skin, causing redness and swelling of the surrounding tissue due to fluid leaking from the circulation. Antihistamines also prevent histamine from irritating the nerve fibres, which causes itching.

Topical corticosteroids are absorbed into the tissues to relieve itching and inflammation. The least potent one that is effective is given. Hydrocortisone 1 per-cent is often used in 1–2-week courses.

Oral or topical antibiotics destroy the bacteria sometimes present in broken, oozing, or blistered skin.

Cyclosporin blocks the action of white blood cells, which are involved in the immune response. The drug is given in

short courses when the immune system responds inappropriately to an allergen.

Risks and special precautions
All types of eczema can become infected, and antibiotics may be needed. Herpes virus may infect atopic eczema, so direct contact with people who have a herpes infection, such as a cold sore, should be avoided. Emollients are generally well tolerated as are short-term topical mild corticosteroids. Cyclosporin, however, may produce some adverse effects.

Preventing eczema
Trigger substances can be identified using patch testing (see above) and avoided. PVC gloves should be worn to protect the hands from detergents. Cotton clothing, rather than wool or synthetic garments, should be worn next to the skin. Cosmetic moisturizers should be avoided because they usually contain perfumes and other sensitizers.

COMMON DRUGS

Emollient and cooling preparations	**Antihistamines** See also p.124
Aqueous cream	Antazoline
Cold cream	Chlorphenamine *
Emulsifying ointment	Diphenhydramine *
Calamine lotion	Mepyramine
	Trimeprazine
Corticosteroids See also p.174	**Other drugs**
Hydrocortisone *	Coal tar
	Ichthammol
	Ichthammol
* See Part 4	Cyclosporin *

DRUGS FOR DANDRUFF

Dandruff is an irritating, but harmless, condition that involves an acceleration in the normal shedding of skin cells from the scalp (see right). Extensive dandruff is considered to be a mild form of a type of dermatitis known as seborrhoeic dermatitis, which is caused by an overgrowth of a yeast organism that lives in the scalp. In severe cases, a rash and reddish yellow, scaly pimples appear along the hairline and on the face.

Why they are used

Frequent washing with a detergent shampoo usually keeps the scalp free of dandruff, but more persistent dandruff can be treated with shampoos medicated with zinc pyrithione or selenium sulphide (p.445), or with shampoos containing coal tar or salicylic acid. Severe cases of seborrheic dermatitis are best treated with shampoo containing the antifungal, ketoconazole (p.314). Ointments containing coal tar and salicylic acid are also available. Corticosteroid gels and lotions may be needed to treat an itchy rash, especially in cases of severe seborrhoeic dermatitis or psoriasis on the scalp (p.178).

How they work

Coal tar and salicylic acid preparations reduce the overproduction of new skin

WHAT HAPPENS IN DANDRUFF

All skin cells are replaced regularly as new cells grow from the epidermis. They gradually flatten as they die, and are shed on reaching the surface. Increased rate of production and sticking together of the cells produces dandruff. In children, dandruff may produce thick scaly flakes that can be 1–2 cm across. In adults, smaller flakes are produced.

Normal shedding

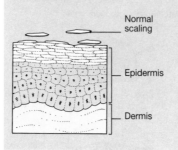

Normal scaling

Epidermis

Dermis

Dandruff

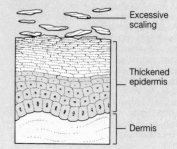

Excessive scaling

Thickened epidermis

Dermis

cells and break down scales which are then washed off while shampooing. Antifungals (p.138) reduce the overgrowth of yeast on the scalp by altering the permeability of the fungal cell walls. Corticosteroids (p.141) help to relieve an itchy rash by reducing inflammation of the underlying skin.

COMMON DRUGS

Antifungals
Ketoconazole ✽
Zinc pyrithione

✽ See Part 4

Other drugs
Coal tar
Corticosteroids
Salicylic acid
Selenium sulphide ✽

DRUGS FOR HAIR LOSS

Hair loss (alopecia) is the result of greater than normal shedding of hairs, or reduced hair production. Hair loss can be caused by a skin condition such as scalp ringworm or scalp psoriasis.

Other forms of hair loss are due to a disorder of the follicles themselves and may be a response to illness, malnutrition, or a reaction to some drugs, such as anticancer drugs or anticoagulants. The hair loss may be diffuse or in a pattern, as in male-pattern baldness which is caused by oversensitivity to testosterone.

Why they are used

If the hair loss is caused by a skin disorder such as scalp ringworm, an antifungal will be used to kill the fungal growth. If male-pattern baldness is a response to the male hormone, testosterone, finasteride could be used to reduce the effect of the hormone. The antihypertensive drug minoxidil can be applied to the scalp to promote hair growth.

How they work

Hair loss can be reversed when the underlying illness is treated, or the drug treatment is stopped. Finasteride, taken by mouth, inhibits conversion of testosterone to its more active form and reduces sensitivity to androgens. The role of minoxidil (p.350) in hair growth is not fully understood, although it is thought to stimulate the hair follicles (see left).

Risks and special precautions

Finasteride can lead to loss of libido or impotence. Anyone with a history of heart disease or hypertension should consult their doctor before using minoxidil, as the drug can be absorbed through the skin.

HAIR REGROWTH IN MALE-PATTERN BALDNESS

Follicles on the scalp have periods of activity and rest. During the rest phase, the bottom of the hair detaches from the follicle and the hair falls out. Regular applications of minoxidil, the antihypertensive drug, stimulate follicles to produce new hair growth.

Normal hair growth
Healthy hair
Skin surface
Follicle

Thinning hair
Inactive hair follicle shrinks and no new hair is produced.

Hair regrowth
Drug is applied to the surface of the scalp.
Drug is absorbed and stimulates the hair follicle.
New hair grows from the follicle.

COMMON DRUGS

Antifungals
Itraconazole
Griseofulvin

✽ See Part 4

Other drugs
Minoxidil ✽
Finasteride ✽

SUNSCREENS

Sunscreens and sunblocks are chemicals, usually formulated as creams or oils, that protect the skin from the damaging effects of ultraviolet radiation from the sun.

People vary in their sensitivity to sunlight. Fair-skinned people generally have the least tolerance and tend to burn easily when exposed to the sun, while those with darker skin, especially brown or black skin, can withstand exposure to the sun for longer periods.

In a few cases, the skin's sensitivity to sunlight is increased by a disease such as pellagra (see p.442) or herpes simplex infection. Some drugs, such as thiazide diuretics, phenothiazine antipsychotics, psoralens, sulphonamide antibacterials, tetracycline antibiotics, and nalidixic acid, can also increase the skin's sensitivity.

Apart from sunburn and premature ageing of the skin, the most serious effect from sunlight is skin cancer. Reducing the skin's exposure to sunlight can help to prevent skin cancers.

How they work

Sunlight consists of different wavelengths of radiation. Of these, ultraviolet (UV) radiation is particularly harmful to the skin. UV radiation ages the skin and causes burning. Excessive exposure to UV radiation also increases the risk of developing skin cancer. UV radiation is mainly composed of UVA and UVB rays, both of which age the skin. In addition, UVA rays cause tanning and UVB rays cause burning. Especially vulnerable are fair-skinned people and those being

ACTION OF SUNSCREENS

Fair skin unprotected by a sunscreen suffers damage as ultraviolet rays pass through to the layers beneath, causing pain and inflammation. Sunscreens act by blocking out some of these ultraviolet rays, while allowing a proportion of them to pass through the skin surface to the epidermis to stimulate the production of melanin, the pigment that gives the skin a tan and helps to protect it during further exposure to the sun.

Skin unprotected

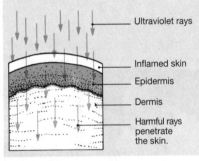

- Ultraviolet rays
- Inflamed skin
- Epidermis
- Dermis
- Harmful rays penetrate the skin.

Skin protected by sunscreen

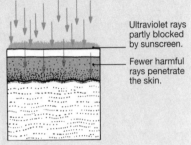

- Ultraviolet rays partly blocked by sunscreen.
- Fewer harmful rays penetrate the skin.

treated with immunosuppressant drugs. Sunscreens absorb some of the UVB radiation, ensuring that less of it reaches the skin. Sunscreens are graded using the Sun Protection Factor (SPF) (see below). Some preparations contain chemicals such as zinc oxide and titanium dioxide, which reflect both UVB and UVA rays; these are often called sunblocks.

A sunscreen is particularly advisable for visitors to tropical, subtropical, and mountainous areas, and for those who wish to sunbathe, because sunscreens can prevent burning while allowing the skin to tan. Sunscreens must be applied before exposure to the sun. People with fair skin should use a sunscreen with a higher SPF than people with darker skin.

Risks and special precautions

Sunscreens only form a physical barrier to the passage of UV radiation. They do not alter the skin to make it more resistant to sunlight. Sunscreen lotions must be applied frequently during exposure to the sun to maintain protection. People who are very fair skinned or are known to be very sensitive to sunlight should never expose their skin to direct sunlight, even if they are using a sunscreen, since not even sunscreens with high SPF values give complete protection.

Sunscreens can irritate the skin and some preparations may cause an allergic rash. People who are sensitive to some drugs, such as procaine and benzocaine and some hair dyes, might develop a rash after applying a sunscreen containing aminobenzoic acid or a benzophenone derivative such as oxybenzone.

SUN PROTECTION FACTORS

Sun protection factor (SPF) refers to the degree of protection given by a sunscreen against sunburn. It is a measure of the amount of UVB radiation a sunscreen absorbs. The higher the number, the greater the protection. The table below shows the major skin types and the minimum SPF recommended for each skin type.

This number only describes the protection against UVB radiation. Some sunscreens protect against UVA radiation as well and these are often called sunblocks. Some preparations carry a "star" classification for the UVA protection they give. The stars do not describe an absolute measure, but indicate a ratio of UVA to UVB protection. Four stars means that the product gives balanced protection against both UVA and UVB. Ratings of 1, 2, or 3 stars mean that the sunscreen has more protection again UVB than UVA.

COMMON DRUGS

Ingredients in sunscreens and sunblocks	
Aminobenzoic acid	Mexenone
Benzones	Methylbenzylidene camphor
Dibenzoylmethanes	Oxybenzone
Ethylhexyl methoxy-cinnamate	Padimate-O
	Titanium dioxide
	Zinc oxide *

Skin type	Type 1	Type 2	Type 3	Type 4	Type 5/6
Skin/hair tone	White or light skin, blue eyes, freckles	White or fair skin, fair hair	Medium white skin, brown hair	Olive skin, dark hair and eyes	Brown/black skin, dark hair and eyes
Sun sensitivity	Always burns, never tans	Burns easily, tans eventually	Tans slowly, burns sometimes	Tans easily, burns occasionally	Very rarely burns
Minimum SPF	SPF 50	SPF 25 + SPF 50 for vulnerable areas	SPF 25	SPF 15 + SPF 25 for vulnerable areas	May not need; SPF 15 if at risk of burning

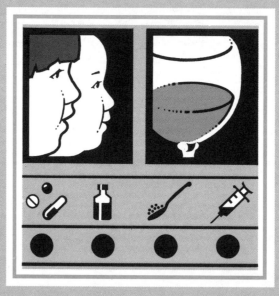

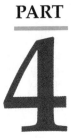
A–Z
OF DRUGS

A–Z OF MEDICAL DRUGS
A–Z OF VITAMINS AND MINERALS
DRUGS OF ABUSE
ALTERNATIVE MEDICINES
DRUGS IN SPORT
MEDICINES AND TRAVEL

A–Z OF MEDICAL DRUGS

The drug profiles in this section provide information and practical advice on 249 individual drugs. It is intended that the profiles should provide reference and guidance for non-medical readers taking drug treatment. However, it is impossible for this kind of book to take into account every variation in individual circumstances; readers should always follow their doctor's or pharmacist's instructions in instances where these differ from the advice in this section.

The drugs have been selected in order to provide representative coverage of the principal classes of drugs in medical use today. For disorders for which a number of drugs are available, the most commonly used drugs have been selected. Emphasis has also been placed on the drugs likely to be used in the home, although in a few cases drugs administered only in hospital have been included when the drug has been judged to be of sufficient general interest. At the end of this section, there are supplementary profiles on vitamins and minerals (pp.437–449), drugs of abuse (pp.450–459), alternative medicine (pp.460–461), drugs in sport (p.462), and medicine and travel (pp.463–465). In addition, there is a useful guide to further information (pp.468–469).

Each drug profile is organized in the same way, using standard headings (see sample page, below). To help you make the most of the information provided, the terms used and the instructions given under each heading are discussed and explained on the following pages.

HOW TO UNDERSTAND THE PROFILES

For ease of reference, the information on each drug is arranged in a consistent format under standard headings.

Drug name
Tells you the drug's generic name, brand names under which the drug is marketed, and combined preparations that contain the drug.

General information
Gives you a brief summary of the drug's important characteristics.

Information for users
Practical information on how and when to take the drug, the usual recommended dosage, how soon it takes effect, how long it is active, and advice on diet, storage, and missed doses.

Possible adverse effects
Indicates adverse effects that you may experience with the drug.

Interactions
Tells you how the drug may interact with other drugs or substances taken at the same time.

Quick reference
Summarizes important facts regarding the drug.

Special precautions
Describes circumstances in which the drug should be taken with special caution or in which it might not be suitable.

Overdose action
Indicates the symptoms that may occur if an overdose has been taken and tells you what immediate action is required.

Prolonged use
Tells you what effects the drug may have when taken over a long period and what monitoring may be advised.

CLOMIPRAMINE

Brand names Anafranil, Anafranil SR
Used in the following combined preparations None

GENERAL INFORMATION

Clomipramine belongs to the class of antidepressant drugs known as the tricyclics. It is used mainly in the long-term treatment of depression. It elevates mood, improves appetite, increases physical activity, and restores interest in everyday activities.

Clomipramine is particularly useful in the treatment of irrational fears and obsessive behaviour. Unlike most other tricyclics, clomipramine can be given by injection in severe illness.

In overdose clomipramine may cause coma and dangerously abnormal heart rhythms.

Tricyclic antidepressant drugs have been linked with an increase in dental caries in long term use.

QUICK REFERENCE

Drug group Tricyclic antidepressant (p.84)
Overdose danger rating High
Dependence rating Low
Prescription needed Yes
Available as generic Yes

INFORMATION FOR USERS

Your drug prescription is tailored for you. Do not alter dosage without checking with your doctor.

How taken
SR-tablets, capsules, liquid, injection.

Frequency and timing of doses
1–4 x daily.

Adult dosage range
10–250mg daily.

Onset of effect
Some effects may be felt within a few days, but full antidepressant effect may not be felt for up to 4 weeks.

Duration of action
During prolonged treatment antidepressant effect may last up to 2 weeks.

Diet advice
None.

Storage
Keep in a closed container in a cool, dry place away from the reach of children.

Missed dose
Take as soon as you remember. If your next dose is due within 3 hours, take a single dose now and skip the next.

Stopping the drug
Stopping abruptly can cause withdrawal symptoms and a recurrence of the original trouble. Consult your doctor, who may supervise a gradual reduction in dosage.

OVERDOSE ACTION

Seek immediate medical advice in all cases. Take emergency action if palpitations are noted or consciousness is lost.

See Drug poisoning emergency guide (p.494).

SPECIAL PRECAUTIONS

Be sure to tell your doctor if:
▼ You have heart problems.
▼ You have had epileptic fits.
▼ You have long-term liver or kidney problems.
▼ You have had glaucoma.
▼ You have thyroid disease.
▼ You have had prostate trouble.
▼ You are taking other medications.

Pregnancy
▼ Safety in pregnancy not established. Discuss with your doctor.

Breast-feeding
▼ The drug passes into the breast milk and may affect the baby. Discuss with your doctor.

Infants and children
▼ Not usually prescribed.

Over 60
▼ Increased likelihood of adverse effects. Reduced dose may therefore be necessary.

Driving and hazardous work
▼ Avoid such activities until you have learned how clomipramine affects you because the drug may cause blurred vision, drowsiness, and dizziness.

Alcohol
▼ Avoid. Alcohol may increase the sedative effects of this drug.

Surgery and general anaesthetics
▼ Clomipramine treatment may need to be stopped before you have a general anaesthetic. Discuss this with your doctor or dentist before any operation.

POSSIBLE ADVERSE EFFECTS

The possible adverse effects of this drug are mainly the result of its anticholinergic action, and include drowsiness and dizziness, dry mouth, and constipation.

Symptom/effect	Frequency		Discuss with doctor		Stop taking drug now	Call doctor now
	Common	Rare	Only if severe	In all cases		
Drowsiness/dizziness	●		■			
Sweating/flushing	●		■			
Dry mouth	●		■			
Blurred vision	●		■			
Constipation	●		■			
Difficulty in passing urine		●		■	▲	
Palpitations		●		■	▲	
Skin reactions/rash		●		■		■

INTERACTIONS

Sedatives All drugs that have a sedative effect may intensify those of clomipramine.

Antihypertensives Clomipramine may enhance the effect of some of these drugs.

Anticonvulsants Clomipramine may reduce the effects of these drugs and vice versa.

Monoamine oxidase inhibitors (MAOIs) A serious reaction may occur if these drugs are given with clomipramine.

Cisapride and quinidine There is an increased risk of abnormal heart rhythms if these drugs are taken with clomipramine.

PROLONGED USE

No problems expected.

Monitoring Regular checks on heart and liver function are recommended. Regular dental check-ups are also advised because prolonged use of clomipramine can cause dental caries.

236

DRUG NAME

Generic name
The main heading on the page is the drug's shortest generic name, unless the short name causes confusion with another drug, in which case the full generic name is given. For example, the antimalarial drug proguanil hydrochloride is listed as proguanil because there is no other generic drug of this name. However, magnesium hydroxide, an antacid, is listed under its full name to avoid confusing it with the mineral magnesium or other compounds, such as magnesium sulphate. If the drug has recently been renamed, the old name appears in brackets after the new one.

Brand names
Under the generic name are the brand names of products in which the drug

is the major single active ingredient. If there are many different brand names of the drug, only the most commonly used ones are given because of limitations of space. The names of the principal preparations, if any, in which the drug is combined with other drugs, are also listed. For more information about brand names and generic names, see page 13.

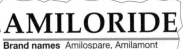

AMILORIDE

Brand names Amilospare, Amilamont
Used in the following combined preparati

GENERAL INFORMATION

GENERAL INFORMATION

The information here gives an overall picture of the drug. It may include notes on the drug's history (for example, when it was first introduced) and the principal disorders for which it is prescribed. This section also discusses the drug's major advantages and disadvantages.

GENERAL INFORMATION

Dexamethasone is a long-acting corticosteroid prescribed for a variety of skin and soft tissue conditions that are caused by allergy or inflammation. The drug can be injected into joints to relieve joint pain and stiffness due to

QUICK REFERENCE

The text in this box summarizes the important facts regarding your drug, and is organized under five headings, which are explained in detail below.

Drug group
This tells you which of the major groups the drug belongs to, and the page on which you can find out more about the drugs in the group and the various disorders or conditions they are used to treat. Where a drug belongs to more than one group, each group mentioned in the book is listed. For example, interferon is listed as an antiviral drug (p.133) and an anticancer drug (p.154).

Overdose danger rating
Gives an indication of the seriousness of the drug's effects if the dosage prescribed by your doctor, or that recommended on the label of an over-the-counter drug, is exceeded. The ratings – low, medium, and high – are

Otomize, Sofradex

QUICK REFERENCE

Drug group Corticosteroid (p.141)
Overdose danger rating Low
Dependence rating Low
Prescription needed Yes
Available as generic Yes

explained below. The rating also determines the advice given under Exceeding the dose.

● **Low** Symptoms unlikely. Death unknown.
● **Medium** Medical advice needed. Death rare.
● **High** Medical attention needed urgently. Potentially fatal.

If you do exceed the dose, advice is given under Exceeding the dose.

Dependence rating
Drugs are rated low, medium, or high on the basis of the risk of dependence.

● **Low** Dependence unknown.
● **Medium** Rare possibility of dependence.
● **High** Dependence is likely in long-term use.

Prescription needed
This tells you whether or not you need a prescription to obtain the drug. Some drugs are currently having their status reviewed and may soon be available without prescription from the pharmacy counter. Certain other prescription drugs are subject to government regulations (see How drugs are classified, page 13).

Available as generic
Tells you if the drug is available as a generic product.

INFORMATION FOR USERS (for common forms of each medication)

This section contains information on the following: administration, dosage frequency and amount, effects and actions, and advice on diet, storage, missed doses, stopping drug treatment, and overdose. All of the information is generalized and should not be taken as a recommendation for an individual dosing schedule. Always follow your doctor's instructions in the case of prescription drugs, and those of the manufacturer or pharmacist for over-the-counter medications.

How taken
The symbols in the box represent the various ways in which drugs can be administered. The dot that appears below

the symbol indicates the form in which a drug is available. This acts as a visual backup to the written information which follows immediately below the box.

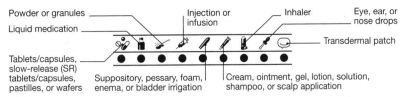

Powder or granules

Liquid medication

Tablets/capsules, slow-release (SR) tablets/capsules, pastilles, or wafers

Suppository, pessary, foam, enema, or bladder irrigation

Injection or infusion

Inhaler

Eye, ear, or nose drops

Transdermal patch

Cream, ointment, gel, lotion, solution, shampoo, or scalp application

A–Z OF MEDICAL DRUGS continued

INFORMATION FOR USERS continued

Frequency and timing of doses

This refers to the standard number of times each day that the drug should be taken and, where relevant, whether it should be taken with liquid, with meals, or on an empty stomach.

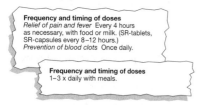

Frequency and timing of doses
Relief of pain and fever Every 4 hours as necessary, with food or milk. (SR-tablets, SR-capsules every 8–12 hours.)
Prevention of blood clots Once daily.

Frequency and timing of doses
1–3 x daily with meals.

Dosage range

This is generally given as the normal oral dosage range for an adult; dosages for injection are not usually given. In cases where the dosages for specific age groups vary significantly from the normal adult dosage, these will also be given. Where dosage varies according to use, the dosage for each is included.

The vast majority of drug dosages are expressed in metric units, usually milligrams (mg) or micrograms (mcg). In a few, dosage is given in units (u) or international units (IU). See also Weights and measures, facing page.

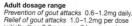

Adult dosage range
Prevention of gout attacks 0.6–1.2mg daily.
Relief of gout attacks 1.0–1.2mg per dose initially, then 0.6mg every 2 hours, up to a maximum of 4–8mg daily until joint is better or gastrointestinal problems arise.

Dosage range
Adults 60–180ml daily (liquid); 1.5–9.5g daily (tablets).
Children over 6 years Reduced dose according to age and weight.

Onset of effect

The onset of effect is the time it takes for the drug to become active in the body. This sometimes coincides with the onset of beneficial effects, but there may sometimes be an interval between the time when a drug is pharmacologically active and when you start to notice improvement in your symptoms or your underlying condition.

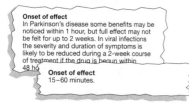

Onset of effect
In Parkinson's disease some benefits may be noticed within 1 hour, but full effect may not be felt for up to 2 weeks. In viral infections the severity and duration of symptoms is likely to be reduced during a 2-week course of treatment if the drug is begun within 48 ho

Onset of effect
15–60 minutes.

Duration of action

The information given here refers to the length of time that one dose of the drug remains active in the body.

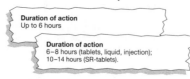

Duration of action
Up to 6 hours

Duration of action
6–8 hours (tablets, liquid, injection); 10–14 hours (SR-tablets).

Diet advice

With some drugs, it is important to avoid certain foods, either because they reduce the effect of the drug or because they interact adversely. This section of the profile tells you what, if any, dietary changes are necessary.

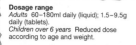

Diet advice
It is necessary to drink plenty of water during the 24 hours following treatment to reduce the risk of kidney damage.

Storage

Drugs will deteriorate and may become inactive if they are not stored under suitable conditions. The advice usually given is to store in a cool, dry place out of the reach of children. Some drugs must also be protected from light. Others, especially liquid medications, need to be kept in a refrigerator, but should not be frozen. For further advice on storing drugs, see p.29.

Storage
Keep in a closed container in a cool, dry place out of the reach of children. Protect from light.

Missed dose

This section gives advice on what to do if you forget a dose of your drug, so that the effectiveness and safety of your treatment is maintained as far as possible. If you forget to take several doses in succession, consult your doctor. You can read more about missed doses on p.28.

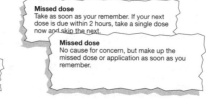

Missed dose
Take as soon as your remember. If your next dose is due within 2 hours, take a single dose now and skip the next.

Missed dose
No cause for concern, but make up the missed dose or application as soon as you remember.

Stopping the drug

If you are taking a drug regularly you should know how and when you can safely stop taking it. Some drugs can be safely stopped as soon as you feel better, or as soon as your symptoms have disappeared. Others must not be stopped until the full course of treatment has been completed, or they must be gradually withdrawn under the supervision of a doctor. Failure to comply with instructions for stopping a drug may lead to adverse effects. It may also cause your condition to worsen or your symptoms to reappear. See also Ending drug treatment, p.28.

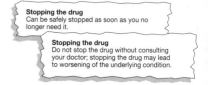

Stopping the drug
Can be safely stopped as soon as you no longer need it.

Stopping the drug
Do not stop the drug without consulting your doctor; stopping the drug may lead to worsening of the underlying condition.

Exceeding the dose

The information in this section expands on that in the quick reference box on the drug's overdose danger rating. It explains possible consequences of exceeding the dose and what to do if an overdose is taken. Examples of wording used for low, medium, and high overdose ratings are as follows:

Low
An occasional extra dose is unlikely to be a cause for concern. But if you notice any unusual symptoms, or if a large overdose has been taken, notify your doctor.

Medium
An occasional extra dose is unlikely to cause problems. Large overdoses may cause [symptoms]. Notify your doctor.

High
Seek immediate medical advice in all cases. Take emergency action if [relevant symptoms] occur.

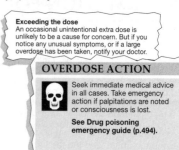

Exceeding the dose
An occasional unintentional extra dose is unlikely to be a cause for concern. But if you notice any unusual symptoms, or if a large overdose has been taken, notify your doctor.

OVERDOSE ACTION

Seek immediate medical advice in all cases. Take emergency action if palpitations are noted or consciousness is lost.

See Drug poisoning emergency guide (p.494).

SPECIAL PRECAUTIONS

Many drugs need to be taken with care by people with a history of particular conditions. The profile lists conditions you should tell your doctor about when you are prescribed a drug, or about which you should consult your doctor or pharmacist before taking an over-the-counter drug. Certain groups of people (pregnant women, breast-feeding mothers, children, and the over 60s) may also be at special risk from drug treatment. Advice for each of these groups is given in every profile. Information is also included about driving, undertaking hazardous work, and drinking alcohol.

Be sure to tell your doctor if:
▼ You have long-term liver or kidney problems.
▼ You have porphyria.
▼ You have previously had an allergic reaction to antifungal drugs.
▼ You are taking other medications.

Pregnancy
▼ Not usually prescribed. May cause defects in the developing baby. Discuss with your doctor.

Breast-feeding
▼ The drug passes into the breast milk and may affect the baby. Discuss with your doctor.

Infants and children
▼ Reduced dose necessary.

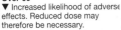

Over 60
▼ Increased likelihood of adverse effects. Reduced dose may therefore be necessary.

Driving and hazardous work
▼ Avoid such activities until you have learned how lisinopril affects you because the drug can cause dizziness and fainting.

Alcohol
▼ Avoid. Alcohol may interact with this drug to cause flushing and nausea.

WEIGHTS AND MEASURES

Metric equivalents of measurements used in this book:

1,000mcg (microgram) = 1mg (milligram)
1,000mg = 1g (gram)
1,000ml (millilitre) = 1l (litre)

Units or international units
Units (u) and international units (IU) are also used to express drug dosages. They represent the biological activity of a drug (its effect on the body). This ability cannot be measured in terms of weight or volume, but must be calculated in a laboratory.

POSSIBLE ADVERSE EFFECTS

The adverse effects discussed in the drug profile are symptoms or reactions that may arise when you take the drug. The emphasis is on symptoms that you, the patient, are likely to notice, rather than on the findings of laboratory tests that your doctor may order. The bulk of the section is in the form of a table that lists the adverse effects and indicates how commonly they occur, when to tell your doctor about them, and when to stop the drug. The headings in the table are explained below.

Frequency
Tells you whether the adverse effect is common or rare. Common effects are listed first.

Discuss with doctor
The marker in this section indicates under what circumstances you need to inform your doctor about an adverse effect you are experiencing.

Only if severe A marker in this column means that the symptom is unlikely to be serious, but that you should seek your doctor's advice if it troubles you.
In all cases Adverse effects marked in this column require prompt, but not necessarily emergency, medical attention. (See also Call doctor now, below.)

Stop taking drug now
In cases where certain unpleasant or dangerous adverse effects of a drug may override its beneficial effects, you are advised to stop taking the drug immediately, if necessary before seeing your doctor.

Call doctor now
Effects marked in this column require immediate medical help. They indicate a potentially dangerous response to the drug treatment, for which you should seek emergency medical attention.

Symptom/effect	Frequency		Discuss with doctor		Stop taking drug now	Call doctor now
	Common	Rare	Only if severe	In all cases		
Nausea/vomiting	●			■		
Headache		●		■		
Abdominal pain		●		■		
Itching/rash		●		■	▲	
Painful breasts (men)		●		■	▲	
Jaundice		●		■	▲	■

INTERACTIONS

The interactions that are discussed here are those that may occur between the drug under discussion and other drugs. Information includes the name of the interacting drug or group of drugs and the effect of the interaction.

INTERACTIONS

Antidepressant drugs Levodopa may interact with monoamine oxidase inhibitors (MAOIs) to cause a dangerous rise in blood

PROLONGED USE

The information given here concerns the adverse, and sometimes beneficial, effects of the drug that may occur during long-term use. These may differ from those listed under Possible adverse effects. This section of the profile also includes information on monitoring the effects of the drug during long-term treatment, explaining the tests you may be given if your doctor thinks they are necessary.

PROLONGED USE

The risk of liver damage increases with use for more than 14 days.

Monitoring Periodic blood tests are usually performed to check the effect of the drug on the liver.

ACICLOVIR

Brand names Boots Avert, Herpetad, Soothelip, Virasorb, Virovir, Zovirax
Used in the following combined preparations None

GENERAL INFORMATION

Aciclovir is an antiviral drug used in the treatment of herpes infections of all types. Most commonly given in the form of a cream, aciclovir reduces the severity of outbreaks of cold sores and herpes. The drug's effectiveness is greatest if it is given when symptoms have just started. Aciclovir may be given by injection or by mouth for severe or recurrent cases of genital herpes.

Herpes zoster (shingles) infections are treated with aciclovir tablets. The drug is prescribed on a regular basis for people who have reduced immunity. It is also administered as ointment for herpes infections affecting the eye.

The injected form is prescribed with caution to those with impaired kidney function because of the risk of aciclovir accumulating in the body.

INFORMATION FOR USERS

Follow instructions on the label. Call your doctor if symptoms worsen.

How taken

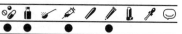

Tablets, liquid, injection, cream, eye ointment.

Frequency and timing of doses
2–5 x daily. Start as soon as possible.

Adult dosage range
Tablets, liquid 1–4g daily (treatment); 800mg daily, occasionally 1.6g daily (prevention).
Cream, eye ointment As directed.

Onset of effect
Within 24 hours.

Duration of action
Up to 8 hours.

Diet advice
It is necessary to drink plenty of water when taking high doses by mouth or injection.

Storage
Keep in a closed container in a cool, dry place out of the reach of children. Protect from light.

Missed dose
Tablets/liquid Take as soon as you remember.
Cream, eye ointment Do not apply the missed dose. Apply your next dose as usual.

Stopping the drug
Complete the full course as directed.

Exceeding the dose
An occasional unintentional extra dose is unlikely to be a cause for concern. But if you notice any unusual symptoms, or if a large overdose has been taken, notify your doctor.

SPECIAL PRECAUTIONS

Be sure to consult your doctor or pharmacist before taking this drug:
▼ You have a long-term kidney problem.
▼ You have reduced immunity.
▼ You are taking other medications.

 Pregnancy
▼ Topical preparations carry no known risk, but oral and injectable forms are not usually prescribed, as the effects on the developing baby are unknown. Discuss with your doctor.

 Breast-feeding
▼ No evidence of risk with topical forms. The drug passes into the breast milk following injection or oral administration. Discuss with your doctor.

 Infants and children
▼ Reduced dose necessary in young children.

 Over 60
▼ Reduced dose may be necessary.

 Driving and hazardous work
▼ Avoid such activities until you know how aciclovir affects you because the drug may cause dizziness if it is taken by mouth.

 Alcohol
▼ No known problems.

POSSIBLE ADVERSE EFFECTS

Serious *adverse effects* are rare. The cream commonly causes discomfort at the site of application. Confusion and hallucinations occur rarely with injections.

Symptom/effect	Frequency		Discuss with doctor		Stop taking drug now	Call doctor now
	Common	Rare	Only if severe	In all cases		
Topical applications						
Burning/stinging/itching	●		■			
Rash		●		■		▲
By mouth						
Nausea/vomiting		●	■			
Headache/dizziness/fatigue		●		■		
Injection						
Inflammation at injection site		●		■		
Confusion/hallucinations		●		■		▲

INTERACTIONS (by mouth or injection only)

General note Any drug that affects the kidneys increases the risk of side effects with aciclovir.

Probenecid This drug may increase the level of aciclovir in the blood.

Mycophenolate mofetil Aciclovir may increase the levels of this drug in the blood and vice versa.

PROLONGED USE

Aciclovir is usually given as single courses of treatment and is not given long term, except for people with reduced immunity.

ALLOPURINOL

Brand names Caplenal, Cosuric, Rimapurinol, Xanthomax, Zyloric
Used in the following combined preparations None

GENERAL INFORMATION

Allopurinol is prescribed as a long-term preventative of recurrent attacks of gout. It acts by halting the formation in the joints of uric acid crystals, which cause the inflammation characteristic of gout. It is also used to lower high uric acid levels (hyperuricaemia) caused by other drugs, such as anticancer drugs.

Allopurinol is not effective in relieving the pain of an acute flare-up. In fact, gout attacks may increase initially, so an anti-inflammatory drug is often given as well.

Unlike the gout drugs that reduce uric acid levels by increasing the quantity excreted in the urine, allopurinol does not raise the risk of kidney stones. This makes it particularly suitable for those with poor kidney function or a tendency to form kidney stones.

INFORMATION FOR USERS

Your drug prescription is tailored for you. Do not alter dosage without checking with your doctor.

How taken

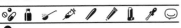

Tablets.

Frequency and timing of doses
1–3 x daily after food.

Adult dosage range
100–300mg daily.

Onset of effect
Within 24–48 hours. Full effect may not be felt for several weeks.

Duration of action
Up to 30 hours. Some effect may last for 1–2 weeks after the drug has been stopped.

Diet advice
A high fluid intake (2 litres of fluid daily) is recommended.

Storage
Keep in a closed container in a cool, dry place out of the reach of children.

Missed dose
If your next dose is not due for another 12 hours or more, take a dose as soon as you remember and take the next one as usual. Otherwise skip the missed dose and take your next dose on schedule.

Stopping the drug
Do not stop the drug without consulting your doctor; symptoms may recur.

Exceeding the dose
An occasional unintentional extra dose is unlikely to cause problems. Large overdoses may cause nausea, vomiting, abdominal pain, diarrhoea, and dizziness. Notify your doctor.

SPECIAL PRECAUTIONS

Be sure to tell your doctor if:
▼ You have long-term liver or kidney problems.
▼ You have had a previous sensitivity reaction to allopurinol.
▼ You have a current attack of gout.
▼ You are taking other medications.

 Pregnancy
▼ Safety in pregnancy not established. Discuss with your doctor.

 Breast-feeding
▼ The drug passes into the breast milk and may affect the baby. Discuss with your doctor.

 Infants and children
▼ Reduced dose necessary.

 Over 60
▼ Reduced dose may be necessary.

 Driving and hazardous work
▼ Avoid such activities until you have learned how allopurinol affects you because the drug can cause drowsiness.

 Alcohol
▼ Avoid. Alcohol may worsen gout.

POSSIBLE ADVERSE EFFECTS

Adverse effects of allopurinol are not very common. The most serious is an allergic rash that may require the drug to be stopped and an alternative treatment substituted. Nausea can be avoided by taking allopurinol after food.

Symptom/effect	Frequency		Discuss with doctor		Stop taking drug now	Call doctor now
	Common	Rare	Only if severe	In all cases		
Nausea	●		■			
Rash/itching	●			■	▲	
Drowsiness/dizziness		●	■			
Headache		●		■		
Sore throat		●		■	▲	
Metallic taste		●		■		
Fever and chills		●		■	▲	

INTERACTIONS

Mercaptopurine and azathioprine Allopurinol blocks the breakdown of these drugs, requiring a reduction in their dosage.

Aspirin Large doses of aspirin may reduce the effects of allopurinol.

Anticoagulant drugs Allopurinol may increase the effects of these drugs.

Chlorpropamide The hypoglycaemic effects of chlorpropamide may be increased.

Cyclosporin Allopurinol may increase the effects of this drug.

ACE inhibitors Allopurinol may increase the effects of these drugs.

PROLONGED USE

Apart from an increased risk of gout in the first weeks or months, no problems are expected.

Monitoring Periodic checks on uric acid levels in the blood are usually performed.

ALPROSTADIL

Brand names Caverject, MUSE, Prostin VR, Viridal
Used in the following combined preparations None

GENERAL INFORMATION

Alprostadil is a member of the prostaglandin group of drugs and is used to treat patent ductus arteriosus, a congenital heart disorder in newborn babies. It works by keeping the ductus blood vessel (which would normally have shut off at birth) open until it can be closed permanently by surgery.

Alprostadil is also used to help men who are impotent to achieve an erection.

It is either injected directly into the penis or applied as a gel into the urethra.

The drug is usually only administered to babies in hospital. *Side effects* such as heart, circulatory, and respiratory problems are common, and there is a risk of unusual bone growth, particularly with long-term use. The most common *side effect* of alprostadil in men is pain in the penis.

QUICK REFERENCE

Drug group Prostaglandin and drug for impotence (p.164)
Overdose danger rating Medium
Dependence rating Low
Prescription needed Yes
Available as generic No

INFORMATION FOR USERS

Your drug prescription is tailored for you. Do not alter dosage without checking with your doctor.

How taken

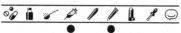

Injection, gel.

Frequency and timing of doses
Up to 3 x per week. Not more than one dose in any 24 hour period.

Dosage range
Starts at 2.5mcg, individually adjusted by your doctor to produce an erection lasting not more than 1 hour.

Onset of effect
Within a few minutes.

Duration of action
Erection should not last more than 1 hour.

Diet advice
None.

Storage
Store in a refrigerator, out of the reach of children. Do not freeze.

Missed dose
Take the next dose when needed. Use no more than one dose in any 24-hour period and no more than 3 doses per week.

Stopping the drug
Can be safely stopped as soon as you no longer need it.

Exceeding the dose
An occasional unintentional extra dose is unlikely to be a cause for concern. But if you notice any unusual symptoms or if a large overdose has been taken, notify your doctor.

SPECIAL PRECAUTIONS

Be sure to tell your doctor if:
▼ You are taking other medications for impotence.

Pregnancy
▼ Not prescribed.

Breast-feeding
▼ Not prescribed.

Infants and children
▼ Other than for newborn babies, not prescribed.

Over 60s
▼ Doses are adjusted individually.

Driving and hazardous work
▼ No special problems.

Alcohol
▼ Excessive use of alcohol with alprostadil can contribute to erectile problems.

POSSIBLE ADVERSE EFFECTS

Breathing difficulties are a side effect of the drug in newborn babies. Less often, it may cause convulsions. In men, there is a risk of prolonged erection. You should report any erection lasting for more than 4 hours to your doctor and stop taking the drug immediately.

Symptom/effect	Frequency		Discuss with doctor		Stop taking drug now	Call doctor now
	Common	Rare	Only if severe	In all cases		
Newborn babies						
Breathing difficulties		●		■		▮
Convulsions		●		■		▮
Men						
Penile pain	●		■			
Bruising/swelling	●			■		
Bleeding	●			■		
Prolonged erection	●			■	▲	▮
Testicular pain/swelling		●		■		
Dizziness/fainting		●		■		
Chest pain/palpitations		●		■		

PROLONGED USE

Prolonged use of alprostadil in newborn babies may cause abnormal bone development and weakening of some blood vessel walls.

Prolonged use for impotence may lead to development of fibrosis of the penis.

Monitoring Regular examinations for penile fibrosis are required.

INTERACTIONS

None.

ALUMINIUM HYDROXIDE

Brand names Alu-Cap, Aludrox
Used in the following combined preparations Asilone, Co-magaldrox, Gaviscon, Maalox, Mucaine, Mucogel, Topal, and others

GENERAL INFORMATION

Aluminium hydroxide is the ingredient basic to many over-the-counter remedies for indigestion and heartburn. Because the drug is constipating (it is sometimes used to treat diarrhoea), it is usually combined with a magnesium-containing antacid with a balancing laxative effect. The combination is sometimes referred to by the generic name of co-magaldrox.

The prolonged action of the drug makes it useful in preventing the pain of stomach and duodenal ulcers or reflux oesophagitis. It can also promote the healing of ulcers.

In the intestine aluminium hydroxide binds with, and thereby reduces the absorption of, phosphate. This makes it helpful in treating high blood phosphate (hyperphosphataemia), which occurs in some people with impaired kidney function. Prolonged heavy use can lead to phosphate deficiency and a consequent weakening of the bones.

Some preparations include large amounts of sodium and should be used with caution by those on low-sodium diets. The drug may be more effective as an antacid in liquid form than in tablets.

INFORMATION FOR USERS

Follow instructions on the label. Call your doctor if symptoms worsen.

How taken

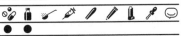

Tablets, capsules, liquid (gel suspension). The tablets should be well chewed.

Frequency and timing of doses
As antacid 4–6 x daily as needed, or 1 hour before and after meals.
Peptic ulcer 6–7 x daily.
Hyperphosphataemia 3–4 x daily with meals.
Diarrhoea 2–6 x daily.

Dosage range
Adults Up to 70ml daily (liquid), 2–10g daily (tablets or capsules).
Children over 6 years Reduced dose according to age and weight.

Onset of effect
Within 15 minutes.

Duration of action
2–4 hours.

Diet advice
For hyperphosphataemia, a low-phosphate diet may be advised in addition to aluminium hydroxide treatment.

Storage
Keep in a closed container in a cool, dry place out of the reach of children.

Missed dose
Do not take the missed dose. Take your next dose as usual.

Stopping the drug
Can be safely stopped as soon as you no longer need it (indigestion). When taken as ulcer treatment or for hyperphosphataemia resulting from kidney failure, do not stop without consulting your doctor.

Exceeding the dose
An occasional unintentional extra dose is unlikely to be a cause for concern. But if you notice any unusual symptoms, or if a large overdose has been taken, notify your doctor.

SPECIAL PRECAUTIONS

Be sure to consult your doctor or pharmacist before taking this drug if:
▼ You have a long-term kidney problem.
▼ You have heart problems.
▼ You have high blood pressure.
▼ You suffer from constipation.
▼ You have a bone disease.
▼ You have porphyria.
▼ You are taking other medications.

Pregnancy
▼ Safety in pregnancy not established. Discuss with your doctor.

Breast-feeding
▼ No evidence of risk.

Infants and children
▼ Not recommended under 6 years except on the advice of a doctor.

Over 60
▼ Increased likelihood of adverse effects. Reduced dose may therefore be necessary.

Driving and hazardous work
▼ No known problems.

Alcohol
▼ No known problems.

POSSIBLE ADVERSE EFFECTS

Constipation is common with aluminium hydroxide; nausea and vomiting may occur due to the granular, powdery nature of the drug. Bone pain occurs only when large doses have been taken regularly for months or years.

Symptom/effect	Frequency		Discuss with doctor		Stop taking drug now	Call doctor now
	Common	Rare	Only if severe	In all cases		
Constipation	●		■			
Nausea		●	■			
Vomiting		●		■		

INTERACTIONS

General note Aluminium hydroxide may interfere with the absorption or excretion of many drugs, including oral anticoagulants, digoxin, many antibiotics, penicillamine, corticosteroids, antipsychotics, and phenytoin.

Enteric-coated tablets Aluminium hydroxide may lead to the break-up of the enteric coating of tablets (e.g., bisacodyl, or enteric-coated prednisolone) before they leave the stomach, causing stomach irritation.

PROLONGED USE

Aluminium hydroxide should not be used for longer than 4 weeks without consulting your doctor. Prolonged use in high doses may deplete blood phosphate and calcium levels, leading to weakening of the bones and fractures.

AMANTADINE

Brand name Symmetrel
Used in the following combined preparations None

GENERAL INFORMATION

Amantadine was first used in the 1960s as an antiviral drug, originally for the prevention and treatment of influenza A. As a preventative against influenza A, it protects some 70 per cent of those not receiving vaccination. As treatment, it is effective in reducing the severity of symptoms when given within 48 hours of the onset of flu. It can also reduce pain following herpes zoster (shingles).

In 1969 amantadine was found to be helpful in *parkinsonism*, except when the condition is caused by drugs. Amantadine usually produces improvement of symptoms during the first few weeks, but its effectiveness wears off over six to eight weeks, requiring replacement by another drug. It is sometimes given with levodopa (see p.319), another drug for parkinsonism.

INFORMATION FOR USERS

Your drug prescription is tailored for you. Do not alter dosage without checking with your doctor.

How taken

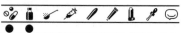

Capsules, liquid.

Frequency and timing of doses
1–2 x daily. The second dose should not be taken later than 4pm.

Adult dosage range
100–200mg daily.

Onset of effect
In parkinsonism the full effect may not be felt for up to 2 weeks. In viral infections the severity and duration of symptoms is likely to be reduced if the drug is begun within 48 hours of the onset of symptoms.

Duration of action
Up to 24 hours.

Diet advice
None.

Storage
Keep in a closed container in a cool, dry place out of the reach of children.

Missed dose
Take as soon as you remember. If your next dose is due within 2 hours, take a single dose now and skip the next.

Stopping the drug
Do not stop taking the drug without consulting your doctor; symptoms may recur.

Exceeding the dose
An occasional unintentional extra dose is unlikely to be a cause for concern. But if you notice any unusual symptoms, or if a large overdose has been taken, notify your doctor.

SPECIAL PRECAUTIONS

Be sure to tell your doctor if:
▼ You have long-term liver or kidney problems.
▼ You have a peptic ulcer.
▼ You have had epileptic fits.
▼ You have heart disease.
▼ You suffer from eczema.
▼ You are taking other medications.

 Pregnancy
▼ Safety in pregnancy not established. Discuss with your doctor.

 Breast-feeding
▼ The drug passes into the breast milk and may affect the baby. Discuss with your doctor.

 Infants and children
▼ Not usually prescribed. Reduced dose necessary.

 Over 60
▼ Increased likelihood of adverse effects. Reduced dose necessary.

 Driving and hazardous work
▼ Avoid such activities until you have learned how amantadine affects you because the drug may cause blurred vision, dizziness, inability to concentrate, hallucinations, agitation, and confusion.

 Alcohol
▼ No known problems.

POSSIBLE ADVERSE EFFECTS

Adverse effects are uncommon and often wear off during continued treatment. They are rarely serious enough to require treatment to be stopped.

Symptom/effect	Frequency		Discuss with doctor		Stop taking drug now	Call doctor now
	Common	Rare	Only if severe	In all cases		
Nervousness/agitation	●		■			
Confusion/hallucinations	●			■		
Insomnia		●	■			
Dizziness		●		■		
Blurred vision		●		■		
Loss of appetite		●		■		
Ankle swelling		●		■		
Rash		●		■		▲

INTERACTIONS

Anticholinergic drugs Amantadine may add to the effects of *anticholinergic* drugs. In that event your doctor will probably reduce the dosage of the anticholinergic drugs.

PROLONGED USE

The beneficial effects of this drug usually diminish during continuous treatment for parkinsonism. When this occurs, another drug may be substituted for or given together with amantadine. Sometimes the effectiveness of amantadine can be restored if it is withdrawn by your doctor for a few weeks and later reintroduced.

AMILORIDE

Brand names Amilospare, Amilamont
Used in the following combined preparations Burinex A, Co-amilofruse, Co-amilozide, Moduretic, Navispare, and others

GENERAL INFORMATION

Amiloride belongs to a class of drugs known as potassium-sparing diuretics. With thiazide or loop diuretics, amiloride is used in the treatment of hypertension, and of oedema (fluid retention) resulting from heart failure or liver disease.

Amiloride's effect on urine flow may be noticed for several hours. For this reason, it should be avoided after about 4 pm; otherwise you may need to pass urine during the night. As with other potassium-sparing diuretics, amiloride can be risky for people who are taking potassium supplements and in those who have unusually high levels of potassium in their blood. The drug is prescribed with caution for people with a kidney disorder.

QUICK REFERENCE

Drug group Potassium-sparing diuretic (p.99)

Overdose danger rating Low

Dependence rating Low

Prescription needed Yes

Available as generic Yes

INFORMATION FOR USERS

Your drug prescription is tailored for you. Do not alter dosage without checking with your doctor.

How taken

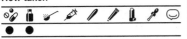

Tablets, liquid.

Frequency and timing of doses
Once daily, usually in the morning.

Adult dosage range
5–20mg daily.

Onset of effect
Within 2–4 hours.

Duration of action
12–24 hours.

Diet advice
Avoid foods that are high in potassium – for example, dried fruit and salt substitutes.

Storage
Keep in a closed container in a cool, dry place out of the reach of children.

Missed dose
Take as soon as you remember. However, if it is late in the day, do not take the missed dose, or you may need to get up at night to pass urine. Take the next scheduled dose as usual.

Stopping the drug
Do not stop the drug without consulting your doctor; symptoms may recur.

Exceeding the dose
An occasional unintentional extra dose is unlikely to be a cause for concern. But if you notice any unusual symptoms, or if a large overdose has been taken, notify your doctor.

SPECIAL PRECAUTIONS

Be sure to tell your doctor if:
▼ You have long-term liver or kidney problems.
▼ You have diabetes.
▼ You are taking other medications.

Pregnancy
▼ Not usually prescribed. May cause a reduction in the blood supply to the developing baby. Discuss with your doctor.

Breast-feeding
▼ Not usually prescribed during breast-feeding. Discuss with your doctor.

Infants and children
▼ Not recommended.

Over 60
▼ Increased likelihood of adverse effects. Reduced dose necessary.

Driving and hazardous work
▼ Avoid such activities until you have learned how amiloride affects you because the drug may cause confusion.

Alcohol
▼ No special problems.

POSSIBLE ADVERSE EFFECTS

Amiloride has few adverse effects; the main problem is the possibility that potassium may be retained by the body, causing muscle weakness and numbness.

Symptom/effect	Frequency		Discuss with doctor		Stop taking drug now	Call doctor now
	Common	Rare	Only if severe	In all cases		
Digestive disturbance	●		■			
Confusion	●			■		
Muscle weakness/cramps	●			■		
Rash	●			■	▲	
Dry mouth/thirst	●			■		

INTERACTIONS

Lithium Amiloride may increase the blood levels of lithium, leading to an increased risk of lithium poisoning.

ACE inhibitors, cyclosporin, and NSAIDs These drugs may increase the risk of potassium retention if taken with amiloride.

PROLONGED USE

Monitoring Blood tests may be carried out to monitor levels of body salts.

AMIODARONE

Brand name Amidox, Cordarone X
Used in the following combined preparations None

GENERAL INFORMATION

Introduced in the 1950s, amiodarone is used to treat a variety of abnormal heart rhythms (arrhythmias). It works by slowing nerve impulses in the heart muscle.

Amiodarone is given to prevent recurrent atrial and ventricular fibrillation and to treat ventricular and supraventricular tachycardias and Wolff-Parkinson-White Syndrome. The drug is often the last

choice, especially when used long term, because of serious *adverse effects* that include liver damage, thyroid problems, and damage to the eyes and lungs.

Treatment should be started only under specialist supervision or in hospital and the dosage carefully controlled in order to achieve the desired effect using the lowest possible dose.

INFORMATION FOR USERS

Your drug prescription is tailored for you. Do not alter dosage without checking with your doctor.

How taken

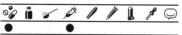

Tablets, injection.

Frequency and timing of doses
3 x daily or by injection initially, then reduced to twice daily, then once daily or every other day (maintenance dose).

Adult dosage range
600mg daily, reduced to 400mg, then 100–200mg daily.

Onset of effect
Taken by mouth, some effects may be noticed within 72 hours, but full benefits may not be felt for some weeks. Taken by injection, effects may be noticed within 30 minutes.

Duration of action
Up to 1 month.

Diet advice
None.

Storage
Keep in a closed container in a cool, dry place out of the reach of children. Protect from light.

Missed dose
Take as soon as you remember. If your next dose is due within 12 hours, do not take the missed dose. Take your next scheduled dose as usual.

Stopping the drug
Do not stop the drug without consulting your doctor; symptoms may recur.

Exceeding the dose
An occasional unintentional extra dose is unlikely to cause problems. But if you notice any unusual symptoms or if a large overdose has been taken, notify your doctor at once.

SPECIAL PRECAUTIONS

Be sure to tell your doctor if:
▼ You have long-term liver or kidney problems.
▼ You have heart disease.
▼ You have eye disease.
▼ You have a lung disorder such as asthma or bronchitis.
▼ You have a thyroid disorder.
▼ You are sensitive to iodine.
▼ You are taking other medications.

 Pregnancy
▼ Not prescribed. Discuss with your doctor.

 Breast-feeding
▼ The drug passes into the breast milk and may affect the baby. Discuss with your doctor.

 Infants and children
▼ Not recommended.

 Over 60
▼ Increased likelihood of adverse effects. Reduced dose necessary.

 Driving and hazardous work
▼ Avoid these activities until you have learned how amiodarone affects you because the drug can cause the eyes to be dazzled by bright light.

 Alcohol
▼ No known problems.

POSSIBLE ADVERSE EFFECTS

Amiodarone has a number of unusual side effects, including a metallic taste in the mouth, increased sensitivity of the skin to sunlight (photosensitivity), and a greyish skin colour.

Symptom/effect	Frequency		Discuss with doctor		Stop taking drug now	Call doctor now
	Common	Rare	Only if severe	In all cases		
Liver damage	●			■		
Photosensitivity	●			■		
Visual disturbances	●			■		
Thyroid problems		●		■		
Heart rate disturbances		●		■		
Numb, tingling extremities		●		■		
Shortness of breath/cough		●		■		
Headache/weakness/fatigue		●		■		
Grey skin colour		●		■		
Nausea/vomiting		●	■			

INTERACTIONS

General note Amiodarone can interact with many drugs. Consult your doctor or pharmacist before taking other medications.

Diuretics The potassium loss caused by these drugs may increase the *toxic* effects of amiodarone.

Other anti-arrhythmic drugs Amiodarone may increase the effects of drugs such as beta blockers, digoxin, diltiazem, or verapamil.

Warfarin Amiodarone may increase the anticoagulant effect of warfarin.

PROLONGED USE

Prolonged use of this drug may cause a number of adverse effects on the eyes, lungs, thyroid gland, and liver.

Monitoring A chest X-ray may be taken before treatment starts. Blood tests are done before treatment starts and then every 6 months to check thyroid and liver function. Regular eye examinations are required.

AMISULPRIDE/SULPIRIDE

Brand names Solian [amisulpride] Dolmatil, Sulparex, Sulpitil [sulpiride]
Used in the following combined preparations None

GENERAL INFORMATION

Amisulpride and sulpiride are antipsychotic drugs used to treat acute and chronic schizophrenia, in which there are "positive" symptoms such as delusions, hallucinations, and thought disorders) and/or "negative" symptoms such as emotional and social withdrawal. Higher doses are needed to control the positive symptoms; lower doses result in increased alertness and elevation of mood. Sulpiride has also been used in the treatment of Tourette's syndrome (an inherited neurological disorder), anxiety disorders, and vertigo.

An advantage of these antipsychotic drugs is that they are less likely than the older drugs to cause parkinsonism or *tardive dyskinesia*.

QUICK REFERENCE

Drug group Antipsychotic drug (p.85)

Overdose danger rating Medium

Dependence rating Low

Prescription needed Yes

Available as generic No

INFORMATION FOR USERS

Your drug prescription is tailored for you. Do not alter dosage without checking with your doctor.

How taken

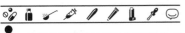

Tablets.

Frequency and timing of doses
1–2 x daily. (doses of up to 300mg may be 1 x daily).

Dosage range
Amisulpride 400–1,200mg daily.
Sulpiride 400–1,200mg daily (acute psychosis); 50–300mg daily (predominantly negative symptoms).

Onset of effect
1 hour.

Duration of action
12–24 hours.

Diet advice
None.

Storage
Keep in a closed container in a cool, dry place out of the reach of children.

Missed dose
Take as soon as you remember. If your next dose is due within 2 hours, take a single dose now and skip the next dose.

Stopping the drug
Do not stop taking the drug without consulting your doctor; symptoms may recur.

Exceeding the dose
An occasional unintentional extra dose is unlikely to cause problems. Large overdoses may cause drowsiness and low blood pressure. Notify your doctor immediately.

SPECIAL PRECAUTIONS

Be sure to tell your doctor if:
▼ You have liver or kidney problems.
▼ You have heart problems or hypertension.
▼ You have epilepsy.
▼ You have Parkinson's disease.
▼ You have phaeochromocytoma.
▼ You have a pituitary tumour or breast cancer.
▼ You have porphyria.
▼ You have had blood problems.
▼ You are taking other medications.

Pregnancy
▼ Safety not established. Discuss with your doctor.

Breast-feeding
▼ Safety not established. Discuss with your doctor.

Infants and children
▼ Not recommended.

Over 60
▼ Reduced dose may be necessary.

Driving and hazardous work
▼ Avoid. Amisulpride and sulpiride can slow reaction times and may occasionally cause drowsiness or loss of concentration.

Alcohol
▼ Avoid. Alcohol increases the sedative effects of these drugs.

POSSIBLE ADVERSE EFFECTS

Most of the *side effects* of antipsychotic drugs like amisulpride and sulpiride are mild; insomnia is the most common problem.

Symptom/effect	Frequency		Discuss with doctor		Stop taking drug now	Call doctor now
	Common	Rare	Only if severe	In all cases		
Sleep disturbances	●		■			
Drowsiness	●		■			
Anxiety/agitation		●	■			
Weight gain		●	■			
Nausea/vomiting		●	■			
Breast swelling		●		■		
Parkinsonism		●		■		
Palpitations/dizziness		●	■		▲	■

INTERACTIONS

Antihypertensive drugs Amisulpride and sulpiride may reduce the blood-pressure lowering effect of certain of these drugs.

Central nervous system depressants These drugs may all increase the sedative effects of amisulpride and sulpiride.

PROLONGED USE

An adverse effect called tardive dyskinesia, in which there are involuntary movements of the tongue and face, may rarely occur during long-term use.

AMITRIPTYLINE

Brand names Domical, Elavil, Lentizol, Tryptizol
Used in the following combined preparation Triptafen

GENERAL INFORMATION

Amitriptyline belongs to the class of antidepressant drugs known as the tricyclics. The drug is used mainly in the long-term treatment of depression. It elevates mood, increases physical activity, improves appetite, and restores interest in everyday activities.
 More sedating than similar drugs, amitriptyline is useful when depression is accompanied by anxiety or insomnia. Taken at night, the drug encourages sleep and helps to eliminate the need for additional sleeping drugs. This drug is sometimes used to treat nocturnal enuresis (bedwetting) in children.
 In overdose, amitriptyline may cause coma, fits, and abnormal heart rhythms.

INFORMATION FOR USERS

Your drug prescription is tailored for you. Do not alter dosage without checking with your doctor.

How taken

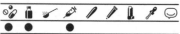

Tablets, SR-capsules, liquid, injection.

Frequency and timing of doses
1–4 x daily, often as a single dose at night.

Adult dosage range
50–150mg daily.

Onset of effect
Sedation can appear within hours, although full antidepressant effect may not be felt for 2–4 weeks.

Duration of action
Antidepressant effect may last for 6 weeks; adverse effects, only a few days.

Diet advice
None.

Storage
Keep in a closed container in a cool, dry place out of the reach of children. Protect from light.

Missed dose
Take as soon as you remember. If your next dose is due within 3 hours, take a single dose now and skip the next.

Stopping the drug
An abrupt stop can cause withdrawal symptoms and a recurrence of the original trouble. Consult your doctor, who may supervise a gradual reduction in dosage.

OVERDOSE ACTION

Seek immediate medical advice in all cases. Take emergency action if palpitations are noted or consciousness is lost.

See Drug poisoning emergency guide (p.494).

SPECIAL PRECAUTIONS

Be sure to tell your doctor if:
▼ You have heart problems.
▼ You have had epileptic fits.
▼ You have long-term liver or kidney problems.
▼ You have glaucoma.
▼ You have prostate trouble.
▼ You have thyroid disease.
▼ You have had mania or a psychotic illness.
▼ You are taking other medications.

Pregnancy
▼ Safety in pregnancy not established. Discuss with your doctor.

Breast-feeding
▼ The drug passes into the breast milk and may affect the baby. Discuss with your doctor.

Infants and children
▼ Not recommended under 16 years for depression, or under 6 years for enuresis.

Over 60
▼ Reduced dose may be necessary.

Driving and hazardous work
▼ Avoid such activities until you have learned how amitriptyline affects you because the drug may cause blurred vision and reduced alertness.

Alcohol
▼ Avoid. Alcohol may increase the sedative effects of this drug.

Surgery and general anaesthetics
▼ Amitriptyline treatment may need to be stopped before you have a general anaesthetic. Discuss this with your doctor or dentist before any operation.

POSSIBLE ADVERSE EFFECTS

The possible adverse effects of this drug are mainly the result of its *anticholinergic* action and its blocking action on the transmission of signals through the heart.

Symptom/effect	Frequency		Discuss with doctor		Stop taking drug now	Call doctor now
	Common	Rare	Only if severe	In all cases		
Drowsiness	●		■			
Sweating	●		■			
Dry mouth	●		■			
Blurred vision	●			■		
Dizziness/fainting	●			■		
Difficulty passing urine		●		■	▲	
Sore throat		●		■	▲	
Palpitations		●		■	▲	■

INTERACTIONS

Monoamine oxidase inhibitors (MAOIs) In the rare cases where these drugs are given with amitriptyline, there is a possibility of serious interactions.

Sedatives All drugs that have *sedative* effects intensify those of amitriptyline.

Antiarrhythmic drugs There is an increased risk of abnormal heart rhythms when these drugs are taken with amitriptyline.

Antiepileptics The effects of these drugs are reduced by amitriptyline.

PROLONGED USE

No problems expected.

AMLODIPINE

Brand name Istin
Used in the following combined preparations None

GENERAL INFORMATION

Amlodipine belongs to a group of drugs known as calcium channel blockers, which interfere with the conduction of signals in the muscles of the heart and blood vessels.

Amlodipine is used in the treatment of angina to help prevent attacks of chest pain. Unlike some other anti-angina drugs (such as beta blockers), it can be used safely by asthmatics and noninsulin-dependent diabetics. It is often successful when other treatments have failed. Amlodipine is also used to reduce raised blood pressure.

In common with other drugs of its class, amlodipine may cause blood pressure to fall too low at the start of treatment. In rare cases, angina may become worse at the start of amlodipine treatment. The drug may sometimes cause mild to moderate leg and ankle swelling.

QUICK REFERENCE

Drug group Anti-angina drug (p.101), antihypertensive drug (p.102)

Overdose danger rating Medium

Dependence rating Low

Prescription needed Yes

Available as generic No

INFORMATION FOR USERS

Your drug prescription is tailored for you. Do not alter dosage without checking with your doctor.

How taken

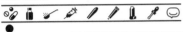

Tablets.

Frequency and timing of doses
Once daily.

Adult dosage range
5–10mg daily.

Onset of effect
6–12 hours.

Duration of action
24 hours.

Diet advice
None.

Storage
Keep in a closed container in a cool, dry place out of the reach of children.

Missed dose
If you miss a dose and you remember it within 12 hours, take it as soon as you remember. However, if you do not remember until later, do not take the missed dose at all and do not double up the next one. Instead, go back to your regular schedule.

Stopping the drug
Do not stop taking the drug without consulting your doctor; stopping the drug may lead to worsening of the underlying condition.

Exceeding the dose
An occasional unintentional extra dose is unlikely to cause problems. Large overdoses may cause a marked lowering of blood pressure. Notify your doctor immediately.

SPECIAL PRECAUTIONS

Be sure to tell your doctor if:
▼ You have long-term liver or kidney problems.
▼ You have heart failure.
▼ You have diabetes.
▼ You are taking other medications.

Pregnancy
▼ Safety in pregnancy not established. Discuss with your doctor.

Breast-feeding
▼ It is not known if the drug passes into the breast milk. Discuss with your doctor.

Infants and children
▼ Not recommended.

Over 60
▼ No special problems.

Driving and hazardous work
▼ Avoid such activities until you have learned how amlodipine affects you because the drug can cause dizziness owing to lowered blood pressure.

Alcohol
▼ Avoid. Alcohol may further reduce blood pressure, causing dizziness or other symptoms.

POSSIBLE ADVERSE EFFECTS

Amlodipine can cause a variety of minor *adverse effects*, including leg and ankle swelling, headache, dizziness, fatigue, and nausea. Dizziness, especially on rising, may be the result of an excessive reduction in blood pressure. The most serious effect is the rare possibility of angina becoming worse after starting amlodipine treatment. This should be reported to your doctor.

Symptom/effect	Frequency		Discuss with doctor		Stop taking drug now	Call doctor now
	Common	Rare	Only if severe	In all cases		
Leg and ankle swelling	●		■			
Headache	●		■			
Dizziness/fatigue	●		■			
Flushing	●		■			
Nausea/abdominal pain		●		■		
Palpitations		●		■		
Worsening of angina		●		■	▲	▮
Skin rash		●		■	▲	
Breathing difficulties		●		■	▲	

INTERACTIONS

Beta blockers Amlodipine may increase the effect of these drugs and vice versa.

Antidiabetic drugs These drugs may reduce the effect of amlodipine.

PROLONGED USE

No problems expected.

AMOXICILLIN

Brand names Almodan, Amix, Amoram, Amoxil, Galenamox, Rimoxallin
Used in the following combined preparations Augmentin, Co-amoxiclav

GENERAL INFORMATION

Amoxicillin is a penicillin antibiotic. It is prescribed to treat a variety of infections, but is particularly useful for treating ear, nose, and throat infections, respiratory tract infections, cystitis, uncomplicated gonorrhea, and certain skin and soft tissue infections. Taken by mouth, the drug is absorbed well by the body, and works quickly and effectively.

The most common *side effect* of this drug is a skin rash, which does not necessarily mean that the patient is allergic to penicillin. It can also provoke a more severe allergic reaction with fever, swelling of the mouth and tongue, itching, and breathing difficulties. This usually means that the patient is allergic to all penicillin antibiotics.

INFORMATION FOR USERS

Your drug prescription is tailored for you. Do not alter dosage without checking with your doctor.

How taken

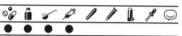

Tablets, capsules, liquid, powder (dissolved in water), injection

Frequency and timing of doses
Normally 3 x daily.

Dosage range
Adults 750mg–1.5g daily. In some cases a short course of up to 6g daily is given. A single dose of 3g may be given as a preventative. *Children* Reduced dose according to age and weight.

Onset of effect
1–2 hours.

Duration of action
Up to 8 hours.

Diet advice
None.

Storage
Keep in a closed container in a cool, dry place out of the reach of children.

Missed dose
Take as soon as you remember. Take your next dose at the scheduled time.

Stopping the drug
Take the full course. Even if you feel better, the original infection may still be present and symptoms may recur if treatment is stopped too soon.

Exceeding the dose
An occasional unintentional extra dose is unlikely to be a cause for concern. But if you notice any unusual symptoms, or if a large overdose has been taken, notify your doctor.

SPECIAL PRECAUTIONS

Be sure to tell your doctor if:
▼ You have a long-term kidney problem.
▼ You have an allergy (for example, asthma, hay fever, or eczema).
▼ You have had a previous allergic reaction to a penicillin or cephalosporin antibiotic.
▼ You have ulcerative colitis.
▼ You have glandular fever.
▼ You have chronic leukaemia.
▼ You are taking other medications.

Pregnancy
▼ No evidence of risk.

Breast-feeding
▼ The drug passes into the breast milk, but at normal doses adverse effects on the baby are unlikely. Discuss with your doctor.

Infants and children
▼ Reduced dose necessary.

Over 60
▼ No known problems.

Driving and hazardous work
▼ No known problems.

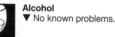

Alcohol
▼ No known problems.

POSSIBLE ADVERSE EFFECTS

If you develop a rash, wheezing, itching, fever, or joint swelling, this may indicate an allergy. Call your doctor, who may prescribe a different antibiotic.

Symptom/effect	Frequency		Discuss with doctor		Stop taking drug now	Call doctor now
	Common	Rare	Only if severe	In all cases		
Rash	●			■		
Diarrhoea	●			■		
Nausea/vomiting		●	■			
Wheezing		●		■	▲	▮
Itching		●		■	▲	▮
Swollen mouth/tongue		●		■	▲	▮

INTERACTIONS

Oral contraceptives Amoxicillin may reduce the effectiveness of the oral contraceptive pill and also increase the risk of breakthrough bleeding. Discuss with your doctor.

PROLONGED USE

Amoxicillin is usually given only for short courses of treatment.

AMPHOTERICIN

Brand names Abelcet, AmBisome, Amphocil, Fungilin, Fungizone
Used in the following combined preparations None

GENERAL INFORMATION

Amphotericin is a highly effective and powerful antifungal drug. When given by injection, it is used to treat serious *systemic* fungal infections. It is also given by mouth to treat candida (thrush) infections of the mouth or intestines, but it is not used in vaginal candidiasis. Treatment administered by injection is carefully supervised, usually in hospital, because of potentially serious *adverse effects*. A test dose for allergy may be given before a full injection. The new, recently introduced formulations of this drug appear to be less toxic than the original injection. Adverse reactions to the oral forms are rare.

INFORMATION FOR USERS

Your drug prescription is tailored for you. Do not alter dosage without checking with your doctor.

How taken

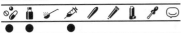

Tablets, lozenges, liquid, injection.

Frequency and timing of doses
Every 6 hours (by mouth); daily, usually over a 6-hour period (injection).

Dosage range
400–800mg daily (tablets and liquid); 40–80mg daily (lozenges); the dosage for injection is determined individually.

Onset of effect
Improvement may be noticed after 2–4 days.

Duration of action
3–6 hours.

Diet advice
When given by injection, this drug may reduce the levels of potassium and magnesium in the blood. To correct this, mineral supplements may be recommended.

Storage
Keep in a closed container in a cool, dry place out of the reach of children.

Missed dose
Take oral dose as soon as you remember. Take your next dose when scheduled.

Stopping the drug
Take the full course as prescribed, Even if symptoms improve, the original infection may still be present and symptoms may recur if treatment is stopped too soon.

Exceeding the dose
An occasional unintentional extra oral dose is unlikely to be a cause for concern. But if you notice unusual symptoms, notify your doctor.

SPECIAL PRECAUTIONS

Be sure to tell your doctor if:
▼ You have a long-term kidney problem.
▼ You have previously had an allergic reaction to amphotericin.
▼ You are taking other medications.

 Pregnancy
▼ There is no evidence of risk from the oral forms of the drug. Injections are given only when the infection very serious.

 Breast-feeding
▼ No evidence of risk from oral forms of the drug. It is not known whether the drug passes into the breast milk when given by injection. Discuss with your doctor.

 Infants and children
▼ Reduced dose may be necessary.

 Over 60
▼ No special problems.

 Driving and hazardous work
▼ No known problems.

 Alcohol
▼ No known problems.

POSSIBLE ADVERSE EFFECTS

Amphotericin is given by injection only under close medical supervision. Adverse effects are thus carefully monitored and promptly treated. Adverse effects from oral administration are rare.

Symptom/effect	Frequency		Discuss with doctor		Stop taking drug now	Call doctor now
	Common	Rare	Only if severe	In all cases		
Injection						
Pain at injection site	●			■		
Nausea/vomiting	●			■		
Headache/fever	●			■		
Unusual bleeding		●		■		
Muscle and joint pain		●		■		

INTERACTIONS (INJECTION ONLY)

Digitalis drugs Amphotericin may increase the *toxicity* of digoxin.

Diuretics Amphotericin increases the risk of low potassium levels with diuretics.

Aminoglycoside antibiotics Taken with amphotericin, these drugs increase the likelihood of kidney damage.

Corticosteroids may increase loss of potassium from the body caused by amphotericin.

Cyclosporin increases the likelihood of kidney damage.

PROLONGED USE

Given by injection, the drug may cause a reduction in blood levels of potassium and magnesium. It may also damage the kidneys and cause blood disorders.

Monitoring Regular blood tests to monitor liver and kidney function, blood cell counts, and potassium and magnesium levels are advised during treatment by injection.

ASPIRIN

Brand names Angettes, Aspro, Caprin, Disprin, Nu-Seals Aspirin, and others
Used in the following combined preparations Anadin, Aspav, Codis, Equagesic, Veganin, and others

GENERAL INFORMATION

In use for over 80 years, aspirin relieves pain, reduces fever, and alleviates the symptoms of arthritis. In low doses, it helps to prevent blood clots, particularly in atherosclerosis or angina due to coronary artery disease, and it reduces the risk of heart attacks and strokes.

It is present in many medicines for colds, flu, headaches, menstrual period pains, and joint or muscular aches.

Aspirin may irritate the stomach and even cause stomach ulcers or bleeding. It can also cause Reye's syndrome, a rare brain and liver disorder usually occurring in children. For this reason, aspirin should not be given to children under 12 except under close medical supervision. Another drawback of aspirin is that it can provoke asthma attacks.

INFORMATION FOR USERS

Follow instructions on the label. Call your doctor if symptoms worsen.

How taken

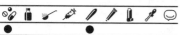

Tablets, SR-capsules, suppositories.

Frequency and timing of doses
Relief of pain or fever Every 4–6 hours, as necessary, with or after food or milk.
Prevention of blood clots Once daily.

Adult dosage range
Relief of pain or fever 300–900mg per dose.
Prevention of blood clots 75–300mg daily.

Onset of effect
30–60 minutes (regular aspirin);
1½–8 hours (coated tablets or SR-capsules).

Duration of action
Up to 12 hours. Effect persists for several days when used to prevent blood clotting.

Diet advice
None.

Storage
Keep in a closed container in a cool, dry place out of the reach of children.

Missed dose
Take as soon as you remember. If your next dose is due within 2 hours, take a single dose now and skip the next.

Stopping the drug
If you have been prescribed aspirin by your doctor for a long-term condition, you should seek medical advice before stopping the drug. Otherwise it can be safely stopped.

OVERDOSE ACTION

Seek immediate medical advice in all cases. Take emergency action if there is restlessness, stomach pain, ringing noises in the ears, blurred vision, or vomiting.

See Drug poisoning emergency guide (p.494).

SPECIAL PRECAUTIONS

Be sure to consult your doctor or pharmacist before taking this drug if:
▼ You have long-term liver or kidney problems.
▼ You have asthma.
▼ You are allergic to aspirin.
▼ You have a blood clotting disorder.
▼ You have had a stomach ulcer.
▼ You are taking other medications.

 Pregnancy
▼ Not usually recommended. An alternative drug may be safer. Discuss with your doctor.

 Breast-feeding
▼ The drug passes into the breast milk. Discuss with your doctor.

 Infants and children
▼ Not recommended under 12 years.

 Over 60
▼ Adverse effects more likely.

 Driving and hazardous work
▼ No special problems.

 Alcohol
▼ Avoid. Alcohol increases the likelihood of stomach irritation with this drug.

Surgery and general anaesthetics
▼ Regular treatment with aspirin may need to be stopped about one week before surgery. Discuss with your doctor or dentist before any operation.

POSSIBLE ADVERSE EFFECTS

Adverse effects are more likely to occur with high doses of aspirin, but may be reduced by taking the drug with food or in buffered or enteric coated forms.

Symptom/effect	Frequency		Discuss with doctor		Stop taking drug now	Call doctor now
	Common	Rare	Only if severe	In all cases		
Indigestion	●		■		▲	
Nausea/vomiting		●		■		
Rash		●		■	▲	
Breathlessness/wheezing		●		■	▲	
Blood in vomit/black faeces		●		■	▲	▮
Ringing in the ears/dizziness		●	■		▲	▮

INTERACTIONS

Anticoagulants Aspirin may add to the anticoagulant effect of such drugs, leading to an increased risk of abnormal bleeding.

Drugs for gout Aspirin may reduce the effect of these drugs.

Corticosteroids These drugs may increase the risk of stomach bleeding with aspirin.

NSAIDs These drugs may increase the likelihood of stomach irritation with aspirin.

Methotrexate Aspirin may increase the *toxicity* of this drug.

Oral antidiabetic drugs Aspirin may increase the effect of these drugs.

PROLONGED USE

Except for low doses to help prevent blood clotting, aspirin should not be taken for longer than 2 days except on your doctor's advice. Prolonged use of aspirin may lead to bleeding in the stomach and to stomach ulcers.

ATENOLOL

Brand names Antipressan, Atenix, Tenormin, Totamol
Used in the following combined preparations Beta-Adalat, Co-tenidone, Kalten, Tenchlor, Tenif, Tenoret, Tenoretic, Totaretic

GENERAL INFORMATION

Atenolol belongs to the group of drugs known as beta blockers. It prevents the heart from beating too quickly and is used mainly to treat irregular heart rhythms, angina, and high blood pressure.

Atenolol is a cardioselective beta blocker (see p.97) and is less likely to provoke breathing difficulties, but it should still be used with caution by people with asthma, bronchitis, or other forms of respiratory disease. Atenolol is sometimes prescribed with a diuretic for high blood pressure, and may also be given after a heart attack to protect the heart from further damage.

Atenolol does not cure heart disease, it only controls the symptoms, so it may have to be taken regularly over a long period, even for life.

QUICK REFERENCE

Drug group Beta blocker (p.97)
Overdose danger rating Medium
Dependence rating Low
Prescription needed Yes
Available as generic Yes

INFORMATION FOR USERS

Your drug prescription is tailored for you. Do not alter dosage without checking with your doctor.

How taken

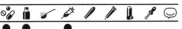

Tablets, liquid, injection.

Frequency and timing of doses
1–2 x daily.

Adult dosage range
25–100mg daily.

Onset of effect
2–4 hours.

Duration of action
20–30 hours.

Diet advice
None.

Storage
Keep in a tightly closed container in a cool, dry place out of the reach of children. Protect from light.

Missed dose
Take as soon as you remember. If your next dose is due within 6 hours, do not take the missed dose but take the next scheduled dose as usual.

Stopping the drug
Do not stop taking the drug without consulting your doctor; sudden withdrawal may lead to dangerous worsening of the underlying condition. It should be withdrawn gradually.

Exceeding the dose
An occasional unintentional extra dose is unlikely to be a cause for concern. But if you notice any unusual symptoms, or if a large overdose has been taken, notify your doctor.

SPECIAL PRECAUTIONS

Be sure to tell your doctor if:
▼ You have a long-term kidney problem.
▼ You have diabetes.
▼ You have a lung disorder such as asthma or bronchitis.
▼ You are taking other medications.

 Pregnancy
▼ Safety in pregnancy not established. Discuss with your doctor.

 Breast-feeding
▼ The drug passes into the breast milk. Discuss with your doctor.

 Infants and children
▼ Not recommended.

 Over 60
▼ No special problems. Reduced dose may be necessary if there is impaired kidney function.

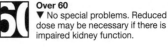 **Driving and hazardous work**
▼ Avoid such activities until you have learned how atenolol affects you because the drug can cause dizziness.

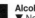 **Alcohol**
▼ No special problems with small intake.

Surgery and general anaesthetics
▼ Atenolol may need to be stopped before you have a general anaesthetic. Discuss this with your doctor or dentist before any surgery.

POSSIBLE ADVERSE EFFECTS

Atenolol has adverse effects that are common to most beta blockers. Symptoms are usually temporary and tend to diminish with long-term use.

Symptom/effect	Frequency		Discuss with doctor		Stop taking drug now	Call doctor now
	Common	Rare	Only if severe	In all cases		
Muscle ache	●		■			
Fatigue/dry eyes	●			■		
Cold hands and feet		●	■			
Nightmares/sleeplessness		●	■			
Headache		●		■		
Rash		●		■	▲	
Breathing difficulties		●		■	▲	■

INTERACTIONS

Anti-arrhythmic drugs When used together with atenolol they may increase the risk of adverse effects on the heart.

Antidiabetic drugs used with atenolol may increase the risk and/or mask many symptoms of low blood sugar.

Decongestants used with atenolol may increase blood pressure and heart rate.

Calcium channel blockers Taken with atenolol, some of these drugs may further decrease blood pressure and/or heart rate. They may also reduce the force of the heart's pumping action.

Non-steroidal anti-inflammatory drugs (NSAIDs) may reduce the antihypertensive effect of atenolol.

PROLONGED USE

No special problems expected.

ATORVASTATIN

Brand name Lipitor
Used in the following combined preparations None

GENERAL INFORMATION

Atorvastatin is a member of the statin group of lipid-lowering drugs. It is used to treat hypercholesterolaemia (high blood cholesterol levels) in patients who have not responded to other treatments, such as a special diet, and are at risk of developing heart disease.

Atorvastatin blocks the action, in the liver, of an enzyme that is needed for the manufacture of cholesterol. As a result, blood levels of cholesterol are lowered, which can help to prevent coronary heart disease.

Rarely, atorvastatin can cause muscle pain, inflammation, and muscle damage. The risk is increased if the drug is given with a fibrate (another kind of lipid-lowering drug).

INFORMATION FOR USERS

Your drug prescription is tailored for you. Do not alter dosage without checking with your doctor.

How taken

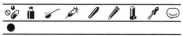

Tablets.

Frequency and timing of doses
Once daily.

Adult dosage range
10–40mg; up to 80mg (inherited hypercholesterolaemia).

Onset of effect
Within 2 weeks. Full beneficial effects may not be felt for 4–6 weeks.

Duration of action
20–30 hours.

Diet advice
A low-fat diet is usually recommended.

Storage
Keep in a closed container in a cool, dry place out of the reach of children.

Missed dose
Take as soon as you remember. If your next dose is due within 8 hours, do not take the missed dose, but take the next one on schedule.

Stopping the drug
Do not stop taking the drug without consulting your doctor. Stopping the drug may lead to a recurrence of the original condition.

Exceeding the dose
An occasional unintentional extra dose is unlikely to cause problems. Large overdoses may cause liver problems. Notify your doctor.

SPECIAL PRECAUTIONS

Be sure to tell your doctor if:
▼ You have had liver problems.
▼ You are a heavy drinker.
▼ You are taking other medications.

Pregnancy
▼ Not usually prescribed. Safety not established. Discuss with your doctor.

Breast-feeding
▼ Safety not established. Discuss with your doctor.

Infants and children
▼ Not recommended.

Over 60
▼ No special problems.

Driving and hazardous work
▼ No special problems.

Alcohol
▼ Avoid excessive amounts. Alcohol may increase the risk of developing liver problems with atorvastatin.

POSSIBLE ADVERSE EFFECTS

Adverse effects of atorvastatin are usually mild and transient. Muscle damage is a rare side effect and muscle aching or weakness should be reported to your doctor at once.

Symptom/effect	Frequency		Discuss with doctor		Stop taking drug now	Call doctor now
	Common	Rare	Only if severe	In all cases		
Nausea	●		■			
Headache	●		■			
Skin rash		●		■	▲	
Muscle pain/weakness		●		■	▲	■
Jaundice		●		■		
Impotence		●		■		
Insomnia		●	■			

PROLONGED USE

Long-term use of atorvastatin can affect liver function.

Monitoring Regular blood tests to check liver and muscle function are needed.

INTERACTIONS

Anticoagulant drugs Atorvastatin may increase the effect of anticoagulants.

Antifungal drugs Itraconazole, ketoconazole, and possibly other antifungals, may increase the risk of muscle damage with atorvastatin.

Other lipid-lowering drugs Taken with atorvastatin, these drugs may increase the risk of muscle damage.

Cyclosporin and other immuno-suppressant drugs Atorvastatin is not usually prescribed with these drugs because of the increased risk of muscle damage.

ATROPINE

Brand name Minims Atropine
Used in the following combined preparations Actonorm, Co-phenotrope, Isopto Atropine, Lomotil

GENERAL INFORMATION

Atropine is an *anticholinergic* drug. Because of its *antispasmodic* action, which relaxes the muscle wall of the intestine, the drug has been used to relieve abdominal cramps in irritable bowel syndrome. Atropine may also be prescribed in combination with diphenoxylate, an antidiarrhoeal drug. However, this combination can be dangerous in overdosage, particularly in young children.

Atropine eye drops, used to enlarge the pupil during eye examinations, are part of the treatment for uveitis.

Atropine may be used as part of the *premedication* before a general anaesthetic. It is occasionally injected to restore normal heart beat in heart block (p.100).

Atropine must be used with caution in children and the elderly due to their sensitivity to the drug's effects.

QUICK REFERENCE

Drug group Anticholinergic drug for irritable bowel syndrome (p.110) and mydriatic drug (p.170)

Overdose danger rating High

Dependence rating Low

Prescription needed Yes

Available as generic Yes

INFORMATION FOR USERS

Your drug prescription is tailored for you. Do not alter dosage without checking with your doctor.

How taken

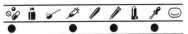

Tablets, injection, eye ointment, eye drops.

Frequency and timing of doses
Once only, or up to 4 times daily according to condition (eye drops); as directed (other forms).

Adult dosage range
1–2 drops as directed (eye drops); as directed (other forms).

Onset of effect
Varies according to method of administration. 30 minutes (eye drops).

Duration of action
7 days or longer (eye drops); several hours (other forms).

Diet advice
None.

Storage
Keep in a closed container in a cool, dry place out of the reach of children. Protect from light.

Missed dose
Take as soon as you remember. If your next dose is due within 2 hours, take a single dose now and skip the next.

Stopping the drug
Do not stop the drug without consulting your doctor.

OVERDOSE ACTION

 Seek immediate medical advice in all cases. Take emergency action if palpitations, tremor, delirium, fits, or loss of consciousness occur.

See Drug poisoning emergency guide (p.494).

POSSIBLE ADVERSE EFFECTS

The use of this drug is limited by the frequency of anticholinergic effects.

In addition to these effects, atropine eye drops may cause stinging.

Symptom/effect	Frequency		Discuss with doctor		Stop taking drug now	Call doctor now
	Common	Rare	Only if severe	In all cases		
Blurred vision/dry mouth/thirst	●		■			
Constipation	●		■			
Flushing/dry skin	●			■		
Difficulty in passing urine		●		■		
Eye pain and irritation		●		■	▲	▌
Palpitations/confusion		●		■	▲	▌
Contact rash		●		■	▲	

INTERACTIONS

Anticholinergic drugs Atropine increases the risk of *side effects* from drugs that also have anticholinergic effects.

Ketoconazole Atropine reduces the absorption of this drug from the digestive tract. Increased dose may be necessary.

SPECIAL PRECAUTIONS

Be sure to tell your doctor if:
▼ You have long-term liver or kidney problems.
▼ You have glaucoma.
▼ You have urinary difficulties.
▼ You have myasthenia gravis.
▼ You have ulcerative colitis.
▼ You wear contact lenses (eye drops).
▼ You have heart problems or high blood pressure.
▼ You are taking other medications.

 Pregnancy
▼ Safety in pregnancy not established. Discuss with your doctor.

 Breast-feeding
▼ The drug passes into the breast milk and may affect the baby. Discuss with your doctor.

 Infants and children
▼ Combination with diphenoxylate not recommended under 4 years; reduced dose necessary in older children.

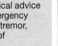 **Over 60**
▼ Increased likelihood of adverse effects.

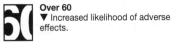 **Driving and hazardous work**
▼ Avoid such activities until you have learned hoeal atropine affects you because the drug can cause blurred vision and may impair concentration.

 Alcohol
▼ Avoid. Alcohol increases the likelihood of confusion when taken with atropine.

PROLONGED USE

No problems expected.

AZATHIOPRINE

Brand names Azamune, Immunoprin, Imuran, Oprisine
Used in the following combined preparations None

GENERAL INFORMATION

Azathioprine is an immunosuppressant drug used to prevent immune system rejection of transplanted organs. The drug is also given for severe rheumatoid arthritis that has failed to respond to conventional drug therapy.

Autoimmune and collagen diseases (including polymyositis, systemic lupus erythematosus, myasthenia gravis, and dermatomyositis) may be treated with azathioprine, usually when corticosteroids have not been effective.

Azathioprine is administered only under close supervision because of the risk of serious *adverse effects*. These include suppression of the production of white blood cells, thereby increasing the risk of infection as well as the risk of excessive or prolonged bleeding.

QUICK REFERENCE

Drug group Antirheumatic drug (p.117) and immunosuppressant drug (p.156)

Overdose danger rating Medium

Dependence rating Low

Prescription needed Yes

Available as generic Yes

INFORMATION FOR USERS

Your drug prescription is tailored for you. Do not alter dosage without checking with your doctor.

How taken

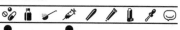

Tablets, injection.

Frequency and timing of doses
Usually once daily with or after food.

Dosage range
Initially according to body weight and the condition being treated and then adjusted according to response.

Onset of effect
2–4 weeks. Antirheumatic effect may not be felt for 8 weeks or more.

Duration of action
Immunosuppressant effects may last for several weeks after the drug is stopped.

Diet advice
None.

Storage
Keep in a closed container in a cool, dry place out of the reach of children. Protect from light.

Missed dose
Take as soon as you remember, then return to your normal schedule. If more than 2 doses are missed, consult your doctor.

Stopping the drug
Do not stop the drug without consulting your doctor. If taken to prevent graft transplant rejection, stopping treatment could provoke the rejection of the transplant.

Exceeding the dose
An occasional unintentional extra dose is unlikely to cause problems. Large overdoses may cause nausea, vomiting, abdominal pains, and diarrhoea. Notify your doctor.

SPECIAL PRECAUTIONS

Be sure to tell your doctor if:
▼ You have long-term liver or kidney problems.
▼ You have had a previous allergic reaction to azathioprine or 6-mercaptopurine.
▼ You have recently had shingles or chickenpox.
▼ You have an infection.
▼ You have a blood disorder.
▼ You are taking other medications.

 Pregnancy
▼ Azathioprine has been taken in pregnancy without problems. Discuss with your doctor.

 Breast-feeding
▼ A small amount of the drug passes into the breast milk. Discuss with your doctor.

 Infants and children
▼ No special problems.

 Over 60
▼ Increased likelihood of adverse effects. Reduced dose necessary.

 Driving and hazardous work
▼ Avoid such activities until you have learned how azathioprine affects you because the drug can cause dizziness.

 Alcohol
▼ No known problems.

POSSIBLE ADVERSE EFFECTS

Digestive disturbances and adverse effects on the blood which could lead to sore throat, fever, and weakness are common with azathioprine. Unusual bleeding or bruising while taking this drug may be a sign of reduced levels of platelets in the blood.

Symptom/effect	Frequency		Discuss with physician		Stop taking drug now	Call physician now
	Common	Rare	Only if severe	In all cases		
Nausea/vomiting	●		■			
Hair loss	●		■			
Loss of appetite	●			■		
Weakness/fatigue		●		■		
Unusual bleeding/bruising		●		■		▮
Jaundice		●		■		▮
Rash		●		■		▮
Fever/chills		●		■		▮
Pain in the side/urinary difficulty		●		■		▮

PROLONGED USE

There may be a slightly increased risk of some cancers with long-term use of azathioprine. Blood changes may also occur. Avoidance of exposure to sunlight may help to prevent adverse skin effects.

Monitoring Regular checks on blood composition are usually carried out.

INTERACTIONS

Allopurinol Azathioprine increases the effects and *toxicity* of allopurinol; dosage of allopurinol will need to be reduced.

Warfarin Azathioprine may reduce the effect of warfarin.

Co-trimoxazole and trimethoprim These drugs may increase the risk of blood problems if taken with azathioprine.

BACLOFEN

Brand names Baclospas, Balgifen, Lioresal
Used in the following combined preparations None

GENERAL INFORMATION

Baclofen is a muscle-relaxant drug that acts on the central nervous system, including the spinal cord. The drug relieves the spasms, cramping, and rigidity of muscles caused by a variety of disorders, including multiple sclerosis and spinal cord injury. Baclofen is also used to treat the spasticity that results from brain injury, cerebral palsy, or stroke. Although this drug does not cure any of these disorders, it increases mobility, allowing other treatment, such as physiotherapy, to be carried out.

Baclofen is less likely to cause muscle weakness than similar drugs, and its *side effects*, such as dizziness or drowsiness, are usually temporary. Elderly people are more susceptible to side effects, especially during early stages of treatment.

QUICK REFERENCE

Drug group Muscle-relaxant drug (p.120)

Overdose danger rating Medium

Dependence rating Low

Prescription needed Yes

Available as generic Yes

INFORMATION FOR USERS

Your drug prescription is tailored for you. Do not alter dosage without checking with your doctor.

How taken

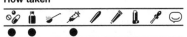

Tablets, liquid, injection (specialist use).

Frequency and timing of doses
3 x daily with food or milk.

Adult dosage range
15mg daily (starting dose). Daily dose may be increased by 15mg every 3 days as necessary. Maximum daily dose: 100mg.

Onset of effect
Some benefits may appear after 1–3 hours, but full beneficial effects may not be felt for several weeks. A dose 1 hour before a specific task will improve mobility.

Duration of action
Up to 8 hours.

Diet advice
None.

Storage
Keep in a closed container in a cool, dry place out of the reach of children. Protect liquid from light.

Missed dose
Take as soon as you remember. If your next dose is due within 2 hours, take a single dose now and skip the next.

Stopping the drug
Do not stop taking the drug without consulting your doctor who will supervise a gradual reduction in dosage. Abrupt cessation may cause hallucinations, fits, and worsening spasticity.

Exceeding the dose
An occasional unintentional extra dose is unlikely to cause problems. Large overdoses may cause weakness, vomiting, and severe drowsiness. Notify your doctor.

SPECIAL PRECAUTIONS

Be sure to tell your doctor if:
▼ You have long-term liver or kidney problems.
▼ You have difficulty in passing urine.
▼ You have had a peptic ulcer.
▼ You have had epileptic fits.
▼ You have diabetes.
▼ You suffer with breathing problems.
▼ You are taking other medications.

Pregnancy
▼ Safety in pregnancy not established. Discuss with your doctor.

Breast-feeding
▼ The drug passes into the breast milk, but at normal doses adverse effects are unlikely. Discuss with your doctor.

Infants and children
▼ Reduced dose necessary.

Over 60
▼ Increased likelihood of adverse effects. Reduced dose may therefore be necessary.

Driving and hazardous work
▼ Avoid such activities until you have learned how baclofen affects you because the drug can cause drowsiness.

Alcohol
▼ Avoid. Alcohol may increase the sedative effects of this drug.

Surgery and general anaesthetics
▼ Be sure to inform your doctor or dentist that you are taking baclofen before you have a general anaesthetic.

POSSIBLE ADVERSE EFFECTS

The common *adverse effects* are related to the sedative effects of the drug. Such effects are minimized by starting with a low dose that is gradually increased.

Symptom/effect	Frequency		Discuss with physician		Stop taking drug now	Call physician now
	Common	Rare	Only if severe	In all cases		
Dizziness	●		■			
Drowsiness	●		■			
Nausea	●		■			
Constipation/diarrhoea		●	■			
Headache		●	■			
Confusion		●		■		
Muscle fatigue/weakness		●		■		
Difficulty in passing urine		●		■		

INTERACTIONS

Antihypertensive and diuretic drugs Baclofen may increase the blood-pressure lowering effect of such drugs.

Drugs for *parkinsonism* Some drugs used for parkinsonism may cause confusion and hallucinations if taken with baclofen.

Sedatives All drugs with a sedative effect on the central nervous system may increase the sedative properties of baclofen.

Tricyclic antidepressants may increase the effects of baclofen, leading to muscle weakness.

PROLONGED USE

No problems expected.

BECLOMETASONE

Brand names Beclazone, Becloforte, Becodisks, Beconase, Becotide, Filair, Qvar, and others
Used in the following combined preparation Ventide

GENERAL INFORMATION

Beclometasone is a corticosteroid drug prescribed to relieve the symptoms of allergic rhinitis (as a nasal spray) and to control asthma (as an inhalant). It controls nasal symptoms by reducing inflammation and mucus production in the nose. It also helps to reduce chest symptoms, such as wheezing and coughing. Asthma sufferers may take it regularly to reduce the severity and frequency of attacks. However, once an attack has started, the drug does not relieve symptoms.

Beclometasone is given primarily to people whose asthma has not responded to bronchodilators alone (p.92). Beclometasone is also used as the main ingredient in some skin creams and ointments but is not usually used on the face.

There are few serious *adverse effects* associated with beclometasone as it is given *topically* by nasal spray or inhaler. Fungal infections causing irritation of the mouth and throat are a possible *side effect* of inhaling beclometasone. These can be avoided to some degree by rinsing the mouth and gargling with water after each inhalation.

INFORMATION FOR USERS

Your drug prescription is tailored for you. Do not alter dosage without checking with your doctor.

How taken

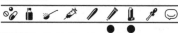

Cream, ointment, inhaler, nasal spray.

Frequency and timing of doses
2–4 x daily.

Dosage range
Adults 1–2 puffs 3–4 x daily according to preparation used (asthma); 1–2 sprays in each nostril 2–4 x daily (allergic rhinitis); as directed (skin conditions).
Children Reduced dose according to age and weight.

Onset of effect
Within 1 week (asthma); 1–3 days (allergic rhinitis). Full benefit may not be felt for up to 4 weeks.

Duration of action
Several days after stopping the drug.

Diet advice
None.

Storage
Keep in a closed container in a cool, dry place out of the reach of children. Protect from light.

Missed dose
Take as soon as you remember. If your next dose is due within 2 hours, take a single dose now and skip the next.

Stopping the drug
Do not stop the drug without consulting your doctor; symptoms may recur. Sometimes a gradual reduction in dosage is recommended.

Exceeding the dose
An occasional unintentional extra dose is unlikely to cause problems. But if you notice any unusual symptoms, or if a large overdose has been taken, notify your doctor. Adverse effects may occur if the recommended dose is regularly exceeded over a prolonged period.

SPECIAL PRECAUTIONS

Be sure to tell your doctor if:
▼ You have had tuberculosis or another nasal or respiratory infection.
▼ You have a skin infection (cream/ointment).
▼ You have varicose ulcers (cream/ointment).
▼ You are taking other medications.

Pregnancy
▼ No evidence of risk.

Breast-feeding
▼ No evidence of risk.

Infants and children
▼ Reduced dose necessary. Avoid prolonged use of ointment in infants and children.

Over 60
▼ No known problems.

Driving and hazardous work
▼ No known problems.

Alcohol
▼ No known problems.

POSSIBLE ADVERSE EFFECTS

The main side effects of the nasal spray and inhaler are irritation of the nasal passages and fungal infection of the throat and mouth. More serious side effects, such as permanent skin changes, may be seen with the ointment, which should not normally be used on the face.

Symptom/effect	Frequency		Discuss with physician		Stop taking drug now	Call physician now
	Common	Rare	Only if severe	In all cases		
Inhaler/nasal spray						
Nasal discomfort/irritation	●		■			
Cough	●		■			
Sore throat/hoarseness	●			■		
Nosebleed	●			■		
Cream/ointment						
Skin changes		●		■		

PROLONGED USE

No problems expected when used for asthma or rhinitis, but high doses of nasal spray can give systemic effects. Prolonged use of cream or ointment should be avoided where possible because it can cause permanent skin changes, especially on the face, and high doses can suppress the body's own corticosteroid production.

Monitoring Periodic checks to ensure that the adrenal glands are functioning healthily may be required if large doses are being used.

INTERACTIONS

None.

BENDROFLUMETHIAZIDE (BENDROFLUAZIDE)

Brand names Aprinox, Berkozide, Neo-Bendromax, Neo-NaClex
Used in the following combined preparations Corgaretic, Inderetic, Inderex, Neo-NaClex-K, Prestim

GENERAL INFORMATION

Bendroflumethiazide belongs to the group of drugs known as the thiazide diuretics, which expel water from the body. It is useful for reducing oedema (water retention) caused by heart conditions, and for treating premenstrual oedema. The drug is frequently used as a treatment for high blood pressure (see Antihypertensive drugs, p.102).

As with all thiazides, this drug increases the loss of potassium in the urine, which can cause a variety of symptoms (see p.99), and increases the likelihood of irregular heart rhythms, particularly if you are taking drugs such as digoxin for heart failure. Potassium supplements are often given with bendroflumethiazide to counteract this effect.

INFORMATION FOR USERS

Your prescription is tailored for you. Do not alter dosage without checking with your doctor.

How taken

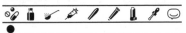

Tablets.

Frequency and timing of doses
Once daily, early in the day. (Sometimes 1–3 x per week.)

Adult dosage range
2.5–10mg daily.

Onset of effect
Within 2 hours.

Duration of action
6–12 hours.

Diet advice
Use of this drug may reduce potassium in the body, so you should eat plenty of fresh fruit and vegetables. Discuss with your doctor the advisability of reducing salt intake as a further precaution for hypertension.

Storage
Keep in a closed container in a cool, dry place out of the reach of children.

Missed dose
No cause for concern, but take as soon as you remember. However, if it is late in the day do not take the missed dose, or you may need to get up during the night to pass urine. Take the next scheduled dose as usual.

Stopping the drug
Do not stop taking the drug without consulting your doctor; symptoms may recur.

Exceeding the dose
An occasional unintentional extra dose is unlikely to be a cause for concern. But if you notice any unusual symptoms, or if a large overdose has been taken, notify your doctor.

SPECIAL PRECAUTIONS

Be sure to tell your doctor if:
▼ You have long-term liver or kidney problems.
▼ You have had gout.
▼ You have diabetes.
▼ You have Addison's disease.
▼ You have systemic lupus erythematosus (SLE)
▼ You are taking other medications.

 Pregnancy
▼ Not usually prescribed. Safety in pregnancy not established. May affect the baby adversely. Discuss with your doctor.

 Breast-feeding
▼ The drug passes into the breast milk and may reduce your milk supply. Discuss with your doctor.

 Infants and children
▼ Not usually prescribed. Reduced dose necessary.

 Over 60
▼ Reduced dose may be necessary.

 Driving and hazardous work
▼ No special problems.

 Alcohol
▼ No problems expected if consumption is kept low.

POSSIBLE ADVERSE EFFECTS

Some adverse effects result from excessive loss of potassium, and these can usually be corrected by taking a potassium supplement. Bendroflumethiazide may precipitate gout in people who are susceptible, and certain forms of diabetes may become more difficult to control. The blood cholesterol level may rise.

Symptom/effect	Frequency		Discuss with doctor		Stop taking drug now	Call doctor now
	Common	Rare	Only if severe	In all cases		
Nausea		●	■			
Lethargy/fatigue		●	■			
Leg cramps		●	■			
Impotence		●		■		
Rash		●		■	▲	

INTERACTIONS

Non-steroidal anti-inflammatory drugs (NSAIDs) may reduce the diuretic effect of bendroflumethiazide, which, conversely, may increase kidney *toxicity* of NSAIDs.

Digoxin The effects of digoxin may be increased if excessive potassium is lost.

Terfenadine Low potassium levels increase the risk of irregular heart beat when bendroflumethiazide is taken with this antihistamine.

Anti-arrhythmic drugs Low potassium levels may increase the toxicity of these drugs.

Lithium Bendroflumethiazide may increase lithium levels in the blood.

Corticosteroids These drugs further increase the loss of potassium from the body when taken with bendroflumethiazide. Potassium supplements may be necessary.

PROLONGED USE

Prolonged use of this drug can lead to excessive loss of potassium and imbalances of other salts.

Monitoring Blood tests may be performed periodically to check kidney function and levels of potassium and other salts.

BENZOYL PEROXIDE

Brand names Acnecide, Nericur, Panoxyl
Used in the following combined preparations Acnidazil, Benzamycin, Quinoderm, Quinoped

GENERAL INFORMATION

Benzoyl peroxide is used in a variety of *topical* preparations for the treatment of acne and some fungal skin infections, particularly of the feet. Available over the counter, it comes in concentrations of varying strengths for moderate acne.

Benzoyl peroxide works by removing the top layer of skin and unblocking the sebaceous glands. The drug reduces inflammation of blocked hair follicles by killing bacteria that infect them.

Benzoyl peroxide may cause irritation due to its drying effect on the skin, but this generally diminishes with time. The drug should be applied to the affected areas as directed on the label. Washing the area prior to application greatly enhances the drug's beneficial effects. *Side effects* are less likely if treatment is started with a preparation containing a low concentration of benzoyl peroxide, and changed to a stronger preparation only if necessary. Marked dryness and peeling of the skin, which may occur, can usually be controlled by reducing the frequency of application. Care should be taken to avoid contact of the drug with the eyes, mouth, and mucous membranes. Preparations of benzoyl peroxide may bleach clothing.

QUICK REFERENCE

Drug group Drug for acne (p.177) and fungal skin infections (p.138)
Overdose danger rating Low
Dependence rating Low
Prescription needed No
Available as generic No

INFORMATION FOR USERS

Follow instructions on the label. Call your doctor if symptoms worsen.

How taken

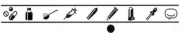

Cream, lotion, gel.

Frequency and timing of doses
1–2 x daily.

Dosage range
Apply sparingly to affected skin, as instructed on the label.

Onset of effect
Reduces oiliness of skin immediately. Acne usually improves within 4–6 weeks.

Duration of action
24–48 hours.

Diet advice
None.

Storage
Keep in a closed container in a cool, dry place out of the reach of children.

Missed dose
Apply as soon as you remember.

Stopping the drug
Can be safely stopped as soon as you no longer need it.

Exceeding the dose
A single extra application is unlikely to cause problems. Regular overuse may result in extensive irritation, peeling, redness, and swelling.

POSSIBLE ADVERSE EFFECTS

Application of benzoyl peroxide may cause temporary burning or stinging of the skin. Redness, peeling, and swelling may result from excessive drying of the skin and usually clears up if the treatment is stopped or used less frequently. If severe burning, blistering, or crusting occur, stop using benzoyl peroxide and consult your doctor.

Symptom/effect	Frequency		Discuss with doctor		Stop taking drug now	Call doctor now
	Common	Rare	Only if severe	In all cases		
Skin irritation	●		■			
Dryness/peeling	●		■			
Stinging/redness	●		■			
Blistering/crusting/swelling		●		■	▲	▮

INTERACTIONS

Skin-drying preparations Medicated cosmetics, soaps, toiletries, and other anti-acne preparations increase the likelihood of dryness and irritation of the skin with benzoyl peroxide.

SPECIAL PRECAUTIONS

Be sure to consult your doctor or pharmacist before using this drug if:
▼ You have eczema.
▼ You have sunburn.
▼ You have had a previous allergic reaction to benzoyl peroxide.
▼ You are taking other medications.

Pregnancy
▼ No evidence of risk.

Breast-feeding
▼ No evidence of risk.

Infants and children
▼ Not recommended under 12 years except under medical supervision.

Over 60
▼ Not usually required.

Driving and hazardous work
▼ No known problems.

Alcohol
▼ No known problems.

PROLONGED USE

Benzoyl peroxide should not be used for longer than 6 weeks except on the advice of your doctor.

BETAHISTINE

Brand name Serc
Used in the following combined preparations None

GENERAL INFORMATION

Betahistine, a drug that resembles the naturally occurring substance histamine in some of its effects, was introduced in the 1970s as a treatment for Ménière's disease, which is caused by the pressure of excess fluid in the inner ear.

Taken regularly, betahistine reduces both the frequency and the severity of the nausea and vertigo attacks that characterize this condition. It is also effective in treating tinnitus (ringing in the ears). Betahistine is thought to work by reducing pressure in the inner ear, possibly by improving blood flow in the small blood vessels. Drug treatment is not successful in all cases, however, and surgery may be needed.

INFORMATION FOR USERS

Your drug prescription is tailored for you. Do not alter dosage without checking with your doctor.

How taken

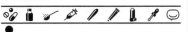

Tablets.

Frequency and timing of doses
3 x daily after food.

Adult dosage range
24–48mg daily.

Onset of effect
Within 1 hour.

Duration of action
6–12 hours.

Diet advice
None.

Storage
Keep in a closed container in a cool, dry place out of the reach of children.

Missed dose
Take as soon as you remember. If your next dose is due within 2 hours, take a single dose now and skip the next.

Stopping the drug
Do not stop the drug without consulting your doctor; symptoms may recur.

OVERDOSE ACTION

 Seek immediate medical advice in all cases. Large overdoses may cause collapse requiring emergency action.

See Drug poisoning emergency guide, p.494.

POSSIBLE ADVERSE EFFECTS

Adverse effects from betahistine are minor and rarely cause problems.

Symptom/effect	Frequency		Discuss with doctor		Stop taking drug now	Call doctor now
	Common	Rare	Only if severe	In all cases		
Nausea	●		■			
Indigestion	●		■			
Headache		●	■			
Rash		●		■		

INTERACTIONS

None.

SPECIAL PRECAUTIONS

Be sure to tell your doctor if:
▼ You have asthma.
▼ You have a peptic ulcer.
▼ You have phaeochromocytoma.
▼ You are taking other medications.

 Pregnancy
▼ Safety in pregnancy not established. Discuss with your doctor.

 Breast-feeding
▼ The drug passes into the breast milk, but at normal doses adverse effects on the baby are unlikely. Discuss with your doctor.

 Infants and children
▼ Not recommended.

 Over 60
No special problems.

 Driving and hazardous work
▼ No special problems.

Alcohol
▼ No special problems.

PROLONGED USE

No special problems.

BETAMETHASONE

Brand names Betacap, Betnelan, Betnesol, Betnovate, Bettamousse, Diprosone, Vista-Methasone
Used in the following combined preparations Betnesol-N, Betnovate-C, Betnovate-N, Diprosalic, Fucibet, Lotriderm

GENERAL INFORMATION

Betamethasone is a corticosteroid drug used to treat a variety of conditions. When injected directly into the joints it relieves joint inflammation and the pain and stiffness of rheumatoid arthritis. It is also given by mouth or injection to treat certain endocrine conditions affecting the pituitary and adrenal glands, and some blood disorders. It is also used *topically* to treat skin complaints, such as eczema and psoriasis.

When taken for short periods, low or moderate doses of betamethasone rarely cause serious *side effects*. High dosages or prolonged use can lead to symptoms such as peptic ulcers, weak bones, muscle weakness, and thin skin, and may retard growth in children.

QUICK REFERENCE

Drug group Corticosteroid (p.141)
Overdose danger rating Low
Dependence rating Low
Prescription needed Yes
Available as generic Yes

INFORMATION FOR USERS

Your drug prescription is tailored for you. Do not alter dosage without checking with your doctor.

How taken

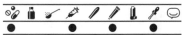

Tablets, injection, cream, ointment, lotion, scalp solution, eye ointment, eye/ear/nose drops.

Frequency and timing of doses
Usually once daily in the morning (*systemic*). Otherwise varies according to disorder being treated.

Dosage range
Varies; follow your doctor's instructions.

Onset of effect
Within 30 minutes (injection); within 48 hours (other forms).

Duration of action
Up to 24 hours.

Diet advice
A low-sodium and high-potassium diet may be recommended when the oral form of the drug is prescribed for extended periods. Follow the advice of your doctor.

Storage
Keep in a closed container in a cool, dry place out of the reach of children. Protect from light.

Missed dose
Take as soon as you remember. If your next dose is due within 2 hours, take a single dose now and skip the next.

Stopping the drug
Do not stop tablets without consulting your doctor, who may supervise a gradual reduction in dosage. Abrupt cessation after long-term treatment may cause problems with the pituitary and adrenal gland system.

Exceeding the dose
An occasional unintentional extra dose is unlikely to cause problems. But if you notice any unusual symptoms, or if a large overdose has been taken, notify your doctor.

SPECIAL PRECAUTIONS

Be sure to tell your doctor if:
▼ You suffer from a mental disorder.
▼ You have a heart condition.
▼ You have glaucoma.
▼ You have high blood pressure.
▼ You have a history of epilepsy.
▼ You have had a peptic ulcer.
▼ You have had tuberculosis.
▼ You have any infection.
▼ You have diabetes.
▼ You have liver or kidney problems.
▼ You are taking other medications.

Avoid exposure to chickenpox, measles, or shingles if you are on systemic treatment.

Pregnancy
▼ No evidence of risk with topical preparations. Taken as tablets in low doses, harm to the baby is unlikely. Discuss with your doctor.

Breast-feeding
▼ No evidence of risk with topical preparations. Taken by mouth in normal doses, the drug is unlikely to have adverse effects on the baby. Discuss with your doctor.

Infants and children
▼ Reduced dose necessary.

Over 60
▼ Reduced dose may be necessary.

Driving and hazardous work
▼ No known problems.

Alcohol
▼ Keep consumption low. Betamethasone tablets increase the risk of peptic ulcers.

POSSIBLE ADVERSE EFFECTS

Serious adverse effects occur only when high doses are taken by mouth for long periods.

Topical preparations are unlikely to cause adverse effects unless overused.

Symptom/effect	Frequency		Discuss with doctor		Stop taking drug now	Call doctor now
	Common	Rare	Only if severe	In all cases		
Indigestion	●			■		
Weight gain		●		■		
Acne		●		■		
Muscle weakness		●		■		
Mood changes		●		■		
Bloody/black faeces		●		■	▲	■

INTERACTIONS

Insulin, antidiabetic drugs, and oral anticoagulant drugs Betamethasone may alter insulin requirements and the effects of these drugs.

Vaccines Serious reactions can occur when certain vaccinations are given during betamethasone treatment.

Antihypertensive drugs and drugs used in myasthenia gravis Betamethasone may reduce the effects of these drugs.

Anticonvulsants These drugs may reduce the effects of betamethasone.

PROLONGED USE

People taking betamethasone tablets regularly should carry a "steroid treatment card". Prolonged use by mouth can lead to peptic ulcers, thin skin, fragile bones, muscle weakness, and adrenal gland suppression; it can also retard growth in children.

BEZAFIBRATE

Brand names Bezalip, Bezalip-Mono
Used in the following combined preparations None

GENERAL INFORMATION

Bezafibrate belongs to a group of drugs, usually called fibrates, that lower lipid levels in the blood. Fibrates are particularly effective in decreasing levels of triglycerides in the blood. They also reduce blood levels of cholesterol. Raised levels of lipids (fats) in the blood are associated with atherosclerosis (deposition of fat in blood vessel walls).

This can lead to coronary heart disease (for example, angina and heart attacks) and cerebrovascular disease (for example, stroke). When bezafibrate is taken with a diet low in saturated fats, there is good evidence that the chances of a heart attack are reduced.

QUICK REFERENCE

Drug group Lipid-lowering drug (p.103)

Overdose danger rating Low

Dependence rating Low

Prescription needed Yes

Available as generic No

INFORMATION FOR USERS

Your drug prescription is tailored for you. Do not alter dosage without checking with your doctor.

How taken

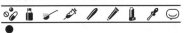

Tablets.

Frequency and timing of doses
1–3 x daily with a little liquid after a meal.

Adult dosage range
400–600mg daily.

Onset of effect
A beneficial effect on blood fat levels may not be produced for some weeks, and it takes months or years for fat deposits in the arteries to be reduced. Treatment should be withdrawn if no adequate response is obtained within 3–4 months.

Duration of action
About 6–24 hours. This may vary according to the individual.

Diet advice
A low-fat diet will have been recommended. Follow the advice of your doctor.

Storage
Keep in a closed container in a cool, dry place out of the reach of children.

Missed dose
Take as soon as you remember. If your next dose is due within 4 hours (and you take it once daily), take a single dose now and skip the next. If you take 2–3 times daily, take the next dose as normal.

Stopping the drug
Do not stop the drug without consulting your doctor.

Exceeding the dose
An occasional unintentional extra dose is unlikely to be a cause for concern. But if you notice unusual symptoms, notify your doctor.

SPECIAL PRECAUTIONS

Be sure to tell your doctor if:
▼ You have long-term liver or kidney problems.
▼ You have a history of gallbladder disease.
▼ You are taking other medications.

Pregnancy
▼ Safety in pregnancy not established. Discuss with your doctor.

Breast-feeding
▼ The drug may pass into the breast milk and may affect the baby. Discuss with your doctor.

Infants and children
▼ Not usually prescribed.

Over 60
▼ No special problems expected.

Driving and hazardous work
▼ No special problems.

Alcohol
▼ No special problems.

POSSIBLE ADVERSE EFFECTS

The most common *adverse effects* are those on the gastrointestinal tract, such as loss of appetite and nausea. These effects normally diminish as treatment continues.

Symptom/effect	Frequency		Discuss with doctor		Stop taking drug now	Call doctor now
	Common	Rare	Only if severe	In all cases		
Nausea	●		■			
Loss of appetite	●		■			
Gastric pain	●		■			
Skin rash		●		■		
Headache		●		■		
Muscular pain/cramp		●		■		
Dizziness/fatigue		●	■			

PROLONGED USE

No problems expected.

Monitoring Blood tests will be performed occasionally to monitor the effect of the drug on lipids in the blood.

INTERACTIONS

Anticoagulants Bezafibrate may increase the effect of anticoagulants such as warfarin. Your doctor will reduce the dosage of your anticoagulant when starting bezafibrate.

Monoamine oxidase inhibitors (MAOIs) There is a risk of liver damage when bezafibrate is taken with an MAOI.

Antidiabetic drugs Bezafibrate may interact with these drugs to lower blood sugar levels.

Pravastatin, simvastatin, and other lipid lowering drugs whose names end in 'statin' There is an increased risk of muscle damage if bezafibrate is taken with these drugs.

BROMOCRIPTINE

Brand name Parlodel
Used in the following combined preparations None

GENERAL INFORMATION

By inhibiting secretion of the hormone prolactin from the pituitary gland, bromocriptine is used in the treatment of conditions associated with excessive prolactin production. Such conditions include some types of female infertility and occasionally male infertility and impotence. It is effective in treating some benign breast conditions and other symptoms of menstrual disorders. Bromocriptine may also be used to suppress lactation in women who do not wish to breast-feed.

Bromocriptine reduces the release of growth hormone, and therefore is used in the treatment of acromegaly (see p.145).

Bromocriptine is also effective for relieving the symptoms of *parkinsonism*. The drug is now widely used to treat people who are in the advanced stages of parkinsonism when other drugs have failed or are unsuitable.

Serious *adverse effects* of the drug are uncommon when it is given in low doses. The most common problems, nausea and vomiting, can be minimized by taking bromocriptine with meals. Bromocriptine may in rare cases cause ulceration of the stomach.

QUICK REFERENCE

Drug group Drug for parkinsonism (p.87) and pituitary agent (p.145)
Overdose danger rating Low
Dependence rating Low
Prescription needed Yes
Available as generic Yes

INFORMATION FOR USERS

Your drug prescription is tailored for you. Do not alter dosage without checking with your doctor.

How taken

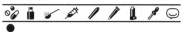

Tablets, capsules.

Frequency and timing of doses
1–4 x daily with food.

Adult dosage range
The dose given depends on the condition being treated and your response. In most cases treatment starts with a daily dose of 1–1.25mg. This is gradually increased until a satisfactory response is achieved.

Onset of effect
Variable depending on the condition.

Duration of action
About 8 hours.

Diet advice
None.

Storage
Keep in a closed container in a cool, dry place out of the reach of children. Protect from light.

Missed dose
Take as soon as you remember. If your next dose is due within 2 hours, take a single dose now and skip the next.

Stopping the drug
Do not stop the drug without consulting your doctor; symptoms may recur.

Exceeding the dose
An occasional unintentional extra dose is unlikely to be a cause for concern. If you notice any unusual symptoms, or if a large overdose has been taken, notify your doctor.

SPECIAL PRECAUTIONS

Be sure to tell your doctor if:
▼ You have poor circulation.
▼ You have a stomach ulcer.
▼ You have a history of psychiatric disorders.
▼ You have heart problems.
▼ You have porphyria.
▼ You are taking other medications.

Pregnancy
▼ Safety in pregnancy not established. Discuss with your doctor.

Breast-feeding
▼ The drug suppresses milk production, and prevents it completely if given within 12 hours of delivery. If you wish to breast-feed, consult your doctor.

Infants and children
▼ Not usually prescribed under 15 years.

Over 60
▼ Reduced dose may be necessary.

Driving and hazardous work
▼ Avoid such activities until you have learned how bromocriptine affects you because the drug may cause dizziness and drowsiness.

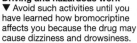

Alcohol
▼ Avoid. Alcohol increases the likelihood of confusion and reduces *tolerance* to bromocriptine.

POSSIBLE ADVERSE EFFECTS

Adverse effects are usually related to the dose being taken. When used for parkinsonism, bromocriptine may cause abnormal movements.

Symptom/effect	Frequency		Discuss with doctor		Stop taking drug now	Call doctor now
	Common	Rare	Only if severe	In all cases		
Confusion/dizziness	●			■		
Circulatory problems	●			■		
Nausea/vomiting	●		■			
Constipation		●	■			
Headache		●		■		
Abnormal movements		●		■		
Drowsiness		●		■	▲	∎

PROLONGED USE

No special problems.

Monitoring Periodic blood tests may be performed to check hormone levels. Gynaecological tests may be carried out annually (or every six months in post-menopausal women). Monitoring for other, rare, adverse effects (e.g. peptic ulcer in acromegaly) may also be carried out.

INTERACTIONS

Antipsychotic drugs These drugs oppose the action of bromocriptine and increase the risk of parkinsonism.

Domperidone and metoclopramide These drugs may reduce some of the effects of bromocriptine.

Sympathomimetic drugs These drugs increase the risk of *toxic* effects caused by bromocriptine.

BUDESONIDE

Brand names Entocort, Pulmicort, Rhinocort Aqua
Used in the following combined preparations None

GENERAL INFORMATION

Budesonide is a corticosteroid drug used in the form of slow-release capsules to relieve the symptoms of Crohn's disease and to treat ulcerative colitis. It is also used as an inhaler to prevent attacks of asthma but will not stop an existing attack. Like other corticosteroids, budesonide is used by people whose asthma is not controlled by bronchodilators (p.92) alone. It is also used as a nasal spray to relieve the symptoms of allergic rhinitis and for nasal polyps.

Budesonide controls symptoms by reducing inflammation, whether it is in the nose, lungs, or intestine.

There are fewer, usually less serious, *side effects* when budesonide is taken by inhaler or nasal spray because the drug is absorbed by the body in much smaller quantities than when it is taken by mouth.

INFORMATION FOR USERS

Your drug prescription is tailored for you. Do not alter dosage without checking with your doctor.

How taken

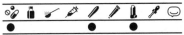

SR-capsules, enema, inhaler, powder for inhalation, nasal spray.

Frequency and timing of doses
Once daily before breakfast (capsules); once daily at bedtime (enema); twice daily (inhaler); once or twice daily (nasal spray).

Dosage range
3–9mg (capsules); 2mg (enema); 200mcg–1,600mcg (inhaler), 100–200mcg (nasal spray).

Onset of effect
Asthma Within 1 week.
Other conditions 1–3 days.

Duration of action
12–24 hours.

Diet advice
None.

Storage
Keep in a closed container in a cool, dry place out of the reach of children.

Missed dose
Take as soon as you remember. If your next dose is due within 2 hours, take a single dose now and skip the next.

Stopping the drug
Do not stop taking the drug without consulting your doctor; symptoms may recur. The SR-capsules used in Crohn's disease should be withdrawn gradually.

Exceeding the dose
An occasional extra dose is unlikely to be a cause for concern. But if you notice any unusual symptoms, or if a large overdose has been taken, notify your doctor.

POSSIBLE ADVERSE EFFECTS

The main side effects of inhalers and nasal spray are irritation of the nasal passages and fungal infection of the mouth and throat. High doses of budesonide by mouth can cause weight gain and high blood pressure as well as other long-term effects.

Symptom/effect	Frequency		Discuss with doctor		Stop taking drug now	Call doctor now
	Common	Rare	Only if severe	In all cases		
Nasal irritation	●		■			
Cough	●		■			
Sore throat/hoarseness	●			■		
Nosebleed		●		■		
Weight gain		●		■		
Pain in the eye		●		■	▲	▮

INTERACTIONS

None.

SPECIAL PRECAUTIONS

Be sure to tell your doctor if:
▼ You have had tuberculosis or another respiratory infection.
▼ You are taking other medications.

 Pregnancy
▼ No special problems.

 Breast-feeding
▼ No evidence of risk.

 Infants and children
▼ Reduced dose necessary.

 Over 60
▼ No special problems.

 Driving and hazardous work
▼ No special problems.

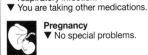 **Alcohol**
▼ No special problems.

PROLONGED USE

Asthma prevention is the condition for which prolonged use may be required. There may be a small risk of glaucoma, cataracts, and effects on bone with high doses inhaled for a prolonged period.

Monitoring If budesonide is being taken in large doses, periodic checks may be needed to make sure that the adrenal glands are working properly. Children using inhalers may have their growth (height) monitored regularly.

BUMETANIDE

Brand names Burinex, Betinex
Used in the following combined preparations Burinex A, Burinex K

GENERAL INFORMATION

Bumetanide is a powerful, short-acting loop diuretic used to treat oedema (fluid retention) resulting from heart failure, nephrotic syndrome, and cirrhosis of the liver. Bumetanide is particularly useful in treating people with impaired kidney function who do not respond well to thiazide diuretics. Because it is fast-acting, it is often injected in an emergency to relieve pulmonary oedema.

Bumetanide increases potassium loss in the urine, which can result in a wide variety of symptoms (see p.99). For this reason, potassium supplements or a diuretic conserving potassium within the body are often given with the drug.

INFORMATION FOR USERS

Your drug prescription is tailored for you. Do not alter dosage without checking with your doctor.

How taken

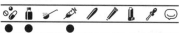

Tablets, liquid, injection.

Frequency and timing of doses
Usually once daily in the morning. In some cases, twice daily.

Dosage range
0.5–5mg daily. Dose may be increased if kidney function is impaired.

Onset of effect
Within 30 minutes by mouth; more quickly by injection.

Duration of action
2–4 hours.

Diet advice
Use of this drug may reduce potassium in the body. Eat plenty of fresh fruit and vegetables.

Storage
Keep in a closed container in a cool, dry place out of the reach of children. Protect from light.

Missed dose
No cause for concern, but take as soon as you remember. However, if it is late in the day do not take the missed dose, or you may need to get up during the night to pass urine. Take the next scheduled dose as usual.

Stopping the drug
Do not stop the drug without consulting your doctor; symptoms may recur.

Exceeding the dose
An occasional unintentional extra dose is unlikely to be a cause for concern. But if you notice any unusual symptoms, or if a large overdose has been taken, notify your doctor.

SPECIAL PRECAUTIONS

Be sure to tell your doctor if:
▼ You have long-term liver or kidney problems.
▼ You have diabetes.
▼ You have prostate trouble.
▼ You have gout.
▼ You are taking other medications.

Pregnancy
▼ Not usually prescribed. May cause a reduction in blood supply to the developing baby. Discuss with your doctor.

Breast-feeding
▼ This drug may reduce your milk supply. Discuss with your doctor.

Infants and children
▼ Not usually prescribed. Reduced dose necessary.

Over 60
▼ Dosage is often reduced.

Driving and hazardous work
▼ Avoid such activities until you have learned how bumetanide affects you because the drug may cause dizziness and faintness.

Alcohol
▼ Keep consumption low. The drug increases the likelihood of dehydration and hangovers after drinking alcohol.

POSSIBLE ADVERSE EFFECTS

Adverse effects are caused mainly by the rapid fluid loss produced by bumetanide. These diminish as the body adjusts to the drug. Bumetanide may precipitate gout in susceptible individuals and can affect the control of diabetes.

Symptom/effect	Frequency		Discuss with doctor		Stop taking drug now	Call doctor now
	Common	Rare	Only if severe	In all cases		
Dizziness/fainting	●		■			
Lethargy/fatigue		●	■			
Muscle cramps		●	■			
Rash/photosensitivity		●		■		
Nausea/vomiting		●		■		
Pain in joints		●		■		

INTERACTIONS

Anti-arrhythmic drugs Low potassium levels may increase these drugs' toxicity.

Terfenadine Low potassium levels increase the risk of irregular heart beat with this antihistamine.

Antibacterials Bumetanide increases the ear damage caused by some antibiotics.

Digoxin Excessive potassium loss may increase the adverse effects of digoxin.

Non-steroidal anti-inflammatory drugs (NSAIDs) These drugs may reduce the diuretic effect of bumetanide.

Lithium Bumetanide may increase the blood levels of lithium, leading to an increased risk of lithium *toxicity*.

Pimozide Low potassium levels increase the risk of abnormal heart rhythms with this antipsychotic drug.

PROLONGED USE

Serious problems are unlikely, but the levels of certain salts in the body may occasionally become abnormal during prolonged use.

Monitoring Regular blood tests may be performed to check on kidney function and levels of body salts.

CALCIPOTRIOL

Brand name Dovonex
Used in the following combined preparations None

GENERAL INFORMATION

Calcipotriol is used in the treatment of plaque psoriasis affecting up to 40 per cent of the patient's skin area, and also for scalp psoriasis.

Calcipotriol is similar to vitamin D. It is thought to work by reducing production of the skin cells that cause skin thickening and scaling, which are the most common symptoms of psoriasis. Because this drug is related to vitamin D, excessive use (more than 100g per week) can lead to a rise in calcium levels in the body; otherwise calcipotriol is unlikely to cause any serious *adverse effects*.

The drug is applied to the affected areas in the form of cream, ointment, or scalp solution. It should not be used on the face, and it is important that the hands are washed following application of this ointment to avoid accidental transfer to unaffected areas. Local irritation may occur during the early stages of treatment.

QUICK REFERENCE

Drug group Drug for psoriasis (p.178)

Overdose danger rating Low

Dependence rating Low

Prescription needed Yes

Available as generic No

INFORMATION FOR USERS

Your drug prescription is tailored for you. Do not alter dosage without checking with your doctor.

How taken

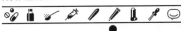

Cream, ointment, scalp solution.

Frequency and timing of doses
1–2 x daily.

Adult dosage range
Maximum 100g each week. Scalp solution, maximum 60ml each week.

Onset of effect
Improvement is seen within 2 weeks.

Duration of action
One application lasts up to 12 hours. Beneficial effects are longer lasting.

Diet advice
None.

Storage
Store at room temperature out of the reach of children.

Missed dose
Apply the next dose at the scheduled time.

Stopping the drug
Do not stop taking the drug without consulting your doctor; symptoms may recur.

Exceeding the dose
Excessive prolonged use may lead to an increase in blood calcium levels, which can cause nausea, constipation, thirst, and frequent urination. Notify your doctor.

SPECIAL PRECAUTIONS

Be sure to tell your doctor if:
▼ You have a metabolic disorder.
▼ You have previously had a hypersensitivity reaction to the drug.
▼ You are taking other medications.

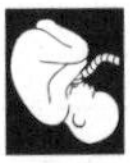

Pregnancy
▼ No evidence of risk, but discuss with your doctor.

Breast-feeding
▼ No evidence of risk, but discuss with your doctor.

Infants and children
▼ Not recommended.

Over 60
▼ No problems expected.

Driving and hazardous work
▼ No problems expected.

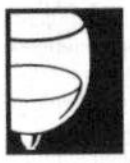

Alcohol
▼ No problems expected.

POSSIBLE ADVERSE EFFECTS

Temporary local irritation may occur when treatment is started. The other effects are usually due to heavy or prolonged use, leading to high calcium levels in the blood.

Symptom/effect	Frequency		Discuss with doctor		Stop taking drug now	Call doctor now
	Common	Rare	Only if severe	In all cases		
Local irritation	●		■			
Rash on face/mouth		●		■		
Thirst/frequent urination		●		■		
Nausea/constipation		●		■		
Light sensitive rash		●		■		

INTERACTIONS

None known.

PROLONGED USE

No problems expected from use of calcipotriol in low doses.

Monitoring Regular checks on calcium levels in the blood or urine are required during prolonged or heavy use.

CAPTOPRIL

Brand names Acepril, Capoten, Kaplon
Used in the following combined preparations Acezide, Capozide

GENERAL INFORMATION

Captopril belongs to the class of drugs called ACE inhibitors, used to treat high blood pressure and heart failure. The drug works by relaxing the muscles around blood vessels, allowing them to dilate and thereby easing blood flow.

Captopril lowers blood pressure rapidly but may require several weeks to achieve maximum effect. People with heart failure may be given captopril in addition to diuretics. It can achieve dramatic improvement, relaxing muscle

in blood vessel walls and reducing the workload of the heart.

The first dose is usually very small and should be taken while lying down as there is a risk of a sudden fall in blood pressure. Diuretics are often prescribed with captopril.

A variety of minor *side effects* may occur. Some people experience upset in their sense of taste, while others get a persistent dry cough. A reduction in dose may help minimize these effects.

QUICK REFERENCE

Drug group ACE inhibitor (p.98)
Overdose danger rating Medium
Dependence rating Low
Prescription needed Yes
Available as generic Yes

INFORMATION FOR USERS

Your drug prescription is tailored for you. Do not alter dosage without checking with your doctor.

How taken

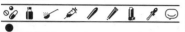

Tablets.

Frequency and timing of doses
2–3 x daily.

Adult dosage range
12.5–25mg daily initially, gradually increased to 50–150mg daily.

Onset of effect
30–60 minutes.

Duration of action
6–8 hours.

Diet advice
None.

Storage
Keep in a closed container in a cool, dry place out of the reach of children.

Missed dose
Take as soon as you remember. If your next dose is due within 2 hours, take a single dose now and skip the next.

Stopping the drug
Do not stop the drug without consulting your doctor; stopping the drug may lead to worsening of the underlying condition.

Exceeding the dose
An occasional unintentional extra dose is unlikely to cause problems. Large overdoses may cause dizziness or fainting. Notify your doctor.

POSSIBLE ADVERSE EFFECTS

Captopril causes a variety of minor adverse effects on the gastrointestinal system. Rashes may occur but usually disappear soon after treatment is begun.

Symptom/effect	Frequency		Discuss with doctor		Stop taking drug now	Call doctor now
	Common	Rare	Only if severe	In all cases		
Loss of taste	●		■			
Rash	●			■		
Persistent dry cough	●			■		
Reduced kidney function	●			■		
Mouth ulcers/sore mouth		●		■		
Dizziness/fainting		●		■		
Sore throat/fever		●		■		

INTERACTIONS

Non-steroidal anti-inflammatory drugs (NSAIDs) Some of these drugs may reduce the effectiveness of captopril. There is also a risk of kidney damage when they are taken with captopril.

Lithium Blood levels of lithium may be raised by captopril.

Vasodilators (e.g., nitrates) These drugs may reduce blood pressure even further.

Potassium supplements and potassium-sparing diuretics These drugs increase the risk of high potassium levels in the blood when they are taken with captopril.

Cyclosporin This drug increases the risk of high potassium levels in the blood when taken with captopril.

Diuretics Taking captopril with these drugs can cause a rapid fall in blood pressure.

SPECIAL PRECAUTIONS

Be sure to tell your doctor if:
▼ You have long-term kidney problems.
▼ You have coronary artery disease.
▼ You are on a low sodium diet.
▼ You are allergic to ACE inhibitors.
▼ You are taking other medications.

Pregnancy
▼ Not usually prescribed. May harm the developing fetus. Discuss with your doctor.

Breast-feeding
▼ The drug passes into the breast milk, but at normal doses adverse effects on the baby are unlikely. Discuss with your doctor.

Infants and children
▼ Not usually prescribed. Reduced dose necessary.

Over 60
▼ Reduced dose may be necessary.

Driving and hazardous work
▼ Avoid such activities until you have learned how captopril affects you because the drug can cause dizziness and fainting.

Alcohol
▼ Avoid. Alcohol may increase the blood-pressure lowering and adverse effects of the drug.

Surgery and general anaesthetics
▼ Captopril may need to be stopped before you have a general anaesthetic. Discuss with your doctor or dentist before any operation.

PROLONGED USE

Rarely, prolonged use can lead to changes in the blood count or kidney function.

Monitoring Periodic checks on potassium levels, white blood cell count, kidney function, and urine are usually performed.

CARBAMAZEPINE

Brand names Tegretol, Epimaz, Teril CR, Timoril Retard
Used in the following combined preparations None

GENERAL INFORMATION

Chemically related to the tricyclic anti-depressant group of drugs (see p.84), carbamazepine reduces the likelihood of fits caused by abnormal nerve signals in the brain (epilepsy).

Carbamazepine is also prescribed to relieve the intermittent severe pain caused by damage to the cranial nerves in trigeminal neuralgia. Carbamazepine is also occasionally prescribed to treat manic depression and diabetes insipidus and is used for pain relief in diabetic neuropathy.

In order to avoid *side effects*, carbamazepine therapy is usually commenced at a low dose and is gradually increased until the required blood level of the drug is achieved.

QUICK REFERENCE

Drug group Anticonvulsant drug (p.86) and antipsychotic drug (p.87)

Overdose danger rating Medium

Dependence rating Low

Prescription needed Yes

Available as generic Yes

INFORMATION FOR USERS

Your drug prescription is tailored for you. Do not alter dosage without checking with your doctor.

How taken

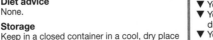
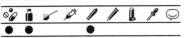

Tablets, chewable tablets, liquid, suppositories.

Frequency and timing of doses
1–4 x daily.

Adult dosage range
Epilepsy 100–1,200mg daily (low starting dose that is slowly increased every 2 weeks).
Pain relief 100–1,600mg daily.
Psychiatric disorders 400–1,600mg daily.

Onset of effect
Within 4 hours.

Duration of action
12–24 hours.

Diet advice
None.

Storage
Keep in a closed container in a cool, dry place out of the reach of children.

Missed dose
Take as soon as you remember. If your next dose is due within 2 hours, take a single dose now and skip the next.

Stopping the drug
Do not stop the drug without consulting your doctor; symptoms may recur.

Exceeding the dose
An occasional unintentional extra dose is unlikely to cause problems. Large overdoses may cause tremor, convulsions, and coma. Notify your doctor.

SPECIAL PRECAUTIONS

Be sure to tell your doctor if:
▼ You have long-term liver or kidney problems.
▼ You have heart problems.
▼ You have had blood problems with other drugs.
▼ You are taking other medications.

Pregnancy
▼ May be associated with abnormalities in the unborn baby. Folic acid supplements are usually recommended. Discuss with your doctor.

Breast-feeding
▼ The drug passes into the breast milk, but at normal doses adverse effects on the baby are unlikely. Discuss with your doctor.

Infants and children
▼ Reduced dose necessary.

Over 60
▼ May cause confused or agitated behaviour in the elderly. Reduced dose may be necessary.

Driving and hazardous work
▼ Discuss with your doctor. Your underlying condition, as well as the possibility of reduced alertness while taking carbamazepine, may make such activities inadvisable.

Alcohol
▼ Avoid. Alcohol may increase the sedative effects of this drug.

POSSIBLE ADVERSE EFFECTS

Most people experience very few adverse effects with this drug, but when blood levels get too high, adverse effects are common and the dose may need to be reduced.

Symptom/effect	Frequency		Discuss with doctor		Stop taking drug now	Call doctor now
	Common	Rare	Only if severe	In all cases		
Dizziness/unsteadiness	●		■			
Drowsiness	●		■			
Nausea/loss of appetite	●		■			
Blurred vision	●			■		
Jaundice		●		■		
Ankle swelling		●		■		
Rash		●		■	▲	■
Sore throat/hoarseness		●		■	▲	

INTERACTIONS

Anticoagulant drugs, analgesic drugs, and oral contraceptives Carbamazepine may reduce the effects of these drugs.

Analgesic drugs, cimetidine, verapamil, co-proxamol, some antibiotics, and isoniazid These drugs may increase the effects of carbamazepine.

Antidepressant and antipsychotic drugs These drugs may antagonize the anticonvulsant effects of carbamazepine.

Other anti-epileptic drugs Complex and variable interactions can occur between these drugs and carbamazepine.

PROLONGED USE

There is a slight risk of changes in liver function or of skin or blood abnormalities occurring during prolonged use.

Monitoring Periodic blood tests are usually performed to monitor levels of the drug, blood cell counts, and liver and kidney function.

CARBARYL

Brand names Carylderm
Used in the following combined preparations None

GENERAL INFORMATION

Carbaryl is an insecticide that is used in the treatment of head and crab lice. It kills the lice by interfering with the functioning of their nervous system, causing paralysis and death.

The drug is applied *topically* either as a water-based liquid or an alcohol-based lotion. Lotion is considered unsuitable for small children and asthmatics, who may be affected by the alcoholic fumes. The lotion is also unsuitable for treating crab lice because it causes genital irritation.

Because lice develop resistance to insecticides, it is possible that carbaryl (or alternatives such as malathion) may not clear the lice. If the drug does not work for you, consult your pharmacist or doctor. You will need a prescription to obtain carbaryl.

QUICK REFERENCE

Drug group Drugs to treat skin parasites (p.176)
Overdose danger rating Low
Dependence rating Low
Prescription needed Yes
Available as generic No

INFORMATION FOR USERS

Your drug prescription is tailored for you. Do not alter dosage without checking with your doctor.

How taken

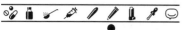

Topical liquid, lotion.

Frequency and timing of doses
Once, repeating after a week.

Adult dosage range
As directed.

Onset of effect
Lotion or liquid should be left on for 12 hours before being washed off.

Duration of action
Until washed off.

Diet advice
None.

Storage
Keep in closed container in a cool, dry place out of the reach of children. Protect from light.

Missed dose
If you forget the second application, use it as soon as you remember.

Stopping the drug
Carbaryl should be applied as a single application or as a short course of treatment.

Exceeding the dose
An occasional unintentional extra application is unlikely to be a cause for concern. Take emergency action if accidentally swallowed.

POSSIBLE ADVERSE EFFECTS

Used correctly, carbaryl preparations are unlikely to produce adverse effects, although the alcoholic fumes given off by some lotions may cause wheezing in asthmatics.

Symptom/effect	Frequency		Discuss with doctor		Stop taking drug now	Call doctor now
	Common	Rare	Only if severe	In all cases		
Skin irritation		●	■			

INTERACTIONS

None.

SPECIAL PRECAUTIONS

Be sure to tell your doctor if:
▼ You have asthma.

Pregnancy
▼ No evidence of risk. It is unlikely that enough carbaryl would be absorbed after occasional application to affect the developing fetus.

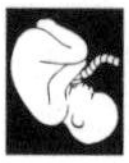

Breast-feeding
▼ No evidence of risk. It is unlikely that enough carbaryl would be absorbed after occasional application to affect the baby.

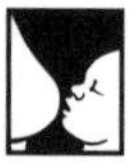

Infants and children
▼ No special problems.

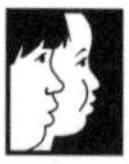

Over 60
▼ No special problems.

Driving and hazardous work
▼ No special problems.

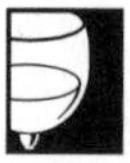

Alcohol
▼ No special problems.

PROLONGED USE

Carbaryl is intended for intermittent use only. It should not be used for prolonged periods.

CARBIMAZOLE

Brand name Neo-Mercazole
Used in the following combined preparations None

GENERAL INFORMATION

Carbimazole is an antithyroid drug used to suppress the formation of thyroid hormones in people with an overactive thyroid gland (hyperthyroidism). In some people, particularly those with Graves' disease (the most common form of hyperthyroidism), drug treatment alone may relieve the disorder.

Carbimazole is also used in more serious cases, for example, to restore the normal function of the thyroid gland before its partial removal by surgery, or to intensify the absorption of the cell-destroying drug radioactive iodine when

that is used. Carbimazole also prevents the harmful release of thyroid hormone that can sometimes follow the use of radioactive iodine. Because the full benefits of this medication are not felt for several weeks, beta blockers may be given during this period to help control symptoms. Maintenance treatment may be continued for as long as 18 months unless surgery or radioactive iodine are used. Occasionally the carbimazole dose is kept high and thyroxine is also prescribed in order to prevent a goitre from developing.

QUICK REFERENCE

Drug group Antithyroid drug (p.144)

Overdose danger rating Medium

Dependence rating Low

Prescription needed Yes

Available as generic No

INFORMATION FOR USERS

Your drug prescription is tailored for you. Do not alter dosage without checking with your doctor.

How taken

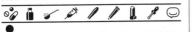

Tablets.

Frequency and timing of doses
2–3 x daily.

Adult dosage range
20–60mg daily. Once control is achieved, dosage is reduced gradually to a maintenance dose of 5–15mg for about 18 months.

Onset of effect
Some improvement is usually felt within 1–3 weeks. Full beneficial effects usually take 4–8 weeks.

Duration of action
12–24 hours.

Diet advice
Your doctor may advise you to avoid foods that are high in iodine.

Storage
Keep in a closed container in a cool, dry place out of the reach of children.

Missed dose
Take as soon as you remember. If your next dose is due, take both doses together.

Stopping the drug
Do not stop the drug without consulting your doctor; symptoms may recur.

Exceeding the dose
An occasional unintentional extra dose is unlikely to cause problems. Large overdoses may cause nausea, vomiting, and headache. Notify your doctor.

SPECIAL PRECAUTIONS

Be sure to tell your doctor if:
▼ You have long-term liver or kidney problems.
▼ You are taking other medications.

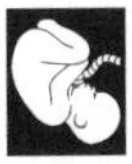

 Pregnancy
▼ May be associated with defects in the baby. However, the risk to the baby of untreated hyperthyroidism is higher. Discuss with your doctor.

 Breast-feeding
▼ The drug passes into the breast milk, but mothers may breast-feed as long as the lowest effective dose is used and the baby is carefully monitored. Discuss with your doctor.

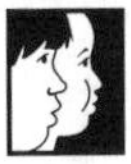

 Infants and children
▼ Reduced dose necessary.

 Over 60
▼ No special problems.

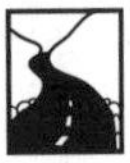

 Driving and hazardous work
▼ Avoid such activities until you have learned how carbimazole affects you because the drug may cause dizziness.

 Alcohol
▼ No known problems.

POSSIBLE ADVERSE EFFECTS

Serious *side effects* are rare. A sore throat or mouth ulcers may indicate adverse effects on the blood and require prompt medical attention.

Symptom/effect	Frequency		Discuss with doctor		Stop taking drug now	Call doctor now
	Common	Rare	Only if severe	In all cases		
Headache/dizziness	●		■			
Joint pain	●		■			
Nausea	●		■			
Rash/Itching	●			■		
Hair loss		●		■		
Sore throat/mouth ulcers		●		■		▮
Jaundice		●		■		▮

INTERACTIONS

None.

PROLONGED USE

Carbimazole may stop or reduce the production of blood cells by the bone marrow.

Monitoring Blood cell counts are carried out, and periodic tests of thyroid function are usually required.

CEFALEXIN

Brand names Ceporex, Keflex, Kiflone, Tenkorex
Used in the following combined preparations None

GENERAL INFORMATION

Cefalexin is a cephalosporin antibiotic that is prescribed for a variety of mild to moderate infections. Cefalexin does not have such a wide range of uses as some other antibiotics, but it is helpful in treating bronchitis, cystitis, and certain skin and soft tissue infections. In some cases it is prescribed as follow-up treatment for severe infections after a

more powerful cephalosporin has been given by injection.

Diarrhoea is the most common *side effect* of cefalexin, although it tends to be less severe than with other cephalosporin antibiotics. In addition, some people may find that they are allergic to this drug, especially if they are sensitive to penicillin.

INFORMATION FOR USERS

Your drug prescription is tailored for you. Do not alter dosage without checking with your doctor.

How taken

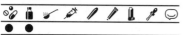

Tablets, capsules, liquid.

Frequency and timing of doses
2–4 x daily.

Dosage range
Adults 1–6g daily.
Children Reduced dose according to age and weight.

Onset of effect
Within 1 hour.

Duration of action
6–12 hours.

Diet advice
None.

Storage
Keep tablets and capsules in a closed container in a cool, dry place out of the reach of children. Refrigerate liquid, but do not freeze, and keep for no longer than 10 days. Protect from light.

Missed dose
Take as soon as you remember. If your next dose is due at this time, take both doses now.

Stopping the drug
Take the full course. Even if you feel better, the original infection may still be present and may recur if treatment is stopped too soon.

Exceeding the dose
An occasional unintentional extra dose is unlikely to be a cause for concern. But if you notice any unusual symptoms, or if a large overdose has been taken, notify your doctor.

SPECIAL PRECAUTIONS

Be sure to tell your doctor if:
▼ You have a long-term kidney problem.
▼ You have had a previous allergic reaction to a penicillin or cephalosporin antibiotic.
▼ You have a history of blood disorders.
▼ You are taking other medications.

Pregnancy
▼ No evidence of risk to the developing baby.

Breast-feeding
▼ The drug passes into the breast milk but at normal doses adverse effects on the baby are unlikely. Discuss with your doctor.

Infants and children
▼ Reduced dose necessary.

Over 60
▼ No special problems.

Driving and hazardous work
▼ No known problems.

Alcohol
▼ No known problems.

POSSIBLE ADVERSE EFFECTS

Most people do not suffer serious adverse effects while taking cefalexin. Diarrhoea is common but it tends not to be severe. The

rarer adverse effects are usually due to an allergic reaction and may necessitate stopping the drug.

Symptom/effect	Frequency		Discuss with doctor		Stop taking drug now	Call doctor now
	Common	Rare	Only if severe	In all cases		
Diarrhoea	●		■			
Nausea/vomiting		●	■			
Abdominal pain		●		■		
Rash		●		■	▲	❚
Itching/swelling/wheezing		●		■	▲	❚

INTERACTIONS

Probenecid This drug increases the level of cefalexin in the blood. The dosage of cefalexin may need to be adjusted accordingly.

Oral contraceptives Cefalexin may reduce the contraceptive effect of these drugs. Discuss with your doctor.

PROLONGED USE

Cefalexin is usually given only for short courses of treatment.

CETIRIZINE

Brand name Zirtek
Used in the following combined preparations None

GENERAL INFORMATION

Cetirizine is a long-acting antihistamine. The drug's main use is in the treatment of allergic rhinitis, particularly hay fever.

Cetirizine is also used to treat allergic skin conditions, such as urticaria (hives).

The principal difference between this drug and traditional antihistamines such as chlorphenamine (chlorpheniramine) is that it has less *sedative* effect on the central nervous system. It may therefore be suitable for people when they need to avoid sleepiness – for example, when driving or at work. However, because cetirizine can cause drowsiness in some people, you should learn how the drug affects you before you undertake any activities that require concentration.

QUICK REFERENCE

Drug group Antihistamine (p.124)

Overdose danger rating Medium

Dependence rating Low

Prescription needed No (tablets); yes (liquid)

Available as generic No

INFORMATION FOR USERS

Follow instructions on the label. Call your doctor if symptoms worsen.

How taken

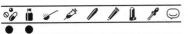

Tablets, liquid.

Frequency and timing of doses
1–2 x daily.

Adult dosage range
10mg daily.

Onset of effect
1–3 hours. Some effects may not be felt for 1–2 days.

Duration of action
Up to 24 hours.

Diet advice
None.

Storage
Keep in a closed container in a cool, dry place out of the reach of children.

Missed dose
No cause for concern, but take as soon as you remember. If your next dose is due within 8 hours, take a single dose now and skip the next.

Stopping the drug
Can be safely stopped as soon as you no longer need it.

Exceeding the dose
An occasional unintentional extra dose is unlikely to cause problems. Large overdoses may cause nausea or drowsiness and have adverse effects on the heart. Notify your doctor.

SPECIAL PRECAUTIONS

Be sure to consult your doctor or pharmacist before taking this drug if:
▼ You have long-term liver or kidney problems.
▼ You have glaucoma.
▼ You are taking other medications.

 Pregnancy
▼ Safety in pregnancy not established. Discuss with your doctor.

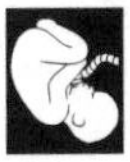

 Breast-feeding
▼ The drug passes into the breast milk. Discuss with your doctor.

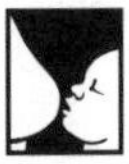

 Infants and children
▼ Not recommended under 2 years.

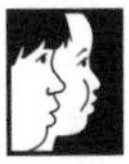

 Over 60
▼ No problems expected.

 Driving and hazardous work
▼ Avoid such activities until you have learned how cetirizine affects you because the drug can cause drowsiness in some people.

 Alcohol
▼ Keep consumption low.

POSSIBLE ADVERSE EFFECTS

The most common adverse effects are drowsiness, dry mouth, and fatigue.

Side effects may be reduced if the dose is taken as 5mg twice a day.

Symptom/effect	Frequency		Discuss with doctor		Stop taking drug now	Call doctor now
	Common	Rare	Only if severe	In all cases		
Drowsiness/fatigue		●	■			
Dry mouth		●	■			

INTERACTIONS

Anticholinergic drugs The *anticholinergic* effects of cetirizine may be increased by all drugs that have anticholinergic effects, including antipsychotics and tricyclic antidepressants.

Sedatives Cetirizine may increase the *sedative* effects of anti-anxiety drugs, sleeping drugs, antidepressants, and antipsychotic drugs.

Allergy tests Antihistamines should be discontinued approximately 48 hours before allergy skin testing.

PROLONGED USE

No problems expected.

CHLORAMPHENICOL

Brand names Chloromycetin, Kemicetine, Minims Chloramphenicol, Sno-Phenicol
Used in the following combined preparation Actinac

GENERAL INFORMATION

Chloramphenicol is an antibiotic used *topically* to treat eye and ear infections. Given by mouth or injection, it is used in the treatment of meningitis and brain abscesses. It is also effective in acute infections such as typhoid, pneumonia, epiglottitis, or meningitis caused by bacteria resistant to other antibiotics.

Although most people experience few *adverse effects*, chloramphenicol occasionally causes serious or even fatal blood disorders. For this reason, chloramphenicol by mouth or injection is normally only given to treat life-threatening infections that do not respond to safer drugs.

QUICK REFERENCE

Drug group Antibiotic (p.128)
Overdose danger rating Low
Dependence rating Low
Prescription needed Yes
Available as generic Yes

INFORMATION FOR USERS

Your drug prescription is tailored for you. Do not alter dosage without checking with your doctor.

How taken

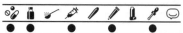

Capsules, liquid, injection, cream, eye and ear drops, eye ointment.

Frequency and timing of doses
Every 6 hours (by mouth or injection); every 2–6 hours (eye preparations); 3 x daily (ear drops).

Adult dosage range
Varies according to preparation and condition. Follow your doctor's instructions.

Onset of effect
1–3 days, depending on the condition and preparation.

Duration of action
6–8 hours.

Diet advice
None.

Storage
Keep in a closed container in a cool, dry place out of the reach of children. Protect from light.

Missed dose
Take as soon as you remember (capsules, liquid). If your next dose is due, double the dose to make up the missed dose. For skin, eye, and ear preparations, apply as soon as you remember.

Stopping the drug
Take the full course. Even if you feel better the infection may still be present and may recur if treatment is stopped too soon.

Exceeding the dose
An occasional unintentional extra dose is unlikely to be a cause for concern. But if you notice any unusual symptoms, or if a large overdose has been taken, notify your doctor.

SPECIAL PRECAUTIONS

Be sure to tell your doctor if:
▼ You have long-term liver or kidney problems.
▼ You have a blood disorder.
▼ You are taking other medications.

Pregnancy
▼ No evidence of risk with eye or ear preparations. Safety in pregnancy, of other methods of administration, not established. Discuss with your doctor.

Breast-feeding
▼ No evidence of risk with eye or ear preparations. Taken by mouth, the drug passes into the breast milk and may increase the risk of blood disorders in the baby. Discuss with your doctor.

Infants and children
▼ Reduced dose necessary.

Over 60
▼ No problems expected.

Driving and hazardous work
▼ No known problems.

Alcohol
▼ No known problems.

POSSIBLE ADVERSE EFFECTS

Transient irritation may occur with eye or ear drops. Sore throat, fever, and unusual tiredness with any form of chloramphenicol may be signs of blood abnormalities and should be reported to your doctor without delay, even if treatment has been stopped.

Symptom/effect	Frequency		Discuss with doctor		Stop taking drug now	Call doctor now
	Common	Rare	Only if severe	In all cases		
Burning/stinging (drops)	●		■			
Nausea/vomiting/diarrhoea	●		■			
Numb/tingling hands/feet	●			■		
Rash/itching	●			■		
Impaired vision	●			■	▲	❚
Sore throat	●			■	▲	❚
Fever/weakness	●			■	▲	❚
Painful mouth/tongue	●			■	▲	❚

INTERACTIONS

General note Chloramphenicol may increase the effect of certain other drugs, including phenytoin, oral anticoagulants, and oral antidiabetics. Phenobarbital or rifampicin may reduce the effect of chloramphenicol.

Antidiabetic drugs Chloramphenicol may increase the effect of antidiabetic drugs.

PROLONGED USE

Prolonged use of this drug may increase the risk of serious blood disorders and eye damage.

Monitoring Periodic blood cell counts and eye tests may be performed. Blood levels of the drug are usually monitored in infants given chloramphenicol by mouth or injection.

CHLORDIAZEPOXIDE

Brand names Librium, Tropium
Used in the following combined preparations None

GENERAL INFORMATION

Chlordiazepoxide was introduced in the mid-1960s and belongs to the group of anti-anxiety drugs known as the benzodiazepines. These drugs are used to help relieve tension and nervousness, relax muscles, and encourage sleep. The actions and the *adverse effects* of this drug group are described more fully on page 83.

Prescribed primarily to treat anxiety, chlordiazepoxide is also used to relieve the symptoms of alcohol withdrawal.
Chlordiazepoxide may lead to mild dependence and withdrawal symptoms if taken regularly over a long period, and it may also lose effectiveness with time. For these reasons, courses of treatment are usually limited to two to four weeks.

INFORMATION FOR USERS

Your drug prescription is tailored for you. Do not alter dosage without checking with your doctor.

How taken

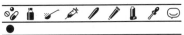

Tablets, capsules.

Frequency and timing of doses
1–4 x daily.

Adult dosage range
10–100mg daily. The dosage varies considerably from person to person.

Onset of effect
1–2 hours.

Duration of action
12–24 hours, but some effect may last up to 4 days.

Diet advice
None.

Storage
Keep in a closed container in a cool, dry place out of the reach of children.

Missed dose
No cause for concern, but take when you remember. If your next dose is due within 2 hours, take a single dose now and skip the next.

Stopping the drug
If you have been taking the drug for less than 2 weeks, it can be safely stopped as soon as you feel you no longer need it. However, if you have been taking the drug for longer, consult your doctor, who may supervise a gradual reduction in dosage. Stopping abruptly may lead to withdrawal symptoms (see p.79).

Exceeding the dose
An occasional unintentional extra dose is unlikely to cause problems. Large overdoses may cause unusual drowsiness or coma. Notify your doctor.

SPECIAL PRECAUTIONS

Be sure to tell your doctor if:
▼ You have long-term liver or kidney problems.
▼ You have a history of breathing problems.
▼ You have had problems with alcohol or drug abuse.
▼ You are taking other medications.

 Pregnancy
▼ Safety in pregnancy not established. Discuss with your doctor.

 Breast-feeding
▼ The drug passes into the breast milk and may affect the baby. Discuss with your doctor.

 Infants and children
▼ Not recommended.

 Over 60
▼ Reduced dose may be necessary.

 Driving and hazardous work
▼ Avoid such activities until you have learned how chlordiazepoxide affects you because the drug can cause reduced alertness and slowed reactions.

 Alcohol
▼ Avoid. Alcohol may increase the sedative effects of this drug.

POSSIBLE ADVERSE EFFECTS

The principal adverse effects of this drug are related to its *sedative* properties. These effects normally diminish after the first few days of treatment.

Symptom/effect	Frequency		Discuss with doctor		Stop taking drug now	Call doctor now
	Common	Rare	Only if severe	In all cases		
Daytime drowsiness	●			■		
Dizziness/unsteadiness	●			■		
Forgetfulness/confusion		●		■		
Headache		●		■		
Blurred vision		●			■	
Rash		●			■	▲

INTERACTIONS

Anticonvulsant drugs The side effects of these drugs may be increased when they are taken with chlordiazepoxide.

Sedatives All drugs that have a *sedative* effect are likely to increase the sedative properties of chlordiazepoxide.

PROLONGED USE

Regular use of this drug over several weeks can lead to a reduction in its effect as the body adapts. It may also be habit-forming when taken for extended periods, especially if it is taken in doses that are larger than average.

CHLOROQUINE

Brand names Avloclor, Nivaquine
Used in the following combined preparation Paludrine/Avloclor

GENERAL INFORMATION

Chloroquine was introduced for the prevention and treatment of malaria. It usually clears an attack of the disease within three days. Injections may be given when an attack is severe. As a preventative treatment, a low dose is given once weekly, starting one week before visiting a high-risk area and continuing for four weeks after leaving. Chloroquine is not suitable for use in all parts of the world as resistance to the drug may have developed in some areas.

The other main use is in the treatment of autoimmune diseases, such as rheumatoid arthritis and lupus erythematosus.

Common *side effects* include nausea, headache, diarrhoea, and abdominal cramps. Occasionally a rash develops. More seriously, chloroquine can damage the retina during prolonged treatment, causing blurred vision that sometimes progresses to blindness. Regular eye examinations are performed to detect early changes.

INFORMATION FOR USERS

Follow instructions on the label. Call your doctor if symptoms worsen.

How taken

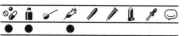

Tablets, liquid, injection.

Frequency and timing of doses
By mouth 1 x weekly (prevention of malaria); 1–4 x daily (treatment of malaria); 1 x daily (arthritis).

Adult dosage range
Prevention of malaria 300mg (2 tablets) as a single dose on the same day each week. Start 1 week before entering endemic area, and continue for 4 weeks after leaving. *Treatment of malaria* Initial dose 600mg (4 tablets) and following doses 300mg. *Rheumatoid arthritis* 150mg (1 tablet) per day.

Onset of effect
2–3 days. In rheumatoid arthritis, full effect may not be felt for up to 6 months.

Duration of action
Up to 1 week.

Diet advice
None.

Storage
Keep in a closed container in a cool, dry, place out of the reach of children. Protect from light.

Missed dose
Take as soon as you remember. If your next dose is due within 24 hours (1 x weekly schedule), or 6 hours (1–2 x daily schedule), take a single dose now and skip the next.

Stopping the drug
Do not stop the drug without consulting your doctor.

OVERDOSE ACTION

 Seek immediate medical advice in all cases. Take emergency action if breathing difficulties, fits, or loss of consciousness occur.

See Drug poisoning emergency guide (p.494).

SPECIAL PRECAUTIONS

Be sure to consult your doctor or pharmacist before taking this drug if:
▼ You have liver or kidney problems.
▼ You have glucose-6-phosphate dehydrogenase (G6PD) deficiency.
▼ You have eye or vision problems.
▼ You have psoriasis.
▼ You have a history of epilepsy.
▼ You suffer from porphyria.
▼ You are taking other medications.

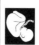 **Pregnancy**
▼ No evidence of risk with low doses. High doses may affect the baby. Discuss with your doctor.

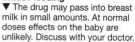 **Breast-feeding**
▼ The drug may pass into breast milk in small amounts. At normal doses effects on the baby are unlikely. Discuss with your doctor.

 **Infants and children**
▼ Reduced dose necessary.

 Over 60
▼ No special problems, except that it may be difficult to tell between changes in eyesight due to ageing, and those that are drug induced.

 Driving and hazardous work
▼ Avoid such activities until you have learned how chloroquine affects you because the drug may cause dizziness.

 Alcohol
▼ Keep consumption low.

POSSIBLE ADVERSE EFFECTS

Side effects such as nausea, diarrhoea, and abdominal pain might be avoided by taking the drug with food. Changes in vision should be reported promptly.

Symptom/effect	Frequency		Discuss with doctor		Stop taking drug now	Call doctor now
	Common	Rare	Only if severe	In all cases		
Nausea	●		■			
Diarrhoea/abdominal pain	●		■			
Headache/dizziness		●	■			
Rash		●		■	▲	▮
Blurred vision		●		■	▲	▮

INTERACTIONS

Anticonvulsant drugs Chloroquine may reduce the anticonvulsant effect of these drugs.

Digoxin The level of digoxin in the blood may be increased by chloroquine.

Cyclosporin Chloroquine increases the blood level of cyclosporin.

Amiodarone Chloroquine may increase the risk of abnormal heart rhythms if taken with this drug.

PROLONGED USE

Prolonged use may cause eye damage and blood disorders.

Monitoring Periodic eye tests and blood counts must be carried out.

CHLORPHENAMINE (CHLORPHENIRAMINE)

Brand names Calimal, Piriton
Used in the following combined preparations Contac 400, Dristan, Expulin, Galpseud Plus, Haymine, Tixylix Cough and Cold

GENERAL INFORMATION

Chlorphenamine has been used for over 30 years to treat allergies such as hay fever, allergic conjunctivitis, urticaria (hives), insect bites and stings, and angioedema (allergic swellings). It is included in several over-the-counter cold remedies (see p.94).

Like other antihistamines, it relieves allergic skin symptoms such as itching, swelling, and redness. It also reduces sneezing and the runny nose and itching eyes of hay fever. Chlorphenamine also has a mild *anticholinergic* action, which suppresses mucus secretion.

Chlorphenamine may also be used to prevent or treat allergic reactions to blood transfusions or X-ray contrast material, and can be given with epinephrine (adrenaline) injections for acute allergic shock (anaphylaxis).

QUICK REFERENCE

Drug group Antihistamine (p.124)

Overdose danger rating Medium

Dependence rating Low

Prescription needed No (tablets and liquid); yes (injection)

Available as generic Yes

INFORMATION FOR USERS

Follow instructions on the label. Call your doctor if symptoms worsen.

How taken

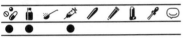

Tablets, liquid, injection.

Frequency and timing of doses
4–6 x daily (tablets, liquid); single dose as needed (injection).

Dosage range
Adults 12–24mg daily (by mouth); up to 40mg daily (injection).
Children Reduced dose according to age and weight.

Onset of effect
Within 60 minutes (by mouth); within 20 minutes (injection).

Duration of action
4–6 hours (tablets, liquid, injection).

Diet advice
None.

Storage
Keep in a closed container in a cool, dry place out of the reach of children.

Missed dose
Take as soon as you remember. If your next dose is due within 2 hours, take a single dose now and skip the next.

Stopping the drug
Can be safely stopped as soon as you no longer need it.

Exceeding the dose
An occasional unintentional extra dose is unlikely to cause problems. Large overdoses may cause drowsiness or agitation. Notify your doctor.

POSSIBLE ADVERSE EFFECTS

Drowsiness is the most common adverse effect of chlorphenamine; other *side effects* are rare. Some of these, such as dryness of the mouth, blurred vision, and difficulty passing urine, are due to its *anticholinergic* effects. Gastrointestinal irritation may be reduced by taking the tablets or liquid with food or drink.

Symptom/effect	Frequency		Discuss with doctor		Stop taking drug now	Call doctor now
	Common	Rare	Only if severe	In all cases		
Drowsiness/dizziness	●		■			
Digestive disturbances		●	■			
Difficulty in passing urine		●	■			
Dry mouth		●	■			
Blurred vision		●		■		
Excitation (children)		●		■	▲	
Rash		●		■	▲	

INTERACTIONS

Sedatives All drugs with a *sedative* effect are likely to increase the sedative properties of chlorphenamine.

Phenytoin The effects of phenytoin may be enhanced by chlorphenamine.

Anticholinergic drugs All drugs, including certain drugs for *parkinsonism*, that have an anticholinergic effect are likely to increase the anticholinergic effect of chlorphenamine.

SPECIAL PRECAUTIONS

Be sure to consult your doctor or pharmacist before taking this drug if:
▼ You have a long-term liver problem.
▼ You have had epileptic fits.
▼ You have glaucoma.
▼ You have urinary difficulties.
▼ You are taking other medications.

 Pregnancy
▼ Safety in pregnancy not established. Discuss with your doctor.

 Breast-feeding
▼ The drug passes into the breast milk, but at normal doses adverse effects on the baby are unlikely. Discuss with your doctor.

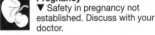 **Infants and children**
▼ Reduced dose necessary.

 Over 60
▼ Reduced dose may be necessary. Increased likelihood of adverse effects.

 Driving and hazardous work
▼ Avoid such activities until you have learned how chlorphenamine affects you because the drug can cause drowsiness, dizziness, and blurred vision.

 Alcohol
▼ Avoid. Alcohol may increase the sedative effects of this drug.

PROLONGED USE

The effect of the drug may become weaker with prolonged use over a period of weeks or months as the body adapts. Transfer to a different antihistamine may be recommended.

CHLORPROMAZINE

Brand names Chloractil, Largactil
Used in the following combined preparations None

GENERAL INFORMATION

The first antipsychotic drug that was marketed, chlorpromazine remains one of the most widely used of this drug group. It is effective in reducing aggression, suppressing abnormal behaviour, and producing a generally tranquillizing effect.

Chlorpromazine is prescribed for the treatment of schizophrenia, mania, and other disorders where confused, aggressive, or abnormal behaviour

may occur and a degree of sedation is required. Other uses of this drug include the treatment of nausea and vomiting, especially when caused by drug or radiation treatment; and treating severe, prolonged hiccoughs.

The main drawback to the use of chlorpromazine is that it can produce many *side effects* (below), some of which may be serious.

QUICK REFERENCE

Drug group Phenothiazine antipsychotic (p.85) and anti-emetic drug (p.90)

Overdose danger rating Medium

Dependence rating Low

Prescription needed Yes

Available as generic Yes

INFORMATION FOR USERS

Your drug prescription is tailored for you. Do not alter dosage without checking with your doctor.

How taken

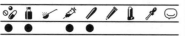

Tablets, liquid, injection, suppositories.

Frequency and timing of doses
1–4 x daily.

Adult dosage range
Mental illness 75–300mg daily; dose is started low and gradually increased. Larger doses may be used in severe illness. *Nausea and vomiting* 40–150mg daily.

Onset of effect
30–60 minutes (by mouth); 15–20 minutes (injection); up to 30 minutes (suppository).

Duration of action
8–12 hours (by mouth or injection); 3–4 hours (suppository). Some effect may

persist for up to 3 weeks when stopping the drug after regular use.

Diet advice
None.

Storage
Keep in a closed container in a cool, dry place out of the reach of children. Protect from light.

Missed dose
Take as soon as you remember. If your next dose is due within 2 hours, do not take the missed dose. Take your next scheduled dose as usual.

Stopping the drug
Do not stop taking the drug without consulting your doctor; symptoms may recur.

Exceeding the dose
An occasional unintentional extra dose is unlikely to cause problems. Larger overdoses may cause unusual drowsiness, fainting, abnormal heart rhythms, muscle rigidity, and agitation. Notify your doctor.

SPECIAL PRECAUTIONS

Be sure to tell your doctor if:
▼ You have long-term liver or kidney problems.
▼ You have had heart problems.
▼ You have had epileptic fits.
▼ You have thyroid disease.
▼ You have Parkinson's disease.
▼ You have glaucoma.
▼ You are taking other medications.

Pregnancy
▼ Not usually prescribed. Taken near the time of delivery it can prolong labour and may cause drowsiness in the newborn baby. Discuss with your doctor.

Breast-feeding
▼ The drug passes into the breast milk and may affect the baby. Discuss with your doctor.

Infants and children
▼ Not recommended for infants under 1 year. Reduced dose necessary for older children.

Over 60
▼ Initial dosage is low; it may be increased if there are no adverse reactions, such as abnormal limb movements or low blood pressure.

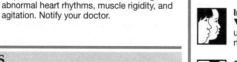

Driving and hazardous work
▼ Avoid such activities until you have learned how chlorpromazine affects you as the drug can cause drowsiness and slowed reactions.

Alcohol
▼ Avoid. Alcohol may increase the sedative effects of this drug.

Surgery and general anaesthetics
▼ Chlorpromazine treatment may need to be stopped before you have a general anaesthetic. Discuss this with your doctor or dentist before any operation.

POSSIBLE ADVERSE EFFECTS

Chlorpromazine commonly causes mild drowsiness and has an *anticholinergic* effect, which can cause symptoms. The most significant adverse effect is *parkinsonism*.

Symptom/effect	Frequency		Discuss with doctor		Stop taking drug now	Call doctor now
	Common	Rare	Only if severe	In all cases		
Drowsiness/lethargy	●		■			
Weight gain	●		■			
Blurred vision	●			■		
Dizziness/fainting	●			■		
Tremor/parkinsonism	●		■			
Infrequent periods		●		■		
Light sensitive rash		●		■	▲	
Jaundice		●		■	▲	

INTERACTIONS

Drugs for parkinsonism Chlorpromazine may reduce the effect of these drugs.

Anticholinergic drugs These drugs may intensify the *anticholinergic* properties of chlorpromazine.

Sedatives All drugs that have a *sedative* effect on the central nervous system are likely to increase the sedative properties of chlorpromazine.

PROLONGED USE

If used for more than a few months, chlorpromazine may cause movement disorders. Occasionally, *jaundice* may occur due to an allergic effect of the drug.

CHORIONIC GONADOTROPHIN

Brand names Choragon, Pregnyl, Profasi
Used in the following combined preparations None

GENERAL INFORMATION

Produced by the placenta, human chorionic gonadotrophin (HCG) is a hormone that stimulates the ovaries to produce two other hormones, oestrogen and progesterone, that are essential to the conception and early growth of the fetus. The hormone is extracted from the urine of pregnant women and has several medical purposes.

Its principal value is in the treatment of female infertility. Given by injection, usually with another hormone, HCG encourages the ovaries to release an egg (known as ovulation) so that it can be fertilized. Ovulation usually occurs 18 hours after injection, and intercourse should follow within 48 hours. The likelihood of multiple births increases because several eggs may be released by the ovaries at once.

In rare cases chorionic gonadotrophin is also given to young boys to treat undescended testes.

The drug is occasionally given to men to improve sperm production; treatment may take as long as six to nine months.

INFORMATION FOR USERS

This drug is given only under medical supervision and is not for self-administration.

How taken

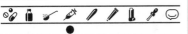

Injection.

Frequency and timing of doses
1–3 x per week.

Dosage range
Dosage varies from person to person, and may need adjustment during treatment.

Onset of effect
1–8 days (female infertility); 6–9 months (male infertility).

Duration of action
2–3 days.

Diet advice
None.

Storage
Not applicable. This drug is not kept in the home.

Missed dose
Arrange to receive the missed dose as soon as possible. Delay of more than 24 hours may reduce the chance of conception.

Stopping the drug
Complete the course of treatment as directed. Stopping the drug prematurely will reduce the chance of conception.

Exceeding the dose
The drug is always injected under close medical supervision. Overdose is unlikely.

POSSIBLE ADVERSE EFFECTS

When taken for fertility problems, the more common *adverse effects* of HCG are rarely severe and tend to diminish with time.

Women who take large doses of the drug may experience abdominal pain or swelling due to overstimulation of the ovaries.

Symptom/effect	Frequency		Discuss with doctor		Stop taking drug now	Call doctor now
	Common	Rare	Only if severe	In all cases		
Headache/tiredness	●		■			
Pain at injection site	●		■			
Mood changes	●			■		
Women only						
Abdominal pain		●		■		
Men only						
Enlarged breasts		●		■	▲	
Swollen feet/ankles		●		■		

INTERACTIONS

None.

SPECIAL PRECAUTIONS

Be sure to tell your doctor if:
▼ You have a long-term kidney problem.
▼ You have asthma.
▼ You have had epileptic fits.
▼ You suffer from migraine.
▼ You have a heart disorder.
▼ You have had a previous allergic reaction to this drug.
▼ You have prostate trouble.
▼ You are taking other medications.

Pregnancy
▼ Not prescribed.

Breast feeding
▼ Not prescribed.

Infants and children
▼ HCG is safely prescribed to treat undescended testes in boys.

Over 60
▼ Not usually required.

Driving and hazardous work
▼ Avoid such activities until you have learned how HCG affects you because the drug can cause tiredness.

Alcohol
▼ Avoid excessive amounts. Alcohol increases tiredness and, if taken in excess, may reduce fertility.

PROLONGED USE

No special problems.

Monitoring Women taking HCG to improve fertility usually have regular pelvic examinations and checks on cervical mucus to confirm that ovulation is taking place. Men are given regular sperm counts.

CIMETIDINE

Brand names Acitak, Dyspamet, Galenamet, Peptimax, Phimetin, Tagamet, Ultec, Zita
Used in the following combined preparations Algitec, Tagamet Dual Action

GENERAL INFORMATION

Introduced in the 1970s, cimetidine was the first of a new group of anti-ulcer drugs. Cimetidine reduces the secretion of gastric acid and of pepsin, an enzyme that helps in the digestion of protein. By reducing levels of acid and pepsin, it promotes healing of ulcers in the stomach and duodenum (see p.109). It is also used for reflux oesophagitis, in which acid stomach contents may flow up the oesophagus. Treatment is usually given in four- to eight-week courses, with further short courses if symptoms recur.

Cimetidine also affects the actions of certain enzymes in the liver, where many drugs are broken down. It is therefore prescribed with caution to people who are receiving other drugs, particularly anticoagulants and anticonvulsants, whose levels need to be carefully controlled. Since cimetidine promotes healing of the stomach lining, it may mask the symptoms of stomach cancer and delay diagnosis. It is therefore prescribed with caution if symptoms persist.

QUICK REFERENCE

Drug group Anti-ulcer drug (p.109)
Overdose danger rating Low
Dependence rating Low
Prescription needed No (some preparations)
Available as generic Yes

INFORMATION FOR USERS

Follow instructions on the label. Call your doctor if symptoms worsen.

How taken

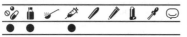

Tablets, liquid, injection.

Frequency and timing of doses
1–4 x daily (after meals and at bedtime).

Adult dosage range
800–1,600mg daily (occasionally increased to 2,400mg daily).

Onset of effect
Within 90 minutes.

Duration of action
2–6 hours.

Diet advice
None.

Storage
Keep in a closed container in a cool, dry place away from the reach of children. Protect from light.

Missed dose
Do not take the missed dose. Take your next dose as usual.

Stopping the drug
If prescribed by your doctor, do not stop taking the drug without consulting him or her because symptoms may recur.

Exceeding the dose
An occasional unintentional extra dose is unlikely to be a cause for concern. But if you notice any unusual symptoms, or if a large overdose has been taken, notify your doctor.

POSSIBLE ADVERSE EFFECTS

Adverse effects of cimetidine are uncommon. They are usually related to dosage level and almost always disappear when the drug is stopped.

Symptom/effect	Frequency		Discuss with doctor		Stop taking drug now	Call doctor now
	Common	Rare	Only if severe	In all cases		
Diarrhoea		●	■			
Dizziness/confusion/tiredness		●		■		
Muscle pain		●		■		
Breast enlargement (men)		●		■		
Impotence		●		■		
Rash		●		■	▲	

INTERACTIONS

Benzodiazepines Cimetidine may increase the blood levels of some of these drugs, increasing the risk of adverse effects.

Theophylline/aminophylline Cimetidine may increase the blood levels of these drugs and their dose may need to be reduced.

Sildenafil Cimetidine may increase the blood level of this drug.

Beta blockers and antiarrhythmic drugs Cimetidine may increase the blood levels of these drugs.

Anticonvulsant drugs Cimetidine may increase the blood levels of these drugs, and their dose may need to be reduced.

Anticoagulant drugs Cimetidine may increase the effect of anticoagulants and their dose may need to be reduced.

SPECIAL PRECAUTIONS

Be sure to consult your doctor or pharmacist before taking this drug if:
▼ You have long-term liver or kidney problems.
▼ You are taking other medications.

 Pregnancy
▼ Safety in pregnancy not established. Discuss with your doctor.

 Breast-feeding
▼ The drug passes into the breast milk, but at normal doses adverse effects on the baby are unlikely. Discuss with your doctor.

 Infants and children
▼ Reduced dose necessary.

 Over 60
▼ No special problems unless kidney function is reduced, in which case dosage is decreased.

 Driving and hazardous work
▼ Avoid such activities until you have learned how cimetidine affects you because the drug may cause dizziness and confusion.

Alcohol
▼ Avoid. Alcohol may aggravate the underlying condition and counter the beneficial effects of cimetidine.

PROLONGED USE

Courses of longer than 8 weeks are not usually necessary.

CINNARIZINE

Brand names Cinaziere, Stugeron, Stugeron Forte
Used in the following combined preparations None

GENERAL INFORMATION

Introduced in the 1970s, cinnarizine is an antihistamine used mainly to control nausea and vomiting, especially motion (travel) sickness. The drug is also used to control the symptoms (nausea and vertigo) of inner ear disorders such as labyrinthitis and Ménière's disease.

Taken in high doses, cinnarizine has a *vasodilator* effect and is used to improve circulation in Raynaud's disease and peripheral vascular disease.

Cinnarizine has adverse effects that are similar to those of most other antihistamines. Drowsiness is the most common problem, but it is usually less severe than with other antihistamines.

QUICK REFERENCE

Drug group Antihistamine anti-emetic drug (p.90)

Overdose danger rating Medium

Dependence rating Low

Prescription needed No

Available as generic Yes

INFORMATION FOR USERS

Follow instructions on the label. Call your doctor if symptoms worsen.

How taken

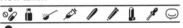

Tablets, capsules.

Frequency and timing of doses
2–3 x daily. For the prevention of motion sickness, the first dose should be taken 2 hours before travel.

Dosage range
Adults 45–90mg daily (nausea/vomiting); 150–225mg daily (circulatory disorders); 30mg, then 15mg every 8 hours as needed (motion sickness).
Children aged 5–12, 15mg, then 7.5mg every 8 hours as needed (motion sickness).

Onset of effect
Within 30 minutes. Several weeks (circulation diseases).

Duration of action
Up to 8 hours.

Diet advice
None.

Storage
Keep in a closed container in a cool, dry place away from the reach of children.

Missed dose
Take as soon as you remember. If your next dose is due within 2 hours, take a single dose now and skip the next.

Stopping the drug
If you are taking cinnarizine to treat an inner ear disorder or a circulatory condition, do not stop the drug without consulting your doctor; symptoms may recur. However, when taken for motion sickness, the drug can be safely stopped as soon as you no longer need it.

Exceeding the dose
An occasional unintentional extra dose is unlikely to cause problems. Large overdoses may cause drowsiness or agitation. Notify your doctor.

SPECIAL PRECAUTIONS

Be sure to consult your doctor or pharmacist before taking this drug if:
▼ You have low blood pressure.
▼ You have glaucoma.
▼ You have an enlarged prostate.
▼ You are taking other medications.

Pregnancy
▼ Safety in pregnancy not established. Discuss with your doctor.

Breast-feeding
▼ Safety not established. Discuss with your doctor.

Infants and children
▼ Reduced dose necessary.

Over 60
▼ No special problems.

Driving and hazardous work
▼ Avoid such activities until you have learned how cinnarizine affects you because the drug can cause drowsiness.

Alcohol
▼ Avoid. Alcohol may increase the sedative effects of this drug.

POSSIBLE ADVERSE EFFECTS

Drowsiness is the main adverse effect of this drug. *Anticholinergic* effects such as blurred vision and dry mouth may also occur occasionally.

Symptom/effect	Frequency		Discuss with doctor		Stop taking drug now	Call doctor now
	Common	Rare	Only if severe	In all cases		
Drowsiness/lethargy	●		■			
Blurred vision		●	■			
Dry mouth		●	■			
Rash		●		■		▲

PROLONGED USE

No special problems.

INTERACTIONS

General note All drugs that have a *sedative* effect on the central nervous system may increase the sedative properties of cinnarizine. Such drugs include sleeping drugs, antidepressants, anti-anxiety drugs, and *opioid* analgesics.

CIPROFLOXACIN

Brand name Ciproxin
Used in the following combined preparations None

GENERAL INFORMATION

Ciprofloxacin, a quinolone antibacterial, is used to treat several types of bacteria resistant to other commonly used antibiotics. It is especially useful for chest, intestine, and urinary tract infections and is also used to treat gonorrhoea.

When taken by mouth, ciprofloxacin is well absorbed by the body and works quickly and effectively. In more severe systemic bacterial infections, however, it may be necessary to administer the drug by injection.

Ciprofloxacin has a long duration of action and needs to be taken only once or twice daily. Its most common *side effect* is gastrointestinal disturbance.

QUICK REFERENCE

Drug group Antibacterial (p.131)
Overdose danger rating Medium
Dependence rating Low
Prescription needed Yes
Available as generic No

INFORMATION FOR USERS

Your drug prescription is tailored for you. Do not alter dosage without checking with your doctor.

How taken

Tablets, liquid, injection.

Frequency and timing of doses
2 x daily with plenty of fluids.

Adult dosage range
500mg–1.5g daily (tablets); 200–400mg daily (injection).

Onset of effect
The drug begins to work within a few hours, although full beneficial effect may not be felt for several days.

Duration of action
About 12 hours.

Diet advice
Do not get dehydrated; ensure that you drink fluids regularly.

Storage
Keep in a closed container in a cool, dry place out of the reach of children. The injection must be protected from light.

Missed dose
Take as soon as you remember, and take your next dose as usual.

Stopping the drug
Take the full course. Even if you feel better the original infection may still be present, and symptoms may recur if treatment is stopped too soon.

Exceeding the dose
An occasional unintentional extra dose is unlikely to cause problems. Large overdoses may cause mental disturbance and fits. Notify your doctor.

SPECIAL PRECAUTIONS

Be sure to tell your doctor if:
▼ You have long-term liver or kidney problems.
▼ You have had epileptic fits.
▼ You have glucose-6-phosphate dehydrogenase (G6PD) deficiency.
▼ You are taking other medications.

Pregnancy
▼ Safety in pregnancy not established. Discuss with your doctor.

Breast-feeding
▼ The drug passes into the breast milk and may affect the baby adversely. Discuss with your doctor.

Infants and children
▼ Not usually recommended.

Over 60
▼ No special problems.

Driving and hazardous work
▼ Avoid such activities until you have learned how ciprofloxacin affects you because the drug can cause dizziness.

Alcohol
▼ Avoid. Alcohol may increase the sedative effects of this drug.

Sunlight
▼ Avoid excessive exposure.

POSSIBLE ADVERSE EFFECTS

Ciprofloxacin commonly causes nausea and vomiting; other side effects are less common, except when very high doses are given. Painful and inflamed tendons should be reported to your doctor at once, treatment should be discontinued, and the affected limbs rested.

Symptom/effect	Frequency		Discuss with doctor		Stop taking drug now	Call doctor now
	Common	Rare	Only if severe	In all cases		
Nausea/vomiting	●		■			
Abdominal pain/diarrhoea	●		■			
Dizziness/headache		●	■			
Joint pain		●	■			
Sleep disturbance		●	■			
Rash		●		■		
Photosensitivity		●		■		
Jaundice		●		■		
Confusion/convulsions		●		■		
Painful, inflamed tendons		●		■	▲	▎

PROLONGED USE

No problems expected.

Monitoring Blood tests may be necessary to monitor kidney and liver function.

INTERACTIONS

Oral iron preparations and antacids containing magnesium or aluminium hydroxide interfere with absorption of ciprofloxacin. Do not take antacids within 2 hours of taking ciprofloxacin tablets.

Anticoagulants and oral antidiabetics Blood levels of these drugs may be increased; their dosage may need adjusting.

Theophylline Ciprofloxacin may increase blood levels of this drug; its dose may need adjusting and its blood levels monitored.

Phenytoin Ciprofloxacin may increase the blood levels of this drug.

Non-steroidal anti-inflammatory drugs These drugs increase the risk of epileptic fits.

CISAPRIDE

Brand name Prepulsid
Used in the following combined preparations None

GENERAL INFORMATION

Cisapride is a drug that stimulates forward movement in the oesophagus and intestines. It is useful in a number of gastrointestinal disorders, including the symptoms of gastro-oesophageal reflux, such as dyspepsia, heartburn, and regurgitation. Cisapride may be useful in cases when emptying of the stomach is delayed, which may occur in some diabetics and in patients suffering from systemic sclerosis (scleroderma) and

autonomic neuropathy. The drug is sometimes used for the short-term treatment of dyspepsia (indigestion) that does not respond to other remedies.

Cisapride works by increasing the release of acetylcholine in the gut wall; this in turn increases the contractions of the muscles in the gut wall. Adverse effects on the gastrointestinal tract rarely require discontinuing the drug and tend to diminish in time.

QUICK REFERENCE

Drug group Motility stimulant (p.111)

Overdose danger rating Medium

Dependence rating Low

Prescription needed Yes

Available as generic No

INFORMATION FOR USERS

Your drug prescription is tailored for you. Do not alter dosage without checking with your doctor.

How taken

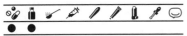

Tablets, liquid.

Frequency and timing of doses
1–4 x daily, 15–30 minutes before meals and/or at bedtime (for symptoms during the night).

Adult dosage range
20–40mg daily in divided doses.

Onset of effect
15–30 minutes.

Duration of action
Up to 10 hours.

Diet advice
Grapefruit juice should be avoided because it increases the amount of cisapride absorbed.

Storage
Keep in a closed container in a cool, dry place out of the reach of children. Protect from light.

Missed dose
Do not take unless you have symptoms. Take the next dose as usual unless you took the last dose less than 2 hours ago.

Stopping the drug
Do not stop taking the drug without consulting your doctor because symptoms may recur.

Exceeding the dose
An occasional unintentional extra dose is unlikely to be a cause for concern. But if you notice any unusual symptoms, or if a large overdose has been taken, notify your doctor.

SPECIAL PRECAUTIONS

Be sure to tell your doctor if:
▼ You have long-term liver or kidney problems.
▼ You have a history of gastrointestinal illness.
▼ You have a history of heart problems.
▼ You are taking other medications.

 Pregnancy
▼ Safety in pregnancy not established. Discuss with your doctor.

 Breast-feeding
▼ The drug passes into the breast milk, but at normal doses adverse effects on the baby are unlikely. Discuss with your doctor.

 Infants and children
▼ Not recommended for children under 12 years.

 Over 60
▼ No special problems.

 Driving and hazardous work
▼ Avoid such activities until you have learned how cisapride affects you because the drug can cause dizziness.

Alcohol
▼ No special problems.

POSSIBLE ADVERSE EFFECTS

The most common *adverse effects* are those on the gastrointestinal system, such as

abdominal cramps and diarrhoea. These usually diminish as treatment continues.

Symptom/effect	Frequency		Discuss with doctor		Stop taking drug now	Call doctor now
	Common	Rare	Only if severe	In all cases		
Abdominal cramps	●		■			
Diarrhoea	●		■			
Dizziness/lightheadedness		●		■		
Headaches		●		■		
Tremor		●		■		
Palpitations		●		■	■	■

INTERACTIONS

Strong analgesics *Opioid* analgesics may reduce the effect of cisapride.

Antibiotics Clarithromycin and erythromycin may increase the blood levels of cisapride, leading to heart problems.

Anticoagulant drugs The effect of anticoagulants such as warfarin may be increased by cisapride.

Tricyclic antidepressants, nefazodone, and terfenadine These drugs may increase blood levels of cisapride, leading to heart problems.

Antifungal drugs Fluconazole, itraconazole, ketoconazole, and, possibly, related antifungals may increase blood levels of cisapride, leading to heart problems.

PROLONGED USE

Cisapride is normally given for a course of treatment lasting between 4 and 12 weeks, after which a maintenance dose may be used once or twice a day, depending on the condition being treated.

CISPLATIN

Brand names None
Used in the following combined preparations None

GENERAL INFORMATION

Cisplatin is one of the most effective drugs available to treat cancer of the ovaries or testes. People with cancer of the head, neck, bladder, cervix, and lung have also responded well to it. Recent research indicates that cisplatin may be an effective treatment against bone cancer in children. It is often given along with other anticancer drugs.

The most common and serious *adverse effect* of cisplatin is impaired kidney function. To reduce the risk of permanent kidney damage, the drug is usually given only once every four weeks, allowing the kidneys time to recover between courses of treatment. Nausea and vomiting may occur after administration of cisplatin. They usually start within an hour and last for up to 24 hours: in some case persisting for up to a week. Because they may be quite severe, anti-emetic drugs are given.

Damage to hearing is common and may be more severe in children. Use of cisplatin may also increase the risk of anaemia, blood clotting disorders, and infection during treatment.

INFORMATION FOR USERS

This drug is given only under medical supervision and is not for self-administration.

How taken

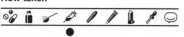

Injection.

Frequency and timing of doses
Once daily for 5 days every 3 weeks (on its own or in combination with other anticancer drugs; once every 3–4 weeks (on its own).

Adult dosage range
Dosage is determined individually according to body height, weight, and response.

Onset of effect
Some adverse effects, such as nausea and vomiting, may appear within 1 hour of starting treatment.

Duration of action
Some adverse effects may last for up to 1 week after treatment has stopped.

Diet advice
Prior to treatment it is important that the body is well hydrated. Therefore, 1–2 litres of fluid are usually given by infusion over 8–12 hours.

Storage
Not applicable. The drug is not normally kept in the home.

Missed dose
Not applicable. The drug is given only in hospital under medical supervision.

Stopping the drug
Not applicable. The drug will be stopped under medical supervision.

Exceeding the dose
Overdosage is unlikely since treatment is carefully monitored, and the drug is given intravenously only under close supervision.

SPECIAL PRECAUTIONS

Cisplatin is prescribed only under close medical supervision, taking account of your present condition and your medical history.

Pregnancy
▼ Not usually prescribed. Cisplatin may cause birth defects or premature birth. Discuss with your doctor.

Breast-feeding
▼ Not advised. The drug passes into the breast milk and may affect the baby adversely. Discuss with your doctor.

Infants and children
▼ The risk of hearing loss is increased. Reduced dose used.

Over 60
▼ Reduced dose may be necessary. Increased likelihood of adverse effects.

Driving and hazardous work
▼ No known problems.

Alcohol
▼ No known problems.

POSSIBLE ADVERSE EFFECTS

Most adverse effects appear within a few hours of injection and are carefully monitored in hospital after each dose. Some effects wear off within 24 hours. Nausea and loss of appetite may last for up to a week.

Symptom/effect	Frequency		Discuss with doctor		Stop taking drug now	Call doctor now
	Common	Rare	Only if severe	In all cases		
Nausea/vomiting	●			■		
Ringing in the ears/hearing loss	●			■		
Loss of appetite/taste	●		■			
Breathing difficulties		●		■		▮
Fits		●		■		▮
Wheezing		●		■		▮
Swollen face/rash		●		■		▮

PROLONGED USE

Prolonged use of this drug increases the risk of damage to the kidneys, nerves, and bone marrow, and to hearing.

Monitoring Hearing tests and blood checks to monitor kidney function and bone marrow activity are carried out regularly.

INTERACTIONS

General note A number of drugs (e.g., antibacterials such as gentamicin) increase the adverse effects of cisplatin. Because cisplatin is given only under close medical supervision, these interactions are carefully monitored and the dosage is adjusted accordingly.

CITALOPRAM

Brand name Cipramil
Used in the following combined preparations None

GENERAL INFORMATION

Citalopram is a member of the selective serotonin re-uptake inhibitor (SSRI) group of antidepressant drugs. It gradually improves the patient's mood, increases physical activity, and restores interest in everyday activities.

Citalopram is generally well tolerated, and any gastrointestinal *adverse effects*, such as nausea, vomiting, or diarrhoea,

are dose related and usually diminish with continued use of the drug.

Like other SSRIs, citalopram causes fewer *anticholinergic side effects* and is less sedating than the tricyclic antidepressants. It is also less likely to be harmful if taken in overdose. It can, however, cause drowsiness and impair performance of tasks such as driving.

INFORMATION FOR USERS

Your drug prescription is tailored for you. Do not alter dosage without checking with your doctor.

How taken

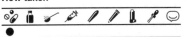

Tablets.

Frequency and timing of doses
Once daily in the morning or evening.

Adult dosage range
Depressive illness 20–60mg.
Panic attacks 10mg (starting dose); 20–30mg (usual range).

Onset of effect
Some benefit may appear within 7 days, but full benefits may not be felt for 2–4 weeks.

Duration of action
Antidepressant effect may persist for some weeks following prolonged treatment.

Diet advice
None.

Storage
Keep in a closed container in a cool, dry place out of the reach of children.

Missed dose
Take as soon as you remember. If your next dose is due within 8 hours, take a single dose now and skip the next.

Stopping the drug
Do not stop taking the drug without consulting your doctor, who will supervise a gradual reduction in dosage. You may experience withdrawal symptoms such as headaches, nausea, dizziness, a "pins-and-needles" sensation, and anxiety.

Exceeding the dose
An occasional unintentional extra dose is unlikely to be a cause for concern. If you notice any unusual symptoms, or if a large overdose has been taken, notify your doctor.

SPECIAL PRECAUTIONS

Be sure to tell your doctor if:
▼ You have epilepsy.
▼ You have liver or kidney problems.
▼ You have had a manic-depressive illness.
▼ You have had heart problems.
▼ You have been taking monoamine oxidase inhibitors (MAOIs) or other antidepressants.
▼ You are taking other medications.

Pregnancy
▼ Safety in pregnancy not established. Discuss with your doctor.

Breast-feeding
▼ The drug may pass into breast milk and may affect the baby. Discuss with your doctor.

Infants and children
▼ Not recommended.

Over 60
▼ Reduced dose necessary.

Driving and hazardous work
▼ Avoid such activities until you have learned how citalopram affects you because the drug can cause drowsiness.

Alcohol
▼ Avoid. Alcohol may increase the sedative effects of citalopram.

POSSIBLE ADVERSE EFFECTS

Common adverse effects such as nausea, indigestion, and diarrhoea usually diminish

with reduction in dosage. If convulsions or a rash occur, consult your doctor immediately.

Symptom/effect	Frequency		Discuss with doctor		Stop taking drug now	Call doctor now
	Common	Rare	Only if severe	In all cases		
Nausea/vomiting/Indigestion	●			■		
Diarrhoea/constipation	●			■		
Anxiety/insomnia		●		■		
Headache/tremor		●		■		
Dizziness/drowsiness		●		■		
Dry mouth/sweating		●		■		
Skin rash		●			■	▲ ∎

PROLONGED USE

No problems expected. However, mild withdrawal symptoms may occur if the drug is not stopped gradually.

INTERACTIONS

Sumatriptan and other 5HT1 agonists and lithium There is an increased risk of adverse effects when citalopram is taken with these drugs.

Monoamine oxidase inhibitors (MAOIs) These drugs may cause a severe reaction if they are taken with citalopram. Avoid taking citalopram if MAOIs have been taken in the last 14 days.

Anticoagulants The effect of these drugs may be increased by citalopram.

Drugs for epilepsy Citalopram may oppose the effect of these drugs.

Terfenadine The risk of arrhythmias is increased when this drug is taken with citalopram.

CLOBETASOL

Brand name Dermovate
Used in the following combined preparation Dermovate-NN

GENERAL INFORMATION

Clobetasol is a corticosteroid drug (p.141) used in the short-term treatment of severe skin conditions such as discoid lupus erythematosus, lichen planus and lichen simplex, eczema, and psoriasis. The drug is generally considered the strongest *topical* corticosteroid and is therefore used only when the disorder has not responded to treatment with another topical corticosteroid.

It is important to apply clobetasol thinly and sparingly to affected areas because it can cause *systemic adverse effects* such as suppression of the pituitary and adrenal glands and Cushing's syndrome. Other side effects include irreversible changes to the structure of the skin in the treated areas. Also, clobetasol can exacerbate eczema infected with a virus such as herpes simplex.

QUICK REFERENCE

Drug group Topical corticosteroid (p.174)

Overdose danger rating Low

Dependence rating Low

Prescription needed Yes

Available as generic No

INFORMATION FOR USERS

Your drug prescription is tailored for you. Do not alter dosage without checking with your doctor.

How taken

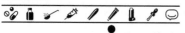

Cream, ointment, scalp application.

Frequency and timing of doses
1 x 2 times daily. If treating the face, use for no more than 5 days.

Dosage range
No more than 50g weekly.

Onset of effect
12 hours. Full beneficial effect after 48 hours.

Duration of action
Up to 24 hours.

Diet advice
None.

Storage
Keep in a closed container, in a cool, dry place out of the reach of children.

Missed dose
Use as soon as you remember. If your next application is due within 8 hours, apply the usual amount now and skip the next application.

Stopping the drug
Do not stop using the drug without consulting your doctor; symptoms may recur.

Exceeding the dose
An occasional unintentional extra application is unlikely to cause problems. But if you notice any unusual symptoms, notify your doctor.

POSSIBLE ADVERSE EFFECTS

Most people who use clobetasol as directed do not have problems. Adverse effects mainly affect the skin. Some of these effects cannot be reversed.

Symptom/effect	Frequency		Discuss with doctor		Stop taking drug now	Call doctor now
	Common	Rare	Only if severe	In all cases		
Thinning of the skin	●			■		
Stretch marks	●			■		
Increased capillary size in skin	●			■		
Acne/dermatitis around mouth	●			■		
Loss of skin pigment	●		■			
Mood changes		●		■		
Weight gain		●		■		

INTERACTIONS

None.

SPECIAL PRECAUTIONS

Be sure to tell your doctor if:
▼ You have a cold sore or chickenpox.
▼ You have any other infection.
▼ You have acne or rosacea.
▼ You are taking other medications.

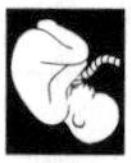

Pregnancy
▼ Safety in pregnancy not established. Discuss with your doctor.

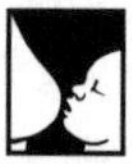

Breast-feeding
▼ The drug passes into the breast milk and may affect the baby. Discuss with your doctor.

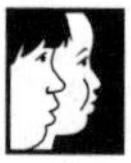

Infants and children
▼ Not recommended for infants under 1 year. Used only with great caution for short periods in older children because overuse can slow growth.

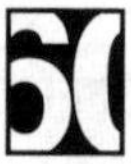

Over 60
▼ No special problems.

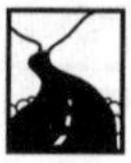

Driving and hazardous work
▼ No special problems.

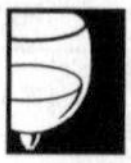

Alcohol
▼ No special problems.

PROLONGED USE

Clobetasol is not normally used for more than 4 weeks. If the condition has not improved in 2 to 4 weeks, you should notify your doctor.

CLOMIFENE

Brand names Clomid, Serophene
Used in the following combined preparations None

GENERAL INFORMATION

Clomifene increases the output of hormones by the pituitary gland, thereby stimulating ovulation (egg release) in women. If hormone levels in the blood fail to rise after the drug is taken, the gland is not working as it should.

For female infertility, tablets are taken within about five days of the onset of each menstrual cycle. This stimulates ovulation. If clomifene does not stimulate ovulation after several months, other drugs may be prescribed.

Multiple pregnancies (usually twins) occur more commonly in women treated with clomifene than in those who have not been treated. Adverse effects include an increased risk of ovarian cysts and ectopic pregnancy.

INFORMATION FOR USERS

Your drug prescription is tailored for you. Do not alter dosage without checking with your doctor.

How taken

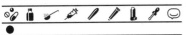

Tablets.

Frequency and timing of doses
Once daily for 5 days during each menstrual cycle.

Dosage range
50mg daily initially; dose may be increased up to 100mg daily.

Onset of effect
Ovulation occurs 4–10 days after the last dose in any cycle. However, ovulation may not occur for several months.

Duration of action
5 days.

Diet advice
None.

Storage
Keep in a closed container in a cool, dry place away from the reach of children. Protect from light.

Missed dose
Take as soon as you remember. If your next dose is due at this time, take the missed dose and the next scheduled dose together.

Stopping the drug
Take as directed by your doctor. Stopping the drug will reduce the chances of conception.

Exceeding the dose
An occasional unintentional extra dose is unlikely to be a cause for concern. But if you notice any unusual symptoms, or if a large overdose has been taken, notify your doctor.

SPECIAL PRECAUTIONS

Be sure to tell your doctor if:
▼ You have a long-term liver problem.
▼ You are taking other medications.

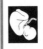
Pregnancy
▼ Not prescribed. The drug is stopped as soon as pregnancy occurs.

Breast-feeding
▼ Not prescribed.

Infants and children
▼ Not prescribed.

Over 60
▼ Not prescribed.

Driving and hazardous work
▼ Avoid such activities until you have learned how clomifene affects you because the drug can cause blurred vision.

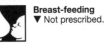
Alcohol
▼ Keep consumption low.

POSSIBLE ADVERSE EFFECTS

Most *side effects* are related to the dose taken. Ovarian enlargement and cyst formation can occur. If this happens the problem usually resolves within a few weeks of stopping the drug.

Symptom/effect	Frequency		Discuss with doctor		Stop taking drug now	Call doctor now
	Common	Rare	Only if severe	In all cases		
Hot flushes	●		■			
Nausea/vomiting	●		■			
"Breakthrough" bleeding	●		■			
Abdominal discomfort	●			■		
Impaired vision		●		■	▲	
Severe pain in chest/abdomen		●		■	▲	■
Breast tenderness		●		■		
Dry skin/hair loss/rash		●		■		
Convulsions		●		■	▲	■
Dizziness		●		■		

PROLONGED USE

Prolonged use of clomifene may cause visual impairment. Also, no more than 6 courses of treatment are recommended since this may lead to an increased risk of ovarian cancer.

Monitoring Eye tests may be recommended if symptoms of visual impairment are noticed. Monitoring of body temperature and blood or urine hormone levels is performed to detect signs of ovulation and pregnancy.

INTERACTIONS

None.

CLOMIPRAMINE

Brand names Anafranil, Anafranil SR
Used in the following combined preparations None

GENERAL INFORMATION

Clomipramine belongs to the class of antidepressant drugs known as the tricyclics. It is used mainly in the long-term treatment of depression. It elevates mood, improves appetite, increases physical activity, and restores interest in everyday activities.

Clomipramine is particularly useful in the treatment of irrational fears and obsessive behaviour. Unlike most other tricyclics, clomipramine can be given by injection in severe illness.

In overdose clomipramine may cause coma and dangerously abnormal heart rhythms.

Tricyclic antidepressant drugs have been linked with an increase in dental caries in long term use.

QUICK REFERENCE

Drug group Tricyclic antidepressant (p.84)
Overdose danger rating High
Dependence rating Low
Prescription needed Yes
Available as generic Yes

INFORMATION FOR USERS

Your drug prescription is tailored for you. Do not alter dosage without checking with your doctor.

How taken

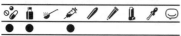

SR-tablets, capsules, liquid, injection.

Frequency and timing of doses
1–4 x daily.

Adult dosage range
10–250mg daily.

Onset of effect
Some effects may be felt within a few days, but full antidepressant effect may not be felt for up to 4 weeks.

Duration of action
During prolonged treatment antidepressant effect may last up to 2 weeks.

Diet advice
None.

Storage
Keep in a closed container in a cool, dry place away from the reach of children.

Missed dose
Take as soon as you remember. If your next dose is due within 3 hours, take a single dose now and skip the next.

Stopping the drug
Stopping abruptly can cause withdrawal symptoms and a recurrence of the original trouble. Consult your doctor, who may supervise a gradual reduction in dosage.

OVERDOSE ACTION

 Seek immediate medical advice in all cases. Take emergency action if palpitations are noted or consciousness is lost.

See Drug poisoning emergency guide (p.494).

SPECIAL PRECAUTIONS

Be sure to tell your doctor if:
▼ You have heart problems.
▼ You have had epileptic fits.
▼ You have long-term liver or kidney problems.
▼ You have had glaucoma.
▼ You have thyroid disease.
▼ You have had prostate trouble.
▼ You are taking other medications.

 Pregnancy
▼ Safety in pregnancy not established. Discuss with your doctor.

 Breast-feeding
▼ The drug passes into the breast milk and may affect the baby. Discuss with your doctor.

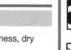 **Infants and children**
▼ Not usually prescribed.

Over 60
▼ Increased likelihood of adverse effects. Reduced dose may therefore be necessary.

Driving and hazardous work
▼ Avoid such activities until you have learned how clomipramine affects you because the drug may cause blurred vision, drowsiness, and dizziness.

Alcohol
▼ Avoid. Alcohol may increase the sedative effects of this drug.

Surgery and general anaesthetics
▼ Clomipramine treatment may need to be stopped before you have a general anaesthetic. Discuss this with your doctor or dentist before any operation.

POSSIBLE ADVERSE EFFECTS

The possible *adverse effects* of this drug are mainly the result of its *anticholinergic* action, and include drowsiness and dizziness, dry mouth, and constipation.

Symptom/effect	Frequency		Discuss with doctor		Stop taking drug now	Call doctor now
	Common	Rare	Only if severe	In all cases		
Drowsiness/dizziness	●			■		
Sweating/flushing	●			■		
Dry mouth	●			■		
Blurred vision	●			■		
Constipation	●			■		
Difficulty in passing urine		●		■	▲	
Palpitations		●		■	▲	■
Skin reactions/rash		●		■		

INTERACTIONS

Sedatives All drugs that have a *sedative* effect may intensify those of clomipramine.

Antihypertensives Clomipramine may enhance the effect of some of these drugs.

Anticonvulsants Clomipramine may reduce the effects of these drugs and vice versa.

Monoamine oxidase inhibitors (MAOIs) A serious reaction may occur if these drugs are given with clomipramine.

Cisapride and quinidine There is an increased risk of abnormal heart rhythms if these drugs are taken with clomipramine.

PROLONGED USE

No problems expected.

Monitoring Regular checks on heart and liver function are recommended. Regular dental check-ups are also advised because prolonged use of clomipramine can cause dental caries.

CLONAZEPAM

Brand name Rivotril
Used in the following combined preparations None

GENERAL INFORMATION

Clonazepam belongs to a group of drugs known as the benzodiazepines, which are mainly used in the treatment of anxiety and insomnia (see p.83). However, clonazepam is used almost exclusively as an anticonvulsant to prevent and treat epileptic fits. It is particularly useful for the prevention of brief muscle spasms and absence seizures (petit mal) in children but other forms of epilepsy, such as sudden flaccidity or fits induced by bright lights, also respond to clonazepam treatment. Being a benzodiazepine, the drug also has tranquillizing and sedative effects.

Clonazepam is used either alone or together with other anticonvulsant drugs. Its anticonvulsant effect may begin to wear off after a few months.

INFORMATION FOR USERS

Your drug prescription is tailored for you. Do not alter dosage without checking with your doctor.

How taken

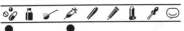

Tablets, injection.

Frequency and timing of doses
1–4 x daily.

Dosage range
Adults 1mg daily (starting dose), increased gradually to 4–8 mg daily (maintenance dose). *Children* Reduced dose according to age and weight.

Onset of effect
Within 1 hour.

Duration of action
Approximately 30 hours.

Diet advice
None.

Storage
Keep in a closed container in a cool, dry place away from the reach of children.

Missed dose
No cause for concern, but take as soon as you remember. Take your next dose when it is due.

Stopping the drug
Do not stop the drug without consulting your doctor because symptoms may recur.

Exceeding the dose
An occasional unintentional extra dose is unlikely to cause problems. Larger overdoses may cause unusual drowsiness and confusion. Notify your doctor.

POSSIBLE ADVERSE EFFECTS

The principal *adverse effects* of this drug are related to its sedative and tranquillizing properties. These effects normally diminish after the first few days of treatment and can often be reduced by medically supervised adjustment of dosage.

Symptom/effect	Frequency		Discuss with doctor		Stop taking drug now	Call doctor now
	Common	Rare	Only if severe	In all cases		
Daytime drowsiness	●		■			
Dizziness/unsteadiness	●		■			
Increased salivation	●		■			
Altered behaviour	●				■	
Forgetfulness/confusion		●			■	
Muscle weakness		●			■	

INTERACTIONS

Sedatives All drugs that have a *sedative* effect on the central nervous system are likely to increase the sedative properties of clonazepam. Such drugs include anti-anxiety and sleeping drugs, antihistamines, opioid analgesics, antidepressants, and antipsychotics.

Other anticonvulsants Clonazepam may alter the effects of other anticonvulsants you are taking, and adjustment of dosage or change of drug may be necessary.

SPECIAL PRECAUTIONS

Be sure to tell your doctor if:
▼ You have severe respiratory disease.
▼ You have long-term liver or kidney problems.
▼ You are taking other medications.

 Pregnancy
▼ Safety in pregnancy not established. Discuss with your doctor.

 Breast-feeding
▼ The drug passes into the breast milk and may affect the baby adversely. Discuss with your doctor.

 Infants and children
▼ Reduced dose necessary.

 Over 60
▼ Reduced dose may be necessary.

 Driving and hazardous work
▼ Your underlying condition, as well as the possibility of drowsiness while taking clonazepam, may make such activities inadvisable. Discuss with your doctor.

Alcohol
▼ Avoid. Alcohol may increase the sedative effects of this drug.

PROLONGED USE

Both beneficial and adverse effects of clonazepam may become less marked during prolonged treatment as the body adapts.

CLOPIDOGREL

Brand name Plavix
Used in the following combined preparations None

GENERAL INFORMATION

Clopidogrel is an antiplatelet drug that is used to prevent blood clots from forming. It is prescribed to patients who have a tendency to form clots in the fast-flowing blood of the arteries and heart, or those who have had a stroke or a heart attack.

The drug may be suitable for people who cannot take aspirin for its anti-platelet effects. It reduces the tendency of platelets to stick together when blood flow is disrupted. However, this can lead to abnormal bleeding. You should, therefore, report any unusual bleeding to your doctor a once, and, if you require dental treatment, you should tell your dentist that you are taking the drug.

Adverse effects are common with clopidogrel and are usually associated with bleeding.

INFORMATION FOR USERS

Your drug prescription is tailored for you. Do not alter dosage without checking with your doctor.

How taken

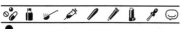

Tablets.

Frequency and timing of doses
Once daily.

Dosage range
75mg.

Onset of effect
1 hour.

Duration of action
24 hours.

Diet advice
None.

Storage
Keep in a closed container in a cool, dry place out of the reach of children.

Missed dose
Take as soon as you remember. If your next dose is due within 4 hours, take a single dose now and skip the next.

Stopping the drug
Do not stop taking the drug without consulting your doctor. Stopping the drug may lead to a recurrence of the original condition.

Exceeding the dose
An occasional unintentional extra dose is unlikely to be a cause for concern. But if you notice any unusual symptoms, or if a large overdose has been taken, notify your doctor.

SPECIAL PRECAUTIONS

Be sure to tell your doctor if:
▼ You have liver or kidney problems.
▼ You have a condition, such as a peptic ulcer, that makes you more likely to bleed.
▼ You are taking other medications.

Pregnancy
▼ Safety in pregnancy not established. Discuss with your doctor.

Breast-feeding
▼ The drug passes into the breast milk and may affect the baby. Discuss with your doctor.

Infants and children
▼ Not recommended.

Over 60
▼ No special problems.

Driving and hazardous work
▼ No special problems.

Alcohol
▼ Excessive intake of alcohol may irritate the stomach and increase the risk of bleeding.

Surgery and general anaesthetics
▼ Clopidogrel may need to be stopped a week before surgery. Discuss this with your doctor or dentist.

POSSIBLE ADVERSE EFFECTS

The most frequent adverse effects of clopidogrel are bleeding and bruising. Nausea and diarrhoea are less common.

Symptom/effect	Frequency		Discuss with doctor		Stop taking drug now	Call doctor now
	Common	Rare	Only if severe	In all cases		
Gastrointestinal bleeding/ulcers		●		■		
Bruising/nosebleeds	●			■		
Blood in urine		●		■		
Nausea/vomiting		●	■			
Diarrhoea/abdominal pain		●	■			
Headache/dizziness		●	■			
Rash/itching		●		■		
Sore throat		●		■		■

INTERACTIONS

Aspirin and other Non steroidal anti-inflammatory drugs (NSAIDs) Clopidogrel increases the effect of aspirin on platelets. The risk of gastrointestinal bleeding is increased when clopidogrel is used with these drugs.

Anticoagulant drugs (e.g., warfarin) The anticoagulant effect of these drugs is increased if they are taken with clopidogrel.

PROLONGED USE

No special problems.

CLOTRIMAZOLE

Brand names Canesten, Masnoderm, Mycil Gold
Used in the following combined preparations Canesten HC, Lotriderm

GENERAL INFORMATION

Clotrimazole is an antifungal drug that is commonly used to treat fungal and yeast infections. It is used for treating tinea (ringworm) infections of the skin, and candida (thrush) infections of the mouth, vagina, or penis. The drug is applied in the form of a cream, spray, topical solution, or dusting powder to the affected area and inserted as pessaries or cream for vaginal conditions such as candida.

Adverse effects from clotrimazole are very rare, although some people may experience burning and irritation on the skin surface in the area where the drug has been applied.

QUICK REFERENCE

Drug group Antifungal drug (p.138)
Overdose danger rating Low
Dependence rating Low
Prescription needed No
Available as generic No

INFORMATION FOR USERS

Follow instructions on the label. Call your doctor if symptoms worsen.

How taken

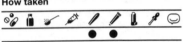

Pessaries, cream, spray, dusting powder, topical solution.

Frequency and timing of doses
2–3 x daily (skin cream, spray, solution); once daily at bedtime (pessaries); 1–2 x daily (vaginal cream).

Dosage range
Vaginal infections One applicatorful (5g) per dose (vaginal cream); 100–500mg per dose (pessaries).
Skin infections (skin cream, spray, solution) as directed.

Onset of effect
Within 2–3 days.

Duration of action
Up to 12 hours.

Diet advice
None.

Storage
Keep in a closed container in a cool, dry place away from the reach of children.

Missed dose
No cause for concern, but make up the missed dose or application as soon as you remember.

Stopping the drug
Apply the full course. Even if symptoms disappear, the original infection may still be present and symptoms may recur if treatment is stopped too soon.

Exceeding the dose
An occasional unintentional extra dose is unlikely to cause problems. But if you notice unusual symptoms or if a large amount has been swallowed, notify your doctor.

SPECIAL PRECAUTIONS

Be sure to tell your doctor or pharmacist if:
▼ You are taking other medications.

Pregnancy
▼ No evidence of risk to developing baby.

Breast-feeding
▼ No evidence of risk.

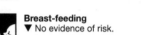

Infants and children
▼ No special problems.

Over 60
▼ No special problems.

Driving and hazardous work
▼ No known problems.

Alcohol
▼ No known problems.

POSSIBLE ADVERSE EFFECTS

Clotrimazole rarely causes adverse effects. Skin preparations and vaginal applications may occasionally cause localized burning and irritation.

Symptom/effect	Frequency		Discuss with doctor		Stop taking drug now	Call doctor now
	Common	Rare	Only if severe	In all cases		
Localized burning or stinging	●		■			
Skin irritation		●	■			
Rash		●	■		▲	

PROLONGED USE

No problems expected.

INTERACTIONS

None known.

CLOZAPINE

Brand name Clozaril
Used in the following combined preparations None

GENERAL INFORMATION

Clozapine is a new type of antipsychotic drug that is used to treat schizophrenia. It is prescribed only for patients who have not responded to other treatments or those patients who have experienced intolerable *side effects* with other drugs. Clozapine helps control severe resistant schizophrenia, helping the patient to re-establish a more normal lifestyle. The improvement is gradual, and relief of severe symptoms can take more than three weeks.

All treatment is started and supervised by a hospital, because all patients must be registered with the Clozaril Patient Monitoring Service (CPMS). The drug can cause a very serious side effect, agranulocytosis (a large decrease in the number of white blood cells). Blood tests are done before treatment and regularly thereafter; the drug is supplied only if results are normal.
Clozapine is less likely than other antipsychotics to cause *parkinsonism*.

INFORMATION FOR USERS

This drug is given only under strict medical supervision and continual monitoring.

How taken

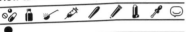

Tablets.

Frequency and timing of doses
1–3 x daily; a larger dose may be given at night.

Adult dosage range
25–900mg daily.

Onset of effect
Gradual. Some effect may appear within 3–5 days, but the full beneficial effect may not be felt for over 3 weeks.

Duration of action
Up to 16 hours.

Diet advice
None.

Storage
Keep in a closed container in a cool, dry place away from the reach of children.

Missed dose
Take as soon as you remember. If your next dose is due within 2 hours, take a single dose now and skip the next.

Stopping the drug
Do not stop the drug without consulting your doctor because symptoms may recur.

Exceeding the dose
An occasional unintentional extra dose is unlikely to cause problems. Large overdoses may cause unusual drowsiness, fits, and agitation. Notify your doctor.

SPECIAL PRECAUTIONS

Be sure to tell your doctor if:
▼ You have long-term liver or kidney problems.
▼ You have a history of blood disorders.
▼ You have had epileptic fits.
▼ You are taking other medications.

Pregnancy
▼ Not usually prescribed. Safety not established. Discuss with your doctor.

Breast-feeding
▼ The drug passes into the breast milk and may affect the baby adversely. Discuss with your doctor.

Infants and children
▼ Not prescribed.

Over 60
▼ Adverse effects are more likely. Initial dose is low and is slowly increased.

Driving and hazardous work
▼ Avoid such activities until you have learned how clozapine affects you because the drug can cause drowsiness, dizziness, and blurred vision.

Alcohol
▼ Avoid. Alcohol may increase the sedative effects of this drug.

POSSIBLE ADVERSE EFFECTS

Clozapine is less likely to cause parkinsonian side effects (tremor and stiffness), which occur with the use of other antipsychotic drugs. The most serious side effect is agranulocytosis, and strict monitoring is necessary.

Symptom/effect	Frequency		Discuss with doctor		Stop taking drug now	Call doctor now
	Common	Rare	Only if severe	In all cases		
Drowsiness/tiredness	●		■			
Excess saliva	●		■			
Dry mouth	●		■			
Fast heartbeat	●			■		
Blurred vision		●		■		
Tremor/muscle rigidity		●		■		
Dizziness/fainting		●		■		
Fever/sore throat		●		■		▮
Fits		●		■		▮

INTERACTIONS

General note A number of drugs increase the risk of adverse effects on the blood. Do not take other medication without checking with your doctor or pharmacist.

Sedatives All drugs that have a *sedative* effect on the central nervous system are likely to increase the sedative properties of clozapine.

PROLONGED USE

Agranulocytosis may occur, and occasionally liver function may be upset.

Monitoring Blood tests are carried out weekly for the first 18 weeks, fortnightly until the end of the first year, and, if blood counts are stable, at four-weekly intervals thereafter. Liver function tests may also be performed.

CODEINE

Used in the following combined preparations Benylin with Codeine, Co-codamol, Codafen Continus, Codis, Diarrest, Migraleve, Panadol Ultra, Solpadeine, Solpadol, Syndol, Terpoin, Tylex, Veganin, and others

GENERAL INFORMATION

Codeine is a mild *opioid* analgesic that is similar to, but weaker than, morphine. It has been in common medical use since the beginning of this century.

Codeine is prescribed primarily to relieve mild to moderate pain, and is often combined with a non-opioid analgesic such as paracetamol. It is also an effective cough suppressant and, for this reason, is included as an ingredient in many non-prescription cough syrups and cold relief preparations.

Like the other opioid drugs, codeine is constipating, a characteristic that sometimes makes it useful in the short-term control of diarrhoea.

Although codeine is habit-forming, addiction seldom occurs if the drug is used for a limited period of time and the recommended dosage is followed.

Constipation is common with codeine. Other, rare, *adverse effects* include breathing difficulties, which should be reported to your doctor without delay.

QUICK REFERENCE

Drug group Opioid analgesic (p.81), antidiarrhoeal drug (p.110), and cough suppressant (p.94)

Overdose danger rating High

Dependence rating Medium

Prescription needed Yes (some preparations)

Available as generic Yes

INFORMATION FOR USERS

Your drug prescription is tailored for you. Do not alter dosage without checking with your doctor.

How taken

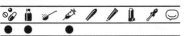

Tablets, liquid, injection.

Frequency and timing of doses
4–6 x daily (pain); 3–4 x daily when necessary (cough); every 4–6 hours when necessary (diarrhoea).

Adult dosage range
120–240mg daily (pain); 45–120mg daily (cough); 30–180mg daily (diarrhoea).

Onset of effect
30–60 minutes.

Duration of action
4–6 hours.

Diet advice
None.

Storage
Keep in a closed container in a cool, dry place out of the reach of children. Protect from light.

Missed dose
Take as soon as you remember if needed for relief of symptoms. If not needed, do not take the missed dose, and return to your normal dose schedule when necessary.

Stopping the drug
Can be safely stopped as soon as you no longer need it.

OVERDOSE ACTION

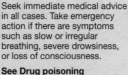 Seek immediate medical advice in all cases. Take emergency action if there are symptoms such as slow or irregular breathing, severe drowsiness, or loss of consciousness.

See Drug poisoning emergency guide (p.494).

SPECIAL PRECAUTIONS

Be sure tell your doctor if:
▼ You have long-term liver or kidney problems.
▼ You have a lung disorder such as asthma or bronchitis.
▼ You are taking other medications.

 Pregnancy
▼ No evidence of risk, but may adversely affect the baby's breathing if taken during labour.

 Breast-feeding
▼ The drug passes into the breast milk, but at normal doses adverse effects on the baby are unlikely. Discuss with your doctor.

 Infants and children
▼ Reduced dose necessary.

 Over 60
▼ Reduced dose may be necessary.

 Driving and hazardous work
▼ Avoid such activities until you have learned how codeine affects you because the drug may cause dizziness and drowsiness.

Alcohol
▼ Avoid. Alcohol may increase the sedative effects of this drug.

POSSIBLE ADVERSE EFFECTS

Serious adverse effects are rare with codeine. Constipation occurs especially with prolonged use, but other side effects, such as nausea, vomiting, and drowsiness, are not usually troublesome at recommended doses, and usually disappear if the dose is reduced.

Symptom/effect	Frequency		Discuss with doctor		Stop taking drug now	Call doctor now
	Common	Rare	Only if severe	In all cases		
Constipation	●		■			
Nausea/vomiting		●		■		
Drowsiness		●		■		
Dizziness		●		■		
Agitation/restlessness		●		■	▲	
Rash/hives		●		■	▲	▮
Wheezing/breathlessness		●		■	▲	▮

PROLONGED USE

Codeine is normally used only for short-term relief of symptoms. It can be habit-forming if taken for extended periods, especially if higher-than-average doses are taken.

INTERACTIONS

Sedatives All drugs, including alcohol, that have a *sedative* effect on the central nervous system are likely to increase sedation with codeine. Such drugs include sleeping drugs, antidepressant drugs, and antihistamines.

COLCHICINE

Brand names None
Used in the following combined preparations None

GENERAL INFORMATION

Colchicine, a drug originally extracted from the autumn crocus flower and later synthesized, has been used since the 18th century for gout. Although it has now, to some extent, been superseded by newer drugs, it is still often used to relieve joint pain and inflammation in flare-ups of gout. Colchicine is most effective when taken at the first sign of symptoms, and almost always produces an improvement. The drug is also often given during the first few months of treatment with allopurinol or probenecid (other drugs used for treating gout), because these may at first increase the frequency of gout attacks.

Colchicine is occasionally prescribed for the relief of the symptoms of familial Mediterranean fever (a rare congenital condition).

INFORMATION FOR USERS

Your drug prescription is tailored for you. Do not alter dosage without checking with your doctor.

How taken

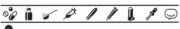

Tablets.

Frequency and timing of doses
Prevention of gout attacks 2–3 x daily.
Relief of gout attacks Every 2–3 hours.

Adult dosage range
Prevention of gout attacks 1–1.5mg daily.
Relief of gout attacks 1mg initially, followed by 0.5mg every 2–3 hours, until relief of pain, vomiting, or diarrhoea occurs, or until a total dose of 10mg is reached. This course must not be repeated within 3 days.

Onset of effect
Relief of symptoms in an attack of gout may be felt in 6–24 hours. Full effect in gout prevention may not be felt for several days.

Duration of action
Up to 2 hours. Some effect may last longer.

Diet advice
Certain foods are known to make gout worse. Discuss with your doctor.

Storage
Keep in a closed container in a cool, dry place out of the reach of children. Protect from light.

Missed dose
Take as soon as you remember. If your next dose is due within 30 minutes, take a single dose now and skip the next.

Stopping the drug
When taking colchicine frequently during an acute attack of gout, stop if diarrhoea or abdominal pain develop. In other cases, do not stop without consulting your doctor.

OVERDOSE ACTION

Seek immediate medical advice in all cases; some reactions can be fatal. Take emergency action if severe nausea, vomiting, bloody diarrhoea, severe abdominal pain, or loss of consciousness occur.

See Drug poisoning emergency guide (p.494).

SPECIAL PRECAUTIONS

Be sure to tell your doctor if:
▼ You have long-term liver or kidney problems.
▼ You have heart problems.
▼ You have a blood disorder.
▼ You have stomach ulcers.
▼ You have chronic inflammation of the bowel.
▼ You are taking other medications.

 Pregnancy
▼ Not usually prescribed. May cause defects in the unborn baby. Discuss with your doctor.

 Breast-feeding
▼ The drug passes into the breast milk and may affect the baby. Discuss with your doctor.

 Infants and children
▼ Not recommended.

 Over 60
▼ Increased likelihood of adverse effects.

 Driving and hazardous work
▼ No special problems.

 Alcohol
▼ Avoid. Alcohol may increase stomach irritation caused by colchicine.

PROLONGED USE

Prolonged use of this drug may lead to hair loss, rashes, tingling in the hands and feet, muscle pain and weakness, and blood disorders.

Monitoring Periodic blood checks are usually required.

POSSIBLE ADVERSE EFFECTS

The appearance of any symptom that may be an *adverse effect* of the drug is a sign that you should stop the drug until you have received further medical advice.

Symptom/effect	Frequency		Discuss with doctor		Stop taking drug now	Call doctor now
	Common	Rare	Only if severe	In all cases		
Nausea/vomiting	●			■	▲	
Diarrhoea/abdominal pain	●			■	▲	
Numbness and tingling		●		■	▲	
Unusual bleeding/bruising		●		■	▲	
Rash		●		■	▲	

INTERACTIONS

Cyclosporin Taking cyclosporin with colchicine may lead to adverse effects on the kidneys.

COLESTYRAMINE

Brand names Questran, Questran Light
Used in the following combined preparations None

GENERAL INFORMATION

Colestyramine is a resin that binds bile acids in the intestine, preventing their reabsorption. Cholesterol in the body is normally converted to bile acids. Therefore, the use of colestyramine results in a reduction of cholesterol levels in the blood. This action on the bile acids makes bowel movements bulkier, creating an antidiarrhoeal effect. The action on cholesterol helps people with hyperlipidaemia (high levels of fat in the blood) who have not responded to dietary measures, and who are at particular risk from heart disease as a result of diabetes or a family history of death from heart attacks.

In liver disorders such as primary biliary cirrhosis, bile salts sometimes accumulate in the bloodstream, and colestyramine may be prescribed to alleviate any accompanying itching.

Taken in large doses, colestyramine often causes bloating, mild nausea, and constipation. It may also interfere with the body's ability to absorb fat and certain fat-soluble vitamins, causing pale, bulky, foul-smelling faeces.

INFORMATION FOR USERS

Your drug prescription is tailored for you. Do not alter dosage without checking with your doctor.

How taken

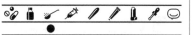

Powder mixed with water, juice, or soft food.

Frequency and timing of doses
1–4 x daily before meals and at bedtime.

Adult dosage range
4–36g daily.

Onset of effect
Full beneficial effects may not be felt for several weeks.

Duration of action
12–24 hours.

Diet advice
A low-fat, low-calorie diet may be advised for patients who are overweight. Use of this drug may deplete levels of certain vitamins. Supplements may be advised.

Storage
Keep in a closed container in a cool, dry place out of the reach of children.

Missed dose
Take as soon as you remember.

Stopping the drug
Do not stop taking the drug without consulting your doctor.

Exceeding the dose
An occasional unintentional extra dose is unlikely to cause problems. But if you notice any unusual symptoms, or if a large overdose has been taken, notify your doctor.

POSSIBLE ADVERSE EFFECTS

Adverse effects are more likely if large doses are taken by people over 60. Minor side effects such as indigestion and abdominal discomfort are rarely a cause for concern. More serious adverse effects are usually the result of vitamin deficiency.

Symptom/effect	Frequency		Discuss with doctor		Stop taking drug now	Call doctor now
	Common	Rare	Only if severe	In all cases		
Indigestion	●		■			
Abdominal discomfort	●		■			
Nausea/vomiting	●		■			
Constipation	●		■			
Bruising/increased bleeding		●		■		
Diarrhoea (high doses)		●		■		

INTERACTIONS

General note Colestyramine reduces the body's ability to absorb other drugs. It may be necessary to organize a schedule in consultation with your doctor whereby you take other medications at a fixed time before you take colestyramine. Usually, taking other medications 30 to 60 minutes prior to colestyramine, or 4 to 6 hours after, solves the problem. The dosage of other drugs may need to be adjusted.

SPECIAL PRECAUTIONS

Be sure to tell your doctor if:
▼ You have *jaundice*.
▼ You have a peptic ulcer.
▼ You suffer from haemorrhoids.
▼ You are taking other medications.

Pregnancy
▼ Safety in pregnancy not established. Discuss with your doctor.

Breast-feeding
▼ Safety not established. The drug binds fat-soluble vitamins long term and may cause vitamin deficiency in the baby. Discuss with your doctor.

Infants and children
▼ Not recommended under 6 years. Reduced dose necessary in older children.

Over 60
▼ Increased likelihood of adverse effects.

Driving and hazardous work
▼ No special problems.

Alcohol
▼ Although this drug does not interact with alcohol, your underlying condition may make it inadvisable to take alcohol.

PROLONGED USE

As this drug reduces vitamin absorption, supplements of vitamins A, D, and K and folic acid may be advised.

Monitoring Periodic blood checks are usually required to monitor the level of cholesterol in the blood.

CONJUGATED ESTROGENS

Brand name Premarin
Used in the following combined preparation Prempak-C

GENERAL INFORMATION

Preparations of conjugated estrogens consist of naturally occurring estrogens similar to those found in the urine of pregnant mares.

Given by mouth, they are used to relieve menopausal symptoms such as hot flushes and sweating. They are also used to prevent osteoporosis (brittle bones), which may occur after the menopause.

As replacement therapy, conjugated estrogens are usually taken on a cyclic dosing schedule, often in conjunction with a progestogen, to simulate the hormonal changes that occur in a normal menstrual cycle. They may also be prescribed in the form of vaginal cream to relieve pain and dryness of the vagina or vulva after the menopause.

INFORMATION FOR USERS

Your drug prescription is tailored for you. Do not alter dosage without checking with your doctor.

How taken

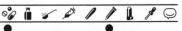

Tablets, cream.

Frequency and timing of doses
1–3 x daily (tablets).
Once daily (cream).

Adult dosage range
Replacement therapy 0.625–1.25mg daily (tablets); 1–2g daily (cream).

Onset of effect
5–20 days.

Duration of action
1–2 days.

Diet advice
None.

Storage
Keep in a closed container in a cool, dry place out of the reach of children.

Missed dose
Take as soon as you remember.

Stopping the drug
Do not stop the drug without consulting your doctor because symptoms may recur.

Exceeding the dose
An occasional unintentional extra dose is unlikely to be a cause for concern. But if you notice any unusual symptoms, or if a large overdose has been taken, notify your doctor.

SPECIAL PRECAUTIONS

Be sure to tell your doctor if:
▼ You have heart failure or high blood pressure.
▼ You have had blood clots or a stroke.
▼ You have a history of breast disease.
▼ You have had fibroids in the uterus.
▼ You suffer from migraine or epilepsy.
▼ You are taking other medications.
▼ You have long-term liver or kidney problems.

Pregnancy
▼ Not prescribed. May affect the baby adversely. Discuss with your doctor.

Breast-feeding
▼ Not prescribed. The drug passes into the breast milk and may inhibit the flow of milk. Discuss with your doctor.

Infants and children
▼ Not prescribed.

Over 60
▼ No special problems.

Driving and hazardous work
▼ No known problems.

Alcohol
▼ No known problems.

Surgery and general anaesthetics
▼ Conjugated estrogens may need to be stopped several weeks before you have surgery. Discuss with your doctor.

POSSIBLE ADVERSE EFFECTS

The most common *adverse effects* of conjugated estrogens are similar to symptoms that occur in the early stages of pregnancy, and generally diminish or disappear after 2–3 months of treatment. Sudden, sharp pain in the chest, groin, or legs may indicate an abnormal blood clot requiring urgent medical attention.

Symptom/effect	Frequency		Discuss with doctor		Stop taking drug now	Call doctor now
	Common	Rare	Only if severe	In all cases		
Nausea/vomiting	●		■			
Breast swelling/tenderness	●		■			
Increase or decrease in weight	●		■			
Reduced sex drive		●	■			
Depression		●		■		
Vaginal bleeding		●		■		
Pain in chest/groin/legs		●		■		■

INTERACTIONS

Tobacco smoking Smoking increases the risk of serious adverse effects on the heart and circulation with conjugated estrogens.

Oral anticoagulant drugs Conjugated estrogens reduce the *anticoagulant* effect of these drugs.

PROLONGED USE

There is a slightly higher risk of cancer of the uterus when estrogens are used long term. The risk of gallbladder disease is also increased. The risk of blood clots is also increased in susceptible people.

Monitoring Physical examinations and blood pressure checks may be needed.

CO-PROXAMOL

Brand names Cosalgesic, Distalgesic
Used in the following combined preparations (Co-proxamol is a combination of two drugs)

GENERAL INFORMATION

Co-proxamol is the generic name for a combination of the non-*opioid* analgesic drug paracetamol and a mild opioid analgesic, dextropropoxyphene. Co-proxamol is used for the relief of mild to moderate pain that has not responded to paracetamol or other non-opioid analgesics alone.

Because the drug contains an opioid, it can cause a variety of *side effects* that are common to drugs of that group:

dizziness, mild euphoria, nausea, and constipation. Co-proxamol may also be habit-forming if taken regularly for an extended period. Overdose with co-proxamol is dangerous because dextropropoxyphene may interfere with breathing if it is taken in excess, and overdose of paracetamol may cause irreversible damage to the liver and kidneys.

QUICK REFERENCE

Drug group Opioid analgesic (p.81)
Overdose danger rating High
Dependence rating Medium
Prescription needed Yes
Available as generic Yes

INFORMATION FOR USERS

Your drug prescription is tailored for you. Do not alter dosage without checking with your doctor.

How taken

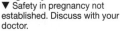

Tablets.

Frequency and timing of doses
3–4 x daily as necessary.

Adult dosage range
2 tablets per dose, up to a maximum of 8 tablets daily.

Onset of effect
30–60 minutes.

Duration of action
6 hours.

Diet advice
None.

Storage
Keep in a closed container in a cool, dry place out of the reach of children.

Missed dose
Take as soon as you remember if needed for the relief of pain. Do not take doses less than 4 hours apart.

Stopping the drug
If you have been taking the drug regularly for less than 4 weeks, it can be safely stopped as soon as you no longer need it. If you have been regularly taking the drug longer than this, your doctor may recommend a gradual reduction in dosage.

OVERDOSE ACTION

Seek immediate medical advice in all cases. Take emergency action if irregular breathing, drowsiness or loss of consciousness occur.

See Drug poisoning emergency guide (p.494).

POSSIBLE ADVERSE EFFECTS

Serious adverse effects are rare with this drug.

Symptom/effect	Frequency		Discuss with doctor		Stop taking drug now	Call doctor now
	Common	Rare	Only if severe	In all cases		
Dizziness/drowsiness	●			■		
Nausea/vomiting	●			■		
Constipation		●		■		
Euphoria/hallucinations		●		■	▲	
Rash		●			■	▲

INTERACTIONS

General note All drugs, including alcohol, that have a *sedative* effect are likely to increase the sedative properties of co-proxamol. These include sleeping drugs, anti-anxiety drugs, and antidepressants.

Carbamazepine Co-proxamol can enhance the effects of carbamazepine.

Oral anticoagulant drugs Co-proxamol may increase the *anticoagulant* effect of these drugs.

SPECIAL PRECAUTIONS

Be sure to tell your doctor if:
▼ You have long-term liver or kidney problems.
▼ You have had problems with drug or alcohol abuse.
▼ You have a lung disorder such as asthma or bronchitis.
▼ You suffer from depression.
▼ You are taking other medications.

Pregnancy
▼ Safety in pregnancy not established. Discuss with your doctor.

Breast-feeding
▼ The drug passes into the breast milk and may affect the baby. Discuss with your doctor.

Infants and children
▼ Not recommended.

Over 60
▼ Reduced dose necessary.

Driving and hazardous work
▼ Avoid such activities until you have learned how co-proxamol affects you because the drug can cause drowsiness and dizziness.

Alcohol
▼ Avoid. Alcohol will dangerously increase the toxicity of this drug.

PROLONGED USE

Co-proxamol is not usually prescribed for long-term use. It can be habit forming if taken for extended periods and a higher dose may be needed to produce the same effect as your body adapts to the drug.

CO-TRIMOXAZOLE

Brand names Bactrim, Chemotrim, Comixco, Fectrim, Laratrim, Septrin
Used in the following combined preparations (Co-trimoxazole is a combination of trimethoprim and sulfamethoxazole)

GENERAL INFORMATION

Co-trimoxazole is a mixture of two antibacterial drugs in the ratio of one part trimethoprim and five parts sulfamethoxazole. It is prescribed for serious respiratory and urinary tract infections only when they cannot be treated with other drugs. Co-trimoxazole is also used to treat pneumocystis pneumonia, toxoplasmosis, and the bacterial infection nocardiasis. The drug may also be used for otitis media in children if no safer drug is suitable.

Although co-trimoxazole was widely prescribed in the past, its use has now greatly declined with the introduction of new, more effective, and safer drugs.

The *side effects* of co-trimoxazole are a combination of those caused by the antibacterial drugs it contains and include nausea, vomiting, rash, sore tongue, and rarely *jaundice*, skin rash, blood disorders, and serious liver or kidney damage.

INFORMATION FOR USERS

Your drug prescription is tailored for you. Do not alter dosage without checking with your doctor.

How taken

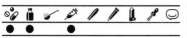

Tablets, liquid, injection.

Frequency and timing of doses
Normally 2 x daily, preferably with food.

Adult dosage range
Usually 4–6 tablets daily (each standard tablet is 480mg). Higher doses are required for the treatment of pneumocystis pneumonia.

Onset of effect
1–4 hours.

Duration of action
12 hours.

Diet advice
Drink plenty of fluids, particularly in warm weather.

Storage
Keep in a closed container in a cool, dry place out of the reach of children. Protect from light.

Missed dose
Take as soon as you remember. If your next dose is due at this time, double the usual dose to make up the missed dose.

Stopping the drug
Take the full course. Even if you feel better, the original infection may still be present and symptoms may recur if treatment is stopped too soon.

Exceeding the dose
An occasional unintentional extra dose is unlikely to be a cause for concern. Large overdoses may cause nausea, vomiting, dizziness, and confusion. Notify your doctor.

SPECIAL PRECAUTIONS

Be sure to tell your doctor if:
▼ You have long-term liver or kidney problems.
▼ You have a blood disorder.
▼ You have glucose-6-phosphate dehydrogenase (G6PD) deficiency.
▼ You are allergic to sulphonamide drugs.
▼ You suffer from porphyria.
▼ You are taking other medications.

Pregnancy
▼ Not usually prescribed. May cause defects in the baby. Discuss with your doctor.

Breast-feeding
▼ The drug passes into the breast milk, but at normal levels adverse effects on the baby are unlikely. Discuss with your doctor.

Infants and children
▼ Not recommended in infants under 6 weeks old. Reduced dose necessary in older children.

Over 60
▼ Side effects are more likely. Used only when necessary, and often in reduced dosage.

Driving and hazardous work
▼ No known problems.

Alcohol
▼ No known problems.

POSSIBLE ADVERSE EFFECTS

Side effects can be caused by either the trimethoprim or the sulfamethoxazole ingredient of this preparation. The most common problems are nausea and rash.

Symptom/effect	Frequency		Discuss with doctor		Stop taking drug now	Call doctor now
	Common	Rare	Only if severe	In all cases		
Nausea/vomiting	●			■		
Rash/itching	●			■	▲	∎
Diarrhoea		●	■			
Sore tongue		●		■		
Headache		●		■		
Jaundice		●		■		∎

INTERACTIONS

Warfarin Co-trimoxazole may increase its *anticoagulant* effect; the dose of warfarin may have to be reduced.

Phenytoin Co-trimoxazole may cause a build-up of phenytoin in the body; the dose of phenytoin may have to be reduced.

Oral antidiabetic drugs Co-trimoxazole may increase the blood sugar lowering effect of these drugs.

Cyclosporin Taking cyclosporin with co-trimoxazole can impair kidney function.

PROLONGED USE

Long-term use of this drug may lead to folic acid deficiency which, in turn, can cause a blood abnormality. Folic acid supplements may be prescribed.

Monitoring Periodic blood tests to monitor blood composition are usually carried out.

CYCLOPENTHIAZIDE

Brand name Navidrex
Used in the following combined preparations Navispare, Trasidrex

GENERAL INFORMATION

Cyclopenthiazide belongs to the thiazide diuretic group of drugs, which remove excess water from the body and reduce oedema (fluid retention) in people with congestive heart failure and liver and kidney disorders. It may occasionally be used on a short-term basis to treat fluid retention in premenstrual syndrome.

Cyclopenthiazide is also used to treat high blood pressure (see Antihypertensive drugs, p.102). The drug increases loss of potassium in the urine, which can cause a variety of symptoms (see p.99) and increases the likelihood of irregular heart rhythms, particularly if you are taking drugs such as digoxin. Therefore, a potassium supplement or a diet rich in potassium is often recommended for patients taking cyclopenthiazide.

INFORMATION FOR USERS

Your drug prescription is tailored for you. Do not alter dosage without checking with your doctor

How taken

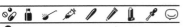

Tablets.

Frequency and timing of doses
Once daily (preferably in the morning).

Adult dosage range
0.25–1mg daily.

Onset of effect
Within 2 hours.

Duration of action
6–12 hours.

Diet advice
Use of this drug may reduce potassium in the body. Eat plenty of fresh fruit and vegetables.

Storage
Keep in a closed container in a cool, dry place out of the reach of children.

Missed dose
No cause for concern, but take as soon as you remember. However, if it is late in the day do not take the missed dose, or you may need to get up during the night to pass urine. Take the next scheduled dose as usual.

Stopping the drug
Do not stop the drug without consulting your doctor; symptoms may recur.

Exceeding the dose
An occasional unintentional extra dose is unlikely to be a cause for concern. But if you notice any unusual symptoms, or if a large overdose has been taken, notify your doctor.

SPECIAL PRECAUTIONS

Be sure to tell your doctor if:
▼ You have long-term liver or kidney problems.
▼ You have had gout.
▼ You have diabetes.
▼ You are taking other medications.

Pregnancy
▼ Safety in pregnancy not established. Discuss with your doctor.

Breast-feeding
▼ The drug passes into the breast milk, but at normal doses adverse effects on the baby are unlikely. Discuss with your doctor.

Infants and children
▼ Not usually prescribed. Reduced dose necessary.

Over 60
▼ Increased likelihood of adverse effects.

Driving and hazardous work
▼ No special problems.

Alcohol
▼ Keep consumption low. Cyclopenthiazide increases the likelihood of dehydration and hangovers after consumption of alcohol.

POSSIBLE ADVERSE EFFECTS

Most *adverse effects* are caused by excessive loss of potassium. This can usually be put right by taking a potassium supplement. In rare cases gout may occur in susceptible people, and certain forms of diabetes may become more difficult to control.

Symptom/effect	Frequency		Discuss with doctor		Stop taking drug now	Call doctor now
	Common	Rare	Only if severe	In all cases		
Loss of appetite	●		■			
Nausea	●			■		
Diarrhoea or constipation		●	■			
Leg cramp/muscle weakness		●		■		
Headache/dizziness		●		■		
Rash		●		■	▲	

INTERACTIONS

Non-steroidal anti-inflammatory drugs Some of these drugs may reduce the diuretic effect of cyclopenthiazide, the dosage of which may need to be adjusted.

ACE inhibitors and other antihypertensive drugs Cyclopenthiazide may cause a further decrease in blood pressure when taken in combination with these drugs.

Corticosteroids These drugs further increase the loss of potassium from the body when taken with cyclopenthiazide.

Lithium Cyclopenthiazide may increase lithium levels in the blood, leading to a risk of serious adverse effects.

Digoxin The effects of digoxin may be increased if excessive potassium is lost.

PROLONGED USE

Excessive loss of potassium may result in irregular heart rhythms. Cyclopenthiazide occasionally causes reduced levels of red blood cells and platelets.

Monitoring Blood tests may be performed periodically to check kidney function and levels of potassium.

CYCLOPHOSPHAMIDE

Brand name Endoxana
Used in the following combined preparations None

GENERAL INFORMATION

Cyclophosphamide belongs to a group of anticancer drugs known as alkylating agents. It is used for a wide range of cancers, including lymphomas (lymph gland cancers), leukaemias, and solid tumours, particularly of the breast and lung. It is commonly given together with radiotherapy or other drugs. Cyclophosphamide has also been used for autoimmune diseases.

Cyclophosphamide causes nausea, vomiting, and hair loss, and can affect the heart, lungs, and liver. It can also cause bladder damage in susceptible people because it produces a toxic substance called acrolein. To reduce *toxicity*, people considered to be at risk may be given a drug called mesna before and after each dose of cyclophosphamide. Also, because the drug often reduces production of blood cells, it may lead to abnormal bleeding, increased risk of infection, and reduced fertility in men.

INFORMATION FOR USERS

Your drug prescription is tailored for you. Do not alter dosage without checking with your doctor.

How taken

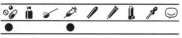

Tablets, injection.

Frequency and timing of doses
Varies from once daily to every 20 days, depending on the condition being treated.

Dosage range
Dosage is determined individually according to the nature of the condition, body weight, and response.

Onset of effect
Some effects may appear within hours of starting treatment. Full beneficial effects may not be felt for up to 6 weeks.

Duration of action
Several weeks.

Diet advice
High fluid intake with frequent bladder emptying is recommended. This will usually prevent the drug causing bladder irritation.

Storage
Keep in a closed container in a cool, dry place out of the reach of children. Protect from light.

Missed dose
Injections are given only in hospital. If you are taking tablets, take the missed dose as soon as you remember. If your next dose is due within 6 hours, take a single dose now and skip the next. Tell your doctor that you missed a dose.

Stopping the drug
The drug will be stopped under medical supervision (injection). Do not stop taking the drug without consulting your doctor (tablets); stopping the drug may lead to worsening of the underlying condition.

Exceeding the dose
An occasional unintentional extra dose is unlikely to cause problems. Large overdoses may cause nausea, vomiting, and bladder damage. Notify your doctor.

SPECIAL PRECAUTIONS

Cyclophosphamide is prescribed only under close medical supervision, taking account of your present condition and medical history.

Pregnancy
▼ Not usually prescribed. May cause birth defects. Discuss with your doctor.

Breast-feeding
▼ Not advised. The drug passes into the breast milk and may affect the baby adversely. Discuss with your doctor.

Infants and children
▼ Reduced dose necessary.

Over 60
▼ No special problems.

Driving and hazardous work
▼ No known problems.

Alcohol
▼ No problems expected, but avoid excessive amounts.

POSSIBLE ADVERSE EFFECTS

Cyclophosphamide often causes nausea and vomiting, which usually diminish as your body adjusts. Also, women often experience irregular periods. Blood in the urine may be a sign of bladder damage and requires prompt medical attention. Those thought to be at risk of bladder damage may be given mesna before and after doses of cyclophosphamide.

Symptom/effect	Frequency		Discuss with doctor		Stop taking drug now	Call doctor now
	Common	Rare	Only if severe	In all cases		
Nausea/vomiting	●		■			
Hair loss	●		■			
Irregular menstruation	●			■		
Mouth ulcers		●		■		
Bloodstained urine		●		■		▪

INTERACTIONS

Allopurinol may increase the risk of *toxic* effects caused by cyclophosphamide.

PROLONGED USE

Prolonged use of this drug may reduce the production of blood cells.

Monitoring Periodic checks on blood composition and on all effects of the drug are usually required.

CYCLOSPORIN

Brand names Neoral, Sandimmun
Used in the following combined preparations None

GENERAL INFORMATION

Introduced in 1984, cyclosporin is one of the immunosuppressants, a group of drugs that suppress the body's natural defences against infection and foreign cells. This action is of particular use following organ transplants, when the recipient's immune system may reject the transplanted organ unless the immune system is controlled.

Cyclosporin is widely used after many types of transplant, such as heart, bone marrow, kidney, liver, and pancreas; its use has considerably reduced the risk of tissue rejection. It is sometimes used to treat rheumatoid arthritis, some severe types of dermatitis, and severe psoriasis when other treatments have failed.

Because cyclosporin reduces the effectiveness of the immune system, people being treated with this drug are more susceptible than usual to infections. Cyclosporin can also cause kidney damage.

It is important not to make dose changes on your own. Ask your pharmacist for a patient information leaflet printed by the manufacturer. Owing to the differences in blood levels of the drug between the brands, it is important that the brand to be used is specified. If your doctor wants to transfer you from one brand to the other, the change will be made in a controlled way.

QUICK REFERENCE

Drug group Immunosuppressant drug (p.156)

Overdose danger rating Medium

Dependence rating Low

Prescription needed Yes

Available as generic No

INFORMATION FOR USERS

Your drug prescription is tailored for you. Do not alter dosage without checking with your doctor.

How taken

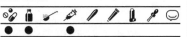

● ● ●

Capsules, liquid, injection.

Frequency and timing of doses
1–2 x daily.

Dosage range
Dosage is calculated on an individual basis according to age and weight.

Onset of effect
Within 12 hours.

Duration of action
Up to 3 days.

Diet advice
Avoid high-potassium foods and potassium supplements.

Storage
Capsules should be left in the blister pack until required. Keep in a closed container in a cool, dry place out of the reach of children. Do not refrigerate.

Missed dose
Take as soon as you remember. If your dose is more than 36 hours late, consult your doctor.

Stopping the drug
Do not stop taking the drug without consulting your doctor; stopping the drug may lead to transplant rejection.

Exceeding the dose
An occasional unintentional extra dose is unlikely to cause problems. Large overdoses may cause vomiting and diarrhoea and may affect kidney function. Notify your doctor.

SPECIAL PRECAUTIONS

Cyclosporin is prescribed only under close medical supervision, taking account of your present condition and medical history.

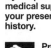

Pregnancy
▼ Not usually prescribed. Safety in pregnancy not established. Discuss with your doctor.

Breast-feeding
▼ Not recommended. The drug passes into the breast milk and safety has not been established. Discuss with your doctor.

Infants and children
▼ Safety not established; used only with great caution.

Over 60
▼ Reduced dose may be necessary.

Driving and hazardous work
▼ No known problems.

Alcohol
▼ No known problems.

Sunlight
▼ Avoid prolonged, unprotected exposure.

POSSIBLE ADVERSE EFFECTS

The most common *adverse effects* are gum swelling, excessive hair growth, nausea and vomiting, and tremor. Headache and muscle cramps may also occur. Less common effects are diarrhoea, facial swelling, flushing, "pins and needles" sensations, rash, and itching.

Symptom/effect	Frequency		Discuss with doctor		Stop taking drug now	Call doctor now
	Common	Rare	Only if severe	In all cases		
Increased body hair	●		■			
Nausea	●			■		
Tremor	●			■		
Swelling of gums	●			■		

PROLONGED USE

Long-term use, especially in high doses, can affect kidney and/or liver function. It may reduce numbers of white blood cells, thus increasing susceptibility to infection.

Monitoring Regular blood tests are normally carried out to measure drug levels and to monitor blood composition, as well as liver and kidney function.

INTERACTIONS

General note Cyclosporin may interact with a large number of drugs. Check with your doctor or pharmacist before taking any new prescription or over-the-counter medications.

DANAZOL

Brand name Danol
Used in the following combined preparations None

GENERAL INFORMATION

Danazol is a synthetic steroid hormone that inhibits hormones called pituitary gonadotrophins.

It is used in a range of conditions, including endometriosis (fragments of endometrial tissue growing outside the uterus), menorrhagia, and, in men, to reduce gynaecomastia (breast swelling). Danazol has also been used, long term, to treat hereditary angioedema (a rare allergic disorder that causes facial swelling).

Danazol is also used to relieve pain, tenderness, and lumpiness in the breasts caused by fibrocystic disease. Treatment commonly disrupts normal menstrual periods and in some cases periods may stop altogether. Women taking high doses may notice unusual hair growth and deepening of the voice.

QUICK REFERENCE

Drug group Drug for menstrual disorders (p.160)

Overdose danger rating Low

Dependence rating Low

Prescription needed Yes

Available as generic Yes

INFORMATION FOR USERS

Your drug prescription is tailored for you. Do not alter dosage without checking with your doctor.

How taken

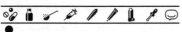

Capsules.

Frequency and timing of doses
2–4 x daily.

Adult dosage range
200–800mg daily, depending on the condition being treated, its severity, and the response to the drug.

Onset of effect
Some effects occur after a few days. Full beneficial effects may take some months.

Duration of action
1–2 days.

Diet advice
None.

Storage
Keep in a closed container in a cool, dry place out of the reach of children.

Missed dose
Take as soon as you remember. If your next dose is due within 2 hours, take a single dose now and skip the next.

Stopping the drug
Do not stop the drug without consulting your doctor; symptoms may recur.

Exceeding the dose
An occasional unintentional extra dose is unlikely to cause problems. But if you notice any unusual symptoms, or if a large overdose has been taken, notify your doctor.

SPECIAL PRECAUTIONS

Be sure to tell your doctor if:
▼ You have long-term liver or kidney problems.
▼ You have heart disease.
▼ You have had epileptic fits.
▼ You suffer from migraine.
▼ You suffer from unexplained vaginal bleeding.
▼ You have diabetes mellitus.
▼ You are taking other medications.

Pregnancy
▼ Not prescribed. May cause masculine characteristics in a female baby. Non-hormonal methods of contraception should be used for women of childbearing age; and pregnancy should be avoided for 3 months after cessation of treatment.

Breast-feeding
▼ The drug passes into the breast milk and may affect the baby. Discuss with your doctor.

Infants and children
▼ Not recommended.

Over 60
▼ Unlikely to be required.

Driving and hazardous work
▼ No known problems.

Alcohol
▼ No known problems.

POSSIBLE ADVERSE EFFECTS

Danazol rarely causes *adverse effects* in low doses. Adverse effects from higher doses, including acne, weight gain, and nausea, are the result of hormonal changes. Voice changes and unusual hair growth in women are largely reversed after treatment.

Symptom/effect	Frequency		Discuss with doctor		Stop taking drug now	Call doctor now
	Common	Rare	Only if severe	In all cases		
Swollen feet/ankles	●		■			
Weight gain	●		■			
Nausea/dizziness	●		■			
Acne/oily skin	●		■			
Backache/cramps	●		■			
Women only						
Unusual hair growth and loss	●			■		
Reduced breast size		●	■			
Voice changes		●		■		
Menstrual disturbances	●			■		

INTERACTIONS

Oral anticoagulant drugs Danazol may increase the effects of these drugs.

Immunosuppressants Danazol may increase the effects of cyclosporin and tacrolimus.

Oral antidiabetic drugs Danazol may reduce the effects of these drugs.

Anticonvulsant drugs The effects of these drugs may be altered by danazol.

PROLONGED USE

The drug is normally taken for 3–9 months depending on the condition being treated. There is a slight risk of liver damage. See also Possible adverse effects, left.

Monitoring Periodic liver function tests may be carried out.

DESMOPRESSIN

Brand names DDAVP, Desmospray, Desmotabs
Used in the following combined preparations None

GENERAL INFORMATION

Desmopressin is a synthetic form of the hormone vasopressin, which is adjusted in response to the concentration of salts in the blood. Deficiency causes diabetes insipidus, in which frequent urination and continual thirst occur because the kidneys cannot concentrate the urine.

Desmopressin controls the production of urine by correcting the deficiency of vasopressin. It is also used to test for diabetes insipidus, to check kidney function, and to treat nocturnal enuresis (bedwetting) in both children and adults. When given by injection, it helps to boost clotting factors in haemophilia.

Side effects of the drug include low blood sodium and fluid retention (which sometimes requires monitoring of body weight and blood pressure to check the body's water balance).

INFORMATION FOR USERS

Your drug prescription is tailored for you. Do not alter dosage without checking with your doctor.

How taken

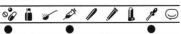

Tablets, injection, nasal solution, nasal spray.

Frequency and timing of doses
Diabetes insipidus 3 x daily (tablets); 1–2 x daily (nasal spray/solution).
Nocturnal enuresis At bedtime (tablets, nasal spray/solution).

Dosage range
Diabetes insipidus: *Adults* 300–600mcg daily (tablets); 1–4 puffs (nasal spray); 10–40mcg daily (nasal solution).
Children 300–600mcg daily (tablets); up to 2 puffs (nasal spray); 20mcg (nasal solution).
Nocturnal enuresis: 200–400mcg for children over 5 years only (tablets); 20–40mcg (nasal solution); 2–4 puffs (nasal spray).

Onset of effect
Begins within a few minutes with full effects in a few hours (injection, nasal solution, and nasal spray); 30–90 minutes (tablets).

Duration of action
Tablets 8 hours; injection and nasal solutions 8–12 hours; nasal spray 10–12 hours.

Diet advice
Your doctor may advise you to monitor your fluid intake.

Storage
Keep in a cool, dry place (tablets) or in a refrigerator, without freezing (nasal solution and nasal spray), out of the reach of children. Protect from light.

Missed dose
Take as soon as you remember. If your next dose is due within 2 hours, take a single dose now and skip the next.

Stopping the drug
Do not stop the drug without consulting your doctor; symptoms of diabetes insipidus may recur.

Exceeding the dose
An occasional unintentional extra dose is unlikely to cause problems. Large overdoses may prevent the kidneys from eliminating fluid, with ensuing problems including convulsions. Notify your doctor immediately.

SPECIAL PRECAUTIONS

Be sure to tell your doctor if:
▼ You have heart problems.
▼ You have high blood pressure.
▼ You have kidney problems.
▼ You have cystic fibrosis.
▼ You have asthma or allergic rhinitis.
▼ You have epilepsy.
▼ You are taking other medications.

Pregnancy
▼ Used with caution in pregnancy.

Breast-feeding
▼ The drug passes into breast milk, in small amounts, but at normal doses adverse effects on the baby are unlikely.

Infants and children
▼ No special problems in children; infants may need monitoring to ensure that fluid balance is correct.

Over 60
▼ May need monitoring to ensure that fluid balance is correct.

Driving and hazardous work
▼ No known problems.

Alcohol
▼ Your doctor may advise on fluid intake.

POSSIBLE ADVERSE EFFECTS

Desmopressin can cause fluid retention and low blood sodium (in serious cases with convulsions). Headache, nausea, vomiting, and epistaxis (nosebleeds) also occur.

Symptom/effect	Frequency		Discuss with doctor		Stop taking drug now	Call doctor now
	Common	Rare	Only if severe	In all cases		
Headache	●		■			
Nausea/vomiting	●		■			
Nasal congestion	●		■			
Nosebleeds	●		■			
Increased body weight	●			■		
Stomach pain	●			■		
Convulsions	●			■	▲	∎

PROLONGED USE

Diabetes insipidus: No problems expected.

Nocturnal enuresis: The drug will be withdrawn for at least a week after 3 months for assessment of the need to continue treatment.

INTERACTIONS

Antidepressants, chlorpropamide, and carbamazepine These drugs may increase the effects of desmopressin.

Indomethacin This anti-inflammatory drug may increase the body's response to desmopressin.

DEXAMETHASONE

Brand name Decadron
Used in the following combined preparations Dexa-Rhinaspray, Maxidex, Maxitrol, Otomize, Sofradex

GENERAL INFORMATION

Dexamethasone is a long-acting corticosteroid prescribed for a variety of skin and soft tissue conditions that are caused by allergy or inflammation. The drug can also be injected into joints to relieve joint pain and stiffness due to rheumatoid arthritis (see p.118). It is injected into a vein for the emergency treatment of shock and brain swelling (due to head injury, stroke, or a tumour), asthma, and emphysema. Eye drops are available to treat eye inflammation.

Low doses of dexamethasone taken for short periods rarely cause serious *side effects*. However, as with other corticosteroids, long-term treatment with high doses can cause unpleasant or dangerous side effects.

INFORMATION FOR USERS

Your drug prescription is tailored for you. Do not alter dosage without checking with your doctor.

How taken

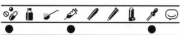

Tablets, injection, eye drops, ear drops/spray.

Frequency and timing of doses
2–4 x daily (with food when taking by mouth); 1–6 hourly (eye drops).

Dosage range
Usually 0.5–10mg daily.

Onset of effect
1–4 days.

Duration of action
Some effects may last several days.

Diet advice
None.

Storage
Keep in a closed container in a cool, dry place out of the reach of children. Protect from light.

Missed dose
Take as soon as you remember. If your next dose is due within 2 hours, take a single dose now and skip the next.

Stopping the drug
Do not stop taking the drug without consulting your doctor. It may be necessary to withdraw the drug gradually.

Exceeding the dose
An occasional unintentional extra dose is unlikely to be a cause for concern. But if you notice any unusual symptoms, or if a large overdose has been taken, notify your doctor.

SPECIAL PRECAUTIONS

Be sure to tell your doctor if:
▼ You have had a peptic ulcer.
▼ You have glaucoma.
▼ You have had tuberculosis.
▼ You have suffered from depression or mental illness.
▼ You have a herpes infection.
▼ You are taking other medications.

Avoid exposure to chickenpox or shingles if you are on *systemic* treatment.

Pregnancy
▼ Safety in pregnancy not established. Discuss with your doctor.

Breast-feeding
▼ The drug passes into the breast milk, but at normal doses adverse effects on the baby are unlikely. Discuss with your doctor.

Infants and children
▼ Reduced dose necessary.

Over 60
▼ No known problems.

Driving and hazardous work
▼ No known problems.

Alcohol
▼ Avoid. Alcohol may increase the risk of peptic ulcer with this drug.

POSSIBLE ADVERSE EFFECTS

The more serious adverse effects only occur when dexamethasone is taken in high doses for long periods of time. These are carefully monitored during prolonged treatment.

Symptom/effect	Frequency		Discuss with doctor		Stop taking drug now	Call doctor now
	Common	Rare	Only if severe	In all cases		
Indigestion	●		■			
Weight gain		●	■			
Acne and other skin effects		●	■			
Fluid retention		●		■		
Muscle weakness		●		■		
Mood changes		●		■		

INTERACTIONS

Antidiabetic drugs Dexamethasone reduces the action of these drugs. Dosage may need to be adjusted accordingly to prevent abnormally high blood sugar.

Barbiturates, phenytoin, rifampicin, and carbamazepine These drugs may reduce the effectiveness of dexamethasone. The dosage may need to be adjusted accordingly.

Oral anticoagulant drugs Dexamethasone may increase the effects of these drugs.

Non-steroidal anti-inflammatory drugs These drugs may increase the likelihood of indigestion from dexamethasone.

Antacids These drugs may reduce the effectiveness of, and should be taken at least 2 hours apart from, dexamethasone.

Vaccines Dexamethasone can interact with some vaccines. Discuss with your doctor before having any vaccinations.

PROLONGED USE

Prolonged use of this drug can lead to glaucoma, cataracts, diabetes, mental disturbances, muscle wasting, fragile bones, and thin skin, and can retard growth in children. People receiving long-term treatment with this drug are advised to carry a 'steroid treatment' card.

DIAZEPAM

Brand names Atensine, Dialar, Diazemuls, Rimapam, Stesolid, Tensium, Valclair, Valium
Used in the following combined preparations None

GENERAL INFORMATION

Introduced in the early 1960s, diazepam is the best known and most widely used of the benzodiazepine group of drugs. The benzodiazepines help relieve tension and nervousness, relax muscles, and encourage sleep. Their actions and *adverse effects* are described more fully on page 83.

Diazepam has a wide range of uses. Besides being commonly used in the treatment of anxiety and anxiety-related insomnia, it is prescribed as a muscle relaxant, in the treatment of alcohol withdrawal, and for the relief of epileptic fits. Given intravenously, it is used to sedate people undergoing certain uncomfortable medical procedures.

Diazepam can be habit-forming if taken regularly over a long period. Its effects may also diminish with time. For these reasons, courses of treatment with diazepam are limited to two weeks whenever possible.

on page 83.

QUICK REFERENCE

Drug group Benzodiazepine anti-anxiety drug (p.83), muscle relaxant (p.120), and anticonvulsant (p.86)

Overdose danger rating Medium

Dependence rating High

Prescription needed Yes

Available as generic Yes

INFORMATION FOR USERS

Your drug prescription is tailored for you. Do not alter dosage without checking with your doctor.

How taken

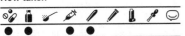

Tablets, liquid, injection, suppositories, rectal solution.

Frequency and timing of doses
1–4 x daily.

Adult dosage range
Anxiety 6–30mg daily.
Muscle spasm 2–60mg daily.

Onset of effect
Immediate effect (injection); 30 minutes–2 hours (other methods of administration).

Duration of action
Up to 24 hours. Some effect may last up to 4 days.

Diet advice
None.

Storage
Keep in a closed container in a cool, dry place out of the reach of children.

Missed dose
Take as soon as you remember. If your next dose is due within 2 hours, take a single dose now and skip the next.

Stopping the drug
If you have been taking the drug continuously for less than 2 weeks, it can be safely stopped as soon as you no longer need it. However, if you have been taking it for longer, consult your doctor, who will supervise a gradual reduction in dosage. Stopping abruptly may lead to withdrawal symptoms (see p.79).

Exceeding the dose
An occasional unintentional extra dose is unlikely to cause problems. Larger overdoses may cause unusual drowsiness. Notify your doctor.

SPECIAL PRECAUTIONS

Be sure to tell your doctor if:
▼ You have severe respiratory disease.
▼ You have long-term liver or kidney problems.
▼ You have had problems with alcohol or drug abuse.
▼ You are taking other medications.

Pregnancy
▼ Safety in pregnancy not established. Discuss with your doctor.

Breast-feeding
▼ The drug passes into the breast milk and may affect the baby. Discuss with your doctor.

Infants and children
▼ Reduced dose necessary.

Over 60
▼ Increased likelihood of adverse effects. Reduced dose may therefore be necessary.

Driving and hazardous work
▼ Avoid such activities until you have learned how diazepam affects you because the drug can cause reduced alertness, slowed reactions, and increased aggression.

Alcohol
▼ Avoid. Alcohol may increase the sedative effects of this drug.

POSSIBLE ADVERSE EFFECTS

The principal adverse effects of this drug are related to its sedative properties. The effects normally diminish after a few days and can often be reduced by adjustment of dosage.

Symptom/effect	Frequency		Discuss with doctor		Stop taking drug now	Call doctor now
	Common	Rare	Only if severe	In all cases		
Daytime drowsiness	●		■			
Dizziness/unsteadiness	●			■		
Headache		●	■			
Blurred vision		●		■		
Forgetfulness/confusion		●		■		
Rash		●		■	▲	

INTERACTIONS

Sedatives All drugs that have a *sedative* effect on the central nervous system can increase the sedative properties of diazepam.

Cisapride The sedative effects of diazepam are increased with this drug.

Cimetidine Breakdown of diazepam in the liver may be inhibited by cimetidine. This can cause a build-up of diazepam in the blood, which increases the likelihood of adverse effects.

PROLONGED USE

Regular use of this drug over several weeks can lead to a reduction in its effect as the body adapts. It may also be habit-forming when taken for extended periods, and severe withdrawal reactions can occur.

DICLOFENAC

Brand names Diclomax SR, Motifene, Rhumalgan, Volraman, Voltarol, and others
Used in the following combined preparation Arthrotec

GENERAL INFORMATION

Taken as a single dose, diclofenac has analgesic properties similar to those of paracetamol. It is taken to relieve mild to moderate headache, menstrual pain, and pain following minor surgery. When diclofenac is given regularly over a long period, it exerts an anti-inflammatory effect and is used to relieve the pain and stiffness associated with rheumatoid arthritis and advanced osteoarthritis.

Diclofenac may also be prescribed to treat acute attacks of gout.

The combined preparation, Arthrotec, contains diclofenac and misoprostol (see p.344). Misoprostol helps prevent gastroduodenal ulceration and may be particularly useful in patients at risk of developing this problem.

INFORMATION FOR USERS

Your drug prescription is tailored for you. Do not alter dosage without checking with your doctor.

How taken

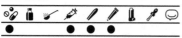

Tablets, dispersible tablets, SR-tablets, capsules, SR-capsules, injection, suppositories, gel.

Frequency and timing of doses
1–3 x daily with food.

Adult dosage range
75–150mg daily.

Onset of effect
Around 1 hour (pain relief); full anti-inflammatory effect may take 2 weeks.

Duration of action
Up to 12 hours; up to 24 hours (SR-preparations).

Diet advice
None.

Storage
Keep in a closed container in a cool, dry place out of the reach of children.

Missed dose
Take as soon as you remember. If your next dose is due within 2 hours, take a single dose now and skip the next.

Stopping the drug
When taken for short-term pain relief, diclofenac can be safely stopped as soon as you no longer need it. If prescribed for long-term treatment (e.g., for arthritis), speak to your doctor before stopping the drug.

Exceeding the dose
An occasional unintentional extra dose is unlikely to be a cause for concern. But if you notice any unusual symptoms or if a large overdose has been taken, notify your doctor.

SPECIAL PRECAUTIONS

Be sure to tell your doctor if:
▼ You have long-term liver or kidney problems.
▼ You have a bleeding disorder.
▼ You have had a peptic ulcer or oesophagitis.
▼ You have porphyria.
▼ You suffer from indigestion.
▼ You are allergic to aspirin.
▼ You suffer from asthma.
▼ You have heart problems or high blood pressure.
▼ You are taking other medications.

Pregnancy
▼ Not usually prescribed in the last 3 months of pregnancy as it may increase the risk of adverse effects on the baby's heart and may prolong labour. Discuss with your doctor.

Breast-feeding
▼ Small amounts of the drug pass into the breast milk, but adverse effects on the baby are unlikely. Discuss with your doctor.

Infants and children
▼ Reduced dose necessary.

Over 60
▼ Increased risk of adverse effects. Reduced dose may therefore be necessary.

Driving and hazardous work
▼ No problems expected.

Alcohol
▼ Keep consumption low. Alcohol may increase the risk of stomach irritation.

Surgery and general anaesthetics
▼ Discuss with your doctor or dentist before any surgery.

POSSIBLE ADVERSE EFFECTS

The most common adverse effects are the result of gastrointestinal disturbances. Black or bloodstained vomit or faeces should be reported to your doctor without delay.

Symptom/effect	Frequency		Discuss with doctor		Stop taking drug now	Call doctor now
	Common	Rare	Only if severe	In all cases		
Gastrointestinal disorders	●		■			
Headache/dizziness		●	■			
Drowsiness		●	■			
Swollen feet/ankles		●		■		
Rash		●		■	▲	
Wheezing/breathlessness		●		■	▲	❚
Black/bloodstained faeces/vomit		●		■	▲	❚

INTERACTIONS

General note Diclofenac interacts with many drugs including other NSAIDs, oral anticoagulants, and corticosteroids.

Antihypertensive drugs and diuretics The beneficial effects of these drugs may be reduced with diclofenac.

Cyclosporin Diclofenac may increase the risk of kidney problems.

Lithium, digoxin, and methotrexate Diclofenac may increase the blood levels of these drugs.

Indigestion remedies These should not be taken at the same time of day as *enteric* coated diclofenac preparations as they disrupt this coating.

PROLONGED USE

There is an increased risk of bleeding from peptic ulcers and in the bowel with prolonged use of diclofenac.

DICYCLOVERINE (DICYCLOMINE)

Brand name Merbentyl
Used in the following combined preparations Diarrest, Kolanticon

GENERAL INFORMATION

Dicycloverine is a mild *anticholinergic* antispasmodic drug that relieves painful abdominal cramps caused by spasm in the gastrointestinal tract. It is used to treat irritable bowel syndrome, indigestion not associated with ulcers, and colicky conditions in babies.

Because the drug has anticholinergic properties, it is also included in some combined preparations used to treat flatulence, indigestion, and diarrhoea.

Dicycloverine relieves symptoms but does not cure the underlying condition. Additional treatment with other drugs and self-help measures, such as dietary changes, may be recommended by your doctor.

Side effects with dicycloverine are rare, but they include headaches, constipation, urinary difficulties, and palpitations.

INFORMATION FOR USERS

Follow instructions on the label. Call your doctor if symptoms worsen.

How taken

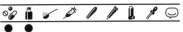

Tablets, liquid.

Frequency and timing of doses
3 x daily before or after meals.

Dosage range
Adults 30–60mg daily.
Children Reduced dose according to age and weight.

Onset of effect
Within 1–2 hours.

Duration of action
4–6 hours.

Diet advice
None.

Storage
Keep in a closed container in a cool, dry place out of the reach of children. Protect from light.

Missed dose
Take as soon as you remember. If your next dose is due within 2 hours, take a single dose now and skip the next.

Stopping the drug
Do not stop the drug without consulting your doctor; symptoms may recur.

Exceeding the dose
An occasional unintentional extra dose is unlikely to cause problems. Large overdoses may cause drowsiness, dizziness, and difficulty in swallowing. Notify your doctor.

SPECIAL PRECAUTIONS

Be sure to consult your doctor or pharmacist before taking this drug if:
▼ You have glaucoma.
▼ You have urinary problems.
▼ You have hiatus hernia.
▼ You are taking other medications.

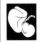

Pregnancy
▼ No evidence of risk.

Breast-feeding
▼ The drug passes into the breast milk, but at normal doses adverse effects on the baby are unlikely. Discuss with your doctor.

Infants and children
▼ Reduced dose necessary.

Over 60
▼ Reduced dose necessary. The elderly are more susceptible to anticholinergic side effects.

Driving and hazardous work
▼ Avoid such activities until you have learned how dicycloverine affects you because the drug can cause drowsiness and blurred vision.

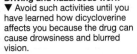

Alcohol
▼ Avoid. Alcohol may increase the sedative effects of this drug.

POSSIBLE ADVERSE EFFECTS

Most people do not notice any *adverse effects* when taking dicycloverine. Those that do occur are related to its anticholinergic properties and include drowsiness and dry mouth. Such symptoms may be overcome by adjusting the dosage, or they may disappear after a few days of usage as your body adjusts to the drug.

Symptom/effect	Frequency		Discuss with doctor		Stop taking drug now	Call doctor now
	Common	Rare	Only if severe	In all cases		
Dry mouth	●		■			
Headache	●		■			
Blurred vision	●		■			
Constipation	●		■			
Drowsiness/dizziness	●		■			
Difficulty in passing urine	●			■		
Palpitations	●			■		

INTERACTIONS

Sedatives All drugs that have a *sedative* effect on the central nervous system may increase the sedative properties of dicycloverine.

Anticholinergic drugs These drug may increase the adverse effects of dicycloverine.

PROLONGED USE

No problems expected.

DIDANOSINE (ddI)

Brand name Videx
Used in the following combined preparations None

GENERAL INFORMATION

Didanosine is an antiviral agent used in the treatment of HIV infection, usually in combination with two other drugs. Like zidovudine (AZT), didanosine works by blocking the action of the reverse transcriptase enzyme.

Didanosine delays the progression of AIDS by temporarily boosting immunity, thereby reducing the frequency and severity of infections, and by helping AIDS patients to gain weight. However, didanosine is not a cure for HIV infection, and patients may continue to be afflicted by the illnesses that are associated with AIDS.

The major *adverse effects* of this drug are pancreatitis (inflammation of the pancreas) and peripheral neuropathy (impaired function of the nerves in the hands and feet).

QUICK REFERENCE

Drug group Antiviral drug for AIDS (p.157)

Overdose danger rating Medium

Dependence rating Low

Prescription needed Yes

Available as generic No

INFORMATION FOR USERS

Your drug prescription is tailored for you. Do not alter dosage without checking with your doctor.

How taken

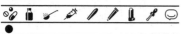

Chewable/dispersible tablets. Tablets should not be swallowed whole: they should be thoroughly chewed, crushed, or dispersed in water or clear apple juice before swallowing.

Frequency and timing of doses
Adults Every 12 hours on an empty stomach.

Adult dosage range
250–400mg daily.

Onset of effect
Usually within 48 hours.

Duration of action
8–12 hours.

Diet advice
None.

Storage
Keep in a closed container in a cool, dry place out of the reach of children. Protect from light.

Missed dose
Take as soon as you remember. If your next dose is due within 4 hours, take a single dose now and skip the next.

Stopping the drug
Do not stop taking the drug without consulting your doctor; symptoms may recur.

Exceeding the dose
An occasional unintentional extra dose is unlikely to cause problems. Large overdoses may cause diarrhoea and abdominal pain. Notify your doctor immediately.

SPECIAL PRECAUTIONS

Be sure to tell your doctor if:
▼ You are taking any other drugs to treat HIV infection or AIDS complications.
▼ You have long-term liver, kidney, or respiratory problems.
▼ You have raised uric acid levels.
▼ You have had pancreatitis.
▼ You are taking other medications.

Pregnancy
▼ Safety in pregnancy not established. Discuss with your doctor.

Breast-feeding
▼ Not recommended. Discuss with your doctor.

Infants and children
▼ Not recommended under 3 months of age. Safety in children not established. Discuss with your doctor.

Over 60
▼ Increased likelihood of adverse effects. Reduced dose may therefore be necessary.

Driving and hazardous work
▼ No special problems.

Alcohol
▼ Avoid. May increase the possibility of adverse effects.

POSSIBLE ADVERSE EFFECTS

The major adverse effects are pancreatitis and peripheral neuropathy. Symptoms of pancreatitis include abdominal pain, nausea, and vomiting. Symptoms of peripheral neuropathy include tingling, burning, pain, or numbness in hands or feet.

Symptom/effect	Frequency		Discuss with doctor		Stop taking drug now	Call doctor now
	Common	Rare	Only if severe	In all cases		
Headache/insomnia	●		■			
Nausea/vomiting/diarrhoea	●		■			
Pallor/fatigue/weakness	●			■		
Breathlessness/cough	●			■		▮
Joint/muscle pain		●		■		
Hives/chills/fever		●		■	▲	▮
Abdominal pain		●		■	▲	▮
Limb burning/numbness		●		■	▲	▮

INTERACTIONS

General note A wide range of drugs may increase the harmful effects or decrease the absorption of didanosine; and didanosine tablets contain antacids which may interfere with the absorption of other drugs. Obtain full information from your doctor or pharmacist.

PROLONGED USE

The long-term effects of didanosine are unknown at this time.

Monitoring Regular blood checks and liver function tests are required during treatment. Eye examinations may be recommended.

DIETHYLSTILBESTROL

Brand name Apstil
Used in the following combined preparation Tampovagan

GENERAL INFORMATION

Diethylstilbestrol is a powerful synthetic oestrogen. Although the drug has been used for many years for a wide range of conditions, including hormone deficiency and menopausal symptoms, its main use these days is in the treatment of prostate cancer and post-menopausal breast cancer. In these conditions it works by suppressing the effects of male sex hormones. Newer drugs are used nowadays for treating the other conditions that were previously treated with diethylstilbestrol.

Side effects are common with this drug, and it is now less widely used because of these potential risks. In men, impotence is often a problem and gynaecomastia (abnormal breast development) can occur. In women, *withdrawal* bleeding often occurs.

QUICK REFERENCE

Drug group Female sex hormone (p.147) and anticancer drug (p.154)

Overdose danger rating Low

Dependence rating Low

Prescription needed Yes

Available as generic Yes

INFORMATION FOR USERS

Your drug prescription is tailored for you. Do not alter dosage without checking with your doctor.

How taken

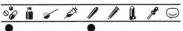

Tablets, pessaries.

Frequency and timing of doses
Tablets Once daily.
Pessaries Once daily.

Adult dosage range
Prostate cancer 1–3mg daily.
Breast cancer 10–20mg daily.

Onset of effect
10–20 days.

Duration of action
Up to 24 hours. Some effects may last a few weeks.

Diet advice
A low sodium diet is advised.

Storage
Keep in a closed container in a cool, dry place out of the reach of children.

Missed dose
Take as soon as you remember. If your next dose is due within 6 hours, take a single dose now and skip the next.

Stopping the drug
Do not stop the drug without consulting your doctor.

Exceeding the dose
An occasional unintentional extra dose is unlikely to be a cause for concern. But if you notice any unusual symptoms, or if a large overdose has been taken, notify your doctor.

SPECIAL PRECAUTIONS

Be sure to tell your doctor if:
▼ You have a long-term liver problem.
▼ You have porphyria.
▼ You have heart failure or high blood pressure.
▼ You have had blood clots or a stroke.
▼ You have diabetes.
▼ You have thyroid disease.
▼ You suffer from migraine or epilepsy.
▼ You are taking other medications.

 Pregnancy
▼ Not prescribed.

 Breast-feeding
▼ The drug passes into the breast milk and may affect the baby. The drug may also have adverse effects on lactation. Discuss with your doctor.

 Infants and children
▼ Not recommended.

 Over 60
▼ No special problems.

 Driving and hazardous work
▼ No known problems.

 Alcohol
▼ No known problems.

POSSIBLE ADVERSE EFFECTS

The most common *adverse effects* are similar to symptoms in early pregnancy, but improve after 2–3 months of treatment. A sudden, sharp pain in the chest, groin, or legs may indicate an abnormal blood clot and requires urgent medical attention. Diethylstilbestrol may also affect the cornea in patients who wear contact lenses.

Symptom/effect	Frequency		Discuss with doctor		Stop taking drug now	Call doctor now
	Common	Rare	Only if severe	In all cases		
Nausea/vomiting	●		■			
Tender, enlarged breasts	●		■			
Swollen feet/ankles	●		■			
Impotence (men only)	●			■		
Pain in chest/groin/legs		●		■	▲	▮

INTERACTIONS

Tobacco smoking Smoking increases the risk of serious adverse effects on the heart and circulation with diethylstilbestrol.

Anticonvulsants, rifampicin, and certain antibiotics These drugs may reduce the effectiveness of diethylstilbestrol.

Antihypertensives and diuretics Diethylstilbestrol may reduce the blood pressure lowering effect of these drugs by causing fluid retention.

PROLONGED USE

The risk of gallstones is increased with long-term use of this drug.

Monitoring Periodic general physical examinations and checks on blood pressure are usually required.

DIGOXIN

Brand name Lanoxin
Used in the following combined preparations None

GENERAL INFORMATION

Digoxin is the most widely used form of digitalis, a drug extracted from the leaves of the foxglove plant. It is sometimes given in the treatment of congestive heart failure and certain alterations of heart rhythm.

Digoxin slows down the rate of the heart so that each beat is more effective in pumping blood. In congestive heart failure it also helps to control tiredness, breathlessness, and fluid retention. Its

effects are not as long lasting as those of other digitalis drugs, but this makes any adverse reactions easier to control.

For digoxin to be effective, the dose must be close to the toxic dose, and the treatment must be monitored carefully. A number of *adverse effects* (see below) may indicate that the toxic level is being reached and should be reported to your doctor immediately.

QUICK REFERENCE

Drug group Digitalis drug (p.96)
Overdose danger rating High
Dependence rating Low
Prescription needed Yes
Available as generic Yes

INFORMATION FOR USERS

Your drug prescription is tailored for you. Do not alter dosage without checking with your doctor.

How taken

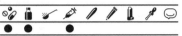

Tablets, liquid, injection.

Frequency and timing of doses
Up to 3 x daily (starting dose); once daily, or divided to reduce nausea, (maintenance dose).

Adult dosage range
0.0625–0.25mg daily (by mouth).

Onset of effect
Within a few minutes (injection); within 1–2 hours (by mouth).

Duration of action
Up to 4 days.

Diet advice
This drug may be more toxic if potassium levels are depleted, so you should include fresh fruit and vegetables in your diet.

Storage
Keep in a closed container in a cool, dry place out of the reach of children. Protect from light.

Missed dose
Take as soon as you remember. If your next dose is due within 8 hours, take a dose now and skip the next.

Stopping the drug
Do not stop the drug without consulting your doctor; stopping the drug may lead to worsening of the underlying condition.

OVERDOSE ACTION

Seek immediate medical advice in all cases. Take emergency action if palpitations, severe weakness, chest pain, or loss of consciousness occur.

See Drug poisoning emergency guide (p.494).

SPECIAL PRECAUTIONS

Be sure to tell your doctor if:
▼ You have a long-term liver problem.
▼ You have thyroid trouble.
▼ You are taking other medications.

Pregnancy
▼ No evidence of risk, but adjustment in dose may be necessary.

Breast-feeding
▼ The drug passes into breast milk, but at normal doses adverse effects on the baby are unlikely. Discuss with your doctor.

Infants and children
▼ Reduced dose necessary.

Over 60
▼ Increased likelihood of adverse effects. Reduced dose may therefore be necessary.

Driving and hazardous work
▼ Special problems are unlikely, but do not undertake these activities until you know how digoxin affects you.

Alcohol
▼ No special problems.

POSSIBLE ADVERSE EFFECTS

The possible adverse effects of digoxin are usually due to increased levels of the drug in the blood. Any symptoms should be reported to your doctor without delay.

Symptom/effect	Frequency		Discuss with doctor		Stop taking drug now	Call doctor now
	Common	Rare	Only if severe	In all cases		
Tiredness	●		■			
Nausea/loss of appetite	●			■		
Confusion	●			■		
Visual disturbance	●			■		
Palpitations	●			■	▲	▮

PROLONGED USE

No problems expected.

Monitoring Periodic checks on blood levels of digoxin and body salts may be advised.

INTERACTIONS

General note Many drugs interact with digoxin. Do not take any medication without your doctor's or pharmacist's advice.

Diuretics may increase the risk of adverse effects from digoxin.

Antacids may reduce the effects of digoxin. The effect of digoxin may increase when such drugs are stopped.

Anti-arrhythmic drugs may increase blood levels of digoxin.

DILTIAZEM

Brand names Adizem, Calcicard, Dilzem, Slozem, Tildiem, and others
Used in the following combined preparations None

GENERAL INFORMATION

Diltiazem belongs to the group of drugs known as calcium channel blockers (p.101). These drugs interfere with the conduction of signals in the muscles of the heart and blood vessels.

Diltiazem is used in the treatment of angina and high blood pressure. When this drug is taken regularly, it reduces the frequency of angina attacks but does not work quickly enough to reduce

the pain of an angina attack that is already in progress.

Diltiazem does not adversely affect breathing and is of particular value for people who suffer from asthma, for whom other anti-angina drugs may not be suitable. *Adverse effects* include headache, ankle swelling, and tiredness.

QUICK REFERENCE

Drug group Calcium channel blocker (p.101) and antihypertensive drug (p.102)

Overdose danger rating Medium

Dependence rating Low

Prescription needed Yes

Available as generic Yes

INFORMATION FOR USERS

Your drug prescription is tailored for you. Do not alter dosage without checking with your doctor.

How taken

Tablets, SR-tablets, capsules, SR-capsules.

Frequency and timing of doses
3 x daily (tablets/capsules); 1–2 x daily (SR-tablets/SR-capsules).

Adult dosage range
180–480mg daily.

Onset of effect
2–3 hours.

Duration of action
6–8 hours.

Diet advice
None.

Storage
Keep in a closed container in a cool, dry place out of the reach of children.

Missed dose
Take as soon as you remember. If your next dose is due within 2 hours, take a single dose now and skip the next.

Stopping the drug
Do not stop taking the drug without consulting your doctor; symptoms may recur. Stopping suddenly may worsen angina.

Exceeding the dose
An occasional unintentional extra dose is unlikely to cause problems. Large overdoses may cause dizziness. Notify your doctor.

SPECIAL PRECAUTIONS

Be sure to tell your doctor if:
▼ You have long-term liver or kidney problems.
▼ You have heart failure.
▼ You are taking other medications.

Pregnancy
▼ Not usually prescribed. Discuss with your doctor.

Breast-feeding
▼ The drug passes into the breast milk and may affect the baby. Discuss with your doctor.

Infants and children
▼ Not recommended.

Over 60
▼ Increased likelihood of adverse effects. Reduced dose may therefore be necessary.

Driving and hazardous work
▼ Avoid such activities until you have learned how diltiazem affects you because the drug can cause dizziness due to lowered blood pressure.

Alcohol
▼ Avoid. Alcohol may lower blood pressure, causing dizziness.

POSSIBLE ADVERSE EFFECTS

Diltiazem can cause various minor symptoms that are common to other calcium channel blockers as well. These include headache and nausea. The most serious effect is the

possibility of a slowed heart beat, which may cause tiredness or dizziness. These effects can sometimes be controlled by an adjustment in dosage.

Symptom/effect	Frequency		Discuss with doctor		Stop taking drug now	Call doctor now
	Common	Rare	Only if severe	In all cases		
Headache	●		■			
Nausea	●		■			
Dry mouth	●		■			
Leg and ankle swelling	●		■			
Tiredness		●		■		
Dizziness		●		■		
Rash		●		■	▲	

INTERACTIONS

Antihypertensive drugs Diltiazem increases the effects of these drugs, leading to a further reduction in blood pressure.

Anticonvulsant drugs Levels of these drugs may be altered by diltiazem.

Anti-arrhythmic drugs There is a risk of side effects on the heart if these are taken with digoxin.

Digoxin Blood levels and adverse effects of this drug may be increased if it is taken with diltiazem. The dosage of digoxin may need to be reduced.

Theophylline/aminophylline Diltiazem may increase the levels of this drug.

Beta blockers increase the risk of the heart slowing.

PROLONGED USE

No problems expected.

DIPHENOXYLATE

Brand names None
Used in the following combined preparations Co-phenotrope, Diarphen, Lomotil, Tropergen

GENERAL INFORMATION

Diphenoxylate is an antidiarrhoeal drug that is chemically related to the opiate analgesics. It reduces bowel contractions and, therefore, the fluidity and frequency of bowel movements. Available in tablet form, it is prescribed for the relief of sudden or recurrent bouts of diarrhoea.

The drug is not suitable for diarrhoea that is caused by infection, poisons, or antibiotics as it may delay recovery by slowing expulsion of harmful substances from the bowel. Diphenoxylate can

cause *toxic* megacolon, a dangerous dilation of the bowel that shuts off the blood supply to the wall of the bowel and increases the risk of perforation.

At recommended doses, serious *adverse effects* are rare. To guard against addiction, atropine is added to diphenoxylate tablets. If these are taken in excessive amounts, the atropine will cause highly unpleasant *anticholinergic* effects. Diphenoxylate is especially dangerous for young children; be sure to store the drug out of their reach.

QUICK REFERENCE

Drug group Opioid antidiarrhoeal drug (p.110)
Overdose danger rating Medium
Dependence rating Medium
Prescription needed Yes
Available as generic No

INFORMATION FOR USERS

Your drug prescription is tailored for you. Do not alter dosage without checking with your doctor.

How taken

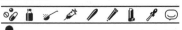

●

Tablets.

Frequency and timing of doses
3–4 x daily.

Dosage range
Adults 10mg initially, followed by doses of 5mg.
Children Reduced dose necessary according to age and weight.

Onset of effect
Within 1 hour. Control of diarrhoea may take some hours.

Duration of action
Up to 24 hours.

Diet advice
Ensure adequate fluid intake during an attack of diarrhoea.

Storage
Keep in a closed container in a cool, dry place out of the reach of children. Protect from light.

Missed dose
Take as soon as you remember. If your next dose is due within 3 hours, take a single dose now and skip the next.

Stopping the drug
Can be safely stopped as soon as you no longer need it.

Exceeding the dose
An occasional unintentional extra dose is unlikely to cause problems. Large overdoses may cause unusual drowsiness, dryness of the mouth and skin, restlessness, and in extreme cases, loss of consciousness. Symptoms of overdose may be delayed. Notify your doctor.

SPECIAL PRECAUTIONS

Be sure to tell your doctor if:
▼ You have a long-term liver problem.
▼ You have severe abdominal pain.
▼ You have bloodstained diarrhoea.
▼ You have recently taken antibiotics.
▼ You have ulcerative colitis.
▼ You have recently travelled abroad.
▼ You are taking other medications.

Pregnancy
▼ Safety in pregnancy not established. Discuss with your doctor.

Breast-feeding
▼ The drug passes into the breast milk and may cause drowsiness in the baby. Discuss with your doctor.

Infants and children
▼ Not recommended under 4 years. Reduced dose necessary for older children.

Over 60
▼ Reduced dose may be necessary.

Driving and hazardous work
▼ Avoid such activities until you have learned how diphenoxylate affects you because the drug may cause drowsiness and dizziness.

Alcohol
▼ Avoid. Alcohol may increase the sedative effects of this drug.

POSSIBLE ADVERSE EFFECTS

Side effects occur infrequently with diphenoxylate. If abdominal pain or distension, nausea, or vomiting occur, notify your doctor.

Symptom/effect	Frequency		Discuss with doctor		Stop taking drug now	Call doctor now
	Common	Rare	Only if severe	In all cases		
Drowsiness	●		■			
Restlessness		●	■			
Headache		●	■			
Skin rash/itching		●		■		
Dizziness		●		■		
Nausea/vomiting		●		■	▲	▌
Abdominal discomfort		●		■	▲	▌

PROLONGED USE

Not usually recommended.

INTERACTIONS

Sedatives All drugs that have a *sedative* effect on the central nervous system may increase the sedative effect of diphenoxylate.

Monoamine oxidase inhibitors (MAOIs) There is a risk of a dangerous rise in blood pressure if MAOIs are taken together with diphenoxylate.

DIPYRIDAMOLE

Brand names Cerebrovase, Modaplate, Persantin
Used in the following combined preparation Asasantin Retard

GENERAL INFORMATION

Dipyridamole was introduced in the late 1970s as an anti-angina drug, to improve the capability of people with angina to exercise. Although more effective drugs are now available for that purpose, dipyridamole is still prescribed as an antiplatelet drug. It "thins" the blood in patients who have had heart valve replacement surgery, a heart attack, or a stroke, reducing the possibility of blood clots in the circulation.

Dipyridamole is usually given together with other drugs such as warfarin or aspirin. The drug can also be given by injection during certain types of diagnostic test on the heart.

Side effects may occur, especially during the early days of treatment. If they persist, your doctor may advise a reduction in dosage.

QUICK REFERENCE

Drug group Antiplatelet drug (p.104)

Overdose danger rating Medium

Dependence rating Low

Prescription needed Yes

Available as generic Yes

INFORMATION FOR USERS

Your drug prescription is tailored for you. Do not alter dosage without checking with your doctor.

How taken

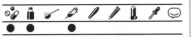

Tablets, capsules, SR-capsules, liquid, injection (for diagnostic tests only).

Frequency and timing of doses
3–4 x daily, 1 hour before meals (tablets, capsules, liquid). 2 x daily with food (SR-capsules).

Adult dosage range
300–600mg daily.

Onset of effect
Within 1 hour. Full therapeutic effect may not be reached for 2–3 weeks.

Duration of action
Up to 8 hours. Up to 12 hours (SR-capsules)

Diet advice
None.

Storage
Keep in a closed container in a cool, dry place out of the reach of children. Protect from light.

Missed dose
Take as soon as you remember. If your next dose is due within 2 hours, take a single dose now and skip the next.

Stopping the drug
Do not stop taking the drug without consulting your doctor; withdrawal of the drug could lead to abnormal blood clotting.

Exceeding the dose
An occasional unintentional extra dose is unlikely to be a cause for concern. Large overdoses may cause dizziness or vomiting. Notify your doctor.

SPECIAL PRECAUTIONS

Be sure to tell your doctor if:
▼ You have low blood pressure.
▼ Your suffer from migraine.
▼ You have angina.
▼ You have had a recent heart attack.
▼ You are taking other medications.

Pregnancy
▼ Safety in pregnancy not established. Discuss with your doctor.

Breast-feeding
▼ The drug passes into the breast milk but at normal doses adverse effects on the baby are unlikely. Discuss with your doctor.

Infants and children
▼ Reduced dose necessary.

Over 60
▼ No special problems.

Driving and hazardous work
▼ Avoid such activities until you have learned how dipyridamole affects you because the drug may cause dizziness and faintness.

Alcohol
▼ No known problems.

POSSIBLE ADVERSE EFFECTS

Adverse effects are rare. Possible symptoms include dizziness, headache, faintness, nausea, and rash. In rare cases, the drug may aggravate angina.

Symptom/effect	Frequency		Discuss with doctor		Stop taking drug now	Call doctor now
	Common	Rare	Only if severe	In all cases		
Nausea	●		■			
Headache		●	■			
Diarrhoea		●	■			
Dizziness/fainting		●		■		
Rash		●		■	▲	

INTERACTIONS

Anticoagulant drugs The effect of these drugs may be increased by dipyridamole, thereby increasing the risk of uncontrolled bleeding. The dosage of the anticoagulant should be reduced accordingly.

Antacids may reduce the effectiveness of dipyridamole.

PROLONGED USE

No known problems.

DISULFIRAM

Brand name Antabuse
Used in the following combined preparations None

GENERAL INFORMATION

Disulfiram is used to help alcoholics abstain from alcohol. It does not cure alcoholism but provides a powerful deterrent to drinking.

If you are taking disulfiram and drink even a small amount of alcohol, highly unpleasant reactions follow, such as flushing, throbbing headache, nausea, thirst, breathlessness, palpitations, dizziness, and fainting. Such reactions may last from 30 minutes to several hours, leaving you feeling drowsy and sleepy. Because the reactions can also include unconsciousness, it is wise to carry a card stating the person to be notified in an emergency.

When disulfiram and alcohol are taken together, acetaldehyde (a *toxic* substance that is manufactured in the body and broken down) rises to higher concentrations in the blood, triggering the unwelcome reactions. It is important not to drink any alcohol for at least 24 hours before beginning disulfiram treatment, and for at least a week after stopping. Foods, medicines, and even toiletries that contain alcohol should also be avoided.

INFORMATION FOR USERS

Your drug prescription is tailored for you. Do not alter dosage without checking with your doctor.

How taken

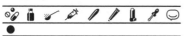

Tablets.

Frequency and timing of doses
Once daily.

Adult dosage range
800mg initially, gradually reduced over 5 days to 100–200mg (maintenance dose).

Onset of effect
Interaction with alcohol occurs within a few minutes of taking alcohol.

Duration of action
Interaction with alcohol can occur for up to 6 days after the last dose of disulfiram.

Diet advice
Avoid all alcoholic drinks, even in very small amounts. Food, fermented vinegar, medicines, mouthwashes, and lotions containing alcohol should also be avoided.

Storage
Keep in a closed container in a cool, dry place out of the reach of children. Protect from light.

Missed dose
Take as soon as you remember. If your next dose is due within 2 hours, take a single dose now and skip the next.

Stopping the drug
Do not stop taking the drug without consulting your doctor.

Exceeding the dose
An occasional unintentional extra dose is unlikely to cause problems. Large overdoses may cause a temporary increase in adverse effects. Notify your doctor.

SPECIAL PRECAUTIONS

Be sure to tell your doctor if:
▼ You have long-term liver or kidney problems.
▼ You have heart problems, coronary artery disease, or high blood pressure.
▼ You have had epileptic fits.
▼ You have diabetes.
▼ You have breathing problems.
▼ You are taking other medications.

Pregnancy
▼ Safety in pregnancy not established. Discuss with your doctor.

Breast-feeding
▼ The drug passes into the breast milk and may affect the baby adversely. Discuss with your doctor.

Over 60
▼ Reduced dose may be necessary.

Driving and hazardous work
▼ Avoid such activities until you have learned how disulfiram affects you because the drug can cause drowsiness and dizziness.

Alcohol
▼ Never drink alcohol while under treatment with disulfiram, and avoid foods, medicines, and toiletries containing alcohol. This drug may interact dangerously with alcohol.

POSSIBLE ADVERSE EFFECTS

Adverse effects of disulfiram usually disappear when you get used to taking the drug. If they persist or become severe, the dosage may need to be adjusted.

Symptom/effect	Frequency		Discuss with doctor		Stop taking drug now	Call doctor now
	Common	Rare	Only if severe	In all cases		
Drowsiness	●		■			
Reduced libido		●	■			
Nausea/vomiting		●	■			

INTERACTIONS

General note A number of drugs can produce an adverse reaction when taken with disulfiram. You are advised to check with your doctor or pharmacist before taking any other medication.

Phenytoin Disulfiram increases the blood levels of this drug.

Anticoagulant drugs Disulfiram increases the effect of these drugs.

Metronidazole A severe reaction can occur if this drug is taken with disulfiram.

Theophylline Disulfiram may increase the toxic effects of this drug.

PROLONGED USE

Not usually prescribed for longer than 6 months without review. It is wise to carry a card indicating you are taking disulfiram with instructions as to who should be notified in an emergency.

DOMPERIDONE

Brand name Motilium
Used in the following combined preparations Domperamol

GENERAL INFORMATION

Domperidone, an anti-emetic drug, was first introduced in the early 1980s. It is particularly effective for treating the nausea and vomiting that are caused by gastrointestinal disorders, such as gastroenteritis, or that occur as a *side effect* of other drug treatment (especially anticancer drugs) or radiation therapy. It is not effective for motion sickness or nausea caused by inner ear disorders such as Ménière's disease.

The main advantage of domperidone over other anti-emetic drugs is that it does not usually cause sedation or other *adverse effects* such as abnormal movement. Domperidone is not suitable, however, for the long-term treatment of gastrointestinal disorders, for which an alternative drug treatment is often prescribed.

Domperidone may also be used to relieve dyspepsia (indigestion and heartburn); and, in combination with paracetamol, it is sometimes used to treat acute attacks of migraine.

INFORMATION FOR USERS

Follow instructions on the label.
Call your doctor if symptoms worsen.

How taken

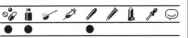

Tablets, liquid, suppositories.

Frequency and timing of doses
Nausea/vomiting Every 4–8 hours as required.
Dyspepsia 3 x daily with water before meals and at night (tablets only).

Adult dosage range
10–20mg (by mouth); 30–60mg (rectally).

Onset of effect
Within 1 hour. The effects of the drug may be delayed if taken after the onset of nausea.

Duration of action
Approximately 6 hours.

Diet advice
None.

Storage
Keep in a closed container in a cool, dry place out of the reach of children. Protect from light.

Missed dose
Take as soon as you remember for dyspepsia. If your next dose is due within 4 hours, take a single dose now and skip the next. Then return to your normal dose schedule.

Stopping the drug
Can be stopped when you no longer need it.

Exceeding the dose
An occasional unintentional extra dose is unlikely to cause problems. Large overdoses may cause dizziness. Notify your doctor.

SPECIAL PRECAUTIONS

Be sure to tell your doctor if:
▼ You have a long-term kidney problem.
▼ You have thyroid disease.
▼ You are taking other medications.

Pregnancy
▼ Safety in pregnancy not established. Discuss with your doctor.

Breast-feeding
▼ The drug may pass into the breast milk, but at normal doses adverse effects on the baby are unlikely. Discuss with your doctor.

Infants and children
▼ Prescribed only to treat nausea and vomiting caused by anticancer drugs or radiation therapy. Reduced dose necessary.

Over 60
▼ No special problems.

Driving and hazardous work
▼ No special problems.

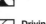

Alcohol
▼ No special problems, but alcohol is best avoided in cases of nausea and vomiting.

POSSIBLE ADVERSE EFFECTS

Adverse effects from this drug are rare.

Symptom/effect	Frequency		Discuss with doctor		Stop taking drug now	Call doctor now
	Common	Rare	Only if severe	In all cases		
Breast enlargement		●		■		
Milk secretion from breast		●		■		
Muscle spasms/tremors		●		■		
Reduced libido		●		■		
Rash		●		■		

INTERACTIONS

Anticholinergic drugs These may reduce the beneficial effects of domperidone.

Opioid analgesics These may reduce the beneficial effects of domperidone.

Bromocriptine and cabergoline Domperidone may reduce the effects of these drugs in some people.

PROLONGED USE

Not prescribed for long-term treatment.

DONEPEZIL

Brand name Aricept
Used in the following combined preparations None

GENERAL INFORMATION

Donepezil is an inhibitor of the enzyme acetylcholinesterase. This enzyme breaks down the natural *neurotransmitter* acetylcholine to limit its effects. Blocking the enzyme raises the levels of acetyl-choline which, in the brain, increases alertness. Donepezil has been found to improve the symptoms of dementia due to Alzheimer's disease and is used to diminish deterioration in that disease. It does not have any effect on dementia due to other causes. It is usual to assess anyone being treated with donepezil after about three months to decide whether the drug is helping and whether it is worth continuing treatment.

Side effects may include bladder outflow obstruction and psychiatric problems, such as agitation and aggression, which might be thought due to the disease.

INFORMATION FOR USERS

Your drug prescription is tailored for you. Do not alter dosage without checking with your doctor.

How taken

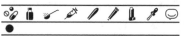

Tablets.

Frequency and timing of doses
Once daily at bedtime.

Adult dosage range
5–10mg.

Onset of effect
1 hour. Full effects might take up to 3 months.

Duration of action
1–2 days.

Diet advice
None.

Storage
Keep in a closed container in a cool, dry place out of the reach of children.

Missed dose
Take as soon as you remember. A carer should be overseeing the taking of the tablets.

Stopping the drug
Do not stop taking the drug without consulting your doctor; symptoms may recur.

Exceeding the dose
An occasional unintentional extra dose is unlikely to be a cause for concern. But if you notice any unusual symptoms, or if a large overdose has been taken, notify your doctor.

POSSIBLE ADVERSE EFFECTS

Adverse effects include such problems as accidents, which are common in this group of people even when not treated.

Symptom/effect	Frequency		Discuss with doctor		Stop taking drug now	Call doctor now
	Common	Rare	Only if severe	In all cases		
Nausea/vomiting	●			■		
Diarrhoea	●			■		
Fatigue/insomnia	●			■		
Muscle cramps	●			■		
Headache		●		■		
Fainting/dizziness		●			■	
Palpitations		●			■	
Difficulty in passing urine		●		■		

INTERACTIONS

Aminoglycoside antibiotics, clindamycin, and colistin These antibiotics block the effect of donepezil.

Antimalarials and anti-arrhythmics Certain drugs from these groups may block the effects of donepezil.

Muscle relaxants used in surgery Donepezil may increase the effect of some muscle relaxants, but it may also block some others.

SPECIAL PRECAUTIONS

Be sure to tell your doctor if:
▼ You have a heart problem.
▼ You have asthma or respiratory problems.
▼ You have had a peptic ulcer.
▼ You are taking an NSAID regularly.
▼ You are taking other medications.

 Pregnancy
▼ Not prescribed.

 Breast-feeding
▼ Not prescribed.

 Infants and children
▼ Not prescribed.

 Over 60
▼ No special problems.

 Driving and hazardous work
▼ Your underlying condition may make such activities inadvisable. Discuss with your doctor.

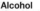 **Alcohol**
▼ Avoid. Alcohol may reduce the effect of donepezil.

Surgery and general anaesthetics
▼ Treatment with donepezil may need to be stopped before you have a general anaesthetic. Discuss this with your doctor or dentist before any operation.

PROLONGED USE

May be continued for as long as there is benefit. Stopping the drug leads to a gradual loss of the improvements.

Monitoring Periodic checks may be performed to test whether the drug is still providing some benefit.

DORZOLAMIDE

Brand name Trusopt
Used in the following combined preparation Cosopt

GENERAL INFORMATION

Dorzolamide is a carbonic anhydrase inhibitor (a kind of diuretic) that is used, in the form of eye drops only, to treat glaucoma. It is also used for ocular hypertension (high blood pressure inside the eye). The drug relieves the pressure by reducing production of aqueous humour, the fluid in the front chamber of the eye.

Dorzolamide may be used with a beta blocker in a combined preparation but is also used on its own by people resistant to the effects of beta blockers or for whom beta blockers are unsuitable.

Most *side effects* of dorzolamide are local to the eye, but *systemic* effects may occur if enough of the drug is absorbed by the body.

QUICK REFERENCE

Drug group Drug for Glaucoma (p.168)

Overdose danger rating Low

Dependence rating Low

Prescription needed Yes

Available as generic No

INFORMATION FOR USERS

Your drug prescription is tailored for you. Do not alter dosage without checking with your doctor.

How taken

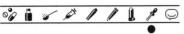

Eye drops.

Frequency and timing of doses
3 x daily (on its own); 2 x daily (combined).

Adult dosage range
1 drop in the affected eye(s) or as directed.

Onset of effect
15–30 minutes.

Duration of action
4–8 hours.

Diet advice
None.

Storage
Keep in a closed container in a cool, dry place out of the reach of children. Protect from light. Discard eye drops 4 weeks after opening.

Missed dose
Take as soon as you remember. If your next dose is due, skip the missed dose and then go back to your normal dosing schedule.

Stopping the drug
Do not stop the drug without consulting your doctor; symptoms may recur.

Exceeding the dose
An occasional unintentional extra application is unlikely to cause problems. Excessive use may provoke side effects as described below.

SPECIAL PRECAUTIONS

Be sure to tell your doctor if:
▼ You have liver or kidney problems.
▼ You are allergic to sulphonamide drugs.
▼ You are allergic to benzalkonium chloride.
▼ You are taking other medications.

 Pregnancy
▼ Not prescribed. Discuss with your doctor.

 Breast-feeding
▼ Not recommended. Discuss with your doctor.

 Infants and children
▼ Not recommended.

 Over 60
▼ No special problems.

 Driving and hazardous work
▼ Avoid such activities until you have learned how dorzolamide affects you because the drug can cause dizziness and blurred vision.

 Alcohol
▼ No special problems.

POSSIBLE ADVERSE EFFECTS

Local side effects of dorzolamide include conjunctivitis and keratitis (inflammation of the cornea, the transparent part of the eye). *Systemic* side effects such as nausea and headache may also occur. If you develop a rash or breathing difficulties, you should consult your doctor urgently.

Symptom/effect	Frequency		Discuss with doctor		Stop taking drug now	Call doctor now
	Common	Rare	Only if severe	In all cases		
Burning/stinging eyes	●		■			
Bitter taste in the mouth	●		■			
Blurred vision/runny eyes	●		■			
Inflamed/sore eyes	●			■		
Headache/tiredness		●	■			
Nausea/dizziness		●	■			
Rash/breathing difficulties		●		■		■

PROLONGED USE

No special problems.

INTERACTIONS

General note Dorzolamide may interact with the following drugs, but there do not appear to be any published reports of problems. Consult your doctor.

Thiazide diuretics Excessive loss of potassium may occur when these drugs are taken with dorzolamide.

Aspirin this drug may increase the levels of dorzolamide and increase the risk of adverse effects.

Lithium Dorzolamide may reduce blood levels of lithium.

DOSULEPIN (DOTHIEPIN)

Brand names Dothapax, Prepadine, Prothiaden
Used in the following combined preparations None

GENERAL INFORMATION

Dosulepin belongs to the tricyclic class of antidepressant drugs, and is used in the long-term treatment of depression. The drug is particularly useful when the depression is accompanied by anxiety and insomnia. Dosulepin has a number of effects – it elevates mood, increases physical activity, improves appetite, and restores interest in everyday activities.

Taken at night, dosulepin encourages sleep and helps eliminate the need to take additional sleeping drugs.

Dosulepin takes several weeks to achieve its full antidepressant effect. It has *adverse effects* that are common to all tricyclic drugs and include a risk of causing dangerous heart rhythms, fits, and coma, if it is taken in overdose.

INFORMATION FOR USERS

Your drug prescription is tailored for you. Do not alter dosage without checking with your doctor.

How taken

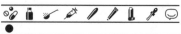

Tablets, capsules.

Frequency and timing of doses
2–3 x daily or once at night.

Adult dosage range
75–150mg daily.

Onset of effect
Full antidepressant effect may not be felt for 2–4 weeks, but adverse effects may be noticed within a day or two.

Duration of action
Several days.

Diet advice
None.

Storage
Keep in a closed container in a cool, dry place out of the reach of children.

Missed dose
Take as soon as you remember. If your next dose is due within 2 hours, take a single dose now and skip the next.

Stopping the drug
Do not stop taking the drug without consulting your doctor, who may supervise a gradual reduction in dosage. Abrupt cessation of the drug may cause withdrawal symptoms and a recurrence of the original problem.

OVERDOSE ACTION

 Seek immediate medical advice in all cases. Take emergency action if palpitations or loss of consciousness occur.

See Drug poisoning emergency guide (p.494).

SPECIAL PRECAUTIONS

Be sure to tell your doctor if:
▼ You have heart problems.
▼ You have had epileptic fits.
▼ You have long-term liver or kidney problems.
▼ You have glaucoma.
▼ You have prostate trouble.
▼ You are taking other medications.

 Pregnancy
▼ Safety in pregnancy not established. Discuss with your doctor.

Breast-feeding
▼ The drug passes into the breast milk, but effects on the baby are unlikely. Discuss with your doctor.

Infants and children
▼ Not recommended.

Over 60
▼ Reduced dose may be necessary.

Driving and hazardous work
▼ Avoid such activities until you have learned how dosulepin affects you because the drug can reduce alertness and may cause blurred vision, dizziness, and drowsiness.

Alcohol
▼ Avoid. Alcohol may increase the sedative effects of this drug.

Surgery and general anaesthetics
▼ Treatment with dosulepin may need to be stopped before you have a general anaesthetic. Discuss this with your doctor or dentist before any operation.

POSSIBLE ADVERSE EFFECTS

The adverse effects of this drug are mainly the result of its *anticholinergic* action. These effects are more common in the early days of treatment.

Symptom/effect	Frequency		Discuss with doctor		Stop taking drug now	Call doctor now
	Common	Rare	Only if severe	In all cases		
Drowsiness	●		■			
Dry mouth	●		■			
Sweating	●		■			
Blurred vision	●			■		
Dizziness/fainting		●		■		
Rash		●		■	▲	
Difficulty passing urine		●		■	▲	
Palpitations		●		■	▲	■

INTERACTIONS

Sedatives All drugs that have a *sedative* effect on the central nervous system increase the sedative properties of dosulepin.

Heavy smoking This may reduce the antidepressant effect of dosulepin.

Antiepileptic drugs dosulepin may reduce the effectiveness of these drugs.

Monoamine oxidase inhibitors (MAOIs) In the rare cases where these drugs are given with dosulepin, serious interactions may occur.

PROLONGED USE

No problems expected.

Monitoring Elderly people experiencing drowsiness, confusion, or convulsions should be monitored for low sodium levels in the blood.

DOXAZOSIN

Brand name Cardura
Used in the following combined preparations None

GENERAL INFORMATION

Doxazosin is an antihypertensive vaso-dilator drug that relieves hypertension (high blood pressure) by relaxing the muscles in the blood vessel walls, which dilates them and thereby eases the flow of blood. As doxazosin is eliminated slowly from the body, it is usually given only once daily. It may be administered together with other antihypertensive drugs, including beta blockers, since its effects on blood pressure are increased when it is combined with most other antihypertensives.

Given in low doses, doxazosin is also used to relieve symptoms caused by an enlarged prostate gland.

Dizziness and fainting may occur at the onset of treatment with doxazosin, because the first dose may cause a marked fall in blood pressure. For this reason, the initial dose is usually low.

INFORMATION FOR USERS

Your drug prescription is tailored for you. Do not alter dosage without checking with your doctor.

How taken

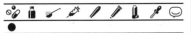

Tablets.

Frequency and timing of doses
Once daily.

Adult dosage range
Hypertension 1mg (starting dose), increased gradually as necessary up to 16mg.
Enlarged prostate 1mg (starting dose), increased gradually at 1–2-week intervals up to 8mg.

Onset of effect
Within 2 hours.

Duration of action
24 hours.

Diet advice
None.

Storage
Keep in a closed container in a cool, dry place out of the reach of children.

Missed dose
Take as soon as you remember. If your next dose is due within 6 hours, take a single dose now and skip the next.

Stopping the drug
Do not stop taking the drug without consulting your doctor; stopping the drug may lead to a rise in blood pressure.

Exceeding the dose
An occasional unintentional extra dose is unlikely to be a cause for concern. Larger overdoses may cause dizziness or fainting. Notify your doctor.

SPECIAL PRECAUTIONS

Be sure to tell your doctor if:
▼ You have long-term liver or kidney problems.
▼ You are taking other medications.

 Pregnancy
▼ Safety in pregnancy not established. Discuss with your doctor.

 Breast-feeding
▼ The drug passes into the breast milk. Discuss with your doctor.

 Infants and children
▼ Not recommended.

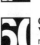 **Over 60**
▼ Reduced dose may be necessary. Take extra care when standing up until you have learned how the drug affects you.

 Driving and hazardous work
▼ Avoid such activities until you have learned how doxazosin affects you because the drug can cause drowsiness, dizziness, and fainting.

 Alcohol
▼ Avoid excessive amounts. Alcohol may increase some of the *adverse effects* of this drug, such as dizziness, drowsiness, and fainting.

POSSIBLE ADVERSE EFFECTS

Nausea, headache, and weakness are common with doxazosin, but the main problem is that it may cause dizziness or fainting when you stand up.

Symptom/effect	Frequency		Discuss with doctor		Stop taking drug now	Call doctor now
	Common	Rare	Only if severe	In all cases		
Nausea	●			■		
Weakness/drowsiness	●			■		
Headache	●			■		
Dizziness/fainting		●		■		
Stuffy nose		●		■		
Palpitations/chest pain		●			■	■
Rash		●			■	

INTERACTIONS

Hypotensive drugs Any drugs that can reduce the blood pressure are likely to have an increased effect when taken with doxazosin.

PROLONGED USE

No known problems.

DOXORUBICIN

Brand name Caelyx
Used in the following combined preparations None

GENERAL INFORMATION

Doxorubicin is one of the most effective anticancer drugs. It is prescribed to treat a wide variety of cancers, usually in conjunction with other anticancer drugs. It is used in acute leukaemia and cancer of the lymph nodes (Hodgkin's disease), lung, breast, bladder, stomach, thyroid, and reproductive organs. It is also used to treat Kaposi's sarcoma in AIDS patients.

Nausea and vomiting after injection are the most common *side effects* of doxorubicin. Although these symptoms are unpleasant, they tend to be less severe as the body adjusts to treatment. The drug may stain the urine bright red, but this is not harmful. More seriously, because doxorubicin interferes with the production of blood cells, blood clotting disorders, *anaemia*, and infections may occur. Therefore, effects on the blood are carefully monitored. Hair loss is also a common side effect. Rarely, heart rhythm disturbance and heart failure are dose-dependent side effects that may also occur.

INFORMATION FOR USERS

This drug is given only under medical supervision and is not for self-administration.

How taken

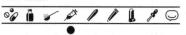

Injection, *bladder instillation*.

Frequency and timing of doses
Every 1–3 weeks.

Adult dosage range
Dosage is determined individually according to body height, weight, and response.

Onset of effect
Some adverse effects may appear within one hour of starting treatment, but full beneficial effects may not be felt for up to 4 weeks.

Duration of action
Adverse effects can persist for up to 2 weeks after stopping treatment.

Diet advice
None.

Storage
Not applicable. The drug is not normally kept in the home.

Missed dose
The drug is administered in hospital under close medical supervision. If for some reason you skip your dose, contact your doctor as soon as you can.

Stopping the drug
Discuss with your doctor. Stopping the drug prematurely may lead to a worsening of the underlying condition.

Exceeding the dose
Overdosage is unlikely since treatment is carefully monitored and supervised.

POSSIBLE ADVERSE EFFECTS

Nausea and vomiting generally occur within an hour of injection. Many people also experience hair loss and loss of appetite. Palpitations may indicate an adverse effect of the drug on the heart. Since treatment is closely supervised in hospital, all adverse effects are monitored.

Symptom/effect	Frequency		Discuss with doctor		Stop taking drug now	Call doctor now
	Common	Rare	Only if severe	In all cases		
Nausea/vomiting	●			■		
Loss of appetite	●			■		
Hair loss	●			■		
Diarrhoea		●		■		
Mouth ulcers		●		■		
Palpitations		●		■		■
Skin irritation/ulcers		●		■		

INTERACTIONS

Cyclosporin Administration of cyclosporin while receiving doxorubicin can lead to adverse effects on the nervous system.

SPECIAL PRECAUTIONS

Doxorubicin is prescribed only under close medical supervision, taking account of your present condition and medical history.

Pregnancy
▼ Not usually prescribed. Doxorubicin may cause birth defects or premature birth. Discuss with your doctor.

Breast-feeding
▼ Not advised. The drug passes into the breast milk and may affect the baby adversely. Discuss with your doctor.

Infants and children
▼ Reduced dose necessary.

Over 60
▼ Increased risk of adverse effects. Reduced dose may be necessary.

Driving and hazardous work
▼ No known problems.

Alcohol
▼ No known problems.

PROLONGED USE

Prolonged use of doxorubicin may reduce the activity of the bone marrow, leading to reduced production of all types of blood cell. It may also affect the heart adversely.

Monitoring Periodic checks on blood composition are usually required. Regular heart examinations are also carried out.

DOXYCYCLINE

Brand names Cyclodox, Demix, Doxylar, Ramysis, Vibramycin
Used in the following combined preparations None

GENERAL INFORMATION

Doxycycline, a tetracycline antibiotic, is longer acting than some drugs in this group. It is used mainly in the treatment of infections of the urinary, respiratory, and gastrointestinal tracts and of the skin, eye, and prostate. It is often used in the treatment of acne and may be recommended for malaria prevention in some parts of the world (see p.137).

Doxycycline is less likely to cause diarrhoea as a *side effect* than other tetracyclines, and its absorption is not significantly impaired by milk and food. It can therefore be taken with meals to reduce side effects such as nausea or indigestion. It is also safe (unlike most other tetracyclines) for people with impaired kidney function. Like other tetracyclines, it can stain developing teeth and may affect bone development; it is therefore usually avoided in young children or pregnant women.

QUICK REFERENCE

Drug group Tetracycline antibiotic (p.128)

Overdose danger rating Low

Dependence rating Low

Prescription needed Yes

Available as generic Yes

INFORMATION FOR USERS

Your drug prescription is tailored for you. Do not alter dosage without checking with your doctor.

How taken

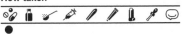

Tablets, capsules.

Frequency and timing of doses
1–2 x daily with water, or with or after food, in a sitting or standing position.

Dosage range
100–200mg daily.

Onset of effect
4–12 hours; several weeks (acne).

Duration of action
Up to 24 hours; several weeks (acne).

Diet advice
None.

Storage
Keep in closed container in a cool, dry place out of the reach of children.

Missed dose
Take as soon as you remember. If your next dose is due within 6 hours, take a single dose now and skip the next.

Stopping the drug
Take the full course. Even if you feel better, the original infection may still be present and symptoms may recur if treatment is stopped too soon.

Exceeding the dose
An occasional unintentional extra dose is unlikely to be a cause for concern. But if you notice any unusual symptoms, or if a large overdose has been taken, notify your doctor.

SPECIAL PRECAUTIONS

Be sure to tell your doctor if:
▼ You have a long-term liver problem.
▼ You have previously suffered an allergic reaction to a tetracycline antibiotic.
▼ You have porphyria.
▼ You are taking other medications.

Pregnancy
▼ Not usually prescribed. May discolour the teeth of the developing baby. Discuss with your doctor.

Breast-feeding
▼ The drug passes into the breast milk and may lead to discoloration of the baby's teeth and may also have other adverse effects. Discuss with your doctor.

Infants and children
▼ Not recommended under 12 years. Reduced dose necessary for older children.

Over 60
▼ No special problems. Dispersible tablets should be used because they are less likely to cause oesophageal irritation or ulceration.

Driving and hazardous work
▼ No known problems.

Alcohol
▼ No known problems, but avoid excessive amounts.

POSSIBLE ADVERSE EFFECTS

Adverse effects from doxycycline are rare, although some people may experience nausea, vomiting, or diarrhoea. Other rare adverse effects include rash, itching, and increased sensitivity of the skin to sunlight, which may cause a rash to develop.

Symptom/effect	Frequency		Discuss with doctor		Stop taking drug now	Call doctor now
	Common	Rare	Only if severe	In all cases		
Nausea/vomiting	●		■			
Mouth ulcers	●		■			
Diarrhoea	●		■			
Rash/itching	●			■	▲	
Photosensitivity	●			■	▲	
Headache/visual disturbances	●			■		

INTERACTIONS

Oral anticoagulant drugs Doxycycline may increase the anticoagulant action of these drugs.

Penicillin antibiotics Doxycycline interferes with the antibacterial action of these drugs.

Barbiturates, carbamazepine, and phenytoin All of these drugs reduce the effectiveness of doxycycline. Doxycycline dosage may need to be increased.

Oral contraceptives A slight risk exists of doxycycline reducing the effectiveness of oral contraceptives. Discuss with your doctor.

Antacids and preparations containing iron, calcium, or magnesium may impair absorption of this drug. Do not take within 2–3 hours of doxycycline.

Cyclosporin Doxycycline may increase the blood levels of this drug.

PROLONGED USE

Not usually prescribed long term, except for acne.

DYDROGESTERONE

Brand names Duphaston, Duphaston HRT
Used in the following combined preparations Femoston, Femapak

GENERAL INFORMATION

Dydrogesterone is a progestogen, a synthetic hormone similar to the natural female sex hormone progesterone. The drug is widely used to treat a variety of menstrual disorders that are thought to result from a deficiency of progesterone. These include premenstrual syndrome and absent, irregular, or painful periods (see also p.160).

Dydrogesterone is also prescribed together with an oestrogen as part of hormone replacement therapy following the menopause. It may be prescribed for endometriosis (p.160), and is also given to prevent miscarriage in women who have already suffered repeated miscarriages.

Dydrogesterone is usually taken on selected days during the menstrual cycle, depending on the disorder that is being treated.

INFORMATION FOR USERS

Your drug prescription is tailored for you. Do not alter dosage without checking with your doctor.

How taken

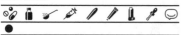

Tablets.

Frequency and timing of doses
1–3 x daily. In many conditions, this drug is taken at certain times in the menstrual cycle.

Adult dosage range
10–30mg daily.

Onset of effect
Beneficial effects of this drug may not be felt for several months.

Duration of action
12 hours.

Diet advice
None.

Storage
Keep in a closed container in a cool, dry place out of the reach of children. Protect from light.

Missed dose
Take as soon as you remember. If your next dose is due within 2 hours, take a single dose now and skip the next.

Stopping the drug
Do not stop the drug without consulting your doctor; symptoms may recur.

Exceeding the dose
An occasional unintentional extra dose is unlikely to be a cause for concern. But if you notice any unusual symptoms, or if a large overdose has been taken, notify your doctor.

SPECIAL PRECAUTIONS

Be sure to tell your doctor if:
▼ You have a long-term liver or kidney problem.
▼ You have heart or circulatory problems.
▼ You have diabetes.
▼ You have high blood pressure.
▼ You have porphyria.
▼ You are taking other medications.

 Pregnancy
▼ No evidence of risk at normal dosage. The drug is used to prevent miscarriage.

 Breast-feeding
▼ The drug passes into the breast milk, but at normal doses adverse effects on the baby are unlikely. High doses may suppress milk production.

 Infants and children
▼ Not prescribed.

 Over 60
▼ No special problems.

 Driving and hazardous work
▼ Avoid such activities until you have learned how dydrogesterone affects you because the drug may rarely cause dizziness.

 Alcohol
▼ No special problems.

POSSIBLE ADVERSE EFFECTS

Irregular periods and "breakthrough" bleeding are the most common adverse effects of this drug. These symptoms may be helped by dosage adjustment.

Symptom/effect	Frequency		Discuss with doctor		Stop taking drug now	Call doctor now
	Common	Rare	Only if severe	In all cases		
Swollen feet/ankles	●		■			
Rash	●		■			
Weight gain	●		■			
Irregular vaginal bleeding	●			■		
Nausea/vomiting		●	■			
Breast tenderness		●	■			
Headache/dizziness		●		■		

INTERACTIONS

Cyclosporin Dydrogesterone increases the effects of this drug.

PROLONGED USE

No special problems.

ENALAPRIL

Brand names Innovace, Innovace Melt
Used in the following combined preparation Innozide

GENERAL INFORMATION

Enalapril belongs to the ACE inhibitor group of *vasodilator* drugs (see p.98), which are used to treat hypertension (high blood pressure) and heart failure (inability of the heart to cope with its workload). It is also given to patients following a heart attack. Enalapril is often given with a diuretic to increase its effect.

The first dose of enalapril may cause a sudden drop in blood pressure. For this reason, you should be resting at the time and be able to lie down for 2 to 3 hours afterwards.

The more common *adverse effects* such as dizziness and headache, usually diminish with long-term treatment. Rashes can also occur but usually disappear when the drug is stopped. In some cases, they clear up on their own despite continued treatment.

QUICK REFERENCE

Drug group Vasodilator (p.98) and antihypertensive drug (p.102)

Overdose danger rating Medium

Dependence rating Low

Prescription needed Yes

Available as generic No

INFORMATION FOR USERS

Your drug prescription is tailored for you. Do not alter dosage without checking with your doctor.

How taken

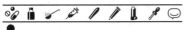

Tablets, wafers.

Frequency and timing of doses
1–2 x daily.

Adult dosage range
2.5–5mg daily (starting dose), increased to 10–40mg daily (maintenance dose).

Onset of effect
Within 1 hour.

Duration of action
24 hours.

Diet advice
None.

Storage
Keep in a closed container in a cool, dry place out of the reach of children. Protect from light.

Missed dose
Take as soon as you remember. If your next dose is due within 8 hours, take a single dose now and skip the next.

Stopping the drug
Do not stop the drug without consulting your doctor; stopping the drug may lead to worsening of the underlying condition.

Exceeding the dose
An occasional unintentional extra dose is unlikely to be a cause for concern. Large overdoses may cause dizziness or fainting. Notify your doctor.

POSSIBLE ADVERSE EFFECTS

The more common adverse effects, such as dizziness and headache, usually diminish with long-term treatment. The less common effects may also diminish during long-term treatment, but an adjustment in dosage may be necessary.

Symptom/effect	Frequency		Discuss with doctor		Stop taking drug now	Call doctor now
	Common	Rare	Only if severe	In all cases		
Dizziness/feeling faint	●		■			
Headache	●		■			
Nausea		●		■		
Diarrhoea		●		■		
Rash/urticaria		●		■		
Muscle cramps		●		■		
Cough/voice changes		●		■	▲	▮
Wheezing/swelling		●		■	▲	▮

SPECIAL PRECAUTIONS

Be sure to tell your doctor if:
▼ You have a long-term kidney problem.
▼ You have a heart problem.
▼ You have had a previous allergic reaction to an ACE inhibitor drug.
▼ You have porphyria.
▼ You are taking other medications.

 Pregnancy
▼ Not normally prescribed. May cause abnormalities in the fetus. Discuss with your doctor.

 Breast-feeding
▼ The drug passes into the breast milk, but at normal doses adverse effects on the baby are unlikely. Discuss with your doctor.

 Infants and children
▼ Not recommended.

 Over 60
▼ Reduced dose may be necessary.

 Driving and hazardous work
▼ Avoid such activities until you have learned how enalapril affects you because the drug can cause dizziness and fainting.

 Alcohol
▼ Avoid. Alcohol increases the likelihood of an excessive drop in blood pressure.

Surgery and general anaesthetics
▼ Discuss with your doctor or dentist before any operation.

INTERACTIONS

Antihypertensive drugs and NSAIDs These drugs are likely to enhance the blood pressure-lowering effect of enalapril.

Lithium Enalapril increases the levels of lithium in the blood, and serious adverse effects from lithium excess may occur.

Cyclosporin Taken with enalapril, this drug may increase levels of potassium in the blood.

Potassium supplements and potassium-sparing diuretics Enalapril may add to the effect of these drugs, leading to raised levels of potassium in the blood.

Non-steroidal anti-inflammatory drugs (NSAIDs) Some of these drugs may reduce the effectiveness of enalapril. There is also risk of kidney damage when they are taken with enalapril.

PROLONGED USE

No problems expected.

Monitoring Periodic tests on blood and urine should be performed.

EPHEDRINE

Brand name CAM
Used in the following combined preparations Do-Do, Do-Do Chesteze, Expulin, Franol, Haymine, and others

GENERAL INFORMATION

In use for more than 50 years, ephedrine promotes the release of norephedrine, a *neurotransmitter*. It was once widely prescribed as a bronchodilator to relax the muscles surrounding the airways, easing the breathing difficulty caused by asthma, bronchitis, and emphysema. Newer, more effective drugs have largely replaced ephedrine for these purposes. Its main use now is as a decongestant in nasal drops and cough preparations.

Adverse effects are unusual from nasal drops used in moderation, but taken by mouth the drug may stimulate the heart and central nervous system, causing palpitations and anxiety. It is not recommended for the elderly, who are more sensitive to ephedrine's effects on the heart, and the drug may also cause urinary retention in elderly men.

INFORMATION FOR USERS

Follow instructions on the label. Call your doctor if symptoms worsen.

How taken

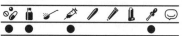

Tablets, syrup, injection, nasal drops.

Frequency and timing of doses
By mouth 3 x daily.
Nasal drops 3–4 x daily.

Dosage range
Adults 45–180mg daily (by mouth); 1–2 drops into each nostril per dose (drops).
Children Reduced dose according to age and weight.

Onset of effect
Within 15–60 minutes.

Duration of action
3–6 hours.

Diet advice
None.

Storage
Keep in a closed container in a cool, dry place out of the reach of children. Protect from light.

Missed dose
Do not take the missed dose. Take your next dose as usual.

Stopping the drug
Can be safely stopped as soon as you no longer need it.

Exceeding the dose
An occasional unintentional extra dose is unlikely to cause problems. Large overdoses may cause shortness of breath, high fever, fits, or loss of consciousness. Notify your doctor immediately.

SPECIAL PRECAUTIONS

Be sure to consult your doctor or pharmacist before taking this drug if:
▼ You have a long-term kidney problem.
▼ You have heart disease.
▼ You have high blood pressure.
▼ You have diabetes.
▼ You have an overactive thyroid gland.
▼ You have had glaucoma.
▼ You have urinary difficulties.
▼ You are taking other medications.

Pregnancy
▼ Safety in pregnancy not established. Discuss with your doctor.

Breast-feeding
▼ The drug passes into the breast milk and may affect the baby. Discuss with your doctor.

Infants and children
▼ Reduced dose necessary.

Over 60
▼ Not usually prescribed.

Driving and hazardous work
▼ Avoid such activities until you have learned how ephedrine affects you. No special problems with nasal drops.

Alcohol
▼ No special problems.

Surgery and general anaesthetics
▼ Ephedrine may need to be stopped before you have a general anaesthetic. Discuss this with your doctor or dentist before surgery.

POSSIBLE ADVERSE EFFECTS

Adverse effects from ephedrine nasal drops are uncommon, although local irritation can occur. When taken by mouth, the drug may have adverse effects on the central nervous system (for example, insomnia and anxiety) and the cardiovascular system (palpitations). Taking the last dose before 4 pm may prevent insomnia.

Symptom/effect	Frequency		Discuss with doctor		Stop taking drug now	Call doctor now
	Common	Rare	Only if severe	In all cases		
Anxiety/restlessness	●		■			
Insomnia	●		■			
Confusion		●	■			
Dry mouth		●	■			
Tremor		●	■			
Urinary difficulties		●		■		
Palpitations/chest pain		●	■		▲	■

INTERACTIONS

Monoamine oxidase inhibitors (MAOIs) Ephedrine may interact with these drugs to cause a dangerous rise in blood pressure.

Beta blockers Ephedrine may interact with these drugs to cause a dangerous rise in blood pressure.

Antihypertensive drugs Ephedrine may counteract the effects of some antihypertensive drugs.

PROLONGED USE

Prolonged use is not recommended except on medical advice. When used as nasal drops, decongestant effects may lessen and rebound congestion may occur.

EPINEPHRINE (ADRENALINE)

Brand names Ana-Guard, EpiPen, Eppy, Mini-I-Jet Epinephrine, Simplene
Used in the following combined preparations Brovon, Ganda, several local anaesthetics (e.g., Xylocaine with epinephrine)

GENERAL INFORMATION

Epinephrine is a *neurotransmitter* that is produced in the centre (medulla) of the adrenal glands. Synthetic epinephrine has been made since 1900. The drug is given in an emergency to stimulate heart activity and raise low blood pressure. It also narrows blood vessels in the skin and intestine.

Epinephrine is injected to counteract cardiac arrest, or to relieve severe allergic reactions (anaphylaxis) to drugs, food, or insect stings. For patients who are at risk of anaphylaxis, it is provided as a pre-filled syringe for immediate self-injection at the start of an attack.

Given as eye drops, the drug lowers the pressure within the eye, making it useful in glaucoma and eye surgery.

Because it constricts blood vessels, epinephrine is used to control bleeding and to slow the dispersal, and thereby prolong the effect, of local *anaesthetics*.

QUICK REFERENCE

Drug group Drug for glaucoma (p.168), cardiac resuscitation, and anaphylaxis

Overdose danger rating High

Dependence rating Low

Prescription needed Yes

Available as generic Yes

INFORMATION FOR USERS

Your drug prescription is tailored for you. Do not alter dosage without checking with your doctor.

How taken

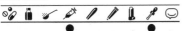

Injection, eye drops.

Frequency and timing of doses
As directed according to method of administration and underlying disorder.

Dosage range
As directed according to method of administration and underlying disorder.

Onset of effect
Within 5 minutes (injection); within 1 hour (eye drops).

Duration of action
Up to 4 hours (injection); up to 24 hours (eye drops).

Diet advice
None.

Storage
Keep in a closed container in a cool, dry place out of the reach of children. Protect from light.

Missed dose
Do not take the missed dose. Take the next dose as usual.

Stopping the drug
Do not stop using the eye drops without consulting your doctor; stopping the drug may lead to worsening of the underlying condition.

OVERDOSE ACTION

Seek immediate medical advice in all cases. Take emergency action if palpitations, breathing difficulties, or loss of consciousness occur.

See Drug poisoning emergency guide (p.494).

SPECIAL PRECAUTIONS

Be sure to tell your doctor if:
▼ You have a heart problem.
▼ You have diabetes.
▼ You have an overactive thyroid gland.
▼ You have a nervous system problem.
▼ You have high blood pressure.
▼ You are taking other medications.

Pregnancy
▼ Not usually prescribed. May cause defects in the fetus and prolong labour. Discuss with your doctor.

Breast-feeding
▼ Adverse effects on the baby are unlikely. Discuss with your doctor.

Infants and children
▼ Reduced dose necessary.

Over 60
▼ Increased likelihood of adverse effects. Reduced dose may therefore be necessary.

Driving and hazardous work
▼ No known problems.

Alcohol
▼ No known problems.

Surgery and general anaesthetics
▼ Epinephrine may need to be stopped before you have a general anaesthetic. Discuss this with your doctor or dentist before surgery.

POSSIBLE ADVERSE EFFECTS

The principal *adverse effects* of this drug are related to its stimulant action on the heart and central nervous system. Eye drops may cause local burning or inflammation.

Symptom/effect	Frequency		Discuss with doctor		Stop taking drug now	Call doctor now
	Common	Rare	Only if severe	In all cases		
Dry mouth	●		■			
Nervousness/restlessness	●		■			
Palpitations	●				■	
Headache/blurred vision	●				■	

INTERACTIONS

General note A variety of drugs interact with epinephrine to increase the risk of palpitations and/or high blood pressure. Such drugs include monoamine oxidase inhibitors (MAOIs) and tricyclic antidepressants.

Beta blockers Epinephrine can produce a dangerous rise in blood pressure with certain beta blockers, such as propranolol.

Antidiabetic drugs Epinephrine may reduce the effectiveness of these drugs.

PROLONGED USE

Long-term use of epinephrine eye drops with soft contact lenses is not recommended.

EPOETIN (ERYTHROPOIETIN)

Brand names Eprex, NeoRecormon
Used in the following combined preparations None

GENERAL INFORMATION

Epoetin is a form of erythropoietin, a naturally occurring hormone produced by the kidneys. Available in two forms (alpha and beta), epoetin stimulates the body to produce red blood cells. The drug is manufactured by a special technique that uses bacteria to make human erythropoietin.

Epoetin is used to treat *anaemia* in people with chronic kidney failure, including patients on dialysis. People with kidney failure produce very little erythropoietin themselves, so the number of red blood cells is very low. This was previously treatable only by giving regular blood transfusions. When epoetin is injected regularly, more red cells are made by the bone marrow,

and this relieves the anaemia, making blood transfusions unnecessary. Since it is a natural hormone, epoetin has few *side effects*, but treatment must be carefully monitored, otherwise patients may produce too many red blood cells, causing high blood pressure, or the blood may start clotting too easily.

The drug has also been given to patients with cancer and AIDS who have anaemia due to these diseases or their treatment; however, this is a trial use and is not yet widely available. Epoetin has also been tried by athletes who wish to improve their performance; but this is not a recognized use and is regarded as an illegal use of drugs by the sports authorities.

QUICK REFERENCE

Drug group Kidney hormone (p.140)

Overdose danger rating Low

Dependence rating Low

Prescription needed Yes

Available as generic No

INFORMATION FOR USERS

Your drug prescription is tailored for you. Do not alter dosage without checking with your doctor.

How taken

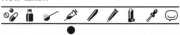

Injection.

Frequency and timing of doses
2–3 x weekly.

Dosage range
Dosage is calculated on an individual basis according to body weight. The dosage also varies depending on the form of epoetin used.

Onset of effect
Active inside the body within 4 hours, but effects may not be noted for 2–3 months.

Duration of action
Some effects may persist for several days.

Diet advice
None. However, if you have kidney failure, you may have to follow a special diet.

Storage
Store at 2–8°C, out of the reach of children. Do not freeze or shake. Protect from light.

Missed dose
Do not make up any missed doses.

Stopping the drug
Discuss with your doctor.

Exceeding the dose
A single excessive dose is unlikely to be a cause for concern. Too high a dose over a long period can increase the likelihood of adverse effects.

SPECIAL PRECAUTIONS

Be sure to tell your doctor if:
▼ You have high blood pressure.
▼ You have a long-term liver problem.
▼ You have previously suffered allergic reactions to any drugs.
▼ You have peripheral vascular disease.
▼ You have had epileptic fits.
▼ You are taking other medications.

Pregnancy
▼ Not usually prescribed. Safety in pregnancy not established. Discuss with your doctor.

Breast-feeding
▼ Safety not established. Discuss with your doctor.

Infants and children
▼ Reduced dose necessary.

Over 60
▼ No known problems.

Driving and hazardous work
▼ Not applicable.

Alcohol
▼ Follow your doctor's advice regarding alcohol.

POSSIBLE ADVERSE EFFECTS

The most common effects are increased blood pressure and problems at the site of the injection; all unusual symptoms should be discussed with your doctor immediately.

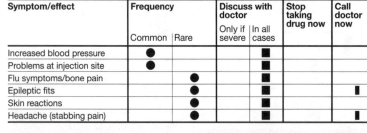

Symptom/effect	Frequency		Discuss with doctor		Stop taking drug now	Call doctor now
	Common	Rare	Only if severe	In all cases		
Increased blood pressure	●			■		
Problems at injection site	●			■		
Flu symptoms/bone pain		●		■		
Epileptic fits		●		■		▮
Skin reactions		●		■		
Headache (stabbing pain)		●		■		▮

INTERACTIONS

ACE inhibitor drugs These drugs may increase the level of potassium in the blood and epoetin may enhance their blood pressure-lowering effect.

Iron supplements These may increase the effect of epoetin if you have a low level of iron in your blood.

PROLONGED USE

The long-term effects of the drug are still under investigation, but problems are unlikely if treatment is carefully monitored.

Monitoring Regular blood tests to monitor blood composition and blood pressure monitoring are required.

ERGOTAMINE

Brand names Lingraine, Medihaler-Ergotamine
Used in the following combined preparations Cafergot, Migril

GENERAL INFORMATION

Ergotamine is used in the treatment of migraine. It constricts blood vessels around the skull and is used only when *analgesics* such as paracetamol or aspirin do not provide enough relief. It is most effective if taken at the first sign of a migraine (the "aura"); once nausea and headache are established, it is less likely to be effective and may cause stomach upset and increase nausea. Ergotamine is also combined with caffeine as tablets and suppositories. These may be more effective for some patients.

Ergotamine causes temporary narrowing of blood vessels throughout the body and is therefore not prescribed to those with poor circulation. If taken too frequently, the drug can dangerously reduce circulation to the hands and feet; it should never be taken regularly. Frequent migraine attacks may indicate the need for a drug to prevent migraine.

INFORMATION FOR USERS

Your drug prescription is tailored for you. Do not alter dosage without checking with your doctor.

How taken

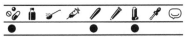

Tablets (held under the tongue or swallowed), suppositories, inhaler.

Frequency and timing of doses
Once at the onset (all forms), repeated if needed after 30 minutes (tablets) or 5 minutes (inhaler), up to the maximum dose (below).

Adult dosage range
Varies according to product. Generally 1–2mg per dose. Take no more than 6mg in 24 hours or 10mg in 1 week (by mouth); 6 inhalations in 24 hours or 15 inhalations in 1 week (inhaler); 4mg in 24 hours or 8mg in 1 week (rectally). Treatment should not be repeated within 4 days or more than twice a month.

Onset of effect
15–30 minutes.

Duration of action
Up to 24 hours.

Diet advice
Changes in diet are unlikely to affect the action of this drug, but certain foods may provoke migraine attacks in some people.

Storage
Keep in a closed container in a cool, dry place out of the reach of children. Protect from light.

Missed dose
Regular doses of this drug are not necessary and may be dangerous. Take only when you have symptoms of migraine.

Stopping the drug
Can be safely stopped as soon as you no longer need it.

Exceeding the dose
An occasional unintentional extra dose is unlikely to cause problems. Large overdoses may cause vomiting, dizziness, fits, or coma. Notify your doctor immediately.

POSSIBLE ADVERSE EFFECTS

Digestive disturbances and nausea (for which an anti-emetic may be given) are common with ergotamine treatment. Rare but serious *adverse effects* may result from arterial spasm.

Symptom/effect	Frequency		Discuss with doctor		Stop taking drug now	Call doctor now
	Common	Rare	Only if severe	In all cases		
Nausea and vomiting	●		■			
Diarrhoea		●	■			
Vertigo		●		■		
Muscle pain and stiffness		●		■		
Chest pain		●		■	▲	▮
Leg/groin pain		●		■	▲	▮
Cold/numb fingers/toes		●		■	▲	▮

INTERACTIONS

Beta blockers These drugs may increase circulatory problems with ergotamine.

Sumatriptan and related drugs There is an increased risk of adverse effects on the blood circulation if ergotamine is used with these drugs.

Erythromycin taken with ergotamine increases the likelihood of adverse effects.

Oral contraceptives There is an increased risk of blood clotting in women taking these drugs with ergotamine.

SPECIAL PRECAUTIONS

Be sure to tell your doctor if:
▼ You have long-term liver or kidney problems.
▼ You have heart problems.
▼ You have poor circulation.
▼ You have high blood pressure.
▼ You have had a recent stroke.
▼ You have an overactive thyroid gland.
▼ You are taking other medications.

Pregnancy
▼ Not usually prescribed. Ergotamine can cause contractions of the uterus.

Breast-feeding
▼ Not recommended. The drug passes into the milk and may have adverse effects on the baby. It may also reduce your milk supply.

Infants and children
▼ Not usually prescribed.

Over 60
▼ Use with caution. Hidden heart or circulatory problems may be aggravated.

Driving and hazardous work
▼ Avoid such activities until you have learned how ergotamine affects you because the drug can cause vertigo.

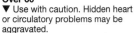

Alcohol
▼ No special problems, but some spirits may provoke migraine in some people.

Surgery and general anaesthetics
▼ Notify your doctor if you have used ergotamine within 48 hours prior to surgery.

PROLONGED USE

Reduced circulation to the hands and feet may result if doses near to the maximum are taken for too long. The recommended dosage and length of treatment should not be exceeded. Rebound headache may occur if it is taken too frequently.

ERYTHROMYCIN

Brand names Arpimycin, Erycen, Erymax, Erythrocin, Erythromid, Erythroped, Ilosone, Rommix, Stiemycin
Used in the following combined preparation Zineryt

GENERAL INFORMATION

One of the safest and most widely used antibiotics, erythromycin is effective against many bacteria. It is used instead of penicillins and tetracyclines for people allergic to these drugs.

Erythromycin is used to treat throat, middle ear, and chest infections (including some rare types of pneumonia such as Legionnaires' disease). It is also used for sexually transmitted diseases such as chlamydial infections, and in some forms of gastroenteritis.

Erythromycin may also be included as part of the treatment for diphtheria and is sometimes given to treat, and reduce the likelihood of infecting others with, pertussis (whooping cough).

When taken by mouth, erythromycin may sometimes cause nausea and vomiting. Other possible *adverse effects* include rash as well as a rare risk of liver disorders. Oral administration or local application of the drug is sometimes helpful in treating acne.

QUICK REFERENCE

Drug group Antibiotic (p.128)
Overdose danger rating Low
Dependence rating Low
Prescription needed Yes
Available as generic Yes

INFORMATION FOR USERS

Your drug prescription is tailored for you. Do not alter dosage without consulting your doctor.

How taken

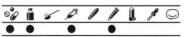

Tablets, capsules, liquid, injection, topical solution.

Frequency and timing of doses
Every 6–12 hours before or with meals.

Dosage range
1–4g daily.

Onset of effect
1–4 hours.

Duration of action
6–12 hours.

Diet advice
None.

Storage
Keep in a closed container in a cool, dry place out of the reach of children.

Missed dose
Take as soon as you remember. If your next dose is due within 2 hours, take a single dose now and skip the next.

Stopping the drug
Take the full course. Even if you feel better, the original infection may still be present and symptoms may recur if treatment is stopped too soon.

Exceeding the dose
An occasional unintentional extra dose is unlikely to be a cause for concern. But if you notice any unusual symptoms, or if a large overdose has been taken, notify your doctor.

SPECIAL PRECAUTIONS

Be sure to tell your doctor if:
▼ You have a long-term liver problem.
▼ You have had a previous allergic reaction to erythromycin.
▼ You have porphyria.
▼ You are taking other medications.

 Pregnancy
▼ No evidence of risk to the developing fetus.

 Breast-feeding
▼ The drug passes into the breast milk, but at normal doses adverse effects on the baby are unlikely. Discuss with your doctor.

 Infants and children
▼ Reduced dose necessary.

 Over 60
▼ No special problems.

 Driving and hazardous work
▼ No known problems.

Alcohol
▼ No known problems.

POSSIBLE ADVERSE EFFECTS

Nausea and vomiting are the most common adverse effects and are most likely to occur with large doses taken by mouth. Symptoms such as fever, rash, and *jaundice* may be a sign of a liver disorder and should always be reported to your doctor.

Symptom/effect	Frequency		Discuss with doctor		Stop taking drug now	Call doctor now
	Common	Rare	Only if severe	In all cases		
Nausea/vomiting	●		■			
Diarrhoea	●		■			
Rash/itching	●			■	▲	
Deafness		●				▮
Jaundice		●		■	▲	▮
Unexplained fever		●		■	▲	▮

PROLONGED USE

Courses of longer than 14 days may increase the risk of liver damage.

INTERACTIONS

General note Erythromycin interacts with a number of other drugs, particularly:

Carbamazepine Erythromycin may increase blood levels of this drug.

Digoxin Erythromycin may increase blood levels of this drug.

Warfarin Erythromycin increases the risk of bleeding with warfarin.

Terfenadine and mizolastine Erythromycin increases the risk of adverse effects on the heart with these drugs.

Ergotamine Erythromycin increases the risk of side effects with this drug.

Theophylline/aminophylline Erythromycin increases the risk of adverse effects with these drugs.

ESTRADIOL

Brand names Climaval, Estraderm, FemSeven, Menorest, Oestrogel, Progynova, Zumenon, and others
Used in the following combined preparations Climagest, Climesse, Estracombi, Femapak, Trisequens, and others

GENERAL INFORMATION

Estradiol is a naturally occurring oestrogen (a female sex hormone). It is mainly used as hormone replacement therapy (HRT) to treat menopausal and post-menopausal symptoms such as hot flushes, night sweats, and vaginal atrophy. Other beneficial effects of HRT include prevention of the loss of bone tissue that occurs in osteoporosis and reduction of the risk of heart attacks. Estradiol is often given together with a progestogen, either as separate drugs or as a combined product. In certain cases, treatment is taken for a specific number of days each month; follow your doctor's instructions carefully.

Estradiol is available in a variety of forms, including implants and skin patches. Implants of estradiol need to be replaced only after four to eight months. Skin patches of the drug may cause a local rash and itching at the site of application.

QUICK REFERENCE

Drug group Female sex hormone (p.147)

Overdose danger rating Low

Dependence rating Low

Prescription needed Yes

Available as generic No

INFORMATION FOR USERS

Your drug prescription is tailored for you. Do not alter dosage without checking with your doctor.

How taken

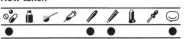

Tablets, pessaries, vaginal rings, skin gel, patches, implants.

Frequency and timing of doses
Once daily (tablets, gel); every 1–7 days (skin patches); every 4–8 months (implants); every 1–7 days (pessaries); every 3 months (vaginal ring).

Adult dosage range
1–4mg daily (tablets); 2–4 measures daily (skin gel); 25–100mcg daily (skin patches); 25–100mcg per dose (implants); 25mcg per dose (pessaries); 7.5mcg daily (vaginal ring).

Onset of effect
10–20 days.

Duration of action
Up to 24 hours; some effects may be longer lasting.

Diet advice
None.

Storage
Keep in a closed container in a cool, dry place out of the reach of children.

Missed dose
Take as soon as you remember. If your next daily treatment is due within 4 hours, take a single dose now and skip the next.

Stopping the drug
Do not stop the drug without consulting your doctor; symptoms may recur.

Exceeding the dose
An occasional unintentional extra dose is unlikely to be a cause for concern. But if you notice any unusual symptoms, or if a large overdose has been taken, notify your doctor.

SPECIAL PRECAUTIONS

Be sure to tell your doctor if:
▼ You have a long-term liver problem.
▼ You have heart or circulation problems.
▼ You have porphyria.
▼ You have had blood clots or a stroke.
▼ You have diabetes.
▼ You are a smoker.
▼ You suffer from migraine or epilepsy.
▼ You are taking other medications.

Pregnancy
▼ Not prescribed.

Breast-feeding
▼ Not prescribed. The drug passes into breast milk and may inhibit its flow. Discuss with your doctor.

Infants and children
▼ Not usually prescribed.

Over 60
▼ No special problems.

Driving and hazardous work
▼ No problems expected.

Alcohol
▼ No known problems.

Surgery and general anaesthetics
▼ You may need to stop taking estradiol several weeks before having major surgery. Discuss this with your doctor.

POSSIBLE ADVERSE EFFECTS

The most common *adverse effects* with estradiol are similar to symptoms in the early stages of pregnancy, and generally diminish with time. Sudden sharp pain in the chest, groin, or legs may indicate an abnormal blood clot that needs attention.

Symptom/effect	Frequency		Discuss with doctor		Stop taking drug now	Call doctor now
	Common	Rare	Only if severe	In all cases		
Nausea/vomiting	●		■			
Breast swelling/tenderness	●			■		
Weight gain	●		■			
Headache		●	■			
Depression		●		■		
Pain in chest/groin/legs		●		■	▲	❚

INTERACTIONS

Tobacco smoking This increases the risk of serious adverse effects on the heart and circulation with estradiol.

Rifampicin This drug may reduce the effects of estradiol.

Anticonvulsants The effects of estradiol are reduced by carbamazepine, phenytoin, and phenobarbital.

Anticoagulant drugs The effects of these drugs are reduced by estradiol.

PROLONGED USE

In some circumstances, prolonged use of estradiol may slightly increase the risk of cancer of the uterus and breast. The risk of gallstones may also be higher.

Monitoring Blood pressure checks and physical examinations, including regular mammograms, may be performed.

ETHAMBUTOL

Brand name Myambutol
Used in the following combined preparations None

GENERAL INFORMATION

Ethambutol is used in the treatment of tuberculosis. Given in conjunction with other antituberculous drugs, it helps to boost their effects.

If resistance to more commonly used drugs is suspected, ethambutol may be used early in treatment. This may apply if the disease might have been caught by contact with a recent immigrant from Africa or Asia, where resistance to other drugs has been increasing.

Although the drug has few common *adverse effects*, it may occasionally cause optic neuritis, a type of eye damage leading to blurring and fading of vision. As a result, ethambutol is not usually prescribed for children under six years of age or for other patients who are unable to communicate their symptoms adequately. Patients taking this drug are normally advised to have periodic eye checks.

QUICK REFERENCE

Drug group Antituberculous drug (p.132)

Overdose danger rating Medium

Dependence rating Low

Prescription needed Yes

Available as generic Yes

INFORMATION FOR USERS

Your drug prescription is tailored for you. Do not alter dosage without checking with your doctor.

How taken

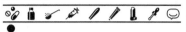

Tablets.

Frequency and timing of doses
Once daily.

Adult dosage range
According to body weight.

Onset of effect
It may take several days for symptoms to improve.

Duration of action
Up to 24 hours.

Diet advice
None.

Storage
Keep in a closed container in a cool, dry, place out of the reach of children.

Missed dose
Take as soon as you remember. If your next dose is due within 6 hours, take a single dose now and skip the next.

Stopping the drug
Take the full course. Even if you feel better the original infection may still be present and may recur if treatment is stopped too soon.

Exceeding the dose
An occasional unintentional extra dose is unlikely to cause problems. Large overdoses may cause headache and abdominal pain. Notify your doctor.

SPECIAL PRECAUTIONS

Be sure to tell your doctor if:
▼ You have a long-term kidney problem.
▼ You have cataracts or other eye problems.
▼ You have gout.
▼ You have had a previous allergic reaction to this drug.
▼ You are taking other medications.

Pregnancy
▼ Safety in pregnancy not established. Discuss with your doctor.

Breast-feeding
▼ The drug passes into the breast milk, but at normal doses adverse effects on the baby are unlikely. Discuss with your doctor.

Infants and children
▼ Not prescribed under 6 years.

Over 60
▼ Increased likelihood of adverse effects. Reduced dose may therefore be necessary.

Driving and hazardous work
▼ Avoid such activities until you have learned how ethambutol affects you because the drug may cause dizziness.

Alcohol
▼ No known problems.

POSSIBLE ADVERSE EFFECTS

Side effects are uncommon with this drug but are more likely after prolonged treatment at high doses. Blurred vision or eye pain require prompt medical attention.

Symptom/effect	Frequency		Discuss with doctor		Stop taking drug now	Call doctor now
	Common	Rare	Only if severe	In all cases		
Nausea/vomiting		●	■			
Dizziness		●	■			
Numb/tingling hands/feet		●		■		
Blurred vision		●		■	▲	■
Eye pain		●		■	▲	
Loss of colour vision		●		■	▲	■
Rash/itching		●		■	▲	

INTERACTIONS

None.

PROLONGED USE

Prolonged use may increase the risk of eye damage.

Monitoring Periodic eye tests are usually necessary.

ETHINYLESTRADIOL

Used in the following combined preparations Combined oral contraceptives (e.g., Brevinor, Eugynon 30, Femodene, Loestrin, Microgynon 30, Norimin, Ovran 30, Ovranette, Ovysmen), Dianette, Schering PC4

GENERAL INFORMATION

Ethinylestradiol is a synthetic oestrogen similar to estradiol, a natural female sex hormone. It is widely used in oral contraceptives, in combination with a synthetic progestogen. The drug is also very occasionally used (often with a progestogen) to supplement oestrogen during the menopause.

Ethinylestradiol is occasionally given to control abnormally heavy bleeding from the uterus and to treat delayed sexual development (hypogonadism) in females. Certain breast and prostate cancers respond to ethinylestradiol. The drug is sometimes given, in high doses, for postcoital contraception. It is used in conjunction with cyproterone to treat severe acne in women.

INFORMATION FOR USERS

Your drug prescription is tailored for you. Do not alter dosage without checking with your doctor.

How taken

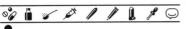

Tablets.

Frequency and timing of doses
Once daily. Often at certain times of the menstrual cycle.

Adult dosage range
Menopausal symptoms 10–20mcg daily.
Hormone deficiency 10–50mcg daily.
Combined contraceptive pills 20–50mcg daily depending on preparation.
Acne 35mcg daily.
Breast and prostate cancer up to 3mg daily.

Onset of effect
10–20 days. Contraceptive protection is effective after 7 days in most cases.

Duration of action
1–2 days.

Diet advice
None.

Storage
Keep in a closed container in a cool, dry place out of the reach of children.

Missed dose
Take as soon as you remember. If your next dose is due within 4 hours, take a single dose now and skip the next. If you are taking the drug for contraceptive purposes, see What to do if you miss a pill (p.163).

Stopping the drug
Do not stop the drug without consulting your doctor. Contraceptive protection is lost unless an alternative is used.

Exceeding the dose
An occasional unintentional extra dose is unlikely to be a cause for concern. But if you notice any unusual symptoms, or if a large overdose has been taken, notify your doctor.

SPECIAL PRECAUTIONS

Be sure to tell your doctor if:
▼ You have heart failure or high blood pressure.
▼ You or a close relative have had blood clots or a stroke.
▼ You have a long-term liver problem.
▼ You are a smoker.
▼ You have diabetes.
▼ You suffer from migraine or epilepsy.
▼ You are taking other medications.

Pregnancy
▼ Not prescribed. May adversely affect the baby. Discuss with your doctor.

Breast-feeding
▼ The drug passes into the breast milk; it may also inhibit milk flow. Discuss with your doctor.

Infants and children
▼ Not usually prescribed.

Over 60
▼ No special problems.

Driving and hazardous work
▼ No known problems.

Alcohol
▼ No known problems.

Surgery and general anaesthetics
▼ Ethinylestradiol may need to be stopped several weeks before you have major surgery. Discuss this with your doctor.

POSSIBLE ADVERSE EFFECTS

The most common *adverse effects* with ethinylestradiol are similar to symptoms in the early stages of pregnancy and generally diminish with time. Sudden, sharp pain in the chest, groin, or legs may indicate an abnormal blood clot and requires urgent attention.

Symptom/effect	Frequency		Discuss with doctor		Stop taking drug now	Call doctor now
	Common	Rare	Only if severe	In all cases		
Nausea/vomiting	●		■			
Breast swelling/tenderness	●		■			
Weight gain	●		■			
Headache		●	■			
Depression		●		■		
Pain in chest/groin/legs		●		■	▲	∎

INTERACTIONS

Tobacco smoking This increases the risk of serious adverse effects on the heart and circulation with ethinylestradiol.

Rifampicin and anticonvulsant drugs These drugs significantly reduce the effectiveness of oral contraceptives containing ethinylestradiol, for which a higher dose will be needed.

Antihypertensive drugs and diuretics Ethinylestradiol may reduce the effectiveness of these drugs.

Other antibiotics These drugs may reduce the effectiveness of oral contraceptives containing ethinylestradiol.

PROLONGED USE

Prolonged use of ethinylestradiol slightly increases the risk of cancer of the uterus after the menopause when used without a progestogen. The risk of gallstones may also be higher.

Monitoring Physical examinations and periodic checks on blood pressure may be performed.

ETHOSUXIMIDE

Brand names Emeside, Zarontin
Used in the following combined preparations None

GENERAL INFORMATION

Ethosuximide was introduced in 1960 and belongs to a group of drugs known as anticonvulsants, which are used in the treatment of epilepsy. Ethosuximide is most commonly prescribed for long-term prevention of absence seizures (daydream-like episodes, also known as petit mal). Ethosuximide is also used to treat myoclonic seizures. Other types of epilepsy do not respond well to the drug. The major drawback to its use is that it can reduce production of blood cells. Minor *adverse effects* often occur in the early days of treatment, but these diminish with time.

INFORMATION FOR USERS

Your drug prescription is tailored for you. Do not alter dosage without checking with your doctor.

How taken

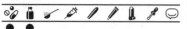

Capsules, liquid.

Frequency and timing of doses
1–2 x daily.

Dosage range
Adults and children over 6 years 500mg daily (starting dose), gradually increased up to a maximum of 1.5g daily.
Children up to 6 years 250mg daily (starting dose) gradually increased up to a maximum of 20mg/kg of body weight daily.

Onset of effect
Within 1 hour.

Duration of action
Approximately 2 days.

Diet advice
None.

Storage
Keep in a closed container in a cool, dry place out of the reach of children.

Missed dose
Take as soon as you remember. If your next dose is due within 6 hours, take a single dose now and skip the next.

Stopping the drug
Do not stop the drug without consulting your doctor; symptoms may recur.

Exceeding the dose
An occasional unintentional extra dose is unlikely to be a cause for concern. Larger overdoses may cause unusual drowsiness. Notify your doctor.

SPECIAL PRECAUTIONS

Be sure to tell your doctor if:
▼ You have long-term liver or kidney problems.
▼ You have porphyria.
▼ You are taking other medications.

 Pregnancy
▼ Safety in pregnancy not established. Discuss with your doctor.

 Breast-feeding
▼ The drug passes into breast milk and may have effects on the baby. Poor suckling may occur. Discuss with your doctor.

 Infants and children
▼ Reduced dose necessary.

 Over 60
▼ Not usually prescribed.

 Driving and hazardous work
▼ Your underlying condition, as well as the sedative effects of ethosuximide, may make such activities inadvisable. Discuss with your doctor.

 Alcohol
▼ Avoid. Alcohol may increase the sedative effect of this drug.

POSSIBLE ADVERSE EFFECTS

Most people experience few adverse effects with this drug, but when blood levels get too high, adverse effects are common and the dosage may need to be reduced.

Symptom/effect	Frequency		Discuss with doctor		Stop taking drug now	Call doctor now
	Common	Rare	Only if severe	In all cases		
Drowsiness	●		■			
Loss of appetite	●		■			
Dizziness	●		■			
Nausea/vomiting	●			■		
Headache		●	■			
Depression		●		■		
Paranoia		●		■		
Sore throat/mouth ulcers		●		■		▌
Easy bruising/bleeding		●		■		▌
Rash		●		■		

PROLONGED USE

A slight risk of blood abnormalities exists with prolonged use of ethosuximide.

Monitoring Periodic blood counts, liver function tests, and urine examinations may be carried out.

INTERACTIONS

Sedatives All drugs that have a sedative effect on the central nervous system are likely to increase the sedative properties of ethosuximide. Such drugs include sleeping drugs, antihistamines, opioid analgesics, antipsychotics, and antidepressants.

Carbamazepine This drug may reduce levels of ethosuximide in the blood.

Phenytoin and sodium valproate These drugs may alter levels of ethosuximide in the blood.

ETIDRONATE

Brand names Didronel, Didronel PMO
Used in the following combined preparations None

GENERAL INFORMATION

Etidronate is given for the treatment of bone disorders such as Paget's disease. It acts only on the bones, reducing the activity of the bone cells and thereby stopping the progress of the disease. This action also stops calcium from being released from the bones into the bloodstream, so it reduces the amount of calcium in the blood. Etidronate is also used together with calcium tablets to treat osteoporosis in post-menopausal women and to prevent and treat steroid-induced osteoporosis. Generally, the drug's *side effects* are mild. The most common is diarrhoea, which is more likely to occur with higher doses. If taken at high doses (20mg/kg body weight daily), the drug stops new bone from being formed properly, which can lead to thinning of the bones and fractures. For this reason, high doses must be carefully monitored and used for as short a time as possible. The effect is reversed on stopping the drug.

INFORMATION FOR USERS

Your drug prescription is tailored for you. Do not alter dosage without checking with your doctor.

How taken

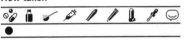

Tablets.

Frequency and timing of doses
Once daily on an empty stomach, 2 hours before or after food.

Dosage range
Paget's disease 5–20mg/kg body weight daily for a maximum of 3–6 months. There may be repeated cycles.
Osteoporosis 400mg daily for 2 weeks, repeated every 3 months.

Onset of effect
Paget's disease/osteoporosis Beneficial effects may not be felt for several months.

Duration of action
Some effects may persist for several weeks or months.

Diet advice
Absorption of etidronate is reduced by foods, especially those containing calcium (e.g., dairy products), so the drug should be taken on an empty stomach. The diet must contain adequate calcium and vitamin D; supplements may be given.

Storage
Keep in a closed container in a cool, dry place out of the reach of children. Protect from light.

Missed dose
Take as soon as you remember. If your next dose is due within 6 hours, take a single dose now and skip the next.

Stopping the drug
Do not stop the drug without consulting your doctor. Stopping the drug may lead to worsening of the underlying condition.

Exceeding the dose
An occasional unintentional extra dose is unlikely to cause problems. Large overdoses may cause numbness and muscle spasm. Notify your doctor.

POSSIBLE ADVERSE EFFECTS

The most common side effect, diarrhoea, is more likely if the dose is increased above 5mg/kg daily. In some patients with Paget's disease, bone pain may be increased initially, but this symptom usually disappears with further treatment.

Symptom/effect	Frequency		Discuss with doctor		Stop taking drug now	Call doctor now
	Common	Rare	Only if severe	In all cases		
Diarrhoea	●			■		
Nausea	●			■		
Constipation/abdominal pain		●		■		
Rash/itching		●	■			
Bone pain		●	■			▮

INTERACTIONS

Antacids and iron Antacids or iron should be given at least 2 hours before or after etidronate to minimize effects on absorption.

SPECIAL PRECAUTIONS

Be sure to tell your doctor if:
▼ You have a long-term kidney problem.
▼ You have had a previous allergic reaction to etidronate or other bisphosphonates.
▼ You have colitis.
▼ You are taking other medications.

Pregnancy
▼ Safety in pregnancy not established. Discuss with your doctor.

Breast-feeding
▼ Safety in breast-feeding not established. Discuss with your doctor.

Infants and children
▼ Not recommended.

Over 60
▼ No special problems.

Driving and hazardous work
▼ No special problems.

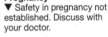
Alcohol
▼ No special problems.

PROLONGED USE

Courses of treatment longer than 3 to 6 months are not usually prescribed, but repeat courses may be required. Continuous use of etidronate is not recommended because it may lead to an increased risk of bone fractures.

Monitoring Blood and urine tests may be carried out.

FELBINAC

Brand name Traxam
Used in the following combined preparations None

GENERAL INFORMATION

Felbinac is a member of the non-steroidal anti-inflammatory (NSAID) group of drugs and similar to aspirin in the way in which it works (as an analgesic as well as reducing inflammation).

Felbinac is prescribed for the relief of pain and inflammation in soft-tissue injuries, such as sprains, strains, and bruising. The drug is applied topically,

as gel or aerosol foam, by being gently massaged into the affected areas of skin.

Felbinac is usually only prescribed for short-term treatment because there is an increased risk of adverse effects with prolonged use. Your doctor will usually review the treatment after two weeks.

Rarely, felbinac may cause indigestion, rash, or breathing difficulties.

INFORMATION FOR USERS

Your drug prescription is tailored for you. Do not alter dosage without checking with your doctor.

How taken

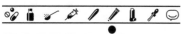

Gel, aerosol foam.

Frequency and timing of doses
2–4 times daily.

Adult dosage range
1g per application massaged in. This is 2.5cm (1in) of gel or a 4-cm (1.5-in) ball of foam. Maximum 25 grams daily for all areas being treated.

Onset of effect
Pain relief begins in 30 minutes. Full anti-inflammatory effect begins in 1–2 days.

Duration of action
4–6 hours.

Diet advice
None.

Storage
Keep in a cool dry place, out of the reach of children. Protect the aerosol canister from sunlight. Do not spray foam near naked flame or while smoking.

Missed dose
Use as soon as you remember. If it is almost time for your next application, skip the missed application and resume your normal schedule with the next one.

Stopping the drug
The drug can be safely stopped as soon as it is no longer needed.

Exceeding the dose
An occasional unintentional extra application is unlikely to cause problems. But if you notice any unusual symptoms, notify your doctor.

SPECIAL PRECAUTIONS

Be sure to tell your doctor if:
▼ You have asthma.
▼ You are allergic to aspirin or NSAIDs.
▼ You are taking other medications.

Pregnancy
▼ Not recommended. Discuss with your doctor.

Breast-feeding
▼ Safety in breast feeding not established. Discuss with your doctor.

Infants and children
▼ Safety not established. Discuss with your doctor.

Over 60
▼ No special problems.

Driving and hazardous work
▼ No special problems.

Alcohol
▼ No special problems.

POSSIBLE ADVERSE EFFECTS

Side effects of felbinac are usually localized to the skin, but systemic effects may sometimes occur because small amounts of the drug are absorbed through the skin.

Symptom/effect	Frequency		Discuss with doctor		Stop taking drug now	Call doctor now
	Common	Rare	Only if severe	In all cases		
Skin irritation/redness	●		■			
Itching/dermatitis	●		■			
Heartburn/indigestion		●		■		
Rash		●		■	▲	▌
Wheezing/breathing difficulties		●		■	▲	▌

INTERACTIONS

Interactions with other drugs are unlikely because amounts of felbinac in the blood are usually very low.

PROLONGED USE

There is an increased risk of stomach ulceration or intestinal bleeding with prolonged use of felbinac.

FILGRASTIM

Brand name Neupogen
Used in the following combined preparations None

GENERAL INFORMATION

Filgrastim is a synthetic form of G-CSF (granulocyte-colony stimulating factor), a naturally occurring protein responsible for the manufacture of white blood cells. Deficiency of G-CSF increases the risk of bacterial infection. The drug works by stimulating bone marrow to produce white blood cells, thus reducing the risk of infection. It also causes bone marrow cells to move into the bloodstream, where they can be collected to use in the treatment of bone marrow disease, or to replace bone marrow lost during intensive cancer treatment.

Filgrastim is used to treat patients with congenital neutropenia (deficiency of G-CSF from birth), some AIDS patients, and those who have recently received high doses of chemo- or radiotherapy during bone-marrow transplantation or cancer treatment. Such patients are prone to frequent and severe infections.
Bone pain is a common *adverse effect* of filgrastim treatment, but can be controlled using painkillers. There is an increased risk of leukaemia if filgrastim is given to patients with certain rare blood disorders.

INFORMATION FOR USERS

Your drug prescription is tailored for you. Do not alter dosage without checking with your doctor.

How taken

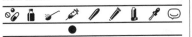

Injection.

Frequency and timing of doses
Once daily.

Adult dosage range
5–12mcg/kg body weight, depending upon condition being treated and response.

Onset of effect
24 hours (increase); several weeks (recovery of normal numbers).

Duration of action
Approximately 2 days.

Diet advice
None.

Storage
Store in a refrigerator out of the reach of children.

Missed dose
Take as soon as you remember. If your next dose is due within 6 hours, do not take the missed dose. Take the next scheduled dose as usual.

Stopping the drug
Do not stop taking the drug without consulting your doctor; stopping the drug may lead to worsening of the underlying condition.

Exceeding the dose
An occasional unintentional extra dose is unlikely to cause problems. But if you notice any unusual symptoms or if a large overdose has been taken, notify your doctor.

POSSIBLE ADVERSE EFFECTS

Adverse effects resulting from short courses of filgrastim are unusual. Most common is bone pain, which is probably linked to the stimulant effect of the drug on bone marrow.

Symptom/effect	Frequency		Discuss with doctor		Stop taking drug now	Call doctor now
	Common	Rare	Only if severe	In all cases		
Bone/muscle pain	●		■			
Difficulty passing urine		●	■			
Skin rash		●			■	

INTERACTIONS

Cytotoxic chemotherapy or radiotherapy should not be administered within 24 hours of taking filgrastim because of the risk of increasing the damage these treatments inflict on the bone marrow.

SPECIAL PRECAUTIONS

Be sure to tell your doctor if:
▼ You suffer from any blood disorders.
▼ You are taking other medications.

Pregnancy
▼ Safety in pregnancy not established. Discuss with your doctor.

Breast-feeding
▼ Safety in breast-feeding not established. Discuss with your doctor.

Infants and children
▼ No special problems.

Over 60
▼ No special problems.

Driving and hazardous work
▼ No known problems.

Alcohol
▼ No known problems.

PROLONGED USE

Prolonged use may lead to a slightly increased risk of certain leukaemias. Cutaneous vaculitis (inflammation of blood vessels of the skin), osteoporosis (weakening of the bones), hair thinning, enlargement of the spleen and liver, and bleeding due to reduction in platelet numbers may also occur.

Monitoring Blood checks and regular physical examinations are performed, as well as X-rays or bone scans to check for bone thinning.

FINASTERIDE

Brand name Proscar
Used in the following combined preparations None

GENERAL INFORMATION

Finasteride is an an anti-androgen drug (see Male sex hormones, p.146) used to treat benign prostatic hyperplasia (BPH), in which the prostate gland increases in size, making urination difficult. The drug works by gradually shrinking the prostate gland, which improves urine flow and other symptoms such as difficulty in starting urination.

Because finasteride is excreted in semen and can feminize a male foetus, you should use a condom if your sexual partner may be, or is likely to become, pregnant. Also, women of childbearing age should not handle broken or crushed tablets because small quantities of the drug are absorbed through the skin.

The symptoms of BPH are similar to those of prostate cancer. Therefore the drug is used only when the possibility of that disease has been ruled out.

Finasteride is also used, at a lower dose, to reverse male-pattern baldness by preventing the hair follicles from becoming inactive. Noticeable improvements may take about three months but will disappear within a year of treatment being stopped.

INFORMATION FOR USERS

Your drug prescription is tailored for you. Do not alter dosage without checking with your doctor.

How taken

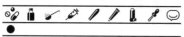

Tablets.

Frequency and timing of doses
Once daily.

Adult dosage range
5mg.

Onset of effect
Within 1 hour, but full beneficial effects may take several months.

Duration of action
24 hours.

Diet advice
None.

Storage
Keep in a closed container, in a cool, dry place out of the reach of children. Protect from light.

Missed dose
Do not take the missed dose, but take your next scheduled dose as usual.

Stopping the drug
Do not stop taking the drug without consulting your doctor; stopping the drug may lead to worsening of the underlying condition.

Exceeding the dose
An occasional unintentional extra dose is unlikely to cause problems. But if you notice any unusual symptoms, or if a large overdose has been taken, notify your doctor.

POSSIBLE ADVERSE EFFECTS

Most people experience very few adverse effects when taking finasteride.

Symptom/effect	Frequency		Discuss with doctor		Stop taking drug now	Call doctor now
	Common	Rare	Only if severe	In all cases		
Impotence/decreased libido	●			■		
Reduced ejaculate volume	●			■		
Breast swelling or tenderness		●		■		
Rash/lip swelling/wheezing		●			■	▲	▮

INTERACTIONS

None.

SPECIAL PRECAUTIONS

Be sure to tell your doctor if:
▼ You are taking other medications.

 Pregnancy
▼ Not prescribed.

 Breast-feeding
▼ Not applicable.

 Infants and children
▼ Not prescribed.

 Over 60
▼ No special problems.

 Driving and hazardous work
▼ No special problems.

 Alcohol
▼ No special problems.

PROLONGED USE

Treatment is reviewed after about six months to see if it has been effective.

FLUCONAZOLE

Brand name Diflucan
Used in the following combined preparations None

GENERAL INFORMATION

Fluconazole is an antifungal drug that is used to treat *systemic* candida infections as well as local candida infections ("thrush") affecting the vagina, mouth, and skin. The drug is also used to treat some more unusual fungal infections, including cryptococcal meningitis. It may also be used to prevent fungal infections in patients with defective immunity. The dosage and length of course will depend on the condition being treated.

The drug is generally well tolerated, although *side effects* such as nausea and vomiting, diarrhoea, and abdominal discomfort are common.

INFORMATION FOR USERS

Your drug prescription is tailored for you. Do not alter dosage without checking with your doctor.

How taken

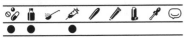

Capsules, liquid, injection.

Frequency and timing of doses
Once daily.

Adult dosage range
50–400mg daily.

Onset of effect
Within a few hours, but full beneficial effects may take several days.

Duration of action
Up to 24 hours.

Diet advice
None.

Storage
Keep in a closed container in a cool, dry place out of the reach of children. Store liquid in a refrigerator (do not freeze) for no longer than 14 days.

Missed dose
Take as soon as you remember. If your next dose is due within 6 hours, take a single dose now and skip the next.

Stopping the drug
Take the full course. Even if you feel better, the original infection may still be present and may recur if treatment is stopped too soon.

Exceeding the dose
An occasional unintentional extra dose is unlikely to be a cause for concern. But if you notice any unusual symptoms, or if a large overdose has been taken, notify your doctor.

SPECIAL PRECAUTIONS

Be sure to tell your doctor if:
▼ You have long-term liver or kidney problems.
▼ You have previously had an allergic reaction to antifungal drugs.
▼ You are taking other medications.

 Pregnancy
▼ Safety in pregnancy not established. Discuss with your doctor.

 Breast-feeding
▼ Not recommended. The drug passes into the breast milk. Discuss with your doctor.

 Infants and children
▼ Reduced dose necessary.

 Over 60
▼ Normal dose used as long as kidney function is not impaired.

 Driving and hazardous work
▼ No known problems.

 Alcohol
▼ No known problems.

POSSIBLE ADVERSE EFFECTS

Fluconazole is generally well tolerated. Most side effects affect the gastrointestinal tract.

Rarely, a rash may occur and should be reported to your doctor.

Symptom/effect	Frequency		Discuss with doctor		Stop taking drug now	Call doctor now
	Common	Rare	Only if severe	In all cases		
Nausea/vomiting	●		■			
Abdominal discomfort	●		■			
Diarrhoea	●		■			
Flatulence	●		■			
Rash		●		■		▲

INTERACTIONS

Anticoagulant drugs Fluconazole may increase the effect of oral anticoagulants such as warfarin.

Oral antidiabetic drugs Fluconazole may increase the risk of hypoglycaemia with oral sulphonylureas, such as gliclazide, glibenclamide, chlorpropamide, and tolbutamide.

Phenytoin Fluconazole may increase the blood level of phenytoin.

Theophylline/aminophylline Fluconazole may increase the blood level of this drug.

Cyclosporin Fluconazole may increase the blood level of cyclosporin.

Rifampicin The effect of fluconazole may be reduced by rifampicin.

Terfenadine When this antihistamine is taken with fluconazole there is an increased risk of adverse effects on the heart.

Cisapride This drug may cause adverse effects on the heart when taken with fluconazole.

PROLONGED USE

Fluconazole is usually given for short courses of treatment. However, for prevention of relapse of cryptococcal meningitis in patients with defective immunity, it may be administered indefinitely.

FLUOXETINE

Brand name Prozac
Used in the following combined preparations None

GENERAL INFORMATION

Fluoxetine belongs a relatively new group of antidepressants called selective serotonin re-uptake inhibitors (SSRIs). These drugs tend to cause less sedation and have different *side effects* to older antidepressants. Fluoxetine elevates mood, increases physical activity, and restores interest in everyday activities.

Fluoxetine is broken down slowly and remains in the body for several weeks after treatment is stopped. Headache, nausea, restlessness, and insomnia are common side effects. It is used to treat depression, to reduce binge eating and purging activity (bulimia nervosa), and to treat obsessive-compulsive disorder.

QUICK REFERENCE

Drug group Antidepressant (p.84)
Overdose danger rating Medium
Dependence rating Low
Prescription needed Yes
Available as generic No

INFORMATION FOR USERS

Your drug prescription is tailored for you. Do not alter dosage without checking with your doctor.

How taken

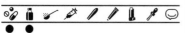

Capsules, liquid.

Frequency and timing of doses
Once daily in the morning.

Adult dosage range
20–60mg daily.

Onset of effect
Some benefits may appear within 14 days, but full benefits may not be felt for 4 weeks or more.

Duration of action
Beneficial effects may last for up to 6 weeks following prolonged treatment. Adverse effects may wear off within a few days.

Diet advice
None.

Storage
Keep in a closed container in a cool, dry place out of the reach of children.

Missed dose
Take as soon as you remember. If your next dose is due within 8 hours, take a single dose now and skip the next.

Stopping the drug
Do not stop the drug without consulting your doctor, who may supervise a gradual reduction in dosage.

Exceeding the dose
An occasional unintentional extra dose is unlikely to cause problems. Large overdoses may cause adverse effects. Notify your doctor.

SPECIAL PRECAUTIONS

Be sure to tell your doctor if:
▼ You have long-term liver or kidney problems.
▼ You have heart problems.
▼ You have diabetes.
▼ You have had epileptic fits.
▼ You have previously had an allergic reaction to fluoxetine or other SSRIs.
▼ You are taking other medications.

Pregnancy
▼ Safety in pregnancy not established. Discuss with your doctor.

Breast-feeding
▼ The drug passes into the breast milk. Discuss with your doctor.

Infants and children
▼ Safety and effectiveness not established.

Over 60
▼ No special problems.

Driving and hazardous work
▼ Avoid such activities until you have learned how fluoxetine affects you because the drug can cause drowsiness and can affect your judgment and coordination.

Alcohol
▼ No special problems.

POSSIBLE ADVERSE EFFECTS

The most common adverse effects of this drug are restlessness, insomnia, and intestinal irregularities. Fluoxetine produces fewer *anticholinergic* side effects than the tricyclics.

Symptom/effect	Frequency		Discuss with doctor		Stop taking drug now	Call doctor now
	Common	Rare	Only if severe	In all cases		
Headache/nervousness	●		■			
Insomnia/anxiety	●			■		
Nausea/diarrhoea	●			■		
Weight loss	●			■		
Drowsiness		●	■			
Sexual dysfunction		●	■			
Rash		●		■	▲	▮

INTERACTIONS

Sedatives All drugs having a *sedative* effect may increase the sedative effects of fluoxetine.

Monoamine oxidase inhibitors (MAOIs) Fluoxetine should not be started less than 14 days after stopping an MAOI (except moclobemide) as serious adverse effects can occur. An MAOI should not be started less than 5 weeks after stopping fluoxetine.

Lithium Fluoxetine increases blood levels and *toxicity* of lithium.

Other antidepressants Fluoxetine reduces the breakdown of tricyclics and may result in sedation, dry mouth, and constipation.

Tryptophan Taken together, tryptophan and fluoxetine may produce agitation, restlessness, and gastric distress.

Terfenadine Taken together, terfenadine and fluoxetine increase the risk of adverse effects on the heart.

PROLONGED USE

No problems expected. Side effects tend to decrease with time.

FLUPENTIXOL

Brand names Depixol, Fluanxol
Used in the following combined preparations None

GENERAL INFORMATION

Flupentixol is an antipsychotic drug that is prescribed to treat schizophrenia and similar illnesses. It is also used as an antidepressant for mild to moderate depression. Flupentixol's *side effects* are similar to those of phenothiazines, but it is less sedating. The drug is not suitable for patients with mania as it may worsen symptoms.

The drug has fewer *anticholinergic* effects than the phenothiazines but is more likely to cause side effects such as *parkinsonism*. Control of severe symptoms may take up to six months, after which a lower maintenance dose is prescribed.

QUICK REFERENCE

Drug group Antipsychotic drug (p.85)

Overdose danger rating Medium

Dependence rating Low

Prescription needed Yes

Available as generic No

INFORMATION FOR USERS

Your drug prescription is tailored for you. Do not alter dosage without checking with your doctor.

How taken

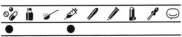

Tablets, injection.

Frequency and timing of doses
1–2 x daily no later than 4 pm (tablets); every 2–4 weeks (injection).

Adult dosage range
Psychosis 6–18mg daily (tablets); 50mg every 4 weeks 300–400mg every 2 weeks (injection). *Depression* 1–3mg daily.

Onset of effect
10 days (side effects may appear much sooner).

Duration of action
Up to 12 hours (by mouth); 2–4 weeks (by injection).

Diet advice
None.

Storage
Store at room temperature out of the reach of children. Protect injections from light.

Missed dose
Take as soon as you remember. If your next dose is due within 2 hours, do not take the missed dose, but take your next scheduled dose as usual.

Stopping the drug
Do not stop taking the drug without consulting your doctor, who will supervise a gradual reduction in dosage. Abrupt cessation of the drug may cause withdrawal symptoms and a recurrence of the original problem.

Exceeding the dose
An occasional unintentional extra dose is unlikely to cause problems. Larger overdoses may cause severe drowsiness, fits, low blood pressure, high or low body temperature, or shock. Notify your doctor.

SPECIAL PRECAUTIONS

Be sure to tell your doctor if:
▼ You have long-term liver or kidney problems.
▼ You have heart problems.
▼ You have porphyria.
▼ You have had epileptic fits.
▼ You have thyroid disease.
▼ You have Parkinson's disease.
▼ You have glaucoma.
▼ You are taking other medications.

Pregnancy
▼ Not usually prescribed. May cause lethargy in the baby during labour. Discuss with your doctor.

Breast-feeding
▼ The drug passes into the breast milk and may affect the baby. Discuss with your doctor.

Infants and children
▼ Not recommended.

Over 60
▼ Reduced dose necessary. Increased risk of late-appearing movement disorders or confusion.

Driving and hazardous work
▼ Avoid such activities until you have learned how flupentixol affects you because the drug can cause drowsiness and slowed reactions.

Alcohol
▼ Avoid. Flupentixol enhances the sedative effect of alcohol.

Surgery and general anaesthetics
▼ Treatment may need to be stopped before you have any surgery. Discuss this with your doctor or dentist.

POSSIBLE ADVERSE EFFECTS

The possible adverse effects of this drug are mainly the result of its anticholinergic action and its blocking action on the transmission of signals through the heart.

Symptom/effect	Frequency		Discuss with doctor		Stop taking drug now	Call doctor now
	Common	Rare	Only if severe	In all cases		
Blurred vision	●			■		
Weight gain	●		■			
Nausea	●		■			
Drowsiness	●		■			
Rapid heartbeat/palpitations	●			■		▮
Dizziness/fainting/confusion	●			■		▮
Parkinsonism/tremor	●			■		
Epileptic fits		●		■	▲	▮
Rash		●		■	▲	
Persistent infection/sore throat		●		■		
Jaundice		●		■	▲	

INTERACTIONS

Antiarrhythmic drugs Taken with these drugs, flupentixol may increase the risk of arrhythmias.

Anticholinergic drugs Flupentixol may increase the effects of these drugs.

Anticonvulsant drugs Flupentixol may reduce the effects of these drugs.

Sedatives Flupentixol enhances the effect of all sedative drugs.

PROLONGED USE

The risk of late-appearing movement disorders increases as treatment with flupentixol continues. Blood disorders, as well as *jaundice* and other liver disorders, are occasionally seen.

Monitoring Blood tests may be performed, particularly if there is persistent infection.

FLUTAMIDE

Brand names Chimax, Drogenil
Used in the following combined preparations None

GENERAL INFORMATION

Flutamide is an anti-androgen drug used in the treatment of advanced prostate cancer, often in combination with gonadorelin analogues, such as goserelin, that control the production of the male sex hormones (androgens). Both drugs are effective because the cancer is dependent on androgens for its continued development. Treatment with gonadorelin analogues causes an initial increase in release of the hormone testosterone, leading to a growth spurt of the cancer ('tumour flare'), which

flutamide is prescribed to stop. In the UK, flutamide treatment is begun three days before the gonadorelin analogue. Flutamide is also used to treat prostate cancer when gonadorelin analogues are not prescribed.

Flutamide may discolour the urine amber or yellow-green, but this is harmless and is not an adverse effect. However, you should notify your doctor straight away if your urine becomes dark coloured, because this may be an indication of liver damage.

INFORMATION FOR USERS

Your drug prescription is tailored for you. Do not alter dosage without checking with your doctor.

How taken

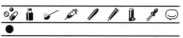

Tablets.

Frequency and timing of doses
3 x daily, starting 3 days before the gonadorelin analogue and continuing for 3 weeks.

Adult dosage range
250mg.

Onset of effect
1 hour.

Duration of action
8 hours.

Diet advice
None.

Storage
Keep in a closed container in a cool, dry place out of the reach of children.

Missed dose
Take as soon as you remember. If your next dose is due within 2 hours, take a single dose now and skip the next.

Stopping the drug
Do not stop taking the drug without consulting your doctor because the condition may worsen rapidly.

Exceeding the dose
An occasional unintentional extra dose is unlikely to be a cause for concern. But if you notice any unusual symptoms, or if a large overdose has been taken, notify your doctor.

SPECIAL PRECAUTIONS

Be sure to tell your doctor if:
▼ You have heart problems.
▼ You have liver problems.
▼ You are taking other medications.

Pregnancy
▼ Not prescribed.

Breast-feeding
▼ Not prescribed.

Infants and children
▼ Not prescribed.

Over 60
▼ No special problems.

Driving and hazardous work
▼ Do not undertake such activities until you have learned how flutamide affects you because the drug can cause blurred vision and dizziness.

Alcohol
▼ No special problems.

POSSIBLE ADVERSE EFFECTS

Nausea and tiredness are common. Breast swelling also occurs when the drug is given in an effective dose; this is usually reversible when treatment stops or dosage is reduced.

Symptom/effect	Frequency		Discuss with doctor		Stop taking drug now	Call doctor now
	Common	Rare	Only if severe	In all cases		
Breast swelling/tenderness	●		■			
Nausea/vomiting/diarrhoea	●		■			
Insomnia/tiredness/headache	●		■			
Dizziness/blurred vision		●	■			
Skin reactions		●		■		
Jaundice/dark urine		●		■	▲	▮

INTERACTIONS

Warfarin Flutamide increases the effect of this drug.

PROLONGED USE

Prolonged use of flutamide may cause liver damage. Because it is an anti-androgen, the drug also reduces sperm count.

Monitoring Periodic liver-function tests are usually performed.

FLUTICASONE

Brand names Cutivate, Flixonase, Flixotide
Used in the following combined preparation Seretide

GENERAL INFORMATION

Fluticasone is a corticosteroid drug used to control asthma and relieve the symptoms of allergic rhinitis. The drug acts mainly by reducing inflammation. Fluticasone does not produce relief immediately, so it is important to take the drug regularly. For allergic rhinitis, treatment with the nasal spray needs to begin two to three weeks before the hay fever season commences. People who suffer from asthma should take fluticasone regularly by inhaler in order to prevent attacks. Proper instruction is essential to ensure that the inhaler

is used correctly. Fluticasone is also prescribed in the form of an ointment or cream to treat dermatitis and eczema (see Topical corticosteroids, p.174).

There are few serious *adverse effects* associated with fluticasone because it is administered directly into the lungs (by the inhaler) or nasal mucosa (by the nasal spray). Fungal infection causing irritation of the mouth and throat is a possible side effect of the inhaled form but can be minimized by thoroughly rinsing the mouth and gargling with water after each inhalation.

QUICK REFERENCE

Drug group Corticosteroid (p.141)
Overdose danger rating Low
Dependence rating Low
Prescription needed Yes
Available as generic No

INFORMATION FOR USERS

Your drug prescription is tailored for you. Do not alter dosage without checking with your doctor.

How taken

Ointment, cream, inhaler, nasal spray.

Frequency and timing of doses
Allergic rhinitis 1–2 x daily; *asthma* 2 x daily.

Adult dosage range
Allergic rhinitis 2 sprays into each nostril per dose; *asthma* 100–1,000mcg per dose.

Onset of effect
4–7 days (asthma); 3–4 days (allergic rhinitis).

Duration of action
The effects can last for several days after stopping the drug.

Diet advice
None.

Storage
Keep in a cool, dry place out of the reach of children.

Missed dose
Take as soon as you remember.

Stopping the drug
Do not stop the drug without consulting your doctor; symptoms may recur.

Exceeding the dose
An occasional unintentional extra dose is unlikely to be a cause for concern. Adverse effects may occur if the recommended dose is regularly exceeded over a prolonged period.

SPECIAL PRECAUTIONS

Be sure to tell your doctor if:
▼ You have chronic sinusitis.
▼ You have had nasal ulcers or surgery.
▼ You have had tuberculosis or another respiratory infection.
▼ You are taking other medications.

Pregnancy
▼ Safety in pregnancy not established. Discuss with your doctor.

Breast-feeding
▼ Safety in breast-feeding not established. However, fluticasone is unlikely to pass into breast milk. Discuss with your doctor.

Infants and children
▼ Not recommended under 4 years. Reduced dose necessary in older children. Avoid prolonged use of ointment in children.

Over 60
▼ No known problems.

Driving and hazardous work
▼ No known problems.

Alcohol
▼ No known problems.

POSSIBLE ADVERSE EFFECTS

Adverse effects are unlikely to occur. The main side effects are irritation of the nasal passages (nasal spray) and fungal infection of the throat and mouth (inhaler). This can be minimized by thoroughly rinsing the mouth, brushing the teeth, or gargling with water.

Symptom/effect	Frequency		Discuss with doctor		Stop taking drug now	Call doctor now
	Common	Rare	Only if severe	In all cases		
Nasal irritation	●		■			
Sore throat/mouth/hoarseness	●			■		
Skin changes (ointment/cream)	●			■		
Taste/smell disturbances		●	■			
Nosebleeds		●		■		
Breathing difficulties		●		■		■
Rash/facial swelling		●		■		■

INTERACTIONS

None.

PROLONGED USE

No problems expected when used for asthma or rhinitis. Prolonged use of ointment and cream can lead to adrenal suppression and can cause permanent skin changes, particularly in facial skin, and should be avoided whenever possible.

Monitoring Periodic checks to confirm that the adrenal glands are functioning properly may be required if large doses are being taken.

FOSINOPRIL

Brand name Staril
Used in the following combined preparations None

GENERAL INFORMATION

Fosinopril belongs to the ACE inhibitor group of *vasodilator* drugs, which are used in the treatment of high blood pressure, heart failure, and after heart attacks. The drug works by relaxing the muscles around blood vessel walls, allowing the vessels to dilate, and thereby easing blood flow.

Fosinopril can cause a rapid fall in blood pressure at the start of treatment, especially if a diuretic is also being taken. For this reason, treatment with the drug for severe heart failure is usually begun in hospital, under close medical supervision. The first dose is usually very small, and should be taken while lying down, preferably at bedtime.

Among the more unusual *side effects* common with fosinopril (and other ACE inhibitors) are persistent dry cough and an altered sense of taste. Reducing the dose may minimize these effects.

INFORMATION FOR USERS

Your drug prescription is tailored for you. Do not alter dosage without checking with your doctor.

How taken

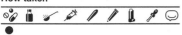
●

Tablets.

Frequency and timing of doses
Once daily.

Adult dosage range
10–40mg.

Onset of effect
1 hour.

Duration of action
Up to 24 hours.

Diet advice
None.

Storage
Keep in a closed container in a cool, dry place out of the reach of children.

Missed dose
Take as soon as you remember. If your next dose is due within 4 hours, take a single dose now and skip the next.

Stopping the drug
Do not stop taking the drug without consulting your doctor; symptoms may recur.

Exceeding the dose
An occasional unintentional extra dose is unlikely to cause problems. Large overdoses may cause dizziness, fainting, and a fall in blood pressure. Notify your doctor immediately.

SPECIAL PRECAUTIONS

Be sure to tell your doctor if:
▼ You are allergic to other ACE inhibitors.
▼ You have a history of angioedema.
▼ You have kidney problems or are on dialysis.
▼ You are taking a diuretic drug.
▼ You are on a low sodium diet.
▼ You are taking other medications.

Pregnancy
▼ Not prescribed. May harm the developing foetus.

Breast-feeding
▼ Not recommended. The drug passes into the breast milk and may affect the baby. Discuss with your doctor.

Infants and children
▼ Not usually prescribed.

Over 60
▼ No special problems.

Driving and hazardous work
▼ Avoid such activities until you have learned how fosinopril affects you because the drug can cause dizziness and fainting.

Alcohol
▼ Avoid. Alcohol may increase the blood pressure lowering and adverse effects of this drug.

POSSIBLE ADVERSE EFFECTS

Dizziness is unlikely to occur after the first dose has been taken. A dry cough is the most common long-term effect.

Symptom/effect	Frequency		Discuss with doctor		Stop taking drug now	Call doctor now
	Common	Rare	Only if severe	In all cases		
Diarrhoea/abdominal pain	●		■			
Nausea/vomiting	●		■			
Rash/itching	●			■		
Dry cough	●			■		
Dizziness/fainting	●			■		
Chest pain/palpitations		●		■		
Severe abdominal pain		●		■		
Persistent sore throat		●		■		
Jaundice		●		■		■

PROLONGED USE

Rarely, prolonged use of fosinopril can lead to changes in blood count or kidney function.

Monitoring Periodic checks on potassium levels, white blood cell counts, and urine are usually performed.

INTERACTIONS

Antacids These drugs may impair absorption of fosinopril and should be taken at least 2 hours before or after.

NSAIDs Some of these drugs may reduce the effect of fosinopril. Used together, there may be a greater risk of kidney damage.

Lithium Blood lithium levels may be increased by fosinopril.

Vasodilators, diuretics, and other drugs to lower blood pressure These drugs increase the effect of fosinopril.

Potassium supplements, potassium-sparing diuretics, and cyclosporin When taken with fosinopril, these drugs increase the risk of high blood levels of potassium.

FUROSEMIDE (FRUSEMIDE)

Brand names Dryptal, Froop, Lasix, Rusyde, Frusol
Used in the following combined preparations Co-Amilofruse, Diumide-K Continus, Fru-Co, Frumil, Lasikal, and others

GENERAL INFORMATION

Furosemide is a powerful, short-acting loop diuretic that has been in use for over 20 years. Like other diuretics, it is used to treat oedema (fluid retention) caused by heart failure, and certain lung, liver, and kidney disorders.

Because it is fast acting, furosemide is often used in emergencies to relieve pulmonary oedema. Furosemide is particularly useful for people who have impaired kidney function because they do not respond well to thiazide diuretics (see p.99).

Furosemide increases potassium loss, which can produce a wide variety of symptoms. For this reason, potassium supplements or a potassium-sparing diuretic are often given with the drug.

QUICK REFERENCE

Drug group Loop diuretic (p.99) and antihypertensive drug (p.102)

Overdose danger rating Low

Dependence rating Low

Prescription needed Yes

Available as generic Yes

INFORMATION FOR USERS

Your drug prescription is tailored for you. Do not alter dosage without checking with your doctor.

How taken

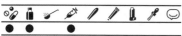

Tablets, liquid, injection.

Frequency and timing of doses
Once daily, usually in the morning; 4–6 x hourly (high dose therapy).

Adult dosage range
20–80mg daily. Dose may be increased to a maximum of 2g daily if kidney function is impaired.

Onset of effect
Within 1 hour (by mouth); within 5 minutes (by injection).

Duration of action
Up to 6 hours.

Diet advice
Use of this drug may reduce potassium in the body. Eat plenty of potassium-rich fresh fruits and vegetables.

Storage
Keep in a closed container in a cool, dry place out of the reach of children. Protect from light.

Missed dose
No cause for concern, but take as soon as you remember. However, if it is late in the day do not take the missed dose, or you may need to get up during the night to pass urine. Take the next scheduled dose as usual.

Stopping the drug
Do not stop the drug without consulting your doctor; symptoms may recur.

Exceeding the dose
An occasional unintentional extra dose is unlikely to be a cause for concern. But if you notice any unusual symptoms, or if a large overdose has been taken, notify your doctor.

SPECIAL PRECAUTIONS

Be sure to tell your doctor if:
▼ You have long-term liver problems.
▼ You have gout.
▼ You have diabetes.
▼ You have previously had an allergic reaction to furosemide or sulphonamides.
▼ You have prostate trouble.
▼ If you are taking laxatives.
▼ You are taking other medications.

Pregnancy
▼ Safety in pregnancy not established. Discuss with your doctor.

Breast-feeding
▼ The drug may reduce milk supply, but the amount in the milk is unlikely to affect the baby. Discuss with your doctor.

Infants and children
▼ Reduced dose necessary.

Over 60
▼ Reduced dose may be necessary.

Driving and hazardous work
▼ Avoid such activities until you have learned how furosemide affects you because the drug may reduce mental alertness and cause dizziness.

Alcohol
▼ Keep consumption low. Furosemide increases the likelihood of dehydration and hangovers after the consumption of alcohol.

POSSIBLE ADVERSE EFFECTS

Adverse effects are caused mainly by the rapid fluid loss produced by furosemide. These tend to diminish as the body adjusts to taking the drug. The disturbance in body salts and water balance can result in muscle cramps, headaches, and dizziness.

Symptom/effect	Frequency		Discuss with doctor		Stop taking drug now	Call doctor now
	Common	Rare	Only if severe	In all cases		
Dizziness/nausea	●			■		
Lethargy		●		■		
Noise in ears (high dose)		●		■		
Muscle cramps		●		■		
Rash/photosensitivity		●			■	▲

INTERACTIONS

Non-steroidal anti-inflammatory drugs (NSAIDs) Some of these drugs may reduce the diuretic effect of furosemide.

Lithium Furosemide may increase blood levels of lithium, leading to an increased risk of lithium poisoning.

Digoxin Loss of potassium may lead to digoxin *toxicity* when furosemide is taken with this drug.

Aminoglycoside antibiotics The risk of hearing and kidney problems may be increased when these drugs are taken with furosemide.

Angiotensin-converting enzyme inhibitors There is a risk of low blood pressure when these drugs are taken with furosemide.

PROLONGED USE

Serious problems are unlikely, but levels of salts, such as potassium, sodium, and calcium, may become depleted. Low blood pressure, headaches, problems passing urine, or muscle cramps may develop, particularly in the elderly.

Monitoring Periodic tests may be performed to check on kidney function and levels of body salts.

GAMOLENIC ACID

Brand names Efamast, Epogam
Used in the following combined preparations Many preparations containing evening primrose oil, including Efamol and EPOC

GENERAL INFORMATION

Gamolenic acid is an essential fatty acid that is found in evening primrose oil and starflower oil (borage oil). Essential fatty acids are found in some foods and are necessary for full health. The beneficial effects of evening primrose oil include improving the hair and skin condition and strengthening the nails. Essential fatty acids have numerous functions and contribute to the manufacture of cells and certain important chemicals, such as *prostaglandins*. Administration of gamolenic acid enhances production of these chemicals in the body.

The drug has been investigated for use in a variety of conditions, including multiple sclerosis and premenstrual syndrome. Gamolenic acid may also be obtained by prescription for treating eczema and mastitis (breast pain).

QUICK REFERENCE

Overdose danger rating Low
Dependence rating Low
Prescription needed No
Available as generic No

INFORMATION FOR USERS

Follow instructions on the label. Call your doctor if symptoms worsen.

How taken

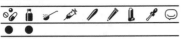

Capsules, liquid.

Frequency and timing of doses
2 x daily, if desired. The capsules may be cut open and the contents swallowed.

Adult dosage range
Epogam 8–12 capsules daily (eczema); Efamast 6–8 capsules daily (breast pain). For other brands, follow the instructions on the packet.

Onset of effect
Normally 8–12 weeks, but some effects may take longer.

Duration of action
12–24 hours, although the beneficial effects will last longer.

Diet advice
None.

Storage
Keep in a closed container in a cool, dry, place out of the reach of children.

Missed dose
Take as soon as you remember.

Stopping the drug
Symptoms may eventually recur if the drug is stopped.

Exceeding the dose
An occasional unintentional extra dose is unlikely to be a cause for concern. Large overdoses may cause loose faeces and abdominal pain. If you notice any unusual symptoms, or if a large overdose has been taken, notify your doctor.

SPECIAL PRECAUTIONS

Be sure to tell your doctor if:
▼ You have a history of epilepsy.
▼ You have ever had a psychiatric illness.
▼ You are taking other medications.

Pregnancy
▼ Safety in pregnancy not established. Discuss with your doctor.

Breast-feeding
▼ No known problems.

Infants and children
▼ Not recommended under 1 year. Reduced dose necessary in older children.

Over 60
▼ No special problems.

Driving and hazardous work
▼ No known problems.

Alcohol
▼ No known problems.

POSSIBLE ADVERSE EFFECTS

Gamolenic acid does not usually cause problems with adverse effects.

Symptom/effect	Frequency		Discuss with doctor		Stop taking drug now	Call doctor now
	Common	Rare	Only if severe	In all cases		
Nausea	●		■			
Headache	●		■			

INTERACTIONS

Phenothiazine antipsychotics (e.g., chlorpromazine and prochlorperazine)
There is an increased risk of convulsions in people taking phenothiazines with gamolenic acid.

PROLONGED USE

No problems expected.

GENTAMICIN

Brand names Cidomycin, Garamycin, Genticin, Minims gentamicin
Used in the following combined preparations Gentisone HC

GENERAL INFORMATION

Gentamicin is one of the aminoglycoside antibiotics. The injectable form is usually reserved for treatment, in hospital, of serious or complicated infections. These include lung, urinary tract, bone, joint, and wound infections, as well as peritonitis, septicaemia, and meningitis. This form is also used together with a penicillin for prevention and treatment of heart valve infections (endocarditis).

Also available as drops and ointment, gentamicin is commonly used to treat eye and ear infections. The ointment may in some cases be prescribed for infected burns or ulcers. Resistance is a common problem following treatment with skin preparations.

Gentamicin given by injection can have serious *adverse effects* on the ears, which may lead to damage to the balance mechanism and deafness, and on the kidneys. Courses of treatment are therefore limited to seven days when possible. Treatment is monitored with particular care when high doses are needed or kidney function is poor.

INFORMATION FOR USERS

Your drug prescription is tailored for you. Do not alter dosage without checking with your doctor.

How taken

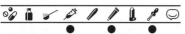

Injection, cream, ointment, eye ointment, eye and ear drops.

Frequency and timing of doses
1–3 x daily (injection); 3–4 x daily or as directed (skin preparations, eye and ear drops, eye ointments).

Adult dosage range
According to condition and response (injection); according to your doctor's instructions (eye, ear, and skin preparations).

Onset of effect
Within 1–2 hours.

Duration of action
8–12 hours.

Diet advice
None.

Storage
Keep in closed container in a cool, dry place out of the reach of children.

Missed dose
Apply skin, eye, and ear preparations as soon as you remember.

Stopping the drug
Complete the course. Even if you feel better, the original infection may still be present and may recur if treatment is stopped too soon.

Exceeding the dose
Although overdose by injection is dangerous, it is unlikely because treatment is carefully monitored. For other preparations of the drug, an occasional unintentional extra dose is unlikely cause concern. But if you notice any unusual symptoms, notify your doctor.

SPECIAL PRECAUTIONS

Be sure to tell your doctor if:
▼ You have a long-term kidney problem.
▼ You have a hearing disorder.
▼ You have myasthenia gravis.
▼ You have Parkinson's disease.
▼ You have previously had an allergic reaction to aminoglycosides.
▼ You are taking other medications.

 Pregnancy
▼ No evidence of risk with *topical* preparations. Injections are not prescribed, as they may cause hearing defects in the baby. Discuss with your doctor.

 Breast-feeding
▼ No evidence of risk with topical preparations. Given by injection, the drug may pass into the breast milk. Discuss with your doctor.

 Infants and children
▼ Reduced dose necessary for injections.

 Over 60
▼ Increased likelihood of adverse effects. Reduced dose may therefore be necessary.

 Driving and hazardous work
▼ No known problems from preparations for the skin, eye, or ear.

 Alcohol
▼ No known problems.

POSSIBLE ADVERSE EFFECTS

Adverse effects are rare but those that occur with the injectable form of gentamicin may be serious. Dizziness, loss of balance (vertigo), impaired hearing, and changes in the urine should be reported promptly. The drug may be absorbed if the ointment or cream is applied to large areas, and could cause hearing loss. Allergic reactions, including rash and itching, may occur with all preparations that contain gentamicin. Blurred vision or eye irritation may occur with the eye preparations and should be reported to your doctor.

Symptom/effect	Frequency		Discuss with doctor		Stop taking drug now	Call doctor now
	Common	Rare	Only if severe	In all cases		
Nausea/vomiting		●	■			
Dizziness/vertigo		●		■	▲	▮
Rash/itching		●		■	▲	▮
Ringing in the ears		●		■	▲	▮
Loss of hearing		●		■	▲	▮
Bloody/cloudy urine		●		■	▲	▮

INTERACTIONS

General note A wide range of drugs, including furosemide, vancomycin, and cephalosporins, increase the risk of hearing loss and/or kidney failure with gentamicin.

PROLONGED USE

Not usually given for longer than 10 days. When given by injection, there is a risk of adverse effects on hearing and balance.

Monitoring Blood levels of the drug are usually checked if it is given by injection. Tests on kidney function are also usually carried out.

GLIBENCLAMIDE

Brand names Daonil, Euglucon, Semi-Daonil
Used in the following combined preparations None

GENERAL INFORMATION

Glibenclamide is an oral antidiabetic drug belonging to the sulphonylurea class. Like other drugs of this type, glibenclamide stimulates the production and secretion of insulin from the islet cells in the pancreas and promotes the uptake of sugar into body cells, thereby lowering the level of sugar in the blood.

This drug is used in the treatment of adult (maturity-onset) diabetes mellitus, in conjunction with a diabetic diet low in carbohydrates and fats.

In conditions of severe illness, injury, or stress, glibenclamide may lose its effectiveness, making insulin injections necessary. *Adverse effects* are generally mild. Symptoms of poor diabetic control will occur if the dosage of glibenclamide is not appropriate.

QUICK REFERENCE

Drug group Oral antidiabetic drug (p.142)

Overdose danger rating High

Dependence rating Low

Prescription needed Yes

Available as generic Yes

INFORMATION FOR USERS

Your drug prescription is tailored for you. Do not alter dosage without checking with your doctor.

How taken

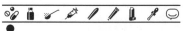

Tablets.

Frequency and timing of doses
Once daily in the morning with breakfast.

Adult dosage range
5–15mg daily.

Onset of effect
Within 3 hours.

Duration of action
10–15 hours.

Diet advice
A low-carbohydrate, low-fat diet must be maintained in order for the drug to be fully effective. Follow the advice of your doctor.

Storage
Keep in a closed container in a cool, dry place out of the reach of children. Protect from light.

Missed dose
Take before your next meal.

Stopping the drug
Do not stop the drug without consulting your doctor; stopping the drug may lead to worsening of your diabetes.

OVERDOSE ACTION

 Seek immediate medical advice in all cases. If any early warning symptoms of excessively low blood sugar (such as fainting, sweating, trembling, confusion, or headache) occur, eat or drink something sugary. Take emergency action if fits or loss of consciousness occur.

See Drug poisoning emergency guide (p.494).

SPECIAL PRECAUTIONS

Be sure to tell your doctor if:
▼ You have long-term liver or kidney problems.
▼ You are allergic to sulphonamide drugs.
▼ You have thyroid problems.
▼ You have ever had problems with your adrenal glands.
▼ You are taking other medications.

 Pregnancy
▼ Not usually prescribed. Insulin is generally substituted in pregnancy because it gives better diabetic control.

Breast-feeding
▼ The drug passes into the breast milk, but at normal doses adverse effects on the baby are unlikely. Discuss with your doctor.

Infants and children
▼ Not prescribed.

 Over 60
▼ Reduced dose may be necessary. Greater likelihood of low blood sugar exists when glibenclamide is used.

 Driving and hazardous work
▼ Usually no problems. Avoid these activities if you have warning signs of low blood sugar.

Alcohol
▼ Avoid. Alcoholic drinks may upset diabetic control.

Surgery and general anaesthetics
▼ Surgery may alter the effect of this drug on diabetes; insulin treatment may need to be substituted.

POSSIBLE ADVERSE EFFECTS

Serious adverse effects with glibenclamide are rare. More common symptoms, often accompanied by hunger, may be signs of low blood sugar due to lack of food or too high a dose of the drug.

Symptom/effect	Frequency		Discuss with doctor		Stop taking drug now	Call doctor now
	Common	Rare	Only if severe	In all cases		
Faintness/confusion	●			■		
Weakness/tremor	●			■		
Sweating	●			■		
Nausea/vomiting		●		■		
Rash/itching		●		■		
Jaundice		●	■			■
Weight changes		●		■		

PROLONGED USE

No problems expected.

Monitoring Regular monitoring of levels of sugar in the urine or blood is required. Periodic assessment of the eyes, heart, and kidneys may also be advised.

INTERACTIONS

General note A variety of drugs may reduce the effect of glibenclamide and so may raise blood sugar levels. These include corticosteroids, oestrogens, diuretics, and rifampicin. Other drugs increase the risk of low blood sugar. These include warfarin, sulphonamides and other antibacterials, aspirin, beta blockers, and ACE inhibitors.

GLICLAZIDE

Brand name Diamicron
Used in the following combined preparations None

GENERAL INFORMATION

Gliclazide is an antidiabetic drug that lowers blood sugar by stimulating insulin secretion from the pancreas. It is used to treat adult (maturity-onset) diabetes mellitus in conjunction with a balanced diet that limits carbohydrate and fat intake to promote weight loss. Regular exercise is an important part of the treatment of diabetes.

In conditions of severe illness, injury, stress, or surgery, the drug may lose its effectiveness, causing loss of diabetic control and necessitating the use of insulin injections. *Adverse effects* of gliclazide are generally mild. However, symptoms of poor diabetic control will occur if the dosage is not appropriate.

QUICK REFERENCE

Drug group Oral antidiabetic drug (p.142)

Overdose danger rating High

Dependence rating Low

Prescription needed Yes

Available as generic No

INFORMATION FOR USERS

Your drug prescription is tailored for you. Do not alter dosage without checking with your doctor.

How taken

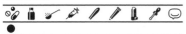

Tablets.

Frequency and timing of doses
1–2 x daily (in the morning and evening with a meal).

Dosage range
80–320mg daily.

Onset of effect
Within 1 hour.

Duration of action
12–24 hours.

Diet advice
An individualized, low-fat, low-carbohydrate diet must be maintained for the drug to be fully effective. Follow the advice of your doctor.

Storage
Keep in a closed container in a cool, dry place out of the reach of children.

Missed dose
Take as soon as you remember with the next meal.

Stopping the drug
Do not stop the drug without consulting your doctor; stopping the drug may lead to worsening of the underlying condition.

OVERDOSE ACTION

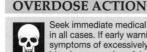

Seek immediate medical advice in all cases. If early warning symptoms of excessively low blood sugar such as fainting, sweating, trembling, confusion, or headache occur, eat or drink something sugary at once. Take emergency action if fits or loss of consciousness occur.

See Drug poisoning emergency guide (p.494).

SPECIAL PRECAUTIONS

Be sure to tell your doctor if:
▼ You have or have recently had a serious trauma or infection.
▼ You have long-term liver or kidney problems.
▼ You have thyroid problems.
▼ You do not eat properly.
▼ You are planning a pregnancy.
▼ You have Addison's disease.
▼ You have an allergy to sulphonylureas.
▼ You are taking other medications.

Pregnancy
▼ Not recommended. May cause abnormally low blood sugar in the newborn baby. Insulin is generally substituted in pregnancy because it gives better diabetic control.

Breast-feeding
▼ The drug passes into the breast milk and may cause low blood sugar in the baby. Discuss with your doctor.

Infants and children
▼ Not prescribed.

Over 60
▼ Signs of low blood sugar may be more difficult to recognize. Reduced dose may be necessary.

Driving and hazardous work
▼ Avoid such activities until you have learned how gliclazide affects you because it can cause dizziness, drowsiness, and confusion.

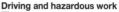

Alcohol
▼ Avoid. Alcoholic drinks upset diabetic control and gliclazide may cause intolerance to alcohol.

Surgery and general anaesthetics
▼ Notify your doctor or dentist that you are diabetic before undergoing any type of surgery.

POSSIBLE ADVERSE EFFECTS

Serious adverse effects are rare. Dizziness, confusion, tremors, sweating, and weakness may be signs of low blood sugar due to lack of food or too high a dose of gliclazide.

Symptom/effect	Frequency		Discuss with doctor		Stop taking drug now	Call doctor now
	Common	Rare	Only if severe	In all cases		
Dizziness/drowsiness/confusion	●			■		
Weakness/lack of energy	●			■		
Tremors/chilliness	●			■		
Sweating/flushing	●			■		
Headache/nervousness	●			■		
Rash/itching		●		■		
Nausea/vomiting/heartburn		●		■		
Prolonged bleeding/bruising		●		■		
Sore throat and fever		●		■		
Thirst		●		■		
Weight changes		●	■			

INTERACTIONS

General note Many drugs (such as corticosteroids and barbiturates) may oppose the effects of gliclazide, thereby raising blood sugar levels. Other drugs (such as warfarin and aspirin) increase the risk of low blood sugar.

PROLONGED USE

No problems expected.

Monitoring Regular testing of sugar levels in the blood and/or urine is required. Periodic assessment of the eyes, heart, and kidneys may also be advised.

GLYCERYL TRINITRATE

Brand names Coro-Nitro, Deponit, Minitran, Nitro-Dur, Nitrolingual, Suscard, Sustac, Transiderm-Nitro, and others
Used in the following combined preparations None

GENERAL INFORMATION

Introduced in the late 1800s, glyceryl trinitrate is one of the oldest drugs in continual use. It belongs to a group of vasodilator drugs called nitrates that are used to relieve the pain of angina attacks. It is available in short-acting forms (sublingual or buccal tablets and spray) and in long-acting forms (slow-release tablets and skin patches). The short-acting forms act very quickly to relieve angina. It is also given by injection in hospital for severe angina and for controlling blood pressure.

Glyceryl trinitrate may cause a variety of minor symptoms, such as flushing and headache, most of which can be controlled by adjusting the dosage. The drug is best taken for the first time while you are sitting, as fainting may follow the drop in blood pressure caused by this medication.

QUICK REFERENCE

Drug group Anti-angina drug (p.101)

Overdose danger rating Medium

Dependence rating Low

Prescription needed Yes

Available as generic Yes

INFORMATION FOR USERS

Your drug prescription is tailored for you. Do not alter dosage without checking with your doctor.

How taken

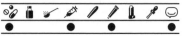

SR-tablets, buccal tablets, sublingual tablets, injection, ointment, skin patches, spray.

Frequency and timing of doses
Prevention 3 x daily (buccal and SR-tablets); once daily (patches); every 3–4 hours (ointment).
Relief Use buccal or sublingual tablets or spray at the onset of an attack or immediately prior to exercise. Dose may be repeated within 5 minutes if further relief is required.

Adult dosage range
Prevention 5.2–30mg daily (SR-tablets); 3–15mg daily (buccal tablets); 2.5–15mg daily (patches); as directed (ointment).
Relief 0.3–1mg per dose (sublingual tablets); 1–3mg per dose (buccal tablets); 1–2 sprays per dose (spray).

Onset of effect
Within minutes (buccal and sublingual tablets and spray); 1–3 hours (SR-tablets, patches, and ointment).

Duration of action
20–30 minutes (sublingual tablets and spray); 3–5 hours (buccal tablets and ointment); 8–12 hours (SR-tablets); up to 24 hours (patches).

Diet advice
None.

Storage
Keep buccal and sublingual tablets in a tightly closed glass container fitted with a foil-lined, screw-on cap in a cool, dry place out of the reach of children. Protect from light. Do not expose to heat. Discard tablets within 8 weeks of opening. Check label of other preparations for storage conditions.

Missed dose
Take as soon as you remember, or when needed. If your next dose is due within 2 hours, take a single dose now and skip the next.

Stopping the drug
Do not stop taking the drug without consulting your doctor.

Exceeding the dose
An occasional unintentional extra dose is unlikely to cause problems. Large overdoses may cause dizziness, vomiting, severe headache, fits, or loss of consciousness. Notify your doctor.

POSSIBLE ADVERSE EFFECTS

The most serious *adverse effect* is lowered blood pressure, and this may need to be monitored periodically. Other adverse effects usually decrease in severity after regular use and they can also be controlled by an adjustment in dosage.

Symptom/effect	Frequency		Discuss with doctor		Stop taking drug now	Call doctor now
	Common	Rare	Only if severe	In all cases		
Headache	●		■			
Flushing	●		■			
Dizziness	●			■		

INTERACTIONS

Antihypertensive drugs These drugs increase the possibility of lowered blood pressure or fainting when taken with glyceryl trinitrate.

SPECIAL PRECAUTIONS

Be sure to tell your doctor if:
▼ You have any other heart condition.
▼ You have a lung condition.
▼ You have long-term liver or kidney problems.
▼ You have any blood disorders.
▼ You have glaucoma.
▼ You have thyroid disease.
▼ You are taking other medications.

Pregnancy
▼ Safety in pregnancy not established. Discuss with your doctor.

Breast-feeding
▼ It is not known whether the drug passes into the breast milk. Discuss with your doctor.

Infants and children
▼ Not usually prescribed.

Over 60
▼ No special problems.

Driving and hazardous work
▼ Avoid such activities until you have learned how glyceryl trinitrate affects you because the drug can cause dizziness.

Alcohol
▼ Avoid excessive intake. Alcohol may increase dizziness due to lowered blood pressure.

PROLONGED USE

The effects of the drug usually become slightly weaker during prolonged use as the body adapts.

Monitoring Periodic checks on blood pressure are usually required.

GOSERELIN

Brand name Zoladex
Used in the following combined preparations None

GENERAL INFORMATION

Goserelin is a synthetic drug chemically related to the hormone gonadorelin. Like gonadorelin, it stimulates the release of other hormones from the pituitary gland, which in turn control production of the sex hormones.

Goserelin is used to suppress the production of sex hormones in cancers of the breast and prostate. It is usually given with an anti-androgen drug (see p.146) at the start of treatment for cancer of the prostate in order to control an initial growth spurt of the tumour – a condition known as 'tumour flare'.

The drug is also used in the management of fibroids, infertility, and endometriosis. The first dose is normally given during menstruation to avoid the possibility that the patient may be pregnant. It is advisable for women of childbearing age to use barrier methods of contraception during treatment.

The injections are usually given by a general practitioner or district nurse.

Loss of bone density is an important *side effect* in women. Therefore, repeat courses of of the drug are given only for cancerous conditions.

INFORMATION FOR USERS

Your drug prescription is tailored for you. Do not alter dosage without checking with your doctor

How taken

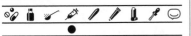

Implant injection, long-acting implant injection.

Frequency and timing of doses
Endometriosis Every 28 days, maximum of a single 6-month treatment only (implant).
Fibroids Implant every 28 days, maximum 3 months' treatment.
Prostate cancer Every 12 weeks (LA implant).

Adult dosage range
3.6mg every 28 days (endometriosis/fibroids); 10.8mg every 3 months (prostate).

Onset of effect
Within 24 hours (endometriosis/fibroids); 1–2 weeks after tumour flare (prostate).

Duration of action
28 days (implant); 12 weeks (long-acting implant).

Diet advice
None.

Storage
Not applicable. The drug is not kept in the home.

Missed dose
No cause for concern. Treatment can be resumed when possible.

Stopping the drug
Do not stop treatment without consulting your doctor.

Exceeding the dose
Overdosage is unlikely since treatment is not self-administered.

SPECIAL PRECAUTIONS

Be sure to tell your doctor if:
▼ You have osteoporosis.
▼ You have previously been treated with goserelin (or another gonadorelin analogue) for endometriosis or fibroids.
▼ You have polycystic ovarian disease.
▼ You are allergic to gonadorelin analogues.
▼ You are taking other medications.

Pregnancy
▼ Not prescribed.

Breast-feeding
▼ Not recommended. Discuss with your doctor.

Infants and children
▼ Not recommended.

Over 60
▼ No special problems.

Driving and hazardous work
▼ No special problems.

Alcohol
▼ No special problems.

POSSIBLE ADVERSE EFFECTS

Symptoms similar to those of the menopause, such as hot flushes and changes in breast size are common. Rare adverse effects should be reported to your doctor straight away.

Symptom/effect	Frequency		Discuss with doctor		Stop taking drug now	Call doctor now
	Common	Rare	Only if severe	In all cases		
Hot flushes	●		■			
Headache	●		■			
Bleeding on stopping drug	●		■			
Rash/wheezing		●		■		
Reaction at injection site		●		■		
Ovarian cysts		●		■		
Dizziness/fainting		●		■		

INTERACTIONS

None.

PROLONGED USE

Goserelin is only used in the long term for treatment of prostate or breast cancer. Bone density is lost over time in women taking the drug, but this may be partly recoverable once treatment stops.

Monitoring Women are usually monitored for changes in bone density.

HALOPERIDOL

Brand names Dozic, Haldol, Serenace
Used in the following combined preparations None

GENERAL INFORMATION

Introduced in the 1960s, haloperidol, is used to reduce the violent, aggressive manifestations of mental illnesses such as schizophrenia, mania, dementia, and other disorders in which hallucinations are experienced. The drug is also used in the short term for severe anxiety. It does not cure the underlying disorder but relieves the distressing symptoms.

Haloperidol is also used in the control of Tourette's syndrome and may be of benefit in children who have severe behavioural problems for which other drugs are ineffective.
The main drawback of haloperidol is that it produces the disturbing *side effect* of abnormal, involuntary movements and stiffness of the face and limbs.

INFORMATION FOR USERS

Your drug prescription is tailored for you. Do not alter dosage without checking with your doctor.

How taken

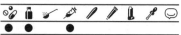

Tablets, capsules, liquid, injection, *depot* injection.

Frequency and timing of doses
2–4 x daily.

Adult dosage range
Mental illness 1.5–20mg daily initially, increased gradually, if necessary, up to a maximum of 100mg daily (or rarely up to 120mg daily). *Severe anxiety* 1mg daily.

Onset of effect
2–3 hours (by mouth); 20–30 minutes (by injection).

Duration of action
6–24 hours (by mouth); 2–4 hours (injection); up to 4 weeks (depot injection).

Diet advice
None.

Storage
Keep in a closed container in a cool, dry place out of the reach of children.

Missed dose
Take as soon as you remember. If your next dose is due within 3 hours, take a single dose now and skip the next.

Stopping the drug
Do not stop the drug without consulting your doctor; symptoms may recur.

Exceeding the dose
An occasional unintentional extra dose is unlikely to cause problems. Larger overdoses may cause unusual drowsiness, muscle weakness or rigidity, and/or faintness. Notify your doctor.

SPECIAL PRECAUTIONS

Be sure to tell your doctor if:
▼ You have long-term liver or kidney problems.
▼ You have heart or circulation problems.
▼ You have had epileptic fits.
▼ You have an overactive thyroid gland.
▼ You have Parkinson's disease.
▼ You have had glaucoma.
▼ You have asthma, bronchitis, or another lung disorder.
▼ You have ever had phaeochromocytoma.
▼ You are taking other medications.

Pregnancy
▼ Safety in pregnancy not established. Discuss with your doctor.

Breast-feeding
▼ The drug passes into the breast milk and may affect the baby. Discuss with your doctor.

Infants and children
▼ Rarely required. Reduced dose necessary.

Over 60
▼ Reduced dose may be necessary.

Driving and hazardous work
▼ Avoid such activities until you have learned how haloperidol affects you because the drug may cause drowsiness and slowed reactions.

Alcohol
▼ Avoid. Alcohol may increase the sedative effect of this drug.

POSSIBLE ADVERSE EFFECTS

Haloperidol can cause a variety of minor *anticholinergic* symptoms that often become less marked with time. The most significant adverse effect, abnormal movements of the face and limbs (parkinsonism), may be controlled by dosage adjustment.

Symptom/effect	Frequency		Discuss with doctor		Stop taking drug now	Call doctor now
	Common	Rare	Only if severe	In all cases		
Drowsiness/lethargy	●		■			
Loss of appetite	●		■			
Parkinsonism	●			■		
Dizziness/fainting		●		■		
Rash		●		■	▲	
High fever/confusion		●		■	▲	■

INTERACTIONS

Sedatives *Sedatives* are likely to increase the sedative properties of haloperidol.

Rifampicin and anticonvulsant drugs These drugs may reduce the effects of haloperidol, the dosage of which may need to be increased.

Lithium This drug may increase the risk of parkinsonism and effects on the nerves.

Methyldopa This drug may increase the risk of parkinsonism and low blood pressure.

Terfenadine This drug may have adverse effects on the heart if taken with haloperidol.

Anticholinergic drugs Haloperidol may increase the side effects of these drugs.

PROLONGED USE

Use of this drug for more than a few months may lead to *tardive dyskinesia* (abnormal, involuntary movements of the eyes, face, and tongue). Occasionally, *jaundice* may occur.

HEPARIN

Brand names Calciparine, Minihep, Monoparin, Multiparin, Uniparin; [LMWH] Alphaparin, Clexane, Fragmin, Innohep
Used in the following combined preparations None

GENERAL INFORMATION

Heparin is an anticoagulant drug used to prevent the formation of, and aid in the dispersion of, blood clots. Because the drug acts quickly, it is particularly useful in emergencies, for instance, to prevent further clotting when a clot has already reached the lungs or the brain. People undergoing open heart surgery or kidney dialysis are also given heparin to prevent clotting. A low dose of the drug is sometimes given following surgery to prevent deep vein thrombosis (clots from forming in the leg veins). Heparin is often given in conjunction with other slower-acting anticoagulants, such as warfarin. It is also used to treat unstable angina.

The most serious *adverse effect* of heparin as with all anticoagulants, is the risk of excessive bleeding, so the ability of the blood to clot is watched very carefully. Bruising may occur around the site of the injection.

New forms of heparin called "low molecular weight heparins" (LMWH) are now widely used and do not have to be given in hospital.

INFORMATION FOR USERS

This drug is given only under medical supervision and is not for self-administration.

How taken

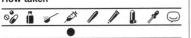

Injection.

Frequency and timing of doses
Every 8–12 hours (continuous intravenous infusion); once daily (LMWH).

Dosage range
Treatment 5,000 units initially, followed by 40,000 units over 24 hours (heparin); treatment depends on bodyweight (LMWH).
Prevention 5,000 units.

Onset of effect
Within 15 minutes.

Duration of action
4–12 hours after treatment is stopped.

Diet advice
None.

Storage
Keep in a cool, dry place out of the reach of children.

Missed dose
Notify your doctor.

Stopping the drug
Do not stop taking the drug without consulting your doctor. Stopping the drug may lead to clotting of blood.

OVERDOSE ACTION

Seek immediate medical advice in all cases. Take emergency action if bleeding, severe headache, or loss of consciousness occur. Overdose can be reversed under medical supervision by a drug called protamine.

See Drug poisoning emergency guide (p.494).

POSSIBLE ADVERSE EFFECTS

As with all anticoagulants, bleeding is the most common adverse effect of heparin. The less common effects may occur during long-term treatment.

Symptom/effect	Frequency		Discuss with doctor		Stop taking drug now	Call doctor now
	Common	Rare	Only if severe	In all cases		
Bleeding/bruising	●			■		▮
Alopecia		●		■		
Aching bones		●		■		
Rash		●		■	▲	▮
Breathing difficulties		●		■		▮
Jaundice/vomiting blood		●		■		▮

SPECIAL PRECAUTIONS

Be sure to tell your doctor if:
▼ You have long-term liver or kidney problems.
▼ You have high blood pressure.
▼ You bleed easily.
▼ You have any allergies.
▼ You have stomach ulcers.
▼ You are taking other medications.

Pregnancy
▼ Careful monitoring is necessary as it may cause the mother to bleed excessively if taken near delivery. Discuss with your doctor.

Breast-feeding
▼ No evidence of risk.

Infants and children
▼ Reduced dose necessary according to age and weight.

Over 60
▼ No special problems.

Driving and hazardous work
▼ Avoid risk of injury, since excessive bruising and bleeding may occur.

Alcohol
▼ No special problems.

Surgery and general anaesthetics
▼ Heparin may need to be stopped. Discuss this with your doctor or dentist before having any surgery.

INTERACTIONS

Aspirin Do not take aspirin, which may increase the anticoagulant effect of this drug and the risk of bleeding in the intestines or joints.

Dipyridamole The anticoagulant effect of heparin may be increased when it is taken with this drug. The dosage of heparin may need to be adjusted accordingly.

PROLONGED USE

Osteoporosis and hair loss may occur; tolerance to heparin may develop.

Monitoring Periodic blood and liver function tests will be required.

HYDROCHLOROTHIAZIDE

Brand name HydroSaluric
Used in the following combined preparations Acezide, Capozide, Co-Betaloc, Dyazide, Moducren, Moduretic, and others

GENERAL INFORMATION

Hydrochlorothiazide belongs to the thiazide group of diuretic drugs, which remove excess water from the body and reduce oedema (fluid retention) in people with congestive heart failure, kidney disorders, cirrhosis of the liver, and premenstrual syndrome. This drug is used to treat high blood pressure (see Antihypertensive drugs, p.102).

Hydrochlorothiazide increases the loss of potassium in the urine, which can cause a variety of symptoms (see p.99), and increases the likelihood of irregular heart rhythms, particularly in patients who are taking drugs such as digoxin. For this reason, potassium supplements are often given with hydrochlorothiazide.

INFORMATION FOR USERS

Your drug prescription is tailored for you. Do not alter dosage without checking with your doctor.

How taken

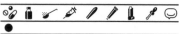

Tablets.

Frequency and timing of doses
Once daily, or every 2 days, early in the day.

Adult dosage range
25–50mg daily.

Onset of effect
Within 2 hours.

Duration of action
6–12 hours.

Diet advice
Use of this drug may reduce potassium in the body. Eat plenty of fresh fruit and vegetables. Discuss with your doctor the advisability of reducing your salt intake.

Storage
Keep in a closed container in a cool, dry place out of the reach of children. Protect from light.

Missed dose
No cause for concern, but take as soon as you remember. However, if it is late in the day do not take the missed dose, or you may have to get up during the night to pass urine. Take the next scheduled dose as usual.

Stopping the drug
Do not stop the drug without consulting your doctor; symptoms may recur.

Exceeding the dose
An occasional unintentional extra dose is unlikely to be a cause for concern. But if you notice any unusual symptoms, or if a large overdose has been taken, notify your doctor.

SPECIAL PRECAUTIONS

Be sure to tell your doctor if:
▼ You have long-term liver or kidney problems.
▼ You have had gout.
▼ You have diabetes.
▼ You have Addison's disease or systemic lupus erythematosus.
▼ You are taking other medications.

 Pregnancy
▼ Not usually prescribed. May cause *jaundice* in the newborn baby. Discuss with your doctor.

 Breast-feeding
▼ The drug passes into the breast milk, but at normal doses adverse effects on the baby are unlikely. Discuss with your doctor.

 Infants and children
▼ Not usually prescribed. Reduced dose necessary.

 Over 60
▼ Increased likelihood of adverse effects.

 Driving and hazardous work
▼ Avoid such activities until you have learned how hydrochlorothiazide affects you because the drug may reduce mental alertness and cause dizziness.

 Alcohol
▼ Keep consumption low. Hydrochlorothiazide increases the likelihood of dehydration and hangovers after consumption of alcohol.

POSSIBLE ADVERSE EFFECTS

Most effects are caused by excessive loss of potassium. This can usually be put right by taking a potassium supplement. In rare cases, gout may occur in susceptible people, and certain forms of diabetes may become more difficult to control.

Symptom/effect	Frequency		Discuss with doctor		Stop taking drug now	Call doctor now
	Common	Rare	Only if severe	In all cases		
Muscle cramps	●		■			
Lethargy		●	■			
Dizziness		●	■			
Digestive disturbance		●	■			
Temporary impotence		●	■			
Rash		●		■	▲	

INTERACTIONS

Non-steroidal anti-inflammatory drugs (NSAIDs) Some NSAIDs may reduce the diuretic effect of hydrochlorothiazide, whose dosage may need to be adjusted.

Digoxin Adverse effects may be increased if excessive potassium is lost.

Corticosteroids These drugs further increase loss of potassium from the body when taken with hydrochlorothiazide.

Lithium Hydrochlorothiazide may increase lithium levels in the blood, leading to a risk of serious *adverse effects*.

PROLONGED USE

Excessive loss of potassium and imbalances of other salts may result.

Monitoring Blood tests may be performed periodically to check kidney function and levels of potassium and other salts.

HYDROCORTISONE

Brand names Colifoam, Corlan, Dioderm, Efcortelan, Efcortesol, Hydrocortistab, Hydrocortisyl, Hydrocortone, Solu-Cortef
Used in the following combined preparations Alphaderm, Tarcortin, Xyloproct, and many others

GENERAL INFORMATION

Hydrocortisone is chemically identical to the hormone cortisol, which is produced by the adrenal glands. For this reason, the drug is prescribed to replace natural hormones in adrenal insufficiency (Addison's disease).

The main use of hydrocortisone is in the treatment of a variety of allergic and inflammatory conditions. Used in *topical* preparations, it provides prompt relief from inflammation of the skin, eye, and outer ear. Hydrocortisone is used in oral form to relieve asthma, inflammatory bowel disease, and many rheumatic and allergic disorders. Injected directly into the joints, the drug relieves pain and stiffness (see p.118). Injections may also be given to relieve severe attacks of asthma.

Overuse of skin preparations with hydrocortisone can lead to permanent thinning of the skin. Taken by mouth, long-term treatment with high doses may cause serious *side effects*.

INFORMATION FOR USERS

Your drug prescription is tailored for you. Do not alter dosage without checking with your doctor.

How taken

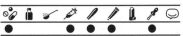

Tablets, lozenges, injection, rectal foam, cream, ointment, eye ointment/drops.

Frequency and timing of doses
Varies according to condition.

Dosage range
Varies according to condition.

Onset of effect
Within 1–4 days.

Duration of action
Up to 12 hours.

Diet advice
Salt intake may need to be restricted when the drug is taken by mouth. It may also be necessary to take potassium supplements.

Storage
Keep in a closed container in a cool, dry place out of the reach of children.

Missed dose
Take as soon as you remember. If your next dose is due within 2 hours, take a single dose now and skip the next.

Stopping the drug
Do not stop taking the drug without consulting your doctor. A gradual reduction in dosage is required following prolonged treatment with oral hydrocortisone.

Exceeding the dose
An occasional unintentional extra dose is unlikely to be a cause for concern. But if you notice any unusual symptoms, or if a large overdose has been taken, notify your doctor.

SPECIAL PRECAUTIONS

Be sure to tell your doctor if:
▼ You have liver or kidney problems.
▼ You have had a peptic ulcer.
▼ You have had a mental illness or epilepsy.
▼ You have glaucoma.
▼ You have had tuberculosis.
▼ You have diabetes or heart problems.
▼ You are taking other medications.

Avoid exposure to chickenpox, shingles, or measles if you are on systemic treatment.

Pregnancy
▼ No evidence of risk with topical preparations. Oral doses may adversely affect the developing baby. Discuss with your doctor.

Breast-feeding
▼ The drug passes into the breast milk and may affect the baby. Discuss with your doctor.

Infants and children
▼ Reduced dose necessary.

Over 60
▼ Reduced dose may be necessary.

Driving and hazardous work
▼ No special problems.

Alcohol
▼ Avoid. Alcohol may increase the risk of peptic ulcer when this drug is taken by mouth.

POSSIBLE ADVERSE EFFECTS

The most serious adverse effects only occur when hydrocortisone is taken by mouth in high doses for long periods of time. These are carefully monitored during treatment.

Symptom/effect	Frequency		Discuss with doctor		Stop taking drug now	Call doctor now
	Common	Rare	Only if severe	In all cases		
Indigestion	●		■			
Weight gain	●		■			
Acne	●		■			
Fluid retention		●		■		
Muscle weakness		●		■		
Mood changes		●		■		

INTERACTIONS (by mouth only)

Barbiturates, anticonvulsants, and rifampicin These drugs reduce the effectiveness of hydrocortisone.

Antidiabetic drugs Hydrocortisone reduces the action of these drugs.

Antihypertensive drugs Hydrocortisone reduces the effects of these drugs.

Vaccines Severe reactions can occur if this drug is taken with certain vaccines.

PROLONGED USE

Depending on method of administration, prolonged high dosage may cause diabetes, glaucoma, fragile bones, and thin skin, and may retard growth in children. People on long-term treatment are advised to carry a treatment card.

Monitoring Periodic checks on blood pressure are usually required when the drug is taken by mouth.

HYOSCINE

Brand names Buscopan, Joy-Rides, Kwells, Scopoderm TTS, Travel Calm
Used in the following combined preparation Papaveretum and hyoscine

GENERAL INFORMATION

Originally derived from the henbane plant, hyoscine is an *anticholinergic* drug that has both an *antispasmodic* effect on the intestine and a calming action on the nerve pathways that control nausea and vomiting. By its anticholinergic action, hyoscine also dilates the pupil.

The drug is produced in two forms. Hyoscine butylbromide is prescribed to reduce spasm of the gastrointestinal tract in irritable bowel syndrome. The other form, hyoscine hydrobromide, is used to control motion sickness and the giddiness and nausea caused by disturbances of the inner ear (see Vertigo and Ménière's disease, p.90) and can be administered as skin patches as well as in tablets. This form is also used as a *premedication* to dry secretions before operations. Eye drops containing the hydrobromide form are used to dilate the pupil during eye examinations and eye surgery.

INFORMATION FOR USERS

Follow instructions on the label. Call your doctor if symptoms worsen.

How taken

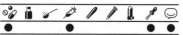

Tablets, injection, eye drops, skin patches.

Frequency and timing of doses
As required up to 4 x daily by mouth (irritable bowel syndrome) or up to 3 x daily (nausea and vomiting); every 3 days (patches).

Adult dosage range
Irritable bowel syndrome 80mg (hyoscine butylbromide) daily.
Nausea and vomiting 0.3mg (hyoscine hydrobromide) per dose.

Onset of effect
Within 1 hour.

Duration of action
Up to 6 hours (by mouth); up to 72 hours (patches).

Diet advice
None.

Storage
Keep in a closed container in a cool, dry place out of the reach of children. Protect from light.

Missed dose
Take when you remember. Adjust the timing of your next dose accordingly.

Stopping the drug
Can be safely stopped as soon as you no longer need it.

Exceeding the dose
An occasional unintentional extra dose is unlikely to cause problems. Large overdoses may cause drowsiness or agitation. Notify your doctor.

POSSIBLE ADVERSE EFFECTS

Taken by mouth or by injection, hyoscine has a strong anticholinergic effect on the body, causing a variety of minor symptoms. These can sometimes be minimized by a reduction in dosage.

Symptom/effect	Frequency		Discuss with doctor		Stop taking drug now	Call doctor now
	Common	Rare	Only if severe	In all cases		
Drowsiness	●		■			
Dry mouth	●		■			
Blurred vision	●			■		
Constipation		●	■			
Difficulty in passing urine		●		■		
Increase in heart rate		●		■		

INTERACTIONS

Sedatives All drugs that have a sedative effect on the central nervous system are likely to increase the sedative properties of hyoscine. Such drugs include anti-anxiety and sleeping drugs, antidepressants, *opioid* analgesics, and antipsychotics.

Anticholinergic drugs Many drugs have either anticholinergic or antimuscarinic effects. Using one of these drugs with hyoscine will increase *side effects* such as dry mouth, difficulty in passing urine, and constipation.

SPECIAL PRECAUTIONS

Be sure to consult your doctor or pharmacist before taking this drug if:
▼ You have long-term liver or kidney problems.
▼ You have heart problems.
▼ You have myasthenia gravis.
▼ You have megacolon or intestinal obstruction problems.
▼ You have had glaucoma.
▼ You have prostate trouble or urinary retention.
▼ You are taking other medications.

 Pregnancy
▼ Safety in pregnancy not established. Discuss with your doctor.

 Breast-feeding
▼ No evidence of risk. Discuss with your doctor.

 Infants and children
▼ Not recommended under 6 years. Reduced dose necessary in older children.

 Over 60
▼ Reduced dose may be necessary.

 Driving and hazardous work
▼ Avoid such activities until you have learned how hyoscine affects you because the drug can cause drowsiness and blurred vision.

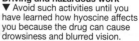 **Alcohol**
▼ Avoid. Alcohol may increase the sedative effect of this drug.

PROLONGED USE

Use of this drug for longer than a few days is unlikely to be necessary.

IBUPROFEN

Brand names Arthrofen, Brufen, Ebufac, Fenbid, Ibufac, Ibugel, Ibuleve, Inoven, Motrin, Nurofen, and many others
Used in the following combined preparation Codafen

GENERAL INFORMATION

Ibuprofen is a non-steroidal anti-inflammatory drug (NSAID) which, like other NSAIDs, reduces pain, stiffness, and inflammation. It is an effective treatment for the symptoms of osteoarthritis, rheumatoid arthritis, and gout. In the treatment of rheumatoid arthritis, ibuprofen may be prescribed with slower-acting drugs. It is also used to relieve mild to moderate headache, menstrual and dental pain, pain resulting from soft tissue injuries, or the pain that may follow an operation.

Ibuprofen has fewer *side effects* than many of the other NSAIDs. Unlike aspirin, it rarely causes bleeding in the stomach. Ibuprofen is also available as a cream or gel that can be applied to the skin for muscular aches and sprains.

QUICK REFERENCE

Drug group Analgesic (p.80) and non-steroidal anti-inflammatory drug (p.116)

Overdose danger rating Low

Dependence rating Low

Prescription needed No

Available as generic Yes

INFORMATION FOR USERS

Follow instructions on the label. Call your doctor if symptoms worsen.

How taken

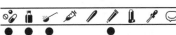

Tablets, SR-tablets, capsules, liquid, granules, cream, gel.

Frequency and timing of doses
1–2 x daily for SR-tablets or 4–6 x daily (general pain relief); 3–4 x daily with food (arthritis).

Adult dosage range
General pain relief 600mg–1.8g daily.
Arthritis 1.2–2.4g daily.

Onset of effect
Pain relief begins in 1–2 hours. The full anti-inflammatory effect in arthritic conditions may not be felt for up to 2 weeks.

Duration of action
5–10 hours.

Diet advice
None.

Storage
Keep in a closed container in a cool, dry place out of the reach of children.

Missed dose
Take as soon as you remember. If your next dose is due within 2 hours, take a single dose now and skip the next.

Stopping the drug
When taken for short-term pain relief, the drug can be safely stopped as soon as you no longer need it. If prescribed for the long-term treatment of arthritis, however, you should seek medical advice before stopping the drug.

Exceeding the dose
An occasional unintentional extra dose is unlikely to be a cause for concern. But if you notice any unusual symptoms, or if a large overdose has been taken, notify your doctor.

SPECIAL PRECAUTIONS

Be sure to consult your doctor or pharmacist before taking this drug if:
▼ You have a long-term kidney problem.
▼ You have a long-term liver problem.
▼ You have high blood pressure.
▼ You have had a peptic ulcer, oesophagitis, or acid indigestion.
▼ You are allergic to aspirin.
▼ You have asthma.
▼ You are taking other medications.

 Pregnancy
▼ Not usually prescribed. May affect the unborn baby and may prolong labour. Discuss with your doctor.

 Breast-feeding
▼ The drug passes into the breast milk, but at normal doses adverse effects on the baby are unlikely. Discuss with your doctor.

 Infants and children
▼ Reduced dose necessary.

 Over 60
▼ Reduced dose may be necessary.

 Driving and hazardous work
▼ No problems expected.

 Alcohol
▼ Avoid. Alcohol may increase the risk of stomach disorders with ibuprofen.

Surgery and general anaesthetics
▼ Ibuprofen may prolong bleeding. Discuss the possibility of stopping treatment temporarily with your doctor or dentist.

POSSIBLE ADVERSE EFFECTS

The most common adverse effects are the result of gastrointestinal disturbances. Black or bloodstained faeces should be reported to your doctor without delay.

Symptom/effect	Frequency		Discuss with doctor		Stop taking drug now	Call doctor now
	Common	Rare	Only if severe	In all cases		
Heartburn/indigestion	●			■		
Nausea/vomiting		●		■		
Rash		●	■		▲	
Wheezing/breathlessness		●	■		▲	∎
Black/bloodstained faeces		●	■		▲	∎
Swollen feet and ankles		●	■			
Ringing in the ears		●	■			

INTERACTIONS

General note Ibuprofen interacts with a wide range of drugs to increase the risk of bleeding and/or peptic ulcers. Such drugs include other non-steroidal anti-inflammatory drugs (NSAIDs), aspirin, oral anticoagulants, and corticosteroids.

Ciprofloxacin This drug and related antibiotics may increase the risk of seizures.

Antihypertensive drugs and diuretics The beneficial effects of these drugs may be reduced by ibuprofen.

Lithium Ibuprofen may raise blood levels of lithium.

Methotrexate Ibuprofen may raise blood levels of methotrexate.

PROLONGED USE

There is an increased risk of bleeding from peptic ulcers and in the bowel with prolonged use of ibuprofen.

IMIPRAMINE

Brand name Tofranil
Used in the following combined preparations None

GENERAL INFORMATION

Imipramine belongs to the tricyclic class of antidepressant drugs. The drug is used mainly in the long-term treatment of depression to elevate mood, improve appetite, increase physical activity, and restore interest in everyday life. Because imipramine is less sedating than some other antidepressants, it is particularly useful when a depressed person is withdrawn or apathetic, although it can aggravate insomnia if it is taken in the evening.

Imipramine is also prescribed to treat night-time enuresis (bedwetting) in children, although proof of its benefit is not conclusive. Imipramine can cause a variety of *side effects*. In overdose the drug may cause coma and dangerous heart rhythms.

QUICK REFERENCE

Drug group Tricyclic anti-depressant (p.84) and drug for urinary disorders (p.166)

Overdose danger rating High

Dependence rating Low

Prescription needed Yes

Available as generic Yes

INFORMATION FOR USERS

Your drug prescription is tailored for you. Do not alter dosage without checking with your doctor.

How taken

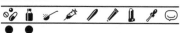

Tablets, liquid.

Frequency and timing of doses
1–4 x daily.

Dosage range
Adults Usually 75–200mg daily.
Children Reduced dose according to age and weight.

Onset of effect
Some benefits and effects may appear within hours, but full antidepressant effect may not be felt for 2–6 weeks.

Duration of action
Following prolonged treatment, antidepressant effect may persist for up to 6 weeks. Any adverse effects may wear off within days.

Diet advice
None.

Storage
Keep in a closed container in a cool, dry place out of the reach of children.

Missed dose
Take as soon as you remember. If your next dose is due within 3 hours, take a single dose now and skip the next.

Stopping the drug
Do not stop taking the drug without consulting your doctor, who will supervise a gradual reduction in dosage. Stopping abruptly may cause withdrawal symptoms.

OVERDOSE ACTION

Seek immediate medical advice in all cases. Take emergency action if consciousness is lost.

See Drug poisoning emergency guide (p.494).

POSSIBLE ADVERSE EFFECTS

The possible adverse effects of this drug are mainly the result of its *anticholinergic* action and its effect on the normal rhythm of the heart.

Symptom/effect	Frequency		Discuss with doctor		Stop taking drug now	Call doctor now
	Common	Rare	Only if severe	In all cases		
Sweating/flushing	●		■			
Dry mouth/constipation	●		■			
Blurred vision	●			■		
Dizziness/drowsiness		●		■		
Rash		●		■	▲	
Palpitations		●		■	▲	■

INTERACTIONS

Sedatives Imipramine may increase the effects of sedative drugs.

Monoamine oxidase inhibitors (MAOIs) There is a possibility of a serious interaction. Such drugs are prescribed with imipramine only under strict supervision.

Antihypertensive drugs Imipramine may reduce the effectiveness of these drugs.

Phenytoin Imipramine may increase levels of phenytoin.

Terfenadine, amiodarone, sotalol, and cisapride These drugs may increase the risk of abnormal heart rhythms.

SPECIAL PRECAUTIONS

Be sure to tell your doctor if:
▼ You have had heart problems.
▼ You have long-term liver or kidney problems.
▼ You have had epileptic fits.
▼ You have had glaucoma.
▼ You have prostate trouble.
▼ You have had mania or a psychotic illness.
▼ You are taking other medications.

 Pregnancy
▼ Safety in pregnancy not established. Discuss with your doctor.

 Breast-feeding
▼ The drug passes into the breast milk, but at normal doses adverse effects on the baby are unlikely. Discuss with your doctor.

 Infants and children
▼ Not recommended under 7 years. Reduced dose necessary in older children.

 Over 60
▼ Increased likelihood of adverse effects. Reduced dose may therefore be necessary.

 Driving and hazardous work
▼ Avoid such activities until you have learned how imipramine affects you because the drug can cause reduced alertness and blurred vision.

 Alcohol
▼ Avoid. Alcohol may increase the sedative effect of imipramine.

Surgery and general anaesthetics
▼ Imipramine treatment may need to be stopped before you have a general anaesthetic. Discuss this with your doctor or dentist before any operation.

PROLONGED USE

No problems expected. Imipramine is not usually prescribed for children as a treatment for bedwetting for longer than three months.

INDAPAMIDE

Brand names Natramid, Natrilix, Nindaxa, Opumide,
Used in the following combined preparations None

GENERAL INFORMATION

Indapamide is a drug related in its effects and uses to the thiazide diuretic group of drugs, but it is used to treat hypertension (high blood pressure).

The drug prevents the hormone norepinephrine (noradrenaline) from constricting blood vessels, thereby allowing them to dilate.

Indapamide is sometimes combined with other antihypertensive drugs but not with other diuretics.

Indapamide's diuretic effects are slight at low doses, but susceptible people need to have their blood levels of potassium and uric acid monitored. These include the elderly, those taking digitalis drugs, or those with gout or hyperaldosteronism (overproduction of the hormone aldosterone).

Unlike the thiazides, indapamide does not affect control of diabetes.

QUICK REFERENCE

Drug group Diuretic (p.99)
Overdose danger rating Low
Dependence rating Low
Prescription needed Yes
Available as generic Yes

INFORMATION FOR USERS

Your drug prescription is tailored for you. Do not alter dosage without checking with your doctor.

How taken

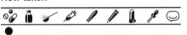

Tablets, SR-tablets.

Frequency and timing of doses
Once daily in the morning.

Adult dosage range
1.5–2.5mg.

Onset of effect
1–2 hours, but the full effect may not be felt for several months.

Duration of action
12–24 hours.

Diet advice
None.

Storage
Keep in a closed container in a cool, dry place out of the reach of children.

Missed dose
Take as soon as you remember. If your next dose is due within 4 hours, take a single dose now and skip the next.

Stopping the drug
Do not stop taking the drug without consulting your doctor; high blood pressure may return.

Exceeding the dose
An occasional unintentional extra dose is unlikely to cause problems. But if you notice any unusual symptoms, or if a large overdose has been taken, notify your doctor.

SPECIAL PRECAUTIONS

Be sure to tell your doctor if:
▼ You have had a stroke.
▼ You have liver or kidney problems.
▼ You have gout.
▼ You have hyperaldosteronism or hyperparathyroidism.
▼ You are allergic to sulphonamide drugs.
▼ You are taking digitalis drugs.
▼ You are taking other medications.

 Pregnancy
▼ Safety not established. Discuss with your doctor.

 Breast-feeding
▼ Safety not established. Discuss with your doctor.

 Infants and children
▼ Not prescribed.

 Over 60
▼ No special problems.

 Driving and hazardous work
▼ No special problems.

 Alcohol
▼ No special problems.

POSSIBLE ADVERSE EFFECTS

Headaches and muscle cramps are common, but other symptoms rarely cause problems.

Symptom/effect	Frequency		Discuss with doctor		Stop taking drug now	Call doctor now
	Common	Rare	Only if severe	In all cases		
Headache/dizziness	●		■			
Fatigue/muscle cramps	●		■			
Diarrhoea/constipation		●	■			
Skin rash		●		■		
Palpitations/fainting		●		■		
Jaundice		●		■		
Sore throat		●		■		
Tingling/"pins and needles"		●		■		
Impotence		●		■		

INTERACTIONS

Diuretics There is a risk of imbalance of salts in the blood if these drugs are taken with indapamide.

Digitalis drugs Loss of potassium may lead to *toxicity* of these drugs with indapamide.

Lithium Blood levels of lithium are increased when it is taken with indapamide.

Antiarrhythmic drugs Loss of potassium may make these drugs less effective if they are taken with indapamide.

PROLONGED USE

Long-term use of indapamide may lead to potassium loss in the elderly and certain other groups.

Monitoring Blood potassium and uric acid levels may be checked periodically.

INDORAMIN

Brand names Baratol, Doralese
Used in the following combined preparations None

GENERAL INFORMATION

Indoramin is a selective alpha blocker drug used to treat hypertension (high blood pressure). It works by relaxing the muscles in the blood vessel walls, dilating (widening) them, thereby easing the flow of blood. Indoramin may be combined with other antihypertensive drugs to achieve better control.

Indoramin is also used, in lower doses, to relieve urinary retention caused by an enlarged prostate gland.

The drug works by relaxing the muscle of the prostate, enabling urine to be passed more easily. Because indoramin can initially cause a rapid fall in blood pressure, the first dose is usually low, and should be taken lying down. The drug can also cause drowsiness at the start of treatment and whenever dosage is increased. If unequal sized daily doses are taken, the largest dose is usually prescribed for bedtime.

QUICK REFERENCE

Drug group Antihypertensive drug (p.102) and drug for urinary retention (p.166)

Overdose danger rating Medium

Dependence rating Low

Prescription needed Yes

Available as generic No

INFORMATION FOR USERS

Your drug prescription is tailored for you. Do not alter dosage without checking with your doctor.

How taken

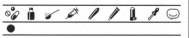

Tablets.

Frequency and timing of doses
Hypertension 2–3 x daily.
Urinary retention: 1–2 x daily.

Adult dosage range
Hypertension 25mg (starting dose), increased if necessary at 2-week intervals. Maximum daily dose 200mg.
Urinary retention 20mg (starting dose), increased if necessary at 2-week intervals. Maximum daily dose 100mg.

Onset of effect
1 hour.

Duration of action
6–12 hours.

Diet advice
None.

Storage
Keep in a closed container in a cool, dry place out of the reach of children.

Missed dose
Take as soon as you remember. If your next dose is due within 2 hours, take a single dose now and skip the next.

Stopping the drug
Do not stop taking the drug without consulting your doctor. Stopping the drug may lead to worsening of the underlying condition.

Exceeding the dose
An occasional unintentional extra dose is unlikely to be a cause for concern. Large overdoses may produce deep sedation and fits. Notify your doctor immediately.

POSSIBLE ADVERSE EFFECTS

Drowsiness and dizziness are the most common *adverse effects*. They are often worse at the start of treatment or following an increase in dosage.

Symptom/effect	Frequency		Discuss with doctor		Stop taking drug now	Call doctor now
	Common	Rare	Only if severe	In all cases		
Drowsiness	●		■			
Dizziness	●		■			
Dry mouth/nasal congestion		●	■			
Headache		●	■			
Fatigue		●	■			
Depression		●			■	
Tremor, abnormal movements		●			■	

INTERACTIONS

Antidepressants, beta-blockers, calcium channel blockers, diuretics, thymoxamine These drugs increase the blood-pressure lowering effect of indoramin.

SPECIAL PRECAUTIONS

Be sure to tell your doctor if:
▼ You have liver or kidney problems.
▼ You have Parkinson's disease.
▼ You have epilepsy.
▼ You have heart failure.
▼ You have a history of depression.
▼ You are taking an MAOI drug.
▼ You are taking other medications.

Pregnancy
▼ Safety not established. Discuss with your doctor.

Breast-feeding
▼ Safety not established. Discuss with your doctor.

Infants and children
▼ Not recommended.

Over 60
▼ Reduced dose may be necessary.

Driving and hazardous work
▼ Avoid such activities until you have learned how indoramin affects you because the drug can cause drowsiness and dizziness.

Alcohol
▼ Avoid. Alcohol increases the amount of indoramin absorbed, which increases its sedative effects.

Surgery and general anaesthetics
▼ Anaesthesia may increase the blood-pressure lowering effect of indoramin. Discuss this with your doctor or dentist before surgery.

PROLONGED USE

No special problems.

INSULIN

Brand names Humalog, Human Actrapid, Human Insulatard, Human Mixtard, Human Monotard, Human Ultratard, Human Velosulin, Humulin, Hypurin, Lentard MC, Pork Insulatard, Pork Mixtard, Pork Velosulin, and others

GENERAL INFORMATION

Insulin is a hormone manufactured by the pancreas and vital to the body's ability to use sugar. It is given by injection to supplement or replace natural insulin in the treatment of diabetes mellitus. It is the only effective treatment in juvenile (insulin-dependent or Type 1) diabetes and may also be prescribed in adult (maturity-onset or Type 2) diabetes. Insulin should be used with a carefully controlled diet. Illness, vomiting, or alterations in diet or in exercise levels may require dosage adjustment.

Insulin is available in a wide variety of preparations, which can be short-, medium-, or long-acting. Combinations of these types are often given. People receiving insulin should carry a warning card or tag.

INFORMATION FOR USERS

Your drug prescription is tailored for you. Do not alter dosage without checking with your doctor.

How taken

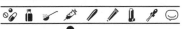

Injection, infusion pump.

Frequency and timing of doses
1–4 x daily. Short-acting insulin is usually given 15–30 minutes before meals. However, the exact time of these injections and the times of administration for longer-acting preparations will be tailored to your individual needs; follow the instructions you are given.

Dosage range
The dose (and type) of insulin is determined according to the needs of the individual.

Onset of effect
30–60 minutes (short-acting); 1–2 hours (medium- and long-acting).

Duration of action
6–8 hours (short-acting); 18–26 hours (medium-acting); 28–36 hours (long-acting).

Diet advice
A low-carbohydrate diet is necessary. Follow your doctor's advice.

Storage
Refrigerate, but do not freeze. Follow the instructions on the container.

Missed dose
Discuss with your doctor. Appropriate action depends on dose and type of insulin.

Stopping the drug
Do not stop taking the drug without consulting your doctor; confusion and coma may occur.

OVERDOSE ACTION

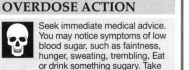

Seek immediate medical advice. You may notice symptoms of low blood sugar, such as faintness, hunger, sweating, trembling, Eat or drink something sugary. Take emergency action if fits or loss of consciousness occur.

See Drug poisoning emergency guide (p.494).

SPECIAL PRECAUTIONS

Be sure to tell your doctor if:
▼ You have had a previous allergic reaction to insulin.
▼ You are taking other medications, or your other drug treatment is changed.

Pregnancy
▼ No evidence of risk to the developing baby from insulin, but poor control of diabetes increases the risk of birth defects. Careful monitoring is required.

Breast-feeding
▼ No evidence of risk. Adjustment in dose may be necessary while breast-feeding.

Infants and children
▼ Reduced dose necessary.

Over 60
▼ No special problems.

Driving and hazardous work
▼ Usually no problem, but strenuous exercise alters your insulin and sugar requirements. Avoid these activities if you have warning signs of low blood sugar.

Alcohol
▼ Avoid. Alcoholic drinks upset diabetic control.

Surgery and general anaesthetics
▼ Insulin requirements may increase during surgery, and blood glucose levels will need to be monitored during and after an operation. Notify your doctor or dentist that you are diabetic before any surgery.

POSSIBLE ADVERSE EFFECTS

Symptoms such as dizziness, sweating, weakness, and confusion indicate low blood sugar. Serious allergic reactions (rash, swelling, and shortness of breath) are rare.

Symptom/effect	Frequency		Discuss with doctor		Stop taking drug now	Call doctor now
	Common	Rare	Only if severe	In all cases		
Injection-site irritation	●			■		
Weakness/sweating	●			■		
Dimpling at injection site		●		■		
Rash/facial swelling		●		■		▮
Shortness of breath		●		■		▮
Eyesight problems		●		■		

INTERACTIONS

General note 1 Many drugs, including some antibiotics, monoamine oxidase inhibitors (MAOIs), and oral antidiabetic drugs, increase the risk of low blood sugar.

Corticosteroids and diuretics may oppose the effect of insulin.

General note 2 Check with your doctor or pharmacist before taking any medicines; some contain sugar and may upset control of diabetes.

Beta blockers may affect insulin needs and mask signs of low blood sugar.

PROLONGED USE

No problems expected.

Monitoring Regular monitoring of levels of sugar in the urine and/or blood is required.

INTERFERON

Brand names Betaferon, Immukin, Intron-A, Roferon-A, Viraferon, Wellferon, Avonex, Rebif
Used in the following combined preparations None

GENERAL INFORMATION

Interferons are a group of substances produced in human and animal cells that have been infected with viruses or stimulated by other substances. They are thought to promote resistance to several types of viral infection (see p.127). Three main types of interferon (alpha, beta, and gamma) are used to treat a range of diseases. Interferon alpha is used for leukaemias, other cancers, and chronic active hepatitis B. Interferon beta reduces the frequency and severity of relapses in multiple sclerosis. Interferon gamma is prescribed in conjunction with antibiotics for patients suffering from chronic granulomatous disease.

Interferons can cause severe *adverse effects* (see below).

INFORMATION FOR USERS

This drug is given only under medical supervision and is not for self-administration.

How taken

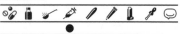

Injection.

Frequency and timing of doses
Once daily or on alternate days.

Adult dosage range
The dosage is calculated taking account of the body surface area of the patient and the condition being treated.

Onset of effect
Active inside the body within 1 hour, but effects may not be noted for 1–2 months.

Duration of action
Effects last for about 12 hours.

Diet advice
None.

Storage
Store in a refrigerator at 2–8°C (36–46°F). Do not let it freeze, and protect from light. Keep out of the reach of children.

Missed dose
Not applicable. This drug is usually given only in hospital under close medical supervision.

Stopping the drug
Discuss with your doctor.

Exceeding the dose
Overdosage is unlikely since treatment is carefully monitored.

SPECIAL PRECAUTIONS

Be sure to tell your doctor if:
▼ You have long-term liver or kidney problems.
▼ You have heart disease.
▼ You have had epileptic fits.
▼ You have previously suffered allergic reactions to any drugs.
▼ You have had asthma or eczema.
▼ You suffer from depression.
▼ You are taking other medications.

 Pregnancy
▼ Not usually prescribed. Safety in pregnancy not established. Discuss with your doctor.

 Breast-feeding
▼ It is not known whether the drug passes into the breast milk. Discuss with your doctor.

 Infants and children
▼ Not usually used.

 Over 60
▼ Increased likelihood of adverse effects. Reduced dose may be necessary.

Driving and hazardous work
▼ Not applicable.

 Alcohol
▼ Avoid. Alcohol may increase the sedative effects of this drug.

POSSIBLE ADVERSE EFFECTS

The symptoms listed below are the most common problems. All unusual symptoms should be brought to your doctor's attention without delay. Some of these symptoms are dose-related, and a reduction in dosage may be necessary to eliminate them.

Symptom/effect	Frequency		Discuss with doctor		Stop taking drug now	Call doctor now
	Common	Rare	Only if severe	In all cases		
Headache	●		■			
Lethargy/depression	●		■			
Dizziness/drowsiness	●			■		
Digestive disturbances	●			■		
Chills, fever, muscle-ache	●			■		
Hair loss		●		■		
Poor appetite and weight loss	●			■		

INTERACTIONS

General note A number of drugs increase the risk of adverse effects on the blood, heart, or nervous system. This is taken into account when prescribing an interferon with other drugs.

Vaccines Interferon may reduce the effectiveness of vaccines.

Theophylline/aminophylline The effects of this drug may be enhanced by interferon.

Sedatives All drugs that have a sedative effect on the central nervous system are likely to increase the sedative properties of interferons. Such drugs include *opioid* analgesics, anti-anxiety and sleeping drugs, antihistamines, antidepressants, and antipsychotics.

PROLONGED USE

There may be an increased risk of liver damage. Blood cell production in the bone marrow may be reduced. Repeated large doses are associated with lethargy, fatigue, collapse, and coma.

Monitoring Frequent blood tests are required to monitor blood composition and liver function.

IPRATROPIUM BROMIDE

Brand names Atrovent, Rinatec, Respontin
Used in the following combined preparations Combivent, Duovent

GENERAL INFORMATION

Ipratropium bromide is an *anticholinergic* bronchodilator that relaxes the muscles surrounding the bronchioles (airways in the lung). It is used primarily in the maintenance treatment of reversible airway disorders, particularly chronic bronchitis. It is given only by inhaler or via a nebulizer for these conditions. Although its effect lasts longer, the drug has a slower onset of action than the *sympathomimetic* bronchodilators. For this reason, it is not as effective in treating acute attacks of wheezing, or

in the emergency treatment of asthma, and it is usually used together with the faster-acting drugs. Ipratropium bromide is also prescribed as a nasal spray for the treatment of a continually runny nose due to allergy.

Unlike other anticholinergic drugs, *side effects* are rare. It is not likely to affect the heart, eyes, bowel, or bladder. Ipratropium bromide must be used with caution by people with glaucoma, but problems are unlikely at normal doses.

QUICK REFERENCE

Drug group Bronchodilator (p.92)
Overdose danger rating Low
Dependence rating Low
Prescription needed Yes
Available as generic Yes

INFORMATION FOR USERS

Your drug prescription is tailored for you. Do not alter dosage without checking with your doctor.

How taken

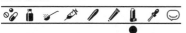

Inhaler, nasal spray, liquid for nebulizer.

Frequency and timing of doses
3–4 x daily.

Adult dosage range
80–320mcg daily (inhaler); 400–2,000mcg daily (nebulizer); 1–2 puffs to the affected nostril 2–3 x daily (nasal spray).

Onset of effect
5–15 minutes.

Duration of action
Up to 8 hours.

Diet advice
None.

Storage
Keep in a cool, dry place out of the reach of children. Do not puncture or burn containers.

Missed dose
Take as soon as you remember. If your next dose is due within 2 hours, take a single dose now and skip the next.

Stopping the drug
Do not stop taking the drug without consulting your doctor; symptoms may recur.

Exceeding the dose
An occasional unintentional extra dose is unlikely to be a cause for concern. But if you notice any unusual symptoms, or if a large overdose has been taken, notify your doctor.

POSSIBLE ADVERSE EFFECTS

Side effects are rare. The most common is dry mouth or throat.

Symptom/effect	Frequency		Discuss with doctor		Stop taking drug now	Call doctor now
	Common	Rare	Only if severe	In all cases		
Dry mouth/throat	●		■			
Constipation		●	■			
Urinary hesitancy		●	■			

INTERACTIONS

None.

SPECIAL PRECAUTIONS

Be sure to tell your doctor if:
▼ You have glaucoma.
▼ You have prostate problems.
▼ You have difficulty in passing urine.
▼ You are taking other medications.

Pregnancy
▼ No evidence of risk, but discuss with your doctor before using in the first 3 months of pregnancy.

Breast-feeding
▼ No evidence of risk, but discuss with your doctor.

Infants and children
▼ Reduced dose necessary.

Over 60
▼ No special problems.

Driving and hazardous work
▼ No special problems.

Alcohol
▼ No known problems.

PROLONGED USE

No special problems.

IRBESARTAN

Brand name Aprovel
Used in the following combined preparations None

GENERAL INFORMATION

Irbesartan is a member of the group of vasodilator drugs called angiotensin-II blockers. Used to treat hypertension, the drug works by blocking the action of angiotensin-II (a naturally occurring substance that constricts blood vessels). This action causes the blood vessel walls to relax, thereby lowering blood pressure.

Unlike ACE inhibitors, irbesartan does not cause a persistent dry cough.

Along with other angiotensin-II blockers, it is being evaluated for the treatment of other conditions, such as heart failure, for which ACE inhibitors are used.

Irbesartan is prescribed with caution to people with stenosis (narrowing) of the arteries to the kidneys because the initial dose causes a sudden drop in blood pressure. It is important to notify your doctor if you know that you have this condition.

QUICK REFERENCE

Drug group Vasodilator (p.98) and antihypertensive drug (p.102)

Overdose danger rating Medium

Dependence rating Low

Prescription needed Yes

Available as generic No

INFORMATION FOR USERS

Your drug prescription is tailored for you. Do not alter dosage without checking with your doctor.

How taken

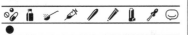

Tablets.

Frequency and timing of doses
Once daily.

Adult dosage range
150–300mg, but 75mg may be used in people over 75 years.

Onset of effect
Within 1 hour. Blood pressure is lowered within 1–2 weeks, and maximum beneficial effect is felt 4–6 weeks from start of treatment.

Duration of action
24 hours.

Diet advice
None.

Storage
Keep in a closed container in a cool, dry place out of the reach of children.

Missed dose
Take as soon as you remember. If your next dose is due within 8 hours, take a single dose now and skip the next.

Stopping the drug
Do not stop the drug without consulting your doctor. Stopping the drug may lead to worsening of the high blood pressure.

Exceeding the dose
An occasional unintentional extra dose is unlikely to be a cause for concern. Large overdoses may cause dizziness and fainting. Notify your doctor.

SPECIAL PRECAUTIONS

Be sure to tell your doctor if:
▼ You have kidney problems or renal artery stenosis.
▼ You have heart problems.
▼ You have congestive heart failure.
▼ You have primary aldosteronism.
▼ You are taking other medications.

 Pregnancy
▼ Not prescribed.

 Breast-feeding
▼ Safety not established. Discuss with your doctor.

 Infants and children
▼ Not prescribed.

 Over 60
▼ Reduced dose may be necessary in people over 75 years.

 Driving and hazardous work
▼ Avoid such activities until you have learned how irbesartan affects you because the drug can cause dizziness and fatigue.

Alcohol
▼ Avoid. Regular intake of alcohol may raise the blood pressure and reduce the effectiveness of irbesartan. Alcohol may also increase the likelihood of an excessive fall in blood pressure.

POSSIBLE ADVERSE EFFECTS

Adverse effects are usually mild.

Symptom/effect	Frequency		Discuss with doctor		Stop taking drug now	Call doctor now
	Common	Rare	Only if severe	In all cases		
Dizziness/fatigue	●		■			
Flushing	●		■			
Headache		●	■			
Rash		●		■		

INTERACTIONS

Diuretics There is a risk of a sudden fall in blood pressure if these drugs are being taken when irbesartan treatment is started.

Potassium supplements, potassium-sparing diuretics, and cyclosporin Irbesartan enhances the effect of these drugs, leading to raised levels of potassium in the blood.

Lithium Irbesartan increases the blood levels and *toxicity* of lithium.

NSAIDs Certain of these drugs may reduce the blood-pressure lowering effects of irbesartan.

PROLONGED USE

No special problems.

Monitoring
Periodic checks on blood potassium levels may be performed.

ISONIAZID

Brand names None
Used in the following combined preparations Rifater, Rifinah, Rimactazid

GENERAL INFORMATION

Isoniazid (also known as INAH and INH) has been in use for over 30 years and remains an effective drug for tuberculosis. It is given alone to prevent tuberculosis and in combination with other drugs for the treatment of the disease. Treatment usually lasts for six months. However, courses lasting nine months or a year may sometimes be prescribed.

One of the *side effects* of isoniazid is the increased loss of pyridoxine (vitamin B_6) from the body. This effect, which is more likely with high doses, is rare in children but common among people with poor nutrition. Since pyridoxine deficiency can lead to irreversible nerve damage, supplements are usually given.

INFORMATION FOR USERS

Your drug prescription is tailored for you. Do not alter dosage without checking with your doctor.

How taken

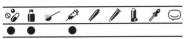

Tablets, liquid, injection.

Frequency and timing of doses
Normally once daily.

Dosage range
Adults 300mg daily.
Children According to age and weight.

Onset of effect
Over 2–3 days.

Duration of action
Up to 24 hours.

Diet advice
Isoniazid may deplete pyridoxine (vitamin B_6) levels in the body, so supplements are usually prescribed.

Storage
Keep in a closed container in a cool, dry place out of the reach of children. Protect from light.

Missed dose
Take as soon as you remember. If your next dose is scheduled within 8 hours, take a single dose now and skip the next.

Stopping the drug
Take the full course. Even if you feel better the infection may still be present and may recur if treatment is stopped too soon.

OVERDOSE ACTION

 Seek immediate medical advice in all cases. Take emergency action if breathing difficulties, fits, or loss of consciousness occur.

See Drug poisoning emergency guide (p.494).

SPECIAL PRECAUTIONS

Be sure to tell your doctor if:
▼ You have long-term liver or kidney problems.
▼ You have had liver damage following isoniazid treatment in the past.
▼ If you have problems with drugs or alcohol abuse.
▼ You have diabetes.
▼ You have had epileptic fits.
▼ You are taking other medications.

 Pregnancy
▼ Safety in pregnancy not established. Discuss with your doctor.

 Breast-feeding
▼ The drug passes into the breast milk and may affect the baby. The infant should be monitored for signs of toxic effects. Discuss with your doctor.

 Infants and children
▼ Reduced dose necessary.

 Over 60
▼ Increased likelihood of adverse effects.

 Driving and hazardous work
▼ No special problems.

Alcohol
▼ Avoid excessive amounts.

POSSIBLE ADVERSE EFFECTS

Although serious problems are uncommon, all adverse effects of this drug should receive prompt medical attention because of the possibility of nerve or liver damage.

Symptom/effect	Frequency		Discuss with doctor		Stop taking drug now	Call doctor now
	Common	Rare	Only if severe	In all cases		
Nausea/vomiting	●		■			
Fatigue/weakness	●			■		
Numbness/tingling	●			■		
Rash	●			■		
Blurred vision	●			■	▲	
Jaundice	●			■	▲	▌
Twitching/muscle weakness	●			■	▲	

INTERACTIONS

Alcohol and rifampicin Large quantities of alcohol may reduce the effectiveness of isoniazid. If the two are taken together, the likelihood of liver damage is increased; if rifampicin is also being taken, the likelihood is increased even further.

Anticonvulsants The effects of these drugs may be increased with isoniazid.

Antacids These drugs may reduce the absorption of isoniazid.

PROLONGED USE

Pyridoxine (vitamin B_6) deficiency may occur with prolonged use and lead to nerve damage. Supplements are usually prescribed. There is also a risk of serious liver damage.

Monitoring Periodic blood tests are usually performed to monitor liver function.

ISOSORBIDE DINITRATE/MONONITRATE

Brand names [Dinitrate] Cedocard, Isocard, Isoket, Isordil, Sorbichew, Sorbid SA, Sorbitrate; [Mononitrate] Elantan, Imdur, Isib 60XL, Ismo, Isotard, Isotrate, MCR-50, Modisal, Monit, Mono-Cedocard, Monomax, Monosorb
Used in the following combined preparation Imazin XL

GENERAL INFORMATION

Isosorbide dinitrate and mononitrate are vasodilator drugs similar to glyceryl trinitrate. They are usually used to treat patients suffering from angina, and are also used in some cases of heart failure.

Unlike glyceryl trinitrate, however, both forms of isosorbide are stable and can be stored for long periods without losing their effectiveness.

Headache, flushing, and dizziness are common *side effects* during the early stages of treatment; small initial doses of the drug minimize these symptoms. The effectiveness of isosorbide dinitrate and mononitrate may be reduced after a few months; if this occurs, an alternative treatment may need to be considered.

INFORMATION FOR USERS

Your drug prescription is tailored for you. Do not alter dosage without checking with your doctor.

How taken

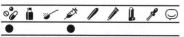

Dinitrate Tablets (held under the tongue, chewed, or swallowed), SR-tablets, SR-capsules, injection, spray.
Mononitrate Tablets, SR-tablets, SR-capsules.

Frequency and timing of doses
Relief of angina attacks Tablets chewed or held under the tongue, or spray, as needed (certain preparations only).
Prevention of angina 2–4 x daily; 1–2 x daily (SR-tablets, capsules).

Adult dosage range
Relief of angina attacks 5–10mg per dose.
Prevention of angina 30–120mg daily.

Onset of effect
2–3 minutes when chewed or held under the tongue or used as spray (certain preparations only); 30 minutes when swallowed.

Duration of action
Up to 2 hours (chewed); up to 5 hours (swallowed); up to 10 hours (SR-capsules).

Diet advice
None.

Storage
Keep in a closed container in a cool, dry place out of the reach of children. Protect from light.

Missed dose
Take as soon as you remember. If your next dose is due within 2 hours, take a single dose now and skip the next.

Stopping the drug
Do not stop taking the drug without consulting your doctor; stopping the drug may lead to worsening of the underlying condition.

Exceeding the dose
An occasional unintentional extra dose is unlikely to cause problems. Large overdoses may cause dizziness and headache. Notify your doctor.

SPECIAL PRECAUTIONS

Be sure to tell your doctor if:
▼ You have long-term liver or kidney problems.
▼ You have any blood disorders or anaemia.
▼ You have had glaucoma.
▼ You have low blood pressure.
▼ You have ever had a heart attack.
▼ You have an underactive thyroid.
▼ You are taking other medications.

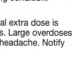

Pregnancy
▼ Safety in pregnancy not established. Discuss with your doctor.

Breast-feeding
▼ Safety not established. Discuss with your doctor.

Infants and children
▼ Not usually prescribed.

Over 60
▼ No special problems.

Driving and hazardous work
▼ Avoid such activities until you have learned how isosorbide dinitrate or mononitrate affects you because these drugs can cause dizziness.

Alcohol
▼ Avoid. Alcohol may further lower blood pressure, depressing the heart and causing dizziness and fainting.

POSSIBLE ADVERSE EFFECTS

The most serious adverse effect is excessively lowered blood pressure, and this may need to be monitored on a regular basis. Other adverse effects of both forms of the drug usually improve after regular use; dose adjustment may help.

Symptom/effect	Frequency		Discuss with doctor		Stop taking drug now	Call doctor now
	Common	Rare	Only if severe	In all cases		
Headache	●		■			
Flushing	●		■			
Dizziness	●			■		
Fainting/weakness		●		■		

INTERACTIONS

Antihypertensives A further lowering of blood pressure occurs when such drugs are taken with isosorbide dinitrate.

PROLONGED USE

The initial adverse effects may disappear with prolonged use. The effects of the drug become weaker as the body adapts, requiring increased dosage or other drugs.

ISOTRETINOIN

Brand names Isotrex, Roaccutane
Used in the following combined preparation Isotrexin

GENERAL INFORMATION

Isotretinoin, a drug that is chemically related to vitamin A, is prescribed for the treatment of severe acne that has failed to respond to other treatments.

The drug reduces production of the skin's natural oils (sebum) and of the horny protein (keratin) in the outer layers of the skin, making it useful in conditions such as ichthyosis, in which the skin thickens abnormally, causing scaling.

A single 16-week course of treatment often clears the acne. The skin may be very dry, flaky, and itchy at first, but this usually improves as treatment continues. Serious *adverse effects* include liver damage and bowel inflammation.

INFORMATION FOR USERS

Your drug prescription is tailored for you. Do not alter dosage without checking with your doctor.

How taken

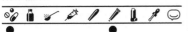

Capsules, gel.

Frequency and timing of doses
1–2 x daily (take capsules with food or milk).

Adult dosage range
Dosage is determined individually.

Onset of effect
2–4 weeks. Acne may worsen during the first few weeks of treatment in some people.

Duration of action
Effects persist for several weeks after the drug has been stopped. Acne is usually completely cleared.

Diet advice
None.

Storage
Keep in a closed container in a cool, dry place out of the reach of children. Protect from light.

Missed dose
Take as soon as you remember. If your next dose is due within 4 hours, take a single dose now and skip the next.

Stopping the drug
Can be safely stopped as soon as you no longer need it, but best results are achieved when the course of treatment is completed as prescribed.

Exceeding the dose
An occasional unintentional extra dose is unlikely to cause problems. Large overdoses may cause headaches, vomiting, abdominal pain, facial flushing, incoordination, and dizziness. Notify your doctor.

SPECIAL PRECAUTIONS

Do not donate blood during, or for at least a month after, taking oral isotretinoin. Be sure to tell your doctor if:
▼ You have long-term liver or kidney problems.
▼ You suffer from arthritis.
▼ You have diabetes.
▼ You wear contact lenses.
▼ You suffer from gout.
▼ You are taking other medications.

Pregnancy
▼ Not prescribed. May cause abnormalities in the developing baby. Effective contraception must be used during treatment and for at least a month before and after.

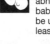

Breast-feeding
▼ The drug passes into the breast milk and may affect the baby. Discuss with your doctor.

Infants and children
▼ Not prescribed.

Over 60
▼ Not usually prescribed.

Driving and hazardous work
▼ Avoid such activities until you have learned how the drug affects you because it can cause vision problems in dim light or darkness.

Alcohol
▼ Regular heavy drinking may raise blood fat levels with isotretinoin.

Sunlight
▼ Avoid exposure to the sun and do not use a sunlamp or sunbed.

POSSIBLE ADVERSE EFFECTS

Dryness of the nose, mouth, and eyes, inflammation of the lips, and flaking of the skin occur in most cases. Temporary loss or increase of hair may also occur. If headache accompanied by symptoms such as nausea and vomiting, abdominal pain with diarrhoea, blood in the faeces, or visual impairment occur, consult your doctor promptly.

Symptom/effect	Frequency		Discuss with doctor		Stop taking drug now	Call doctor now
	Common	Rare	Only if severe	In all cases		
Dry skin/nosebleeds	●		■			
Muscle/joint pain	●		■			
Lip/eye dryness/inflammation	●			■		
Headache		●		■		
Impaired vision		●		■		
Nausea/vomiting		●		■		
Abdominal pain/diarrhoea		●			▲	■
Mood changes		●	■			

INTERACTIONS

Tetracycline antibiotics These may increase the risk of high pressure in the skull, leading to headaches, nausea, and vomiting.

Skin-drying preparations Medicated cosmetics, soaps, toiletries, and anti-acne preparations increase the likelihood of dryness and irritation of the skin with isotretinoin.

Vitamin A Supplements of this vitamin increase the risk of adverse effects from isotretinoin.

PROLONGED USE

A course of treatment rarely exceeds 16 weeks. Prolonged use may raise fat levels in the blood, thereby increasing the risk of heart and blood vessel disease. Bone changes may also occur.

Monitoring Liver function tests and periodic checks on fat levels in the blood are usually performed.

KETOCONAZOLE

Brand name Nizoral
Used in the following combined preparations None

GENERAL INFORMATION

Ketoconazole is prescribed for severe, internal *systemic* fungal infections. It is also given to treat serious infections of the skin and mucous membranes caused by the *Candida* yeast. People with rare fungal diseases (for example, paracoccidioidomycosis, histoplasmosis, and coccidioidomycosis) may also be given this antifungal drug.

Ketoconazole is applied as a cream to treat fungal skin infections, and as a shampoo for the treatment of scalp infections and seborrhoeic dermatitis.

The most common *side effect* with ketoconazole is nausea, which can be reduced by taking the drug at bedtime or with meals. Ketoconazole may also cause liver damage.

QUICK REFERENCE

Drug group Antifungal drug (p.138)
Overdose danger rating Medium
Dependence rating Low
Prescription needed Yes
Available as generic No

INFORMATION FOR USERS

Your drug prescription is tailored for you. Do not alter dosage without checking with your doctor.

How taken

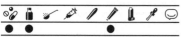

Tablets, liquid, cream, shampoo.

Frequency and timing of doses
Once daily with food (by mouth); 1–2 x daily (cream); 1–2 times weekly (shampoo used for seborrhoeic dermatitis).

Dosage range
Adults 200–400mg daily (by mouth).
Children Reduced dose according to age and weight.

Onset of effect
The drug begins to work within a few hours; full beneficial effect may take several days.

Duration of action
Up to 24 hours.

Diet advice
None.

Storage
Keep in a closed container in a cool, dry place out of the reach of children.

Missed dose (oral)
Take as soon as you remember. If your next dose is due within 6 hours, take a single dose now and skip the next.

Stopping the drug
Take the full course. Even if you feel better, the infection may still be present; symptoms may recur if treatment is stopped too soon.

Exceeding the dose
An occasional unintentional extra dose is unlikely to be a cause for concern. Large overdoses may cause gastric problems. Notify your doctor.

SPECIAL PRECAUTIONS

Be sure to tell your doctor if:
▼ You have long-term liver or kidney problems.
▼ You have porphyria.
▼ You have previously had an allergic reaction to antifungal drugs.
▼ You are taking other medications.

Pregnancy
▼ Not usually prescribed. May cause defects in the developing baby. Discuss with your doctor.

Breast-feeding
▼ The drug passes into the breast milk and may affect the baby. Discuss with your doctor.

Infants and children
▼ Reduced dose necessary.

Over 60
▼ No special problems.

Driving and hazardous work
▼ No special problems.

Alcohol
▼ Avoid. Alcohol may interact with this drug to cause flushing and nausea.

POSSIBLE ADVERSE EFFECTS

Nausea is the most common side effect of ketoconazole; liver damage is a rare but serious adverse effect causing *jaundice* that may necessitate stopping the drug.

Symptom/effect	Frequency		Discuss with doctor		Stop taking drug now	Call doctor now
	Common	Rare	Only if severe	In all cases		
Nausea/vomiting	●		■			
Headache		●	■			
Abdominal pain		●	■			
Itching/rash		●		■	▲	
Painful breasts (men)		●		■	▲	
Jaundice		●		■	▲	■

INTERACTIONS (administration by mouth only)

Antacids, cimetidine, and ranitidine These drugs may reduce the effectiveness of ketoconazole if it they are taken within 2 hours before or after ketoconazole.

Rifampicin This drug reduces the effect of ketoconazole.

Sedatives and warfarin Ketoconazole increases the effects of these drugs.

Cyclosporin, tacrolimus, and theophylline Ketoconazole increases the level of these drugs in the blood.

Phenytoin Levels of ketoconazole may be reduced by phenytoin.

Terfenadine This drug increases the risk of adverse effects on the heart with ketoconazole.

Cisapride This drug may increase the risk of abnormal heart rhythms if it is taken with ketoconazole.

Simvastatin Ketoconazole may increase the risk of muscle damage if it is taken with this drug.

PROLONGED USE

The risk of liver damage increases with use for more than 14 days.

Monitoring Periodic blood tests are usually performed to check the effect of the drug on the liver.

KETOPROFEN

Brand names Fenoket, Ketocid, Ketovail, Ketozip, Larafen, Orudis, Oruvail, Powergel
Used in the following combined preparations None

GENERAL INFORMATION

Ketoprofen is a non-steroidal anti-inflammatory (NSAID) drug which, like other NSAIDs, relieves pain and reduces inflammation and stiffness in rheumatoid arthritis, osteoarthritis, and ankylosing spondylitis. The drug does not cure the underlying disease, however.

Ketoprofen is also given to relieve mild to moderate pain of menstruation and soft tissue injuries, and the pain that occurs following operations.

The most common *adverse reactions* to ketoprofen, as with all NSAIDs, are gastrointestinal disturbances such as nausea and indigestion. Switching to another NSAID may be recommended by your doctor if unwanted effects are persistent or troublesome.

INFORMATION FOR USERS

Follow instructions on the label. Call your doctor if symptoms worsen.

How taken

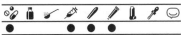

Tablets, capsules, injection, suppositories, gel.

Frequency and timing of doses
2–4 x daily with food (by mouth).
6 x daily for up to 3 days (injection).
2 x daily (suppositories).

Adult dosage range
100–200mg daily.

Onset of effect
Pain relief may be felt in 30 minutes to 2 hours. Full anti-inflammatory effect may not be felt for up to 2 weeks.

Duration of action
Up to 8–12 hours.

Diet advice
None.

Storage
Keep in a closed container in a cool, dry place out of the reach of children.

Missed dose
Take as soon as you remember. If your next dose is due within 4 hours, take a single dose now and skip the next.

Stopping the drug
Seek medical advice before stopping the drug.

Exceeding the dose
An occasional unintentional extra dose is unlikely to be a cause for concern. Large overdoses may cause vomiting, confusion, or irritability. Notify your doctor.

SPECIAL PRECAUTIONS

Be sure to consult your doctor or pharmacist before taking this drug if:
▼ You have long-term liver or kidney problems.
▼ You have heart problems.
▼ You have high blood pressure.
▼ You have asthma.
▼ You have had a peptic ulcer, oesophagitis, or acid indigestion.
▼ You have bleeding problems.
▼ You are allergic to aspirin or other NSAIDs.
▼ You are taking other medications.

Pregnancy
▼ Safety in pregnancy not established. Discuss with your doctor.

Breast-feeding
▼ The drug passes into the breast milk and may affect the baby. Discuss with your doctor.

Infants and children
▼ Not recommended for children under 12 years.

Over 60
▼ Increased likelihood of adverse effects. Reduced dose may therefore be necessary.

Driving and hazardous work
▼ Avoid such activities until you have learned how ketoprofen affects you because the drug can cause dizziness and drowsiness.

Alcohol
▼ Avoid. Alcohol may increase the risk of stomach disorders with ketoprofen.

Surgery and general anaesthetics
▼ Ketoprofen may prolong bleeding. Discuss this with your doctor or dentist before having any surgery.

POSSIBLE ADVERSE EFFECTS

Gastrointestinal disturbances, such as nausea, abdominal pain, and indigestion, commonly occur with ketoprofen when taken by mouth.

Suppositories may cause rectal irritation. Black or bloodstained faeces should be reported promptly.

Symptom/effect	Frequency		Discuss with doctor		Stop taking drug now	Call doctor now
	Common	Rare	Only if severe	In all cases		
Nausea/vomiting	●			■		
Abdominal pain	●			■		
Heartburn	●		■			
Headache		●	■			
Dizziness/drowsiness		●	■			
Swollen feet or legs		●	■			
Weight gain		●	■			
Rash/itching		●		■	▲	❙
Wheezing/breathlessness		●		■	▲	❙
Black/bloodstained faeces		●		■	▲	❙

INTERACTIONS

General note Ketoprofen interacts with a wide range of drugs, such as other NSAIDs including aspirin, oral anticoagulants, and corticosteroids, to increase the risk of bleeding and/or stomach ulcers.

Methotrexate Ketoprofen may raise blood levels of methotrexate, leading to an increased risk of adverse effects.

Phenytoin Ketoprofen may enhance the effects of phenytoin.

Quinolone antibiotics Ketoprofen may increase the risk of seizures if taken with these drugs.

Antihypertensive drugs Ketoprofen may reduce the beneficial effects of these drugs.

PROLONGED USE

There is an increased risk of bleeding from peptic ulcers and in the bowel with prolonged use of ketoprofen.

LACTULOSE

Brand names Duphalac, Lactugal, Laxose, Osmolax, Regulose
Used in the following combined preparations None

GENERAL INFORMATION

Lactulose is an effective laxative that softens faeces by increasing the amount of water in the large intestine. It is used for the relief of constipation and faecal impaction, especially in the elderly. This drug is less likely than some of the other laxatives to disrupt normal bowel action.

Lactulose is also used for preventing and treating brain disturbance associated with liver failure, known as hepatic encephalopathy.

Because lactulose acts locally in the large intestine and is not absorbed into the body, it is safer than many other laxatives. However, the drug can cause stomach cramps and flatulence especially at the start of treatment.

INFORMATION FOR USERS

Follow instructions on the label. Call your doctor if symptoms worsen.

How taken

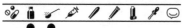

Liquid, powder.

Frequency and timing of doses
2 x daily (chronic constipation);
3–4 x daily (liver failure).

Adult dosage range
15–30ml daily (chronic constipation);
90–150ml daily (liver failure).

Onset of effect
24–48 hours.

Duration of action
6–18 hours.

Diet advice
It is important to maintain an adequate intake of fluid – up to 8 glasses of water daily.

Storage
Keep in a closed container in a cool, dry place out of the reach of children. Do not store after diluting.

Missed dose
Take as soon as you remember. If your next dose is due within 3 hours, take a single dose now and skip the next.

Stopping the drug
In the treatment of constipation, the drug can be safely stopped as soon as you no longer need it.

Exceeding the dose
An occasional unintentional extra dose is unlikely to be a cause for concern. But if you notice any unusual symptoms, or if a large overdose has been taken, notify your doctor.

POSSIBLE ADVERSE EFFECTS

Adverse effects are rarely serious and often disappear when your body adjusts to the medicine. Diarrhoea may indicate that the dosage of lactulose is too high.

Symptom/effect	Frequency		Discuss with doctor		Stop taking drug now	Call doctor now
	Common	Rare	Only if severe	In all cases		
Flatulence/belching	●		■			
Stomach cramps	●		■			
Nausea		●	■			
Abdominal distension		●		■		
Diarrhoea		●		■		

INTERACTIONS

Mesalazine Lactulose may reduce the release of mesalazine at the site of action.

SPECIAL PRECAUTIONS

Be sure to consult your doctor or pharmacist before taking this drug if:
▼ You have severe abdominal pain.
▼ You suffer from lactose intolerance or galactosaemia.
▼ You are taking other medications.

Pregnancy
▼ No evidence of risk. Discuss with your doctor.

Breast-feeding
▼ No evidence of risk.

Infants and children
▼ Reduced dose necessary.

Over 60
▼ No special problems.

Driving and hazardous work
▼ No known problems.

Alcohol
▼ No known problems.

PROLONGED USE

No problems expected.

LAMIVUDINE

Brand names Epivir, Zeffix
Used in the following combined preparation Combivir

GENERAL INFORMATION

Lamivudine is an antiviral drug used in the treatment of HIV. It has also been used for treating hepatitis B virus infections. Lamivudine is a nucleoside reverse transcriptase inhibitor. When used to treat HIV, it is always prescribed with another drug to help prevent resistance from developing. The drug slows the progression of, but does not cure, the illness.

Often, when starting treatment, three drugs are used: two nucleoside reverse transcriptase inhibitors and a third drug from another class, such as ritonavir, a protease inhibitor. However, these combinations may need to be changed during treatment if the patient's condition worsens.

Health workers and other people who are occupationally exposed to HIV may be treated with these antiviral drugs in an attempt to protect them from becoming HIV positive and developing AIDS.

QUICK REFERENCE

Drug group Drug for AIDS and immune deficiency (p.157)

Overdose danger rating Medium

Dependence rating Medium

Prescription needed Yes

Available as generic No

INFORMATION FOR USERS

Your drug prescription is tailored for you. Do not alter dosage without checking with your doctor.

How taken

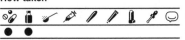

Tablets, oral solution.

Frequency and timing of doses
2 x daily (HIV); once daily (Hepatitis B).

Adult dosage range
HIV 300mg daily.
Hepatitis B 100mg daily.

Onset of effect
1 hour.

Duration of action
12 hours.

Diet advice
None.

Storage
Keep in a closed container in a cool, dry place out of the reach of children.

Missed dose
Take as soon as you remember. If your next dose is due within 2 hours, take a single dose now and skip the next.

Stopping the drug
Do not stop taking the drug without consulting your doctor because of the danger of drug resistance developing.

Exceeding the dose
An occasional unintentional extra dose is unlikely to cause problems. But if you notice any unusual symptoms, or if a large overdose has been taken, notify your doctor.

SPECIAL PRECAUTIONS

Be sure to tell your doctor if:
▼ You have liver or kidney problems.
▼ You have had a previous allergic reaction to lamivudine.
▼ You are taking other medications.

 Pregnancy
▼ Safety not established. Discuss with your doctor.

 Breast-feeding
▼ Safety not established. Discuss with your doctor.

 Infants and children
▼ Safety not established under 3 months. Reduced dose necessary in older infants and children.

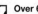 **Over 60**
▼ Increased likelihood of adverse effects. Reduced dose may therefore be necessary.

 Driving and hazardous work
▼ No special problems.

 Alcohol
▼ No special problems.

POSSIBLE ADVERSE EFFECTS

Nausea, vomiting, and diarrhoea are the most common *adverse effects* of lamivudine.

Symptom/effect	Frequency		Discuss with doctor		Stop taking drug now	Call doctor now
	Common	Rare	Only if severe	In all cases		
Nausea/vomiting	●		■			
Diarrhoea/abdominal pain	●		■			
Cough/headache	●		■			
Tingling/"pins and needles"		●	■			
Malaise/fever		●		■		
Jaundice		●		■		
Rash/hair loss		●		■		
Sore throat		●		■		
Severe abdominal pain		●		■		■

INTERACTIONS

Trimethoprim and co-trimoxazole
These drugs increase blood levels of lamivudine.

PROLONGED USE

White blood-cell production may be affected by lamivudine during long-term use.

Monitoring Regular blood counts are usually carried out.

LAMOTRIGINE

Brand name Lamictal
Used in the following combined preparations None

GENERAL INFORMATION

Lamotrigine, introduced in 1993, is an anticonvulsant drug that is prescribed, either alone or in combination with other anticonvulsants, for the treatment of epilepsy. The drug acts by restoring the balance between excitatory and inhibitory *neurotransmitters* in the brain. Lamotrigine may be less sedating than older anticonvulsants, and there is no need for blood tests to determine the level of the drug in the blood.

Lamotrigine may cause a number of minor *adverse effects* (see below), most of which will respond to an adjustment in dosage. Unlike many of the older anticonvulsant drugs, lamotrigine does not interfere with the action of the oral contraceptive pill.

QUICK REFERENCE

Drug group Anticonvulsant drug (p.86)

Overdose danger rating Medium

Dependence rating Low

Prescription needed Yes

Available as generic No

INFORMATION FOR USERS

Your drug prescription is tailored for you. Do not alter dosage without checking with your doctor.

How taken

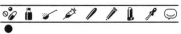

Tablets, dispersible tablets.

Frequency and timing of doses
1–2 x daily.

Adult dosage range
100–500mg (100–200mg if given together with sodium valproate) daily (maintenance dose). Smaller doses are used at the start of treatment.

Onset of effect
Approximately 5 days at a constant dose.

Duration of action
Up to 24 hours.

Diet advice
None.

Storage
Keep in a closed container in a cool, dry place out of the reach of children.

Missed dose
Take as soon as you remember. If your next dose is due within 2 hours, take a single dose now and skip the next.

Stopping the drug
Do not stop taking the drug without consulting your doctor, who will supervise a gradual reduction in dosage over a period of about two weeks. Abrupt cessation increases the risk of rebound fits.

Exceeding the dose
An occasional unintentional extra dose is unlikely to be a cause for concern. Large overdoses may cause sedation, double vision, loss of muscular coordination, nausea, and vomiting. Contact your doctor immediately.

SPECIAL PRECAUTIONS

Be sure to tell your doctor if:
▼ You have long-term liver or kidney problems.
▼ You suffer from thalassaemia.
▼ You have heart disease.
▼ You are taking other medications.

Pregnancy
▼ Safety in pregnancy not established. Discuss with your doctor.

Breast-feeding
▼ Safety in breast-feeding not established. Discuss with your doctor.

Infants and children
▼ Not recommended under 2 years. Not recommended as a single therapy under 12 years. Doses may be relatively higher than adult doses due to increased metabolism.

Over 60s
▼ The dose may need to be reduced.

Driving and hazardous work
▼ Your underlying condition, in addition to the possibility of sedation, dizziness, and vision disturbances while taking lamotrigine, may make such activities inadvisable. Discuss with your doctor.

Alcohol
▼ Alcohol may increase the adverse effects of this drug.

POSSIBLE ADVERSE EFFECTS

Serious adverse effects are rare. The most common side effects are skin rash, nausea, headache, tiredness, insomnia, blurred or double vision, dizziness, agitation, confusion, and poor muscle coordination. These will respond to a dose reduction, and a rash is less likely if the treatment is started at a low dose (25mg), increasing gradually over about 4 weeks. If sore throat or persistent or unusual bruising occur, call your doctor immediately.

Symptom/effect	Frequency		Discuss with doctor		Stop taking drug now	Call doctor now
	Common	Rare	Only if severe	In all cases		
Rash	●			■		▮
Blurred vision/double vision	●		■			
Headache	●		■			
Tremor/incoordination	●			■		
Nausea		●	■			
Flu-like symptoms		●		■		▮
Sore throat/bruising		●		■		▮
Swelling around the face		●		■		▮

PROLONGED USE

No special problems.

INTERACTIONS

Sodium valproate increases and prolongs the effectiveness of lamotrigine. A reduced dose of lamotrigine will be used.

Carbamazepine may reduce lamotrigine blood levels, but lamotrigine may increase the side effects of carbamazepine.

Phenytoin and phenobarbital may decrease blood levels of lamotrigine so a higher dose of lamotrigine may be needed.

LANSOPRAZOLE

Brand name Zoton
Used in the following combined preparations None

GENERAL INFORMATION

Lansoprazole is an anti-ulcer drug belonging to the group called proton pump inhibitors (p.109). It is used to treat peptic ulcers, gastro-oesophageal reflux (in which the stomach acid rises into and irritates the oesophagus), and Zollinger-Ellison syndrome (in which large quantities of stomach acid are produced, leading to ulceration).

Lansoprazole may be used alone or, for peptic ulcers, with two antibiotics, as part of a seven-day regimen to eradicate *Helicobacter pylori* bacteria, the main cause of such ulcers.

Because lansoprazole may mask the symptoms of stomach cancer, it is prescribed only when the possibility of this disease has been ruled out.

QUICK REFERENCE

Drug group Anti-ulcer drug (p.109)
Overdose danger rating Low
Dependence rating Low
Prescription needed Yes
Available as generic No

INFORMATION FOR USERS

Your drug prescription is tailored for you. Do not alter dosage without checking with your doctor.

How taken

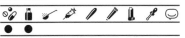

Capsules, oral suspension.

Frequency and timing of doses
1–2 x daily in the morning.

Dosage range
Benign gastric ulcer 30mg daily.
NSAID-associated gastric ulcer 15–30mg daily.
Duodenal ulcer 30mg daily; 15mg daily (maintenance dose).
H. pylori-associated ulcer 60mg daily.

Onset of effect
1–2 hours.

Duration of action
24 hours.

Diet advice
None, although spicy foods and alcohol may exacerbate the condition.

Storage
Keep in a closed container in a cool, dry place out of the reach of children.

Missed dose
Take as soon as you remember. If your next dose is due within 8 hours, take a single dose now and skip the next.

Stopping the drug
Do not stop taking the drug without consulting your doctor; symptoms may recur.

Exceeding the dose
An occasional unintentional extra dose is unlikely to be a cause for concern. But if you notice any unusual symptoms, or if a large overdose has been taken, notify your doctor.

SPECIAL PRECAUTIONS

Be sure to tell your doctor if:
▼ You have liver problems.
▼ You are taking other medications.

 Pregnancy
▼ Safety not established. Discuss with your doctor.

 Breast-feeding
▼ Safety not established. Discuss with your doctor.

 Infants and children
▼ Not recommended.

 Over 60
▼ No special problems.

 Driving and hazardous work
▼ No special problems.

 Alcohol
▼ Avoid. Alcohol may aggravate your condition and reduce the beneficial effects of lansoprazole.

POSSIBLE ADVERSE EFFECTS

Common *side effects* include headache, indigestion, and diarrhoea. A sore throat or breathlessness are rare but should be reported to your doctor at once.

Symptom/effect	Frequency		Discuss with doctor		Stop taking drug now	Call doctor now
	Common	Rare	Only if severe	In all cases		
Headache/dizziness	●		■			
Diarrhoea/constipation	●		■			
Flatulence/abdominal pain	●		■			
Fatigue/malaise		●	■			
Muscle/joint pain		●		■		
Bruising/swollen extremities		●		■		
Rash/itching		●		■	▲	
Sore throat		●		■	▲	▌
Wheeziness/breathing difficulty		●		■	▲	▌

PROLONGED USE

No problems expected.

INTERACTIONS

Oral contraceptives, phenytoin, warfarin, theophylline Lansoprazole may reduce the effect of these drugs.

Antacids and sucralfate These drugs may reduce the absorption of, and should not be taken within an hour of, lansoprazole.

LEVODOPA

Brand names None
Used in the following combined preparations Madopar, Sinemet

GENERAL INFORMATION

The treatment of Parkinson's disease underwent dramatic change in the 1960s with the introduction of levodopa. Since the body can transform levodopa into dopamine, a chemical messenger in the brain the absence or shortage of which causes Parkinson's disease (see p.87), rapid improvements in control were obtained. These improvements were not a cure of the disease but a marked relief of symptoms.

However, it was found that, while levodopa was effective, it produced severe *side effects*, such as nausea, dizziness, and palpitations. Even when treatment was initiated gradually, it was difficult to balance the benefits against the *adverse reactions*.

Today the drug is combined with carbidopa or benserazide, both of which enhance the effects of levodopa in the brain and also help to reduce the side effects of levodopa.

(see p.87)

QUICK REFERENCE

Drug group Drug for parkinsonism (p.87)

Overdose danger rating Medium

Dependence rating Low

Prescription needed Yes

Available as generic Yes

INFORMATION FOR USERS

Your drug prescription is tailored for you. Do not alter dosage without checking with your doctor.

How taken

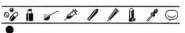

Tablets, capsules.

Frequency and timing of doses
3–6 x daily with food or milk.

Adult dosage range
125–500mg initially, increased until benefits and side effects are balanced.

Onset of effect
Within 1 hour.

Duration of action
2–12 hours.

Diet advice
None.

Storage
Keep in a closed container in a cool, dry place out of the reach of children. Protect from light.

Missed dose
Take as soon as you remember. If your next dose is due within 2 hours, take a single dose now and skip the next.

Stopping the drug
Do not stop taking the drug without consulting your doctor; stopping the drug may lead to severe worsening of the underlying condition.

Exceeding the dose
An occasional unintentional extra dose is unlikely to cause problems. Larger overdoses may cause vomiting or drowsiness. Notify your doctor.

SPECIAL PRECAUTIONS

Be sure to tell your doctor if:
▼ You have heart problems.
▼ You have long-term liver or kidney problems.
▼ You have a lung disorder, such as asthma or bronchitis.
▼ You have an overactive thyroid gland.
▼ You have had glaucoma.
▼ You have a peptic ulcer.
▼ You have diabetes.
▼ You have any serious mental illness.
▼ You have ever had malignant melanoma.
▼ You are taking other medications.

Pregnancy
▼ Unlikely to be required.

Breast-feeding
▼ Unlikely to be required.

Infants and children
▼ Not normally used in children.

Over 60
▼ No special problems.

Driving and hazardous work
▼ Your underlying condition, as well as the possibility of levodopa causing fainting and dizziness, may make such activities inadvisable. Discuss with your doctor.

Alcohol
▼ No known problems.

POSSIBLE ADVERSE EFFECTS

Adverse effects of levodopa are closely related to dosage levels. At the start of treatment, when dosage is usually low, unwanted effects are likely to be mild.

Such effects may increase in severity as dosage is increased to boost the drug's beneficial effects. All adverse effects of this drug should be discussed with your doctor.

Symptom/effect	Frequency		Discuss with doctor		Stop taking drug now	Call doctor now
	Common	Rare	Only if severe	In all cases		
Digestive disturbance	●			■		
Abnormal movement	●			■		
Nervousness/agitation	●			■		
Dark urine	●		■			
Dizziness/fainting		●		■		
Confusion/vivid dreams		●		■		
Palpitations		●		■	▲	∎

INTERACTIONS

Antidepressant drugs Levodopa may interact with monoamine oxidase inhibitors (MAOIs) to cause a dangerous rise in blood pressure. It may also interact with tricyclic antidepressants.

Iron Absorption of levodopa may be reduced by iron.

Antipsychotic drugs Some of these drugs may reduce the effect of levodopa.

Pyridoxine (vitamin B$_6$) Excessive intake of this vitamin may reduce the effect of levodopa.

PROLONGED USE

Effectiveness usually declines in time, necessitating increased dosage. The adverse effects may become so severe that ultimately the drug must be stopped.

LEVOFLOXACIN

Brand name Tavanic
Used in the following combined preparations None

GENERAL INFORMATION

Levofloxacin is a quinolone antibacterial drug used for soft-tissue and respiratory and urinary tract infections that have not responded to other antibiotics.

The drug is usually prescribed in the form of tablets, but it is administered by intravenous *infusion* to people with serious *systemic* infections or to those who cannot take drugs by mouth.

Like other quinolones, levofloxacin may occasionally cause tendon inflammation and damage, especially in the elderly or in people taking corticosteroids. You should, therefore, report tendon pain or inflammation to your doctor immediately and stop taking the drug. The affected limb or limbs should be rested until the symptoms have subsided.

QUICK REFERENCE

Drug group Antibacterial (p.131)
Overdose danger rating Medium
Dependence rating Low
Prescription needed Yes
Available as generic No

INFORMATION FOR USERS

Your drug prescription is tailored for you. Do not alter dosage without checking with your doctor.

How taken

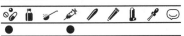

Tablets, injection.

Frequency and timing of doses
1 x 2 times daily for 7–14 days depending on infection (tablets).

Adult dosage range
250–1,000mg daily.

Onset of effect
1 hour.

Duration of action
12–24 hours.

Diet advice
None.

Storage
Keep in a closed container in a cool, dry place out of the reach of children.

Missed dose
Take as soon as you remember, then take your next dose when it is due.

Stopping the drug
Take the full course. Even if you feel better, the original infection may still be present, and symptoms may recur if treatment is stopped too soon.

Exceeding the dose
An occasional unintentional extra dose is unlikely to cause problems. Larger overdoses may cause mental disturbances and fits. Notify your doctor.

SPECIAL PRECAUTIONS

Be sure to tell your doctor if:
▼ You have kidney problems.
▼ You suffer from epilepsy.
▼ You have glucose-6-phosphate dehydrogenase (G6PD) deficiency.
▼ You are taking aspirin or another NSAID.
▼ You have had a previous allergic reaction to a quinolone antibacterial.
▼ You have had a previous tendon problem with a quinolone.
▼ You are taking other medications.

Pregnancy
▼ Safety not established. Discuss with your doctor.

Breast-feeding
▼ Safety not established. Discuss with your doctor.

Infants and children
▼ Not recommended.

Over 60
▼ No special problems, except that tendon damage is more likely over the age of 60.

Driving and hazardous work
▼ Avoid such activities until you have learned how levofloxacin affects you because the drug can cause dizziness, drowsiness, visual disturbances, and hallucinations.

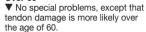

Alcohol
▼ Avoid. Alcohol may increase the sedative effects of levofloxacin.

POSSIBLE ADVERSE EFFECTS

Given by injection, levofloxacin may cause palpitations and a fall in blood pressure.

Nausea and vomiting are the most common *side effects* of the drug taken by mouth.

Symptom/effect	Frequency		Discuss with doctor		Stop taking drug now	Call doctor now
	Common	Rare	Only if severe	In all cases		
Nausea/vomiting	●			■		
Diarrhoea/abdominal pain	●			■		
Headache/dizziness		●		■		
Skin rash/itching		●		■		
Drowsiness/restlessness		●		■		
Jaundice		●			▲	
Confusion/hallucinations		●		■	▲	
Fever/allergic reaction		●		■	▲	
Painful or inflamed tendons		●		■	▲	■

INTERACTIONS

Nonsteroidal anti-inflammatory drugs (NSAIDs) and theophylline There is an increased risk of convulsions when these drugs are taken with levofloxacin.

Anticoagulants The effect of these drugs may be increased by levofloxacin.

Antacids, adsorbents, sucralfate, iron and zinc These drugs may reduce the absorption of levofloxacin.

Cyclosporin There is an increased risk of kidney damage if cyclosporin is taken with levofloxacin.

PROLONGED USE

Levofloxacin is not usually prescribed for long-term use.

LEVONORGESTREL

Brand names Microval, Norgeston
Used in the following combined preparations Cyclo-progynova, Eugynon 30, Microgynon 30, Ovranette, and others

GENERAL INFORMATION

Levonorgestrel is a synthetic hormone similar to progesterone, a natural female sex hormone. The drug's primary use is as an ingredient in oral contraceptives. It performs this function by thickening the mucus at the neck of the uterus (cervix), thereby making it difficult for sperm to enter the uterus.

Levonorgestrel is available both in combined oral contraceptives with an oestrogen drug and in progestogen-only preparations.

It is occasionally given alone or with an oestrogen for emergency, post-coital contraception. It is also given in combination with an oestrogen drug in hormone replacement therapy to treat menopausal symptoms.

Levonorgestrel rarely causes serious *adverse effects*. When it is used without an oestrogen, menstrual irregularities, especially mid-cycle, or "breakthrough", bleeding are common.

QUICK REFERENCE

Drug group Female sex hormone (p.147) and oral contraceptive (p.161)

Overdose danger rating Low

Dependence rating Low

Prescription needed Yes

Available as generic No

INFORMATION FOR USERS

Your drug prescription is tailored for you. Do not alter dosage without checking with your doctor.

How taken

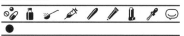

Tablets, implant, intrauterine device (IUD).

Frequency and timing of doses
Once daily, at the same time each day.

Adult dosage range
Progestogen-only pills 30mcg daily.

Onset of effect
Levonorgestrel starts to act within 4 hours, but contraceptive protection may not be fully effective for 14 days, depending on which day of the cycle the tablets are started.

Duration of action
24 hours. Some effects may persist for up to 3 months after levonorgestrel is stopped.

Diet advice
None.

Storage
Keep in a closed container in a cool, dry place out of the reach of children.

Missed dose
If a tablet is delayed by 3 hours or more, regard it as a missed dose. See What to do if you miss a pill (p.163).

Stopping the drug
The drug can be safely stopped as soon as contraceptive protection is no longer required. For treatment of menopausal symptoms, consult your doctor before stopping the drug.

Exceeding the dose
An occasional unintentional extra dose is unlikely to be a cause for concern. But if you notice any unusual symptoms, or if a large overdose has been taken, notify your doctor.

SPECIAL PRECAUTIONS

Be sure to tell your doctor if:
▼ You have a liver problem.
▼ You have heart failure or high blood pressure.
▼ You have diabetes.
▼ You have unexplained abnormal vaginal bleeding.
▼ You have had blood clots or a stroke.
▼ You have ever had migraines or severe headaches.
▼ You are taking other medications.

Pregnancy
▼ Not prescribed. May cause abnormalities in the developing baby. Discuss with your doctor.

Breast-feeding
▼ The drug passes into the breast milk, but at normal doses adverse effects on the baby are unlikely. Discuss with your doctor.

Infants and children
▼ Not prescribed.

Over 60
▼ Not prescribed.

Driving and hazardous work
▼ No known problems.

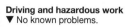
Alcohol
▼ No known problems.

POSSIBLE ADVERSE EFFECTS

Menstrual irregularities (blood spotting between menstrual periods or absence of menstruation) are the most common side effects of levonorgestrel alone.

Symptom/effect	Frequency		Discuss with doctor		Stop taking drug now	Call doctor now
	Common	Rare	Only if severe	In all cases		
Swollen feet/ankles	●		■			
Weight gain	●		■			
Irregular vaginal bleeding	●			■		
Nausea/vomiting		●	■			
Breast tenderness		●	■			
Depression		●		■		
Headache		●		■		

INTERACTIONS

General note The beneficial effects of many drugs, including bromocriptine, oral anticoagulants, anticonvulsants, and antihypertensive and antidiabetic drugs, may be affected by levonorgestrel. Many other drugs may affect the action of oral contraceptives, reducing contraceptive protection. These include anticonvulsants, antituberculous drugs, and antibiotics. Inform your doctor that you are taking this drug before taking additional prescribed medication.

PROLONGED USE

Problems are rare.

LISINOPRIL

Brand names Carace, Zestril
Used in the following combined preparations Carace Plus, Zestoretic

GENERAL INFORMATION

Lisinopril is an ACE inhibitor drug used in the treatment of high blood pressure (including that caused by diabetic kidney problems), heart failure, and following a heart attack. It works by relaxing the muscles in blood vessel walls, allowing them to dilate (widen), thereby easing blood flow.

Lisinopril can initially cause a rapid fall in blood pressure, especially when taken with a diuretic drug. Therefore, treatment for heart failure is usually started under close medical supervision, in hospital in severe cases. The first dose is usually very small, and should be taken while lying down, preferably at bedtime.

QUICK REFERENCE

Drug group ACE inhibitor (p.98)
Overdose danger rating Medium
Dependence rating Low
Prescription needed Yes
Available as generic No

INFORMATION FOR USERS

Your drug prescription is tailored for you. Do not alter dosage without checking with your doctor.

How taken

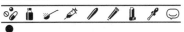

Tablets.

Frequency and timing of doses
Once daily.

Adult dosage range
Hypertension 2.5mg (starting dose) up to 40mg.
Heart failure/diabetic nephropathy 2.5mg (starting dose) up to 20mg.
Prevention of further heart attacks 2.5–5mg (starting dose) up to 10mg.

Onset of effect
1–2 hours; full beneficial effect may take several weeks.

Duration of action
12–24 hours.

Diet advice
None.

Storage
Keep in a closed container in a cool, dry place out of the reach of children.

Missed dose
Take as soon as you remember. If your next dose is due within 8 hours, take a single dose now and skip the next.

Stopping the drug
Do not stop taking the drug without consulting your doctor. Stopping the drug may lead to worsening of the underlying condition.

Exceeding the dose
An occasional unintentional extra dose is unlikely to be a cause for concern. Larger overdoses may cause dizziness or fainting. Notify your doctor.

POSSIBLE ADVERSE EFFECTS

Common but unusual *side effects* of lisinopril are persistent dry cough and an altered sense of taste. A reduction of dosage may minimize these effects.

Symptom/effect	Frequency		Discuss with doctor		Stop taking drug now	Call doctor now
	Common	Rare	Only if severe	In all cases		
Nausea/vomiting	●		■			
Rash/itching		●	■			
Chest pain/palpitations		●			■	
Dry cough/altered sense of taste	●				■	
Dizziness/fainting		●			■	
Runny nose/sore throat		●			■	
Confusion/mood changes		●			■	
Jaundice		●			■	

INTERACTIONS

Potassium supplements, potassium-sparing diuretics, and cyclosporin Taken with lisinopril, these drugs increase the risk of high blood potassium levels.

Nonsteroidal anti-inflammatory drugs (NSAIDs) Some of these drugs may reduce the effect of lisinopril, and the risk of kidney damage is increased.

Vasodilators, diuretics, and other drugs for hypertension These drugs may increase the effect of lisinopril.

Lithium Blood levels of lithium may be increased by lisinopril.

Insulin and antidiabetic drugs Lisinopril may increase the effect of these drugs.

SPECIAL PRECAUTIONS

Be sure to tell your doctor if:
▼ You are allergic to other ACE inhibitors.
▼ You have a history of angioedema.
▼ You have kidney problems or are on dialysis.
▼ You are taking a diuretic drug.
▼ You are on a low sodium diet.
▼ You are taking other medications.

 Pregnancy
▼ Not prescribed. May harm the developing baby.

 Breast-feeding
▼ Safety not established. Discuss with your doctor.

 **Infants and children**
▼ Not recommended.

 Over 60
▼ No special problems.

 Driving and hazardous work
▼ Avoid such activities until you have learned how lisinopril affects you because the drug can cause dizziness and fainting.

 Alcohol
▼ Avoid. Alcohol may increase the blood-pressure lowering and adverse effects of this drug.

PROLONGED USE

Rarely, prolonged use of lisinopril can lead to changes in blood count or kidney function.

Monitoring Periodic checks on potassium levels, white blood cell counts and urine are usually performed.

LITHIUM

Brand names Camcolit, Li-liquid, Liskonum, Litarex, Priadel
Used in the following combined preparation Efalith

GENERAL INFORMATION

Lithium, the lightest known metal, has been used since the 1940s in the form of various salts to treat a severe mental disturbance, manic depressive illness. Lithium decreases the intensity and frequency of the episodic swings from extreme excitement to deep depression that are characteristic of the disorder.

Although preferred for mania alone, it is also sometimes used to prevent and treat severe depression (see p.84). Treatment with lithium may be started in hospital for the more seriously ill. Careful monitoring is required because high blood levels of lithium can cause serious *adverse effects*. Since it may take two to three weeks for any benefit to become apparent, an antipsychotic drug is often given with lithium until the lithium becomes effective.

QUICK REFERENCE

Drug group Antimanic drug (p.85)
Overdose danger rating High
Dependence rating Low
Prescription needed Yes
Available as generic No

INFORMATION FOR USERS

Your drug prescription is tailored for you. Do not alter dosage without checking with your doctor.

How taken

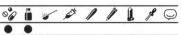

Tablets, SR-tablets, liquid.

Frequency and timing of doses
1–2 x daily with meals. Always take the same brand of lithium to ensure a consistent effect; change of brand must be closely supervised.

Adult dosage range
0.25–2g daily. Dosage may vary according to individual response.

Onset of effect
Some effects may be noticed in 3–5 days, but full benefits may not be felt for 3 weeks.

Duration of action
18–36 hours. Some effect may last for several days.

Diet advice
Lithium levels in the blood are affected by the amount of sodium (present in salt) in the body, so do not suddenly increase or reduce the amount of salt in your diet. Be sure to drink adequate volumes of fluids, especially in hot weather.

Storage
Keep in a closed container in a cool, dry place out of the reach of children.

Missed dose
Take as soon as you remember. If your next dose is due within 4 hours, take a single dose now and skip the next.

Stopping the drug
Do not stop the drug without consulting your doctor; symptoms may recur.

OVERDOSE ACTION

Seek immediate medical advice in all cases. Take emergency action if convulsions or loss of consciousness occur.

See Drug poisoning emergency guide (p.494).

SPECIAL PRECAUTIONS

Be sure to tell your doctor if:
▼ You have long-term liver or kidney problems.
▼ You have heart or circulation problems.
▼ You have an overactive thyroid gland.
▼ You have myasthenia gravis.
▼ You have Addison's disease.
▼ You are taking other medications.

Pregnancy
▼ Not usually prescribed. May cause defects in the unborn baby. Discuss with your doctor.

Breast-feeding
▼ The drug passes into the breast milk and may affect the baby. Discuss with your doctor.

Infants and children
▼ Not recommended.

Over 60
▼ Increased likelihood of adverse effects. Reduced dose may therefore be necessary.

Driving and hazardous work
▼ Avoid such activities until you have learned how lithium affects you because the drug can cause reduced alertness.

Alcohol
▼ Avoid. Alcohol may increase the sedative effects of this drug.

PROLONGED USE

Prolonged use may lead to kidney problems. Treatment for periods of longer than 5 years is not normally advised unless the benefits are significant and tests show no sign of reduced kidney function.

Monitoring Regular monitoring of blood levels of the drug and the composition of the blood is usually carried out. Kidney and thyroid function should also be monitored.

POSSIBLE ADVERSE EFFECTS

Many of the symptoms below are signs of a high lithium level in the blood. Stop taking the drug and seek medical advice promptly if you notice any of these symptoms.

Symptom/effect	Frequency		Discuss with doctor		Stop taking drug now	Call doctor now
	Common	Rare	Only if severe	In all cases		
Nausea/vomiting/diarrhoea	●			■	▲	
Tremor	●			■		
Weight gain		●	■			
Drowsiness/lethargy		●		■	▲	
Blurred vision		●		■	▲	
Rash		●		■	▲	
Muscle weakness		●		■		
Increase in urine/thirst		●		■		

INTERACTIONS

General note Many drugs interact with lithium. Do not take any over-the-counter or prescription drugs without consulting your doctor or pharmacist. Paracetamol should be used in preference to other analgesics for everyday pain relief.

LOFEPRAMINE

Brand name Gamanil
Used in the following combined preparations None

GENERAL INFORMATION

Lofepramine belongs to the tricyclic antidepressant group of drugs. It is used primarily in the long-term treatment of depression. The drug serves to elevate the mood, improve appetite, increase physical activity, and restore interest in everyday activities.

Less sedating than some of the other tricyclic antidepressants, lofepramine is particularly useful when depression is accompanied by lethargy.

The main advantage of lofepramine over other similar drugs is that it seems to have a weaker *anticholinergic* action and therefore has milder *side effects*. In overdose, lofepramine is thought to be less harmful than the older tricyclic antidepressant drugs.

INFORMATION FOR USERS

Your drug prescription is tailored for you. Do not alter dosage without checking with your doctor.

How taken

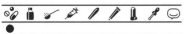

Tablets.

Frequency and timing of doses
2–3 x daily.

Adult dosage range
140–210mg daily.

Onset of effect
Can appear within hours, although full antidepressant effect may not be felt for 2–6 weeks.

Duration of action
Antidepressant effect may last for 6 weeks; adverse effects, only a few days.

Diet advice
None.

Storage
Keep in a closed container in a cool, dry place out of the reach of children. Protect from light.

Missed dose
Take as soon as you remember. If your next dose is due within 3 hours, take a single dose now and skip the next.

Stopping the drug
An abrupt stop can cause withdrawal symptoms and a recurrence of the original problem. Consult your doctor, who may supervise a gradual reduction in dosage.

Exceeding the dose
An occasional unintentional extra dose is unlikely to be a cause for concern. But if you notice any unusual symptoms, or if a large overdose has been taken, notify your doctor.

SPECIAL PRECAUTIONS

Be sure to tell your doctor if:
▼ You have heart problems.
▼ You have had epileptic fits.
▼ You have long-term liver or kidney problems.
▼ You have glaucoma.
▼ You have an overactive thyroid gland.
▼ You have prostate trouble.
▼ You are taking other medications.

Pregnancy
▼ Safety in pregnancy not established. Discuss with your doctor.

Breast-feeding
▼ The drug passes into the breast milk and may affect the baby. Discuss with your doctor.

Infants and children
▼ Not recommended.

Over 60
▼ Reduced dose may be necessary.

Driving and hazardous work
▼ Avoid such activities until you have learned how lofepramine affects you because the drug may cause blurred vision and reduced alertness.

Alcohol
▼ Avoid. Alcohol may increase the sedative effects of this drug.

Surgery and general anaesthetics
▼ Lofepramine may need to be stopped. Discuss with your doctor or dentist before you have any surgery.

POSSIBLE ADVERSE EFFECTS

The possible adverse effects of this drug are mainly the result of its mild anticholinergic action and its blocking action on the transmission of signals though the heart.

Symptom/effect	Frequency		Discuss with doctor		Stop taking drug now	Call doctor now
	Common	Rare	Only if severe	In all cases		
Sweating/flushing	●		■			
Drowsiness		●	■			
Constipation		●	■			
Dry mouth		●	■			
Blurred vision		●		■		
Dizziness/fainting		●		■		
Difficulty in passing urine		●		■		
Palpitations		●		■	▲	∎

INTERACTIONS

Sedatives All drugs that have sedative effects may intensify those of lofepramine.

Heavy smoking This may reduce the antidepressant effect of lofepramine.

Monoamine oxidase inhibitors (MAOIs) Serious interactions are possible. These drugs are only prescribed together under close medical supervision.

Antihypertensive drugs Lofepramine may reduce the effectiveness of some of these drugs.

Antihistamines Terfenadine intensifies some effects of lofepramine.

Anti-arrhythmic drugs, cisapride, and sotalol These drugs may increase the risk of abnormal heart rhythms.

PROLONGED USE

No problems expected.

LOPERAMIDE

Brand names Arret, Diasorb, Diocalm Ultra, Imodium
Used in the following combined preparations None

GENERAL INFORMATION

Loperamide is an antidiarrhoeal drug available in either capsule or liquid form. It reduces the loss of water and salts from the bowel and slows bowel activity, resulting in the passage of firmer bowel movements at less frequent intervals.

A fast-acting drug, loperamide is widely prescribed for both sudden and recurrent bouts of diarrhoea. However, it is not generally recommended for diarrhoea caused by infection because

it may delay the expulsion of harmful substances from the bowel. Loperamide is often prescribed for people who have had a colostomy or an ileostomy, to reduce fluid loss from the stoma (outlet).

Adverse effects from this drug are rare, and there is no risk of abuse, as there may be with the opium-based antidiarrhoeals. It can be purchased over the counter in a pharmacy.

QUICK REFERENCE

Drug group Antidiarrhoeal drug (p.110)

Overdose danger rating Medium

Dependence rating Low

Prescription needed No

Available as generic Yes

INFORMATION FOR USERS

Follow instructions on the label. Call your doctor if symptoms worsen.

How taken

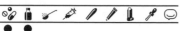

Capsules, liquid.

Frequency and timing of doses
Acute diarrhoea Take a double dose at start of treatment, then a single dose after each loose faeces, up to the maximum daily dose.
Chronic diarrhoea 2 x daily.

Adult dosage range
Acute diarrhoea 4mg (starting dose), then 2mg after each loose faeces (maximum 16mg daily). Use for up to 5 days only (3 days only for children between 4–8 years), then consult your doctor.
Chronic diarrhoea 4–8mg daily.

Onset of effect
Within 1–2 hours.

Duration of action
6–18 hours.

Diet advice
Ensure adequate fluid, sugar, and salt intake during a diarrhoeal illness.

Storage
Keep in a closed container in a cool, dry place out of the reach of children.

Missed dose
Do not take the missed dose. Take your next dose if needed.

Stopping the drug
Can be safely stopped as soon as you no longer need it.

Exceeding the dose
An occasional unintentional extra dose is unlikely to be a cause for concern. Large overdoses may cause constipation, vomiting, or drowsiness, and affect breathing. Notify your doctor.

SPECIAL PRECAUTIONS

Be sure to consult your doctor or pharmacist before taking this drug if:
▼ You have long-term liver or kidney problems.
▼ You have had recent abdominal surgery.
▼ You have an infection or blockage in the intestine, pseudomembranous colitis, or ulcerative colitis.
▼ You are taking other medications.

 Pregnancy
▼ Safety in pregnancy not established. Discuss with your doctor.

 Breast-feeding
▼ The drug passes into the breast milk and may affect the baby. Discuss with your doctor.

 Infants and children
▼ Not to be given to infants and children under 4 years. Reduced dose necessary in older children.

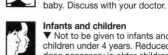 **Over 60**
▼ No special problems.

Driving and hazardous work
▼ No known problems.

Alcohol
▼ No known problems.

POSSIBLE ADVERSE EFFECTS

Adverse effects are rare with loperamide and often difficult to distinguish from the effects of the diarrhoea it is used to treat. If symptoms

such as bloating, abdominal pain, or fever persist or worsen during treatment with loperamide, consult your doctor.

Symptom/effect	Frequency		Discuss with doctor		Stop taking drug now	Call doctor now
	Common	Rare	Only if severe	In all cases		
Constipation		●	■		▲	
Bloating		●	■			
Abdominal pain		●	■			
Dry mouth		●	■			
Drowsiness or dizziness		●	■			
Itching skin		●		■		
Rash		●		■	▲	

INTERACTIONS

None.

PROLONGED USE

Although this drug is not usually taken for prolonged periods (except by persons with a medically diagnosed long-term gastrointestinal condition), special problems are not expected during long-term use.

LORATADINE

Brand name Clarityn
Used in the following combined preparations None

GENERAL INFORMATION

Loratadine, a long-acting antihistamine drug, is used for the relief of symptoms associated with allergic rhinitis, such as sneezing, nasal discharge, and itching and burning of the eyes. Symptoms are normally relieved within an hour of oral administration. Loratadine is also used to treat allergic skin conditions such as chronic urticaria (itching). An advantage of loratadine over older antihistamines, such as chlorphenamine, is that it has fewer sedative and *anticholinergic* effects, so this drug is less likely to cause drowsiness.

Loratadine should be discontinued about four days prior to skin testing for allergy as it may decrease or prevent otherwise positive results.

INFORMATION FOR USERS

Follow instructions on the label. Call your doctor if symptoms worsen.

How taken

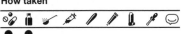

Tablets, liquid.

Frequency and timing of doses
Once daily.

Adult dosage range
10mg daily.

Onset of effect
Usually within 1 hour.

Duration of action
Up to 24 hours.

Diet advice
None.

Storage
Keep in a closed container in a cool, dry place out of the reach of children.

Missed dose
Take as soon as you remember. If your next dose is due within 6 hours, take a single dose now and skip the next.

Stopping the drug
Can be safely stopped as soon as you no longer need it.

Exceeding the dose
An occasional unintentional extra dose is unlikely to be a cause for concern. But if you notice any unusual symptoms, or if a large overdose has been taken, notify your doctor.

POSSIBLE ADVERSE EFFECTS

The incidence of adverse effects with loratadine is low.

Symptom/effect	Frequency		Discuss with doctor		Stop taking drug now	Call doctor now
	Common	Rare	Only if severe	In all cases		
Fatigue		●	■			
Nausea		●	■			
Headache		●	■			
Palpitations		●			■	
Fainting		●			■	

INTERACTIONS

Cimetidine This drug may increase the effects of loratadine.

SPECIAL PRECAUTIONS

Be sure to consult your doctor or pharmacist before taking this drug if:
▼ You are taking other medications.

Pregnancy
▼ Safety in pregnancy not established. Discuss with your doctor.

Breast-feeding
▼ The drug passes into the breast milk, but effects on the baby are unlikely.

Infants and children
▼ Not recommended for children under 2 years. Reduced dose necessary for older children.

Over 60
▼ No problems expected.

Driving and hazardous work
▼ Problems are unlikely.

Alcohol
▼ No known problems, but avoid excessive amounts.

PROLONGED USE

No problems expected.

LOSARTAN

Brand name Cozaar
Used in the following combined preparation Cozaar-Comp

GENERAL INFORMATION

Losartan is a member of the group of vasodilator drugs called angiotensin-II blockers. Used to treat hypertension, the drug works by blocking the action of angiotensin-II (a naturally occurring substance that constricts blood vessels). This action causes the blood vessel walls to relax, thereby easing blood pressure.

Unlike ACE inhibitors, losartan does not cause a persistent dry cough, and its use is now being evaluated in conditions such as heart failure, for which ACE inhibitors are currently being used.

Losartan is prescribed with caution to people with stenosis (narrowing) of the arteries to the kidneys because the initial dose causes a sudden drop in blood pressure. *Adverse effects*, which include diarrhoea, dizziness, and fatigue, are rare.

QUICK REFERENCE

Drug group Vasodilator (p.98) and Antihypertensive drug (p.102)

Overdose danger rating Medium

Dependence rating Low

Prescription needed Yes

Available as generic No

INFORMATION FOR USERS

Your drug prescription is tailored for you. Do not alter dosage without checking with your doctor.

How taken

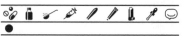

Tablets.

Frequency and timing of doses
Once daily.

Adult dosage range
50–100mg. People over 75 years, and other groups that are especially sensitive to the drug's effects, may start on 25mg.

Onset of effect
Blood pressure 1–2 weeks, with maximum effect in 3–6 weeks from start of treatment.
Other conditions Within 1 hour.

Duration of action
12–24 hours.

Diet advice
None.

Storage
Keep in a closed container in a cool, dry place out of the reach of children.

Missed dose
Take as soon as you remember. If your next dose is due within 8 hours, take a single dose now and skip the next.

Stopping the drug
Do not stop the drug without consulting your doctor. Stopping the drug may lead to worsening of the underlying condition.

Exceeding the dose
An occasional unintentional extra dose is unlikely to cause problems. Large overdoses may cause dizziness and fainting. Notify your doctor.

SPECIAL PRECAUTIONS

Be sure to tell your doctor if:
▼ You have stenosis of the kidney arteries.
▼ You have liver or kidney problems.
▼ You have congestive heart failure.
▼ You have primary aldosteronism.
▼ You are taking other medications.

Pregnancy
▼ Not prescribed.

Breast-feeding
▼ Not prescribed. Safety not established.

Infants and children
▼ Not prescribed. Safety not established.

Over 60
▼ Reduced dose may be necessary over 75 years.

Driving and hazardous work
▼ Do not undertake such activities until you have learned how losartan affects you because the drug can cause dizziness and fatigue.

Alcohol
▼ Avoid. Alcohol may raise blood pressure, reducing the effectiveness of losartan. Alcohol also causes blood vessels to dilate, increasing the likelihood of an excessive fall in blood pressure.

POSSIBLE ADVERSE EFFECTS

Side effects, of which dizziness and fatigue are the most common, are usually mild.

Symptom/effect	Frequency		Discuss with doctor		Stop taking drug now	Call doctor now
	Common	Rare	Only if severe	In all cases		
Dizziness/fatigue	●		■			
Migraine		●	■			
Diarrhoea		●	■			
Taste disturbance		●	■			
Rash/itching		●		■		
Jaundice		●		■		

INTERACTIONS

Diuretics There is a risk of a sudden fall in blood pressure when these drugs are taken with losartan.

Potassium supplements, potassium-sparing diuretics, and cyclosporin Losartan increases the effect of these drugs, leading to raised levels of potassium in the blood.

Lithium Losartan may increase the levels and *toxicity* of lithium.

Non steroidal anti-inflammatory drugs (NSAIDs) Certain NSAIDs may reduce the blood-pressure lowering effect of losartan.

PROLONGED USE

No special problems.

Monitoring Periodic checks on blood potassium levels may be performed.

MAGNESIUM HYDROXIDE

Brand names Cream of Magnesia, Milk of Magnesia
Used in the following combined preparations Carbellon, Maalox, Mucaine, Mucogel, and others

GENERAL INFORMATION

Magnesium hydroxide is a fast-acting antacid given to neutralize stomach acid. The drug is available in a number of over-the-counter preparations for the treatment of indigestion and heartburn. Magnesium hydroxide also prevents pain caused by stomach and duodenal ulcers, gastritis, and reflux oesophagitis, although other drugs are normally used for these problems nowadays. It also

acts as a laxative by drawing water into the intestine from the surrounding blood vessels to soften the faeces.

Magnesium hydroxide is not often used alone as an antacid because of its laxative effect. However, this effect is countered when the drug is used in combination with aluminium hydroxide, which can cause constipation.

QUICK REFERENCE

Drug group Antacid (p.108) and laxative (p.111)

Overdose danger rating Low

Dependence rating Low

Prescription needed No

Available as generic Yes

INFORMATION FOR USERS

Follow instructions on the label. Call your doctor if symptoms worsen.

How taken

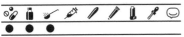

Tablets, liquid, powder.

Frequency and timing of doses
4 x daily with water, preferably an hour after food.

Adult dosage range
Antacid 1–2g per dose (tablets); 5–20ml per dose (liquid).
Laxative 5–20ml per dose (liquid).

Onset of effect
Antacid within 15 minutes.
Laxative 2–8 hours.

Duration of action
2–4 hours.

Diet advice
None.

Storage
Keep in a closed container in a cool, dry place out of the reach of children.

Missed dose
Take as soon as you remember.

Stopping the drug
When used as an antacid, can be safely stopped as soon as you no longer need it. When given as ulcer treatment, follow your doctor's advice.

Exceeding the dose
An occasional unintentional extra dose is unlikely to be a cause for concern. But if you notice any unusual symptoms, or if a large overdose has been taken, notify your doctor.

SPECIAL PRECAUTIONS

Be sure to consult your doctor or pharmacist before taking this drug if:
▼ You have a long-term kidney problem.
▼ You have a bowel disorder.
▼ You are taking other medications.

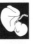
Pregnancy
▼ No evidence of risk.

Breast-feeding
▼ No evidence of risk.

Infants and children
▼ Not recommended under 1 year except on the advice of a doctor. Reduced dose necessary for older children.

Over 60
▼ No special problems.

Driving and hazardous work
▼ No known problems.

Alcohol
▼ Avoid excessive alcohol as it irritates the stomach and may reduce the benefits of the drug.

POSSIBLE ADVERSE EFFECTS

Diarrhoea is the only common adverse effect of this drug. Dizziness and muscle weakness due to absorption of excess magnesium in

the body may occur in people with poor kidney function.

Symptom/effect	Frequency		Discuss with doctor		Stop taking drug now	Call doctor now
	Common	Rare	Only if severe	In all cases		
Diarrhoea	●		■			

INTERACTIONS

General note Magnesium hydroxide interferes with the absorption of a wide range of drugs taken by mouth, including tetracycline antibiotics, iron supplements, diflunisal, phenytoin, and penicillamine.

Enteric-coated tablets As with other antacids, magnesium hydroxide may allow break-up of the *enteric* coating of tablets, sometimes leading to stomach irritation.

PROLONGED USE

Magnesium hydroxide should not be used for prolonged periods without consulting your doctor. If you are over 40 years of age and are experience long-term indigestion or heartburn, your doctor will probably refer you to a specialist. Prolonged use in people with kidney damage may cause drowsiness, dizziness, and weakness, resulting from accumulation of magnesium in the body.

MALATHION

Brand names Derbac M, Prioderm, Suleo-M
Used in the following combined preparations None

GENERAL INFORMATION

Malathion is an insecticide used in the treatment of lice and mite infestations. The drug kills parasites by interfering with their nervous system function, causing paralysis and death.

Malathion is applied *topically*, either as a shampoo or a lotion. Lotion is more convenient to use than shampoo, requiring only a single application. It is also more effective because shampoo is diluted in use. However, lotions with a high alcohol content are unsuitable for small children or asthmatics, who may be affected by the solvent, or for treating crab lice in the genital area. Care should be taken to avoid contact of the drug with the eyes or broken skin.

If resistance occurs during a course of treatment, your pharmacist will recommend an alternative insecticide.

INFORMATION FOR USERS

Follow instructions on the label. Call your doctor if symptoms worsen.

How taken

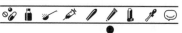

●

Lotion, shampoo.

Frequency and timing of doses
Scabies Once only (lotion).
Lice 3 applications 3 days apart (shampoo); 2 doses, 7 days apart (lotion).

Adult dosage range
As directed. Family members and close contacts should also be treated.

Onset of effect
Lotion leave on for 12 hours (lice), or 24 hours (scabies), before washing off.
Shampoo leave on for 5 minutes, rinse off, repeat, then use fine-toothed comb.

Duration of action
Until washed off.

Diet advice
None.

Storage
Keep in closed container in a cool, dry place out of the reach of children. Protect from light.

Missed dose
When a repeat application of the shampoo has been missed, it should be carried out as soon as is practicable.

Stopping the drug
Malathion should be applied as a single application or as a short course of treatment.

Exceeding the dose
An extra application is unlikely to cause problems. Take emergency action if the insecticide has been swallowed.

SPECIAL PRECAUTIONS

Be sure to consult your doctor or pharmacist before using this drug if:
▼ You have asthma.

 Pregnancy
▼ No evidence of risk. It is unlikely that enough malathion would be absorbed after occasional application to affect the developing fetus.

 Breast-feeding
▼ No evidence of risk. It is unlikely that enough malathion would be absorbed after occasional application to affect the baby.

 Infants and children
▼ No special problems.

 Over 60
▼ No special problems.

Driving and hazardous work
▼ No special problems.

Alcohol
▼ No special problems.

POSSIBLE ADVERSE EFFECTS

Used correctly, malathion preparations are unlikely to produce *adverse effects*, although the alcoholic fumes given off by some lotions may cause wheezing in asthmatics.

Symptom/effect	Frequency		Discuss with doctor		Stop taking drug now	Call doctor now
	Common	Rare	Only if severe	In all cases		
Skin irritation		●	■			

INTERACTIONS

None.

PROLONGED USE

Malathion is intended for intermittent use only. The lotions should not be used more than once a week for three weeks at a time.

MEBEVERINE

Brand names Colofac, Equilon, Fomac
Used in the following combined preparation Fybogel-Mebeverine

GENERAL INFORMATION

Mebeverine is an *antispasmodic* drug used to relieve painful spasms of the intestine (known as colic), such as those that occur as a result of irritable bowel syndrome and other intestinal disorders such as diverticular disease. It has a direct relaxing effect on the muscle in the bowel wall, and may also have an *anticholinergic* action, which reduces the transmission of nerve signals to the smooth muscle of the bowel wall and thereby prevents spasm. Mebeverine does not have serious *side effects*.

In addition to being available in both tablet and liquid form, mebeverine is also produced in a combined form with ispaghula husk to provide roughage in an easily assimilable formulation. Both the drug itself and the combined form are commonly used to improve symptoms in the control of irritable bowel syndrome.

INFORMATION FOR USERS

Follow instructions on the label. Call your doctor if symptoms worsen.

How taken

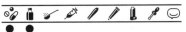

Tablets, SR-capsules, liquid.

Frequency and timing of doses
3 x daily, 20 minutes before meals.

Adult dosage range
405–450mg daily.

Onset of effect
30–60 minutes.

Duration of action
6–8 hours.

Diet advice
None.

Storage
Keep in a closed container in a dry place at room temperature, out of the reach of children. Protect from light.

Missed dose
Take as soon as you remember, then return to your normal dosing schedule.

Stopping the drug
The drug can be stopped as soon as you no longer need it.

Exceeding the dose
An occasional unintentional extra dose is unlikely to be a cause for concern. Larger overdoses will probably cause constipation, and may cause central nervous system excitability.

SPECIAL PRECAUTIONS

Be sure to consult your doctor or pharmacist before taking this drug if:
▼ You have cystic fibrosis.
▼ You have porphyria.

 Pregnancy
▼ Safety in pregnancy not established. Discuss with your doctor.

 Breast-feeding
▼ Safety in breast-feeding not established. Discuss with your doctor.

 Infants and children
▼ Not used in in infants and children under 10 years.

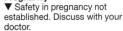 **Over 60**
▼ No special problems.

 Driving and hazardous work
▼ No special problems.

 Alcohol
▼ No special problems.

POSSIBLE ADVERSE EFFECTS

Any side effects are likely to be recognized.

Symptom/effect	Frequency		Discuss with doctor		Stop taking drug now	Call doctor now
	Common	Rare	Only if severe	In all cases		
Constipation	●		■			
Agitation/confusion		●		■	▲	

INTERACTIONS

None.

PROLONGED USE

No problems expected.

MEDROXYPROGESTERONE

Brand names Depo-Provera, Farlutal, Provera,
Used in the following combined preparations Improvera, Premique, Tridestra

GENERAL INFORMATION

Medroxyprogesterone is a progestogen, a synthetic female sex hormone similar to the natural hormone progesterone. This drug is used to treat a variety of menstrual disorders such as mid-cycle bleeding and amenorrhoea (absence of periods).

Medroxyprogesterone is also often used to treat endometriosis, a condition in which there is abnormal growth of the uterine-lining tissue in the pelvic cavity.

Depot injections of the drug are used as a contraceptive. However, since they may cause serious *side effects,* such as persistent bleeding from the uterus, amenorrhoea, and prolonged infertility, their use remains controversial, and they are recommended only under special circumstances in Britain.

Medroxyprogesterone may be used to treat some types of cancer, such as cancer of the breast, uterus, or prostate.

INFORMATION FOR USERS

Your drug prescription is tailored for you. Do not alter dosage without checking with your doctor.

How taken

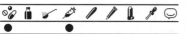

Tablets, depot injection.

Frequency and timing of doses
1–3 x daily with plenty of water (by mouth); tablets may need to be taken at certain times during your cycle; follow the instructions you have been given. Every 3 months (depot injection).

Adult dosage range
Menstrual disorders 2.5–10mg daily.
Endometriosis 30mg daily.
Cancer 100–1,500mg daily.
Contraception 150mg.

Onset of effect
1–2 months (cancer); 1–2 weeks (other conditions).

Duration of action
1–2 days (by mouth); up to some months (depot injection).

Diet advice
None.

Storage
Keep in a closed container in a cool, dry place out of the reach of children.

Missed dose
Take as soon as you remember. If your next dose is due within 3 hours, take a single dose now and skip the next.

Stopping the drug
Do not stop the drug without consulting your doctor; symptoms may recur.

Exceeding the dose
An occasional unintentional extra dose is unlikely to be a cause for concern. But if you notice any unusual symptoms, or if a large overdose has been taken, notify your doctor.

SPECIAL PRECAUTIONS

Be sure to tell your doctor if:
▼ You have high blood pressure.
▼ You have diabetes.
▼ You have had blood clots or a stroke.
▼ You have long-term liver or kidney problems.
▼ You are taking other medications.

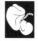 **Pregnancy**
▼ Not prescribed. May cause abnormalities in the unborn baby. Discuss with your doctor.

 Breast-feeding
▼ The drug passes into the breast milk, but at normal doses adverse effects on the baby are unlikely. Discuss with your doctor.

 Infants and children
▼ Not usually prescribed.

 Over 60
▼ No special problems.

 Driving and hazardous work
▼ No known problems.

 Alcohol
▼ No known problems.

POSSIBLE ADVERSE EFFECTS

Medroxyprogesterone rarely causes serious adverse effects. Fluid retention may lead to weight gain, swollen feet or ankles, and breast tenderness.

Symptom/effect	Frequency		Discuss with doctor		Stop taking drug now	Call doctor now
	Common	Rare	Only if severe	In all cases		
Weight gain	●		■			
Swollen ankles	●		■			
Breast tenderness		●	■			
Nausea		●	■			
Fatigue/depression		●		■		
Irregular menstruation		●		■		
Rash/itching/acne		●		■	▲	

INTERACTIONS

None.

PROLONGED USE

Long-term use of this drug may slightly increase the risk of blood clots in the leg veins. Irregular menstrual bleeding or spotting between periods may also occur during long-term use.

Monitoring Periodic checks on blood pressure, yearly cervical smear tests, and breast examinations are usually required.

MEFENAMIC ACID

Brand names Dysman, Ponstan
Used in the following combined preparations None

GENERAL INFORMATION

Mefenamic acid, introduced in 1963, is a non-steroidal anti-inflammatory drug (NSAID). Like other NSAIDs, it relieves pain and inflammation. The drug is an effective analgesic, and is used to treat headache, toothache, and menstrual pains (dysmenorrhoea), as well as to reduce excessive menstrual bleeding (menorrhagia). Mefenamic acid is also prescribed for long-term relief of pain and stiffness in rheumatoid arthritis and osteoarthritis.

The most common *side effects* of mefenamic acid are gastrointestinal: abdominal pain, nausea and vomiting, and indigestion. Other, more serious effects include kidney problems and blood disorders.

INFORMATION FOR USERS

Your drug prescription is tailored for you. Do not alter dosage without checking with your doctor.

How taken

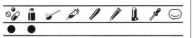

Tablets, capsules, liquid.

Frequency and timing of doses
3 x daily with food.

Adult dosage range
1,500mg daily.

Onset of effect
1–2 hours.

Duration of action
Up to 6 hours.

Diet advice
None.

Storage
Keep in a closed container in a cool, dry place out of the reach of children.

Missed dose
Take as soon as you remember. If your next dose is due within 2 hours, take a single dose now and skip the next.

Stopping the drug
Can be safely stopped as soon as you no longer need it.

Exceeding the dose
An occasional unintentional extra dose is unlikely to be a cause for concern. Large overdoses may cause poor coordination, muscle twitching, or fits. Notify your doctor.

POSSIBLE ADVERSE EFFECTS

Gastrointestinal disturbances are the most common side effects of mefenamic acid. The drug should be stopped if diarrhoea or a rash occur, and not used thereafter. Black or bloodstained bowel movements should be reported to your doctor without delay.

Symptom/effect	Frequency		Discuss with doctor		Stop taking drug now	Call doctor now
	Common	Rare	Only if severe	In all cases		
Indigestion	●		■			
Diarrhoea	●			■	▲	
Dizziness/drowsiness		●	■			
Nausea/vomiting		●	■			
Abdominal pain		●		■		
Rash		●		■	▲	
Wheezing/breathlessness		●		■	▲	▮

INTERACTIONS

General note Mefenamic acid interacts with a wide range of drugs to increase the risk of bleeding and/or peptic ulcers. These drugs include other non-steroidal anti-inflammatory drugs (NSAIDs) such as aspirin, oral anticoagulant drugs, and corticosteroids.

Antihypertensive drugs and diuretics
The beneficial effects of these drugs may be reduced by mefenamic acid.

Lithium Mefenamic acid may raise blood levels of lithium.

Oral antidiabetic drugs Mefenamic acid may increase the blood sugar-lowering effect of these drugs.

ACE inhibitors Mefenamic acid reduces the effectiveness of these drugs, and the chance of experiencing adverse effects from mefenamic acid are increased.

SPECIAL PRECAUTIONS

Be sure to tell your doctor if:
▼ You have liver or kidney problems.
▼ You have had a peptic ulcer, oesophagitis, or acid indigestion.
▼ You have inflammatory bowel disease.
▼ You have asthma.
▼ You have high blood pressure.
▼ You are allergic to aspirin.
▼ You have porphyria.
▼ You are taking other medications.

Pregnancy
▼ Not usually prescribed. May cause defects in the unborn baby and, taken in late pregnancy, may affect the baby's cardiovascular system. Discuss with your doctor.

Breast-feeding
▼ The drug passes into the breast milk, but at normal doses adverse effects on the baby are unlikely. Discuss with your doctor.

Infants and children
▼ Reduced dose necessary.

Over 60
▼ Increased likelihood of adverse effects.

Driving and hazardous work
▼ Avoid such activities until you have learned how mefenamic acid affects you because the drug can cause drowsiness and dizziness.

Alcohol
▼ Avoid. Alcohol may increase the risk of stomach irritation with mefenamic acid.

Surgery and general anaesthetics
▼ Mefenamic acid may prolong bleeding. Discuss the possibility of stopping treatment with your doctor or dentist before any surgery.

PROLONGED USE

Prolonged use increases the risk of bleeding from peptic ulcers and in the bowel. Rarely, the drug may affect the liver and blood. Blood tests may be carried out during prolonged use.

MEFLOQUINE

Brand name Lariam
Used in the following combined preparations None

GENERAL INFORMATION

Mefloquine is used for the prevention and treatment of malaria. It is recommended for use in areas where malaria is resistant to other drugs (e.g., China, Southeast Asia, South America, and Central and Southern Africa).

However, the use of mefloquine is limited by the fact that it can cause, in some patients, serious *side effects* that include depression, suicidal tendencies, anxiety, panic, confusion, hallucinations, paranoid delusions, and convulsions.

For most people, the benefits of the use of mefloquine outweigh the risks, although this should be discussed with your doctor.

INFORMATION FOR USERS

Your drug prescription is tailored for you. Do not alter dosage without checking with your doctor.

How taken

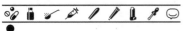

Tablets.

Frequency and timing of doses
Prevention Once weekly.
Treatment Up to 3 x daily, every 6–8 hours.

Adult dosage range
Prevention 1 tablet once weekly starting 1–3 weeks before departure and continuing until 4 weeks after leaving the malarial area.
Treatment Initial dose 3 tablets (750mg) followed by further doses according to body weight.

Onset of effect
2–3 days.

Duration of action
Over 1 week. Low levels of the drug may persist for several months.

Diet advice
None.

Storage
Keep in a cool, dry place out of the reach of children.

Missed dose
Take as soon as you remember. If your next dose is due within 48 hours (if taken once weekly for prevention), take a single dose now and skip the next.

Stopping the drug
Do not stop taking the drug without consulting your doctor about alternative treatment.

OVERDOSE ACTION

 Seek immediate medical advice in all cases. Take emergency action if dizziness, palpitations, collapse, or loss of consciousness occur.

See Drug poisoning emergency guide (p.494).

SPECIAL PRECAUTIONS

Be sure to tell your doctor if:
▼ You have long-term liver or kidney problems.
▼ You have had epileptic fits.
▼ You have had depression or other psychiatric illness.
▼ You have had a previous allergic reaction to mefloquine or quinine.
▼ You have heart problems.
▼ You are taking other medications.

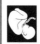

Pregnancy
▼ Not prescribed. Pregnancy must be avoided during and for 3 months after mefloquine use.

Breast-feeding
▼ Not prescribed. The drug passes into the breast milk.

Infants and children
▼ Not used in infants under 3 months old. Reduced dose necessary in older children.

Over 60
▼ Careful monitoring is necessary if liver or kidney problems or heart disease are present.

Driving and hazardous work
▼ Avoid such activities when taking mefloquine for prevention until you know how the drug affects you. Also avoid during treatment and for 3 weeks afterwards as the drug can cause dizziness or disturb balance.

Alcohol
▼ Keep consumption low.

POSSIBLE ADVERSE EFFECTS

Mefloquine commonly causes dizziness, vertigo, nausea, vomiting, and headache. In rare cases, serious adverse effects on the nervous system can occur, including anxiety or panic attacks, depression, hallucinations, and paranoid delusions.

Symptom/effect	Frequency		Discuss with doctor		Stop taking drug now	Call doctor now
	Common	Rare	Only if severe	In all cases		
Dizziness/vertigo	●			■		
Nausea/vomiting	●			■		
Headache	●			■		
Abdominal pain	●			■		
Depression		●		■	▲	
Anxiety/panic attacks		●		■	▲	
Hallucinations/delusions		●		■	▲	
Hearing disorders		●		■	▲	
Palpitations		●		■	▲	

PROLONGED USE

May be taken for prevention of malaria for up to one year.

INTERACTIONS

Anticonvulsant drugs Mefloquine may decrease the effect of these drugs.

Other antimalarial drugs Mefloquine may increase the risk of adverse effects when taken with these drugs.

General note Mefloquine may increase the effects on the heart of drugs such as beta blockers, calcium channel blockers, and digitalis drugs.

MEGESTROL

Brand name Megace
Used in the following combined preparations None

GENERAL INFORMATION

Megestrol is a progestogen, which is a synthetic female sex hormone similar to the natural hormone progesterone. The drug is used in the treatment of certain types of advanced cancer affecting the breast and uterus that are sensitive to hormone treatment. Megestrol is often prescribed when the tumour cannot be removed by surgery, when the disease has recurred after surgery, or when treatment with other anticancer drugs or radiotherapy have failed.

Successful treatment with megestrol reduces the size of the tumour; the drug may also cause secondary growths to disappear. Improvement usually occurs within two months of starting treatment. Because megestrol does not eradicate the cancer completely, the drug may need to be continued indefinitely.

INFORMATION FOR USERS

Your drug prescription is tailored for you. Do not alter dosage without checking with your doctor.

How taken

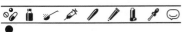

Tablets.

Frequency and timing of doses
1–4 x daily.

Adult dosage range
Breast cancer 160mg daily.
Cancer of the uterus 40–320mg daily.

Onset of effect
Within 2 months.

Duration of action
1–2 days.

Diet advice
None.

Storage
Keep in a closed container in a cool, dry place out of the reach of children.

Missed dose
Take as soon as you remember.

Stopping the drug
Do not stop the drug without consulting your doctor. Stopping the drug may lead to worsening of your underlying condition.

Exceeding the dose
An occasional unintentional extra dose is unlikely to be a cause for concern. But if you notice any unusual symptoms, or if a large overdose has been taken, notify your doctor.

SPECIAL PRECAUTIONS

Be sure to tell your doctor if:
▼ You have long-term liver or kidney problems.
▼ You have had thrombosis.
▼ You have high blood pressure.
▼ You have heart problems.
▼ You are taking other medications.

Pregnancy
▼ Not usually prescribed.

Breast-feeding
▼ Breast-feeding is usually discontinued. Discuss with your doctor.

Infants and children
▼ Not usually required.

Over 60
▼ No special problems.

Driving and hazardous work
▼ No known problems.

Alcohol
▼ No known problems.

POSSIBLE ADVERSE EFFECTS

Adverse effects are rare with megestrol. It may cause weight gain owing to increased appetite and food intake. Stop taking the drug and consult your doctor if a rash occurs.

Symptom/effect	Frequency		Discuss with doctor		Stop taking drug now	Call doctor now
	Common	Rare	Only if severe	In all cases		
Weight gain	●		■			
Swollen feet/ankles		●	■			
Nausea		●	■			
Headache		●			■	
Itching		●			■	
Hair loss		●			■	
Rash		●			■	▲

INTERACTIONS

None known.

PROLONGED USE

Long-term use of this drug may increase the risk of blood clots in the leg veins.

Monitoring Periodic checks on blood pressure may be performed.

MELOXICAM

Brand name Mobic
Used in the following combined preparations None

GENERAL INFORMATION

Meloxicam is a member of the non-steroidal anti-inflammatory (NSAID) group of drugs. It reduces pain, stiffness, and inflammation and is used to relieve the symptoms of rheumatoid arthritis, ankylosing spondylitis, and acute episodes of osteoarthritis. Meloxicam does not cure the underlying condition, however.

Meloxicam does not affect the stomach and is therefore less likely than many other NSAIDs to cause gastrointestinal bleeding, ulceration, and perforation. Because elderly people are more sensitive to the drug's effects, they are usually prescribed only half the normal adult dose.

QUICK REFERENCE

Drug group Nonsteroidal anti-inflammatory drug (p.116)

Overdose danger rating Medium

Dependence rating Low

Prescription needed Yes

Available as generic No

INFORMATION FOR USERS

Your drug prescription is tailored for you. Do not alter dosage without checking with your doctor.

How taken

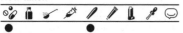

Tablets, suppositories.

Frequency and timing of doses
Once daily.

Adult dosage range
7.5–15mg.

Onset of effect
1 hour.

Duration of action
24 hours.

Diet advice
None.

Storage
Keep in a closed container in a cool, dry place out of the reach of children.

Missed dose
Take as soon as you remember. If your next dose is due within 8 hours, take a single dose now and skip the next.

Stopping the drug
The drug can be safely stopped as soon as you no longer need it (short term). Do not stop taking the drug without consulting your doctor (long term).

Exceeding the dose
An occasional unintentional extra dose is unlikely to cause problems. Large overdoses can cause stomach and intestinal pain and damage. Notify your doctor.

SPECIAL PRECAUTIONS

Be sure to tell your doctor if:
▼ You have asthma.
▼ You are allergic to aspirin or other NSAIDs.
▼ You have had a peptic ulcer, oesophagitis, or acid indigestion.
▼ You have liver or kidney problems.
▼ You have a bleeding disorder, proctitis, or haemorrhoids.
▼ You are taking other medications.

Pregnancy
▼ Safety not established. May affect the developing foetus. Discuss with your doctor.

Breast-feeding
▼ Safety not established. Discuss with your doctor.

Infants and children
▼ Not recommended.

Over 60
▼ Increased likelihood of adverse effects. Reduced doses necessary.

Driving and hazardous work
▼ Avoid such activities until you have learned how meloxicam affects you because the drug can cause vertigo and drowsiness.

Alcohol
▼ Keep consumption low. Alcohol may increase the risk of stomach irritation with meloxicam.

POSSIBLE ADVERSE EFFECTS

Gastrointestinal disturbance, skin rash, and headache are common *adverse effects*. Black or bloodstained faeces and wheezing should be reported to your doctor without delay.

Symptom/effect	Frequency		Discuss with doctor		Stop taking drug now	Call doctor now
	Common	Rare	Only if severe	In all cases		
Abdominal pain/indigestion	●			■		
Headache	●			■		
Diarrhoea or constipation	●			■		
Skin rash/itching	●			■		
Lightheadedness/drowsiness	●			■		
Palpitations		●		■		
Vertigo/ringing in the ears		●		■		
Persistent sore throat		●		■		
Wheezing/breathing difficulties		●		■	▲	▮
Black/bloodstained faeces		●		■	▲	▮

PROLONGED USE

No special problems.

Monitoring Periodic tests on kidney function may be performed.

INTERACTIONS

Anticoagulants, other NSAIDs, oxpentifylline Taken with meloxicam, these drugs increase the risk of gastrointestinal bleeding.

Cyclosporin There is an increased risk of kidney damage when meloxicam is taken with cyclosporin.

Methotrexate Meloxicam may increase the risk of *toxicity* with this drug.

Lithium Meloxicam may increase the effects and risk of toxicity with lithium.

Antibacterials Meloxicam may increase the risk of convulsions with quinolones.

MERCAPTOPURINE

Brand name Puri-Nethol
Used in the following combined preparations None

GENERAL INFORMATION

Mercaptopurine, an anticancer drug, is widely used to prevent the recurrence of certain forms of leukaemia. Used with other anticancer drugs, mercaptopurine is also given to leukaemia victims who have not responded to other treatments.

Nausea and vomiting, mouth ulcers, and loss of appetite are the drug's most common *side effects*. Such symptoms tend to be milder than those of other cytotoxic drugs, and often disappear as the body adjusts to the drug. More seriously, mercaptopurine can interfere with blood cell production, resulting in blood clotting disorders and anaemia, and can also cause liver damage. The likelihood of infections is also increased.

INFORMATION FOR USERS

Your drug prescription is tailored for you. Do not alter dosage without checking with your doctor.

How taken

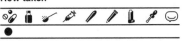

Tablets.

Frequency and timing of doses
Once daily.

Dosage range
Dosage is determined individually according to body weight and response.

Onset of effect
1–2 weeks.

Duration of action
Side effects may persist for several weeks after stopping treatment.

Diet advice
None.

Storage
Keep in a closed container in a cool, dry place out of the reach of children. Protect from light.

Missed dose
If your next dose is due within 6 hours, take a single dose now and skip the next. Tell your doctor that you missed a dose.

Stopping the drug
Do not stop taking the drug without consulting your doctor; stopping the drug may lead to worsening of your underlying condition.

Exceeding the dose
An occasional unintentional extra dose is unlikely to cause problems. Large overdoses may cause nausea and vomiting. Notify your doctor.

SPECIAL PRECAUTIONS

Be sure to tell your doctor if:
▼ You have long-term liver or kidney problems.
▼ You suffer from gout.
▼ You have recently had any infection.
▼ You have porphyria.
▼ You are taking other medications.

Pregnancy
▼ Not usually prescribed. Discuss with your doctor.

Breast-feeding
▼ Not advised. The drug passes into the breast milk and may affect the baby adversely. Discuss with your doctor.

Infants and children
▼ Reduced dose necessary.

Over 60
▼ Reduced dose may be necessary. Increased risk of adverse effects.

Driving and hazardous work
▼ No known problems.

Alcohol
▼ Avoid. Alcohol may increase the adverse effects of this drug.

POSSIBLE ADVERSE EFFECTS

The most common adverse effects are nausea and vomiting, and loss of appetite. *Jaundice* may also occur, but is reversible on stopping the drug. Because mercaptopurine interferes with the production of blood cells, it may cause anaemia and blood clotting disorders; and infections are more likely.

Symptom/effect	Frequency		Discuss with doctor		Stop taking drug now	Call doctor now
	Common	Rare	Only if severe	In all cases		
Nausea/vomiting	●		■			
Loss of appetite	●		■			
Mouth ulcers	●			■		▮
Jaundice		●		■		▮
Black faeces		●		■		▮
Bloodstained vomit		●		■		▮

INTERACTIONS

Allopurinol This drug increases blood levels of mercaptopurine.

Warfarin The effects of warfarin may be decreased by mercaptopurine.

PROLONGED USE

Prolonged use of this drug may reduce bone marrow activity, leading to a reduction of all types of blood cells.

Monitoring Regular blood checks and tests on liver function are required.

MESALAZINE

Brand names Asacol, Pentasa, Salofalk
Used in the following combined preparations None

GENERAL INFORMATION

Mesalazine is prescribed for patients with ulcerative colitis and is sometimes used for Crohn's disease, which affects the large intestine. The drug is given to relieve symptoms in an acute attack and is also taken as a preventative measure. When mesalazine is used to treat severe cases, it is often taken with other drugs such as corticosteroids.

When taken in tablet form, the active component of the drug is released in the large intestine, where its local effect relieves the inflamed mucosa. Enemas and suppositories are also available and are particularly useful when the disease affects the rectum and lower colon.

This drug produces fewer *side effects* than some older treatments, such as sulfasalazine. Patients who are unable to tolerate sulfasalazine may be able to take mesalazine without any problems.

INFORMATION FOR USERS

Your drug prescription is tailored for you. Do not alter dosage without checking with your doctor.

How taken

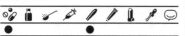

Tablets, suppositories, enema (aerosol).

Frequency and timing of doses
3 x daily, swallowed whole and not chewed (tablets); 3 x daily (suppositories); once daily at bedtime (enema).

Adult dosage range
1.5–2.4g daily (acute attack); 750mg–2.4g daily (maintenance dose).

Onset of effect
Adverse effects may be noticed within a few days, but full beneficial effects may not be felt for a couple of weeks.

Duration of action
Up to 12 hours.

Diet advice
Your doctor may advise you, taking account of the condition affecting you.

Storage
Keep in a closed container in a cool, dry place out of the reach of children. Protect from light. Keep aerosol container out of direct sunlight.

Missed dose
Take as soon as you remember. If your next dose is due within 2 hours, take a single dose now and skip the next.

Stopping the drug
Do not stop taking the drug without consulting your doctor; symptoms may recur.

Exceeding the dose
An occasional unintentional extra dose is unlikely to be a cause for concern. But if you notice any unusual symptoms, or if a large overdose has been taken, notify your doctor.

SPECIAL PRECAUTIONS

Be sure to tell your doctor if:
▼ You have long-term liver or kidney problems.
▼ You are allergic to aspirin.
▼ You are taking other medications.

 Pregnancy
▼ Negligible amounts of the drug cross the placenta. However, safety in pregnancy is not established. Discuss with your doctor.

 Breast-feeding
▼ Negligible amounts of the drug pass into the breast milk. However, safety is not established. Discuss with your doctor.

 Infants and children
▼ Not recommended under 15 years.

 Over 60
▼ Dosage reduction not normally necessary unless there is kidney impairment.

 Driving and hazardous work
▼ No special problems.

 Alcohol
▼ No special problems.

POSSIBLE ADVERSE EFFECTS

The common side effects of mesalazine are on the gastrointestinal tract. Other problems rarely occur. However, unexplained bleeding, bruising, sore throat, fever, or malaise should be reported to your doctor, who will carry out a blood test to eliminate blood disorders.

Symptom/effect	Frequency		Discuss with doctor		Stop taking drug now	Call doctor now
	Common	Rare	Only if severe	In all cases		
Nausea	●		■			
Abdominal pain	●		■			
Diarrhoea	●		■			
Fever/wheezing		●		■	▲	■
Colitis worsening		●		■	▲	
Rash		●		■	▲	
Bleeding/bruising		●		■	▲	
Sore throat/malaise		●		■	▲	

INTERACTIONS

Lactulose The release of mesalazine at its site of action may be reduced by lactulose.

PROLONGED USE

No problems expected.

METFORMIN

Brand names Glucamet, Glucophage, Orabet
Used in the following combined preparations None

GENERAL INFORMATION

Metformin is an antidiabetic drug used to treat adult (maturity-onset or Type 2) diabetes in which some insulin-secreting cells are still active in the pancreas. It is usually prescribed for obese patients.

Metformin lowers blood sugar by reducing the absorption of glucose from the digestive tract into the bloodstream, by reducing the glucose production by cells in the liver and kidneys, and by increasing the sensitivity of cells to insulin so that they take up glucose more effectively from the blood.

The drug is given in conjunction with a special diabetic diet that limits sugar and fat intake. It is often given with another antidiabetic drug that stimulates insulin secretion by the pancreas, or with insulin for treatment of maturity-onset diabetes, especially to obese patients.

INFORMATION FOR USERS

Your drug prescription is tailored for you. Do not alter dosage without checking with your doctor.

How taken

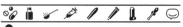

Tablets.

Frequency and timing of doses
2–3 x daily with food.

Adult dosage range
1.5–3g daily.

Onset of effect
Within 2 hours. It may take 2 weeks to achieve control of diabetes.

Duration of action
8–12 hours.

Diet advice
An individualized low-fat, low-sugar diet must be maintained in order for the drug to be fully effective. Follow your doctor's advice.

Storage
Keep in a closed container in a cool, dry place out of the reach of children.

Missed dose
Take as soon as you remember. If your next dose is due within 2 hours, take a single dose now and skip the next.

Stopping the drug
Do not stop taking the drug without consulting your doctor; stopping the drug may lead to worsening of the underlying condition.

OVERDOSE ACTION

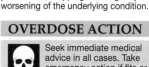

Seek immediate medical advice in all cases. Take emergency action if fits or loss of consciousness occur.

See Drug poisoning emergency guide (p.494).

SPECIAL PRECAUTIONS

Be sure to tell your doctor if:
▼ You have long-term liver or kidney problems.
▼ You have heart failure.
▼ You are a heavy drinker.
▼ You are taking other medications.

 Pregnancy
▼ Not usually prescribed. Insulin is usually substituted because it provides better diabetic control during pregnancy. Discuss with your doctor.

 Breast-feeding
▼ Safety not established. Discuss with your doctor.

 **Infants and children**
▼ Not recommended.

Over 60
▼ Increased likelihood of adverse effects. Reduced dose may therefore be necessary.

 Driving and hazardous work
▼ Usually no problems. Avoid such activities if you have warning signs of low blood sugar.

 Alcohol
▼ Avoid. Alcohol increases the risk of low blood sugar, and can cause coma by increasing the acidity of the blood.

Surgery and general anaesthetics
▼ Surgery may reduce the response to this drug. Notify your doctor that you are diabetic before any surgery; insulin treatment may need to be substituted.

POSSIBLE ADVERSE EFFECTS

Minor gastrointestinal symptoms such as nausea, vomiting, and loss of appetite are often helped by taking the drug with food.

Diarrhoea usually settles after a few days of continued treatment.

Symptom/effect	Frequency		Discuss with doctor		Stop taking drug now	Call doctor now
	Common	Rare	Only if severe	In all cases		
Loss of appetite	●		■			
Nausea/vomiting	●		■			
Diarrhoea		●	■			
Dizziness/confusion		●		■		
Weakness/sweating		●		■		
Rash		●		■		

INTERACTIONS

General note A number of drugs reduce the effects of metformin. These include corticosteroids, oestrogens, and diuretics. Other drugs, notably monoamine oxidase inhibitors (MAOIs) and beta blockers, increase its effects.

Warfarin Metformin may increase the effect of this anticoagulant drug. The dosage of warfarin may need to be adjusted accordingly.

PROLONGED USE

Prolonged treatment with metformin can deplete reserves of vitamin B$_{12}$, and this may cause anaemia.

Monitoring Regular checks on kidney function and on levels of sugar in the urine and/or blood are usually required. Vitamin B$_{12}$ levels may also be checked annually.

METHADONE

Brand names Methadose, Metharose, Methex, Physeptone
Used in the following combined preparations None

GENERAL INFORMATION

Methadone is a synthetic drug belonging to the *opioid* analgesic group. It is used in the control of severe pain and as a cough suppressant, but it is more widely used to replace morphine or heroin in the treatment of *dependence*. In this situation, methadone can be given once daily to prevent *withdrawal symptoms*.

In some cases, dosage can be reduced until the drug is no longer needed.

Tolerance to methadone is marked. Although the initial dose for a person not used to taking opioids is very low, the dose needed by someone who regularly takes the drug could be fatal for a non-user.

QUICK REFERENCE

Drug group Opioid analgesic (p.80)

Overdose danger rating High

Dependence rating High

Prescription needed Yes

Available as generic Yes

INFORMATION FOR USERS

Your drug prescription is tailored for you. Do not alter dosage without checking with your doctor.

How taken

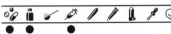

Tablets, liquid, injection.

Frequency and timing of doses
Pain 3–4 x daily; 2 x daily (prolonged use).
Cough 4–6 x daily (starting dose); 2 x daily (prolonged use).
Opioid addiction Once daily.

Adult dosage range
Pain 5–10mg per dose initially, adjusted according to response.
Cough 1–2mg per dose.
Opioid addiction 10–20mg (starting dose); 40–60mg daily (maintenance dose).

Onset of effect
15–60 minutes.

Duration of action
36–48 hours.

Diet advice
None.

Storage
Keep in a closed container in a cool, dry place out of the reach of children. Protect injections and liquids from light.

Missed dose
Take as soon as you remember and return to your normal dosing schedule as soon as possible. If you missed the dose because it caused you to vomit, or if you cannot swallow, consult your doctor.

Stopping the drug
If the reason for taking the drug no longer exists, it can be safely stopped. Discuss with your doctor.

OVERDOSE ACTION

 Seek immediate medical advice in all cases. Take emergency action if symptoms such as slow or irregular breathing, severe drowsiness, or loss of consciousness occur.

See Drug poisoning emergency guide (p.494).

POSSIBLE ADVERSE EFFECTS

Drowsiness and nausea are the most common *side effects* of methadone, but these diminish as the body adapts.

Symptom/effect	Frequency		Discuss with doctor		Stop taking drug now	Call doctor now
	Common	Rare	Only if severe	In all cases		
Nausea/vomiting	●		■			
Drowsiness	●		■			
Constipation	●		■			
Dizziness/confusion	●			■		
Loss of consciousness		●	■		▲	▌
Slow, difficult breathing		●	■		▲	▌

INTERACTIONS

Phenytoin, carbamazepine, and ritonavir These drugs may reduce the effects of methadone.

Monoamine oxidase inhibitors (MAOIs) Taken with methadone, these drugs may produce a rise or fall in blood pressure.

Sedatives The effects of all drugs that have a sedative effect on the central nervous system are likely to be increased by methadone.

SPECIAL PRECAUTIONS

Be sure to tell your doctor if:
▼ You have heart or circulatory problems.
▼ You have liver or kidney problems.
▼ You have lung problems such as asthma or bronchitis.
▼ You have thyroid disease.
▼ You have a history of epileptic fits.
▼ You are an alcoholic.
▼ You are taking other medications.

 Pregnancy
▼ Not prescribed in late pregnancy if possible. May cause breathing difficulties in the newborn baby. Discuss with your doctor.

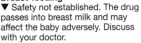 **Breast-feeding**
▼ Safety not established. The drug passes into breast milk and may affect the baby adversely. Discuss with your doctor.

 Infants and children
▼ Not recommended.

 Over 60
▼ Not recommended.

 Driving and hazardous work
▼ Your underlying condition may make such activities inadvisable. Discuss with your doctor.

Alcohol
▼ Avoid. Alcohol increases the sedative effects of the drug and may depress breathing.

PROLONGED USE

Treatment with methadone is always closely monitored. If the drug is being taken long term, the dose must be carefully reduced before the drug is stopped.

METHOTREXATE

Brand name Maxtrex
Used in the following combined preparations None

GENERAL INFORMATION

Methotrexate is an anticancer drug used, together with other anticancer drugs, in the treatment of leukaemia, lymphoma, and solid cancers such as those of the breast, bone, lung, bladder, head, and neck. It is also used to treat severe uncontrolled psoriasis until less potent drugs can be re-introduced. It is also prescribed for people with severe acute rheumatoid arthritis that has not responded to other treatment. Once the condition is under control, the dose of methotrexate is reduced to a minimum.

As with most anticancer drugs, methotrexate affects both healthy and cancerous cells, so that its usefulness is limited by its *adverse effects* and *toxicity*. The drug is usually given with folinic acid to prevent it from destroying bone marrow cells when it is given in high doses.

Methotrexate has been reported to reduce the IQ of children. It may also reduce fertility by depressing sperm and egg development.

QUICK REFERENCE

Drug group Anticancer drug (p.154), antirheumatic drug (p.117), and drug for psoriasis, (p.178)

Overdose danger rating Medium

Dependence rating Low

Prescription needed Yes

Available as generic Yes

INFORMATION FOR USERS

Your drug prescription is tailored for you. Do not alter dosage without checking with your doctor.

How taken

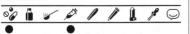

Tablets, injection.

Frequency and timing of doses
Daily or every 2 days, for 4–5 doses, repeating at weekly intervals (some short chemotherapy courses only); once weekly (other conditions).

Adult dosage range
Cancer Dosage is determined individually according to the nature of the condition, body weight, and response.
Rheumatoid arthritis 7.5–20mg weekly.
Psoriasis 10-25mg weekly.

Onset of effect
30–60 minutes.

Duration of action
10–15 hours.

Diet advice
None.

Storage
Keep in a closed container in a cool, dry place out of the reach of children. Wash your hands after handling the tablets.

Missed dose
Take as soon as you remember and consult your doctor.

Stopping the drug
Do not stop taking the drug without consulting your doctor. Stopping the drug may lead to worsening of the underlying condition.

Exceeding the dose
Tell your doctor if you accidentally take an extra tablet. Large overdoses damage the bone marrow and cause nausea and abdominal pain. Notify your doctor immediately.

SPECIAL PRECAUTIONS

Be sure to tell your doctor if:
▼ You have liver or kidney problems.
▼ You have porphyria.
▼ You have a problem with alcohol abuse.
▼ You have a peptic or other digestive-tract ulcer.
▼ You are taking other medications.

 Pregnancy
▼ Not prescribed. Methotrexate may cause birth defects in the unborn baby.

 Breast-feeding
▼ Not advised. The drug passes into the breast milk and may affect the baby adversely.

 Infants and children
▼ For cancer treatment only. Reduced dose necessary.

 Over 60
▼ Increased likelihood of adverse effects. Reduced doses necessary.

 Driving and hazardous work
▼ No special problems.

 Alcohol
▼ Avoid. Alcohol may increase the adverse effects of methotrexate.

POSSIBLE ADVERSE EFFECTS

Nausea and vomiting may occur within a few hours of taking methotrexate. Diarrhoea and mouth ulcers are also common side effects.

Symptom/effect	Frequency		Discuss with doctor		Stop taking drug now	Call doctor now
	Common	Rare	Only if severe	In all cases		
Nausea/vomiting	●			■		
Diarrhoea	●			■		
Dry cough/chest pain	●			■		
Mouth/gum ulcers/inflammation	●			■	▲	▮
Jaundice		●		■		
Mood changes/confusion		●		■		
Sore throat/fever		●		■	▲	▮
Rash		●		■	▲	

PROLONGED USE

Long-term treatment with methotrexate may be needed for rheumatoid arthritis. Once the condition is controlled, the drug is reduced as much as possible to the lowest effective dose.

Monitoring Full blood counts and kidney and liver function tests will be performed before treatment starts and at intervals during treatment. Blood concentrations of methotrexate may also be measured periodically.

INTERACTIONS

General Note Many drugs, including NSAIDs, diuretics, cyclosporin, phenytoin, and probenecid, may increase blood levels and toxicity of methotrexate.

Co-trimoxazole, trimethoprim, and nitrous oxide (including Entonox©) These drugs may enhance the effects of methotrexate.

METHYLCELLULOSE

Brand name Celevac
Used in the following combined preparations None

GENERAL INFORMATION

Methylcellulose is a laxative used for the treatment of constipation, diverticular disease, and irritable bowel syndrome. Taken by mouth, methylcellulose is not absorbed into the bloodstream but remains in the intestine. It absorbs up to 25 times its volume of water, thereby softening faeces and increasing their volume. It is also used to reduce the frequency and increase the firmness of faeces in chronic watery diarrhoea, and to control the consistency of faeces after colostomies and ileostomies.

Methylcellulose preparations are also used with appropriate dieting in some cases of obesity. The bulking agent swells to give a feeling of fullness, thereby encouraging adherence to a reducing diet.

Methylcellulose is found in contact lens irrigation solutions and in various lotions, creams, ointments, and pastes.

QUICK REFERENCE

Drug group Laxative (p.111) and antidiarrhoeal drug (p.110)

Overdose danger rating Low

Dependence rating Low

Prescription needed No

Available as generic No

INFORMATION FOR USERS

Follow instructions on the label. Call your doctor if symptoms worsen.

How taken

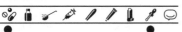

Tablets, eye drops

Frequency and timing of doses
1–4 x daily. Unless otherwise instructed, take with a full glass of water. Use eye drops as directed.

Adult dosage range
1.5–6g daily.

Onset of effect
Within 24 hours.

Duration of action
Up to 3 days.

Diet advice
If taken as a laxative, drink plenty of fluids, at least 6–8 glasses daily.

Storage
Keep in a closed container in a cool, dry place out of the reach of children.

Missed dose
Take as soon as you remember. Take the next dose as scheduled.

Stopping the drug
Can be safely stopped as soon as you no longer need it.

Exceeding the dose
An occasional unintentional extra dose is unlikely to be a cause for concern. But if you notice any unusual symptoms, or if a large overdose has been taken, notify your doctor.

POSSIBLE ADVERSE EFFECTS

When taken by mouth, the drug may cause bloating and excess wind. Insufficient fluid intake may cause blockage of the oesophagus (gullet) or intestine. Consult your doctor if you experience severe abdominal pain or if you have no bowel movement for 2 days after taking methylcellulose. When taken as eye drops, no adverse effects are expected.

Symptom/effect	Frequency		Discuss with doctor		Stop taking drug now	Call doctor now
	Common	Rare	Only if severe	In all cases		
Abdominal distension		●	■			
Flatulence		●	■			
Abdominal pain		●		■		

SPECIAL PRECAUTIONS

Be sure to consult your doctor or pharmacist before taking this drug if:
▼ You have severe constipation and/or abdominal pain.
▼ You have unexplained rectal bleeding.
▼ You have difficulty in swallowing.
▼ You vomit readily.
▼ You are taking other medications.

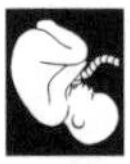

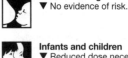

Pregnancy
▼ No evidence of risk to developing baby.

Breast-feeding
▼ No evidence of risk.

Infants and children
▼ Reduced dose necessary.

Over 60
▼ No special problems.

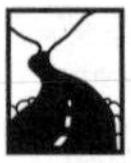

Driving and hazardous work
▼ No known problems.

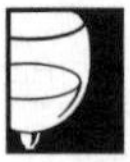

Alcohol
▼ No known problems.

INTERACTIONS

None.

PROLONGED USE

No problems expected.

METHYLDOPA

Brand name Aldomet
Used in the following combined preparations None

GENERAL INFORMATION

Introduced in the 1960s, methyldopa was, for many years, one of the most widely prescribed antihypertensive drugs for the treatment of high blood pressure. In recent years, its use has declined as newer drugs with fewer *side effects* have been introduced. However, it is effective in treating people for whom other, newer drugs are ineffective, and for treating those patients who have taken the drug for many years without experiencing side effects such as drowsiness, which can be a problems for others.

Unlike some other antihypertensives, methyldopa does not reduce blood flow to the kidneys and is therefore used for patients with kidney disorders.

Because methyldopa does not affect unborn babies, it is often prescribed to women who experience high blood pressure during late pregnancy.

QUICK REFERENCE

Drug group Antihypertensive drug (p.102)

Overdose danger rating Medium

Dependence rating Low

Prescription needed Yes

Available as generic Yes

INFORMATION FOR USERS

Your drug prescription is tailored for you. Do not alter dosage without checking with your doctor.

How taken

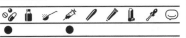

Tablets, injection.

Frequency and timing of doses
2–4 x daily.

Dosage range
Adults 500mg–3g daily.
Children Reduced dose necessary.

Onset of effect
3–6 hours. Full effect begins in 2–3 days.

Duration of action
6–12 hours. Some effect may last for 1–2 days after stopping the drug.

Diet advice
None.

Storage
Keep in a closed container in a cool, dry place out of the reach of children. Protect from light.

Missed dose
Take as soon as you remember. If your next dose is due within 2 hours, take a single dose now and skip the next.

Stopping the drug
Do not stop the drug without consulting your doctor, who will gradually reduce your dose. Suddenly stopping methyldopa may lead to an increase in blood pressure.

Exceeding the dose
An occasional unintentional extra dose is unlikely to cause problems. Large overdoses may cause drowsiness or palpitations. Notify your doctor.

SPECIAL PRECAUTIONS

Be sure to tell your doctor if:
▼ You have long-term liver or kidney problems.
▼ You have anaemia.
▼ You have angina.
▼ You suffer from depression.
▼ You are taking other medications.

 Pregnancy
▼ No evidence of risk.

 Breast-feeding
▼ The drug passes into the breast milk, but at normal doses adverse effects on the baby are unlikely. Discuss with your doctor.

 Infants and children
▼ Reduced dose necessary.

 Over 60
▼ Reduced dose necessary.

 Driving and hazardous work
▼ Avoid such activities until you have learned how methyldopa affects you because the drug can cause drowsiness.

 Alcohol
▼ Avoid. Alcohol may increase the hypotensive and sedative effects of this drug.

Surgery and general anaesthetics
▼ Discuss the possibility of stopping methyldopa with your doctor or dentist before any surgery.

POSSIBLE ADVERSE EFFECTS

Most adverse effects are uncommon and diminish in time. The fluid retention that occurs during treatment with methyldopa is counteracted by taking a diuretic.

Symptom/effect	Frequency		Discuss with doctor		Stop taking drug now	Call doctor now
	Common	Rare	Only if severe	In all cases		
Drowsiness	●		■			
Depression/headaches	●			■		
Fever		●		■		
Stuffy nose		●		■		
Dizziness/fainting		●		■		
Nausea/vomiting		●		■		
Rash		●		■	▲	
Jaundice		●		■	▲	■

INTERACTIONS

Lithium Lithium *toxicity* may occur as methyldopa may raise blood lithium levels.

Tricyclic antidepressants These drugs may reduce the effects of methyldopa.

Levodopa The effects of methyldopa may be enhanced by levodopa.

PROLONGED USE

Liver and blood problems may occur rarely.

Monitoring Periodic checks on blood and urine are usually required.

METOCLOPRAMIDE

Brand names Gastrobid, Gastroflux, Gastromax, Maxolon, Parmid, Primperan
Used in the following combined preparations Migravess, Paramax

GENERAL INFORMATION

Metoclopramide has a direct action on the gastrointestinal tract. It is used for conditions in which there is a need to encourage normal propulsion of food through the stomach and intestine.

The drug has powerful anti-emetic properties and its most common use is in the prevention and treatment of nausea and vomiting. It is particularly effective for the relief of the nausea that sometimes accompanies migraine headaches, and the nausea caused by treatment with anticancer drugs. It is also prescribed to alleviate symptoms of hiatus hernia caused by acid reflux into the oesophagus.

One *side effect* of metoclopramide, muscle spasm of the face and neck, is more likely to occur in children and young adults under 20 years. Other side effects are not usually troublesome.

INFORMATION FOR USERS

Your drug prescription is tailored for you. Do not alter dosage without checking with your doctor.

How taken

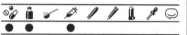

Tablets, SR-tablets/capsules, liquid, injection.

Frequency and timing of doses
Usually 3 x daily; 1–2 x daily (SR-preparations).

Adult dosage range
Usually 15–30mg daily; may be higher for nausea caused by anticancer drugs.

Onset of effect
Within 1 hour.

Duration of action
6–8 hours.

Diet advice
Fatty and spicy foods and alcohol are best avoided if nausea is a problem.

Storage
Keep in a closed container in a cool, dry place out of the reach of children.

Missed dose
Take as soon as you remember. If your next dose is due within 3 hours, take a single dose now and skip the next.

Stopping the drug
Can be safely stopped as soon as you no longer need it.

Exceeding the dose
An occasional unintentional extra dose is unlikely to be a cause for concern. Large overdoses may cause drowsiness and muscle spasms. Notify your doctor.

POSSIBLE ADVERSE EFFECTS

The main adverse effects of metoclopramide are drowsiness and, even less commonly, uncontrolled muscle spasm. Other symptoms rarely occur.

Symptom/effect	Frequency		Discuss with doctor		Stop taking drug now	Call doctor now
	Common	Rare	Only if severe	In all cases		
Drowsiness	●		■			
Restlessness	●			■		
Diarrhoea	●			■		
Muscle tremor/rigidity	●			■		
Muscle spasm of face	●			■	▲	■

INTERACTIONS

Sedatives The sedative properties of metoclopramide are increased by all drugs that have a sedative effect on the central nervous system. Such drugs include anti-anxiety and sleeping drugs, antihistamines, antidepressants, *opioid* analgesics, and antipsychotics.

Phenothiazine antipsychotics The likelihood of adverse effects from these drugs is increased by metoclopramide.

Lithium Metoclopramide increases the risk of central nervous system side effects.

SPECIAL PRECAUTIONS

Be sure to tell your doctor if:
▼ You have long-term liver or kidney problems.
▼ You have acute porphyria.
▼ You are taking other medications.

 Pregnancy
▼ Safety in pregnancy not established. Discuss with your doctor.

 Breast-feeding
▼ The drug passes into the breast milk but at normal doses adverse effects on the baby are unlikely. Discuss with your doctor.

 Infants and children
▼ Reduced dose necessary.

 Over 60
▼ Reduced dose may be necessary.

 Driving and hazardous work
▼ Avoid such activities until you have learned how metoclopramide affects you because the drug can cause drowsiness.

 Alcohol
▼ Avoid. Alcohol may oppose the beneficial effects and increase the sedative effects of this drug.

PROLONGED USE

Not normally used long term, except under specialist supervision for certain gastrointestinal disorders.

METOPROLOL

Brand names Betaloc, Betaloc SA, Lopresor, Lopresor SR, Mepranix
Used in the following combined preparations Co-Betaloc, Co-Betaloc SA

GENERAL INFORMATION

Metoprolol is a member of the beta-blocker group of drugs. It is used to prevent the heart from beating too quickly in conditions such as angina, hypertension (high blood pressure), arrhythmias (abnormal heart rhythms), and hyperthyroidism (overactive thyroid gland). It is also used to prevent migraine attacks and to protect the heart from further damage following a heart attack.

Because the drug is cardioselective (see p.97), it is less likely to provoke breathing difficulties than other, non-cardioselective, beta blockers. However, it should be used with caution by people with respiratory diseases such as asthma or bronchitis.

INFORMATION FOR USERS

Your drug prescription is tailored for you. Do not alter dosage without checking with your doctor.

How taken

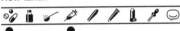

Tablets, SR-tablets, injection.

Frequency and timing of doses
1–2 x daily (hypertension); 2–3 x daily (angina/arrhythmias; 4 x daily for 2 days, then 2 x daily (heart attack prevention); 2 x daily (migraine prevention); 4 x daily (hyperthyroidism).

Adult dosage range
100–300mg daily.

Onset of effect
1–2 hours.

Duration of action
3–7 hours.

Diet advice
None.

Storage
Keep in a closed container in a cool, dry place out of the reach of children.

Missed dose
Take as soon as you remember. If your next dose is due within 2 hours, take a single dose now and skip the next.

Stopping the drug
Do not stop taking the drug without consulting your doctor. Stopping suddenly may lead to worsening of the underlying condition.

OVERDOSE ACTION

Seek immediate medical advice in all cases. Take emergency action if breathing difficulties, collapse, or loss of consciousness occur.

See Drug poisoning emergency guide (p.494).

SPECIAL PRECAUTIONS

Be sure to tell your doctor if:
▼ You have liver or kidney problems.
▼ You have asthma, bronchitis, or emphysema.
▼ You have heart failure.
▼ You have diabetes.
▼ You have hyperthyroidism.
▼ You have phaeochromocytoma.
▼ You have poor circulation in the legs.
▼ You are taking other medications.

 Pregnancy
▼ Not usually prescribed. May affect the baby. Discuss with your doctor.

 Breast-feeding
▼ The drug passes into the breast milk, but at normal doses adverse effects on the baby are unlikely. Discuss with your doctor.

 Infants and children
▼ Not recommended.

 Over 60
▼ There may be an increased risk of adverse effects.

 Driving and hazardous work
▼ Avoid such activities until you have learned how metoprolol affects you because the drug can cause fatigue, dizziness, and drowsiness.

 Alcohol
▼ No special problems.

POSSIBLE ADVERSE EFFECTS

Like all beta blockers, metoprolol is associated with nightmares and cold fingers and toes. Other common *adverse effects* include breathing difficulties and slow heart beat.

Symptom/effect	Frequency		Discuss with doctor		Stop taking drug now	Call doctor now
	Common	Rare	Only if severe	In all cases		
Cold hands and feet	●		■			
Nightmares/drowsiness	●		■			
Fatigue/dizziness/headache	●		■			
Nausea/vomiting/abdominal pain		●	■			
Breathing difficulties/wheezing		●		■		
Fainting		●		■		

INTERACTIONS

Verapamil When first taken with metoprolol, this drug may seriously slow or stop the heart beat and lower the blood pressure.

Decongestants Taken with metoprolol, these drugs may increase blood pressure and heart rate.

Ergotamine Taken with metoprolol, this drug increases the constriction of blood vessels in the extremities.

Antidiabetic drugs Taken with metoprolol, these drugs may increase the risk or mask the symptoms of low blood sugar.

Nonsteroidal anti-inflammatory drugs NSAIDs) These drugs may oppose the blood-pressure lowering effects of metoprolol.

PROLONGED USE

No special problems.

METRONIDAZOLE

Brand names Anabact, Elyzol, Flagyl, Metrogel, Metrolyl, Metrotop, Metrozol, Rozex, Vaginyl, Zadstat
Used in the following combined preparations Flagyl Compak

GENERAL INFORMATION

Metronidazole is prescribed to fight both protozoal infections and a variety of bacterial infections.

It is widely used in the treatment of trichomonas infection of the vagina. Because the organism responsible for this disorder is sexually transmitted and may not cause any symptoms, a simultaneous course of treatment is usually advised for the sexual partner.

Certain infections of the abdomen, pelvis, and gums also respond well to metronidazole. The drug is used to treat septicaemia and infected leg ulcers and pressure sores. Metronidazole may be given to prevent or treat infections after surgery. Because the drug in high doses can penetrate the brain, it is prescribed to treat abscesses occurring there.

Metronidazole is also prescribed for amoebic dysentery and giardiasis, a rare protozoal infection.

Metronidazole may be applied *topically* in the form of a gel to treat some forms of acne, rosacea, infected tumours, and gum disease.

QUICK REFERENCE

Drug group Antibacterial (p.131) and antiprotozoal drug (p.136)

Overdose danger rating Low

Dependence rating Low

Prescription needed Yes

Available as generic Yes

INFORMATION FOR USERS

Your drug prescription is tailored for you. Do not alter dosage without checking with your doctor.

How taken

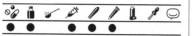

Tablets, liquid, injection, suppositories, gel.

Frequency and timing of doses
3 x daily for 5–10 days, depending on the condition being treated. Sometimes a single large dose is prescribed. Tablets should be taken after meals and swallowed whole with plenty of water.

Adult dosage range
600–1,200mg daily (by mouth); 3g daily (suppositories); 1.5g daily (injection).

Onset of effect
The drug starts to work within an hour or so, but beneficial effects may not be felt for 1–2 days.

Duration of action
6–12 hours.

Diet advice
None.

Storage
Keep in a closed container in a cool, dry place out of the reach of children. Protect from light.

Missed dose
Take as soon as you remember. If your next dose is due within 2 hours, take a single dose now and skip the next.

Stopping the drug
Take the full course. Even if you feel better the infection may still be present and symptoms may recur if treatment is stopped too soon.

Exceeding the dose
An occasional unintentional extra dose is unlikely to be a cause for concern. But if you notice unusual symptoms, especially numbness or tingling, or if a large overdose has been taken, notify your doctor.

SPECIAL PRECAUTIONS

Be sure to tell your doctor if:
▼ You have long-term liver problems.
▼ You have a blood disorder.
▼ You have a disorder of the central nervous system, such as epilepsy.
▼ You are taking other medications.

 Pregnancy
▼ Safety in pregnancy not established. Discuss with your doctor

 Breast-feeding
▼ The drug passes into the breast milk, but at normal doses adverse effects on the baby are unlikely. However, metronidazole may give the milk a bitter taste. Discuss with your doctor.

 Infants and children
▼ Reduced dose necessary.

 Over 60
▼ No special problems.

 Driving and hazardous work
▼ Avoid such activities until you have learned how metronidazole affects you because the drug can cause dizziness and drowsiness.

Alcohol
▼ Avoid. Taken with metronidazole, alcohol may cause flushing, nausea, vomiting, abdominal pain, and headache.

POSSIBLE ADVERSE EFFECTS

Various minor gastrointestinal disturbances are common but tend to diminish with time. The drug may cause a darkening of the urine, which is of no concern. More serious *adverse effects* on the nervous system, causing numbness or tingling, are extremely rare.

Symptom/effect	Frequency		Discuss with doctor		Stop taking drug now	Call doctor now
	Common	Rare	Only if severe	In all cases		
Nausea/loss of appetite	●		■			
Dark urine	●		■			
Dry mouth/metallic taste		●	■			
Headache/dizziness		●	■			
Numbness/tingling		●		■		

INTERACTIONS

Oral anticoagulants Metronidazole may increase the effect of oral anticoagulants.

Lithium Metronidazole increases the risk of adverse effects on the kidneys.

Phenytoin Metronidazole may increase the effects of phenytoin.

Cimetidine This drug may increase the levels of metronidazole in the body.

Phenobarbital This drug may reduce the effects of metronidazole.

PROLONGED USE

Not usually prescribed for longer than 10 days. Prolonged treatment may cause temporary loss of sensation in the hands and feet, and may also reduce production of white blood cells.

MICONAZOLE

Brand names Daktarin, Dumicoat, Femeron, Gyno-Daktarin
Used in the following combined preparation Daktacort

GENERAL INFORMATION

Miconazole is an antifungal drug used to treat candida (yeast) infections of the mouth, candida and bacterial infections of the vagina, and other fungal skin infections. Once given intravenously to treat *systemic* fungal infections, it has now been superseded for this use by newer drugs.

The drug is available for oral infections as a gel and antifungal denture paint.

Cream, dusting powder, or ointment are used for skin infections, and several vaginal preparations are available.

Side effects usually only occur with oral preparations because miconazole is absorbed in only very small quantities following topical or vaginal application.

The pessaries, vaginal capsules, and vaginal cream damage latex condoms and diaphragms.

INFORMATION FOR USERS

Follow instructions on the label. Call your doctor if symptoms worsen.

How taken

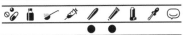

Pessaries, vaginal cream, vaginal capsules, cream, ointment, gel, dusting powder, dental lacquer.

Frequency and timing of doses
4 x daily after food (oral gel); once a week for 3 weeks (dental lacquer); 1–2 x daily (vaginal/skin preparations).

Adult dosage range
Vaginal infections 1 x 5g applicatorful (cream); 1 x 100mg pessary; 1 x 1.2g vaginal capsule. *Oral/skin infections* As directed.

Onset of effect
2–3 days.

Duration of action
Up to 12 hours.

Diet advice
None.

Storage
Keep in a closed container in a cool, dry place out of the reach of children.

Missed dose
No cause for concern, but apply missed dose or application as soon as you remember.

Stopping the drug
Apply the full course. Even if you feel better, the original infection may still be present and may recur if treatment is stopped too soon.

Exceeding the dose
An occasional unintentional extra dose is unlikely to cause problems. But if you notice any unusual symptoms or if a large amount has been swallowed, notify your doctor.

SPECIAL PRECAUTIONS

Be sure to consult your doctor or pharmacist before taking this drug if:
▼ You have porphyria.
▼ You are taking other medications.

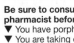 **Pregnancy**
▼ Safety not established. Discuss with your doctor.

 Breast-feeding
▼ Safety not established. Discuss with your doctor.

 Infants and children
▼ Reduced dose necessary (oral gel).

 Over 60
▼ No special problems.

 Driving and hazardous work
▼ No special problems.

 Alcohol
▼ No special problems.

POSSIBLE ADVERSE EFFECTS

Adverse effects are rare with miconazole and usually only occur with oral use.

Symptom/effect	Frequency		Discuss with doctor		Stop taking drug now	Call doctor now
	Common	Rare	Only if severe	In all cases		
Skin irritation		●	■			
Nausea/vomiting		●	■			
Wheezing/blotchy rash		●		■	▲	∎
Vaginal irritation		●		■		

INTERACTIONS

Oral anticoagulants, cyclosporin, phenytoin, antidiabetics, terfenadine, and cisapride Miconazole oral gel may increase the effects and *toxicity* of these drugs.

PROLONGED USE

No problems expected. Miconazole is not usually prescribed long term.

MINOCYCLINE

Brand names Aknemin, Blemix, Cyclomin, Dentomycin, Minocin MR
Used in the following combined preparations None

GENERAL INFORMATION

Minocycline is a member of the tetracycline group of antibiotics but has a substantially longer duration of action than tetracycline itself. The drug is most commonly used to treat acne.

Minocycline may be given to treat pneumonia or to prevent infection in people with chronic bronchitis. It is also used for the treatment of gonorrhea and non-gonococcal urethritis and may be used to treat other sexually transmitted diseases. Minocycline is also used to treat chronic gum disease in adults.

The drug's most frequent *side effects* are nausea, vomiting, and diarrhoea. It also interferes with the functioning of the balance mechanism in the inner ear, with resultant nausea, dizziness, and unsteadiness, but these symptoms generally disappear after the drug is stopped. Minocycline is not prescribed for people with poor kidney function.

QUICK REFERENCE

Drug group Tetracycline antibiotic (p.128)

Overdose danger rating Low

Dependence rating Low

Prescription needed Yes

Available as generic No

INFORMATION FOR USERS

Your drug prescription is tailored for you. Do not alter dosage without checking with your doctor.

How taken

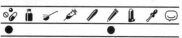

Tablets, capsules, gel.

Frequency and timing of doses
1–2 x daily.

Dosage range
Adults 100–200mg daily.
Children Reduced dose according to age and weight.

Onset of effect
4–12 hours.

Duration of action
Up to 24 hours.

Diet advice
Milk products may impair absorption; avoid from 1 hour before to 2 hours after dosage.

Storage
Keep in a closed container in a cool, dry, well-secured place out of the reach of children.

Missed dose
Take as soon as you remember. If your next dose is due within 4 hours, take a single dose now and skip the next.

Stopping the drug
Use the full course. Even if you feel better, the original infection may still be present and symptoms may recur if treatment is stopped too soon.

Exceeding the dose
An occasional unintentional extra dose is unlikely to be a cause for concern. But if you notice any unusual symptoms, or if a large overdose has been taken, notify your doctor.

POSSIBLE ADVERSE EFFECTS

Minocycline may occasionally cause nausea, vomiting, or diarrhoea. Other less common adverse effects are rashes, an increased sensitivity of the skin to sunlight, and, in some cases, dizziness and loss of balance (vertigo).

Symptom/effect	Frequency		Discuss with doctor		Stop taking drug now	Call doctor now
	Common	Rare	Only if severe	In all cases		
Nausea/vomiting/diarrhoea	●		■			
Dizziness/vertigo	●			■	▲	
Rash/itching		●		■	▲	
Light-sensitive rash		●		■	▲	
Headache/blurred vision		●		■	▲	

INTERACTIONS

Oral anticoagulants Minocycline may increase the anticoagulant action of these drugs.

Penicillin antibiotics Minocycline interferes with the antibacterial action of these drugs.

Oral contraceptives Minocycline can reduce the effectiveness of these drugs.

Iron may interfere with the absorption of minocycline and may reduce its effectiveness.

Antacids and milk interfere with the absorption of minocycline and may reduce its effectiveness. Doses should be separated by 1–2 hours.

SPECIAL PRECAUTIONS

Be sure to tell your doctor if:
▼ You have liver or kidney problems.
▼ You have previously suffered an allergic reaction to a tetracycline antibiotic.
▼ You are taking other medications.

Pregnancy
▼ Not prescribed. May damage the teeth and bones of the developing baby, as well as the mother's liver. Discuss with your doctor.

Breast-feeding
▼ The drug passes into the breast milk and may lead to discoloration of the baby's teeth. Discuss with your doctor.

Infants and children
▼ Not recommended under 13 years. Reduced dose necessary in older children.

Over 60
▼ No special problems.

Driving and hazardous work
▼ Avoid such activities until you have learned how minocycline affects you because the drug can cause dizziness and drowsiness.

Alcohol
▼ No known problems.

How to take your tablets
▼ To prevent retention in the oesophagus, a small amount of water should be taken before, and a full glass of water taken after, each dose of minocycline. Take this medication while sitting or standing and do not lie down immediately afterwards.

PROLONGED USE

Prolonged use of minocycline may occasionally cause skin darkening and discoloration of the teeth.

Monitoring Regular blood tests should be carried out to assess liver function.

MINOXIDIL

Brand names Loniten, Regaine
Used in the following combined preparations None

GENERAL INFORMATION

Minoxidil is a vasodilator drug (see p.98) that works by relaxing the muscles of artery walls and dilating blood vessels. It is effective in controlling dangerously high blood pressure that is rising very rapidly. Because minoxidil is stronger acting than many other antihypertensive drugs, it is particularly useful for people whose blood pressure is not controlled by other treatment.

Because minoxidil can cause fluid retention and increased heart rate, it is usually prescribed with a diuretic and a beta blocker to increase effectiveness and to counteract its *side effects*. Unlike many other drugs in the antihypertensive group, minoxidil rarely causes dizziness and fainting. Its major drawback is that, if it is taken for more than two months, it increases hair growth, especially on the face. Although this effect can be controlled by shaving or depilatories, some people find the abnormal growth distressing. This effect is put to use, however, to treat baldness in men and women, and for this purpose minoxidil is applied locally as a solution.

INFORMATION FOR USERS

Your drug prescription is tailored for you. Do not alter dosage without checking with your doctor.

How taken

Tablets, topical solution.

Frequency and timing of doses
Once or twice daily.

Adult dosage range
5mg daily initially, increasing gradually to a maximum of 50mg daily.

Onset of effect
Blood pressure Within 1 hour (tablets).
Hair growth Up to 1 year (solution).

Duration of action
Up to 24 hours. Some effect may last for 2–5 days after stopping the drug.

Diet advice
None.

Storage
Keep in a closed container in a cool, dry place out of the reach of children.

Missed dose
Take as soon as you remember (tablets). If your next dose is due within 5 hours, take a single dose now and skip the next.

Stopping the drug
Do not stop the drug without consulting your doctor; stopping the drug may lead to worsening of the underlying condition.

Exceeding the dose
An occasional unintentional extra dose is unlikely to cause problems. Large overdoses may cause nausea, vomiting, palpitations, or dizziness. Notify your doctor.

POSSIBLE ADVERSE EFFECTS

Fluid retention is a common adverse effect of minoxidil, which may lead to an increase in weight. Diuretics are often prescribed to control this adverse effect. Side effects with minoxidil lotion are very rare.

Symptom/effect	Frequency		Discuss with doctor		Stop taking drug now	Call doctor now
	Common	Rare	Only if severe	In all cases		
Increased hair growth	●		■			
Fluid retention/ankle swelling	●		■			
Nausea		●	■			
Breast tenderness		●		■		
Dizziness/lightheadedness		●		■		
Rash		●		■		
Palpitations		●		■	▲	■

INTERACTIONS

Antidepressant drugs The hypotensive effects of minoxidil may be enhanced by antidepressant drugs.

Oestrogens and progestogens (including those in some contraceptive pills) may reduce the effects of minoxidil.

SPECIAL PRECAUTIONS

Be sure to tell your doctor if:
▼ You have a long-term kidney problem.
▼ You have heart problems.
▼ You retain fluid.
▼ You are taking other medications.

Pregnancy
▼ Safety in pregnancy not established. Discuss with your doctor.

Breast-feeding
▼ The drug passes into the breast milk, but at normal doses adverse effects on the baby are unlikely. Discuss with your doctor.

Infants and children
▼ Reduced dose necessary.

Over 60
▼ Reduced dose may be necessary.

Driving and hazardous work
▼ Avoid such activities until you have learned how minoxidil affects you because the drug can cause dizziness and lightheadedness.

Alcohol
▼ Avoid. Alcohol may further reduce blood pressure.

Surgery and general anaesthetics
▼ Minoxidil treatment may need to be stopped before you have a general anaesthetic. Discuss this with your doctor or dentist before any surgery.

PROLONGED USE

Prolonged use of this drug may lead to swelling of the ankles and increased hair growth.

MISOPROSTOL

Brand name Cytotec
Used in the following combined preparations Arthrotec, Condrotec, Napratec

GENERAL INFORMATION

Misoprostol reduces the amount of acid secreted in the stomach and promotes healing of gastric and duodenal ulcers. The drug is related to naturally occurring chemicals called prostaglandins. Gastric and duodenal ulcers may be caused by aspirin (p.201) and non-steroidal anti-inflammatory drugs (p.116) that block certain prostaglandins, and misoprostol can be used to prevent or cure these ulcers. The ulcers usually heal after a few weeks' treatment with misoprostol.

In some cases, misoprostol is given during treatment with these drugs as a preventative measure and combined preparations are available that reduce the likelihood of ulcers occurring. The most likely *adverse effects* are diarrhoea and indigestion; if they are severe it may be necessary to stop treatment with the drug. Diarrhoea can be made worse by antacids containing magnesium; these should therefore be avoided.

QUICK REFERENCE

Drug group Anti-ulcer drug (p.109)
Overdose danger rating Low
Dependence rating Low
Prescription needed Yes
Available as generic No

INFORMATION FOR USERS

Your drug prescription is tailored for you. Do not alter dosage without checking with your doctor.

How taken

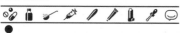

Tablets.

Frequency and timing of doses
2–4 x daily.

Adult dosage range
400–800mcg daily.

Onset of effect
Within 24 hours.

Duration of action
Up to 24 hours; some effects may be longer lasting.

Diet advice
None.

Storage
Keep in a closed container in a cool, dry place out of the reach of children.

Missed dose
Take as soon as you remember. If your next dose is due within 3 hours, take a single dose now and skip the next.

Stopping the drug
Do not stop the drug without consulting your doctor; symptoms may recur.

Exceeding the dose
An occasional unintentional extra dose is unlikely to be a cause for concern. But if you notice any unusual symptoms, or if a large overdose has been taken, notify your doctor.

SPECIAL PRECAUTIONS

Be sure to tell your doctor if:
▼ You are pregnant, or intending to become pregnant.
▼ You have had a stroke.
▼ You have heart or circulation problems.
▼ You have high blood pressure.
▼ You have bowel problems.
▼ You are taking other medications.

 Pregnancy
▼ Misoprostol should not be taken during pregnancy since it can cause the uterus to contract before the baby is due.

 Breast-feeding
▼ Safety not established. Discuss with your doctor.

 Infants and children
▼ Not recommended.

 Over 60
▼ No special problems.

 Driving and hazardous work
▼ No problems expected.

Alcohol
▼ No problems expected, but excessive amounts may undermine the desired effect of the drug.

POSSIBLE ADVERSE EFFECTS

Adverse effects on the gastrointestinal tract can occur. These effects may be reduced by spreading the doses out during the day. Taking the drug with food may be recommended.

Symptom/effect	Frequency		Discuss with doctor		Stop taking drug now	Call doctor now
	Common	Rare	Only if severe	In all cases		
Diarrhoea	●		■			
Indigestion	●		■			
Nausea/vomiting		●	■			
Vaginal/intermenstrual bleeding		●		■		
Abdominal pain		●		■		
Skin rashes		●		■	▲	

INTERACTIONS

Magnesium-containing antacids These may increase the severity of any diarrhoea caused by misoprostol.

PROLONGED USE

No problems expected.

MOMETASONE

Brand names Elocon, Nasonex
Used in the following combined preparations None

GENERAL INFORMATION

Mometasone is a corticosteroid drug used in the form of a nasal spray to relieve the symptoms of allergic rhinitis. The drug is also used *topically* for the treatment of severe inflammatory skin disorders and in conditions such as eczema that have not responded to other corticosteroids (see Topical corticosteroids, p.174).

Serious adverse effects are rare if the drug is used for short periods or in small amounts. However, prolonged or excessive topical use may cause local *side effects* such as thin skin with enlarged capillaries, and *systemic* side effects such as weak bones, muscle weakness, and peptic ulcers. Because corticosteroids can affect growth, children using the nasal spray for prolonged periods may need to have their growth (height) monitored.

INFORMATION FOR USERS

Your drug prescription is tailored for you. Do not alter dosage without checking with your doctor.

How taken

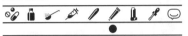

Cream, ointment, scalp lotion, nasal spray.

Frequency and timing of doses
Once daily.

Dosage range
Nasal spray 100mcg (2 puffs) into each nostril.
Topical preparations As directed, applied thinly.

Onset of effect
12 hours. Full beneficial effect after 48 hours.

Duration of action
24 hours.

Diet advice
None.

Storage
Keep in a cool, dry place out of the reach of children.

Missed dose
Take as soon as you remember. If your next dose/application is due within 8 hours, take a single dose or apply the usual amount now and skip the next.

Stopping the drug
Do not stop the drug without consulting your doctor; symptoms may recur.

Exceeding the dose
An occasional unintentional extra dose/application may not be a cause for concern, but if you notice unusual symptoms, notify your doctor.

POSSIBLE ADVERSE EFFECTS

Irritation of, and sometimes bleeding from, the nose are the most common side effects.

Symptom/effect	Frequency		Discuss with doctor		Stop taking drug now	Call doctor now
	Common	Rare	Only if severe	In all cases		
Sore throat	●				■	
Thinning skin	●				■	
Increased capillary size in skin	●				■	
Acne/dermatitis around mouth	●				■	
Nasal irritation/bleeding	●			■		
Loss of skin pigment	●			■		
Weight gain		●			■	
Mood changes		●			■	

INTERACTIONS

None.

SPECIAL PRECAUTIONS

Be sure to tell your doctor if:
▼ You have a cold sore, measles, or chickenpox.
▼ You have any other nasal or skin infection.
▼ You have rosacea or acne.

Avoid exposure to chickenpox, measles, or shingles while using mometasone.

Pregnancy
▼ Safety not established. Discuss with your doctor.

Breast-feeding
▼ No evidence of risk. Discuss with your doctor.

Infants and children
▼ Only used for very short courses in children.

Over 60
▼ No special problems.

Driving and hazardous work
▼ No special problems.

Alcohol
▼ No special problems.

PROLONGED USE

Not advisable. Prolonged use of topical preparations of this drug can cause permanent skin changes and should be avoided whenever possible.

MONTELUKAST

Brand name Singulair
Used in the following combined preparations None

GENERAL INFORMATION

Montelukast belongs to the leukotriene receptor antagonist (blocker) group of anti-allergy drugs and is used in the prevention of asthma. It is thought that stimulation of leukotriene receptors by naturally occurring leukotrienes from the mast cells plays a part in causing asthma. Montelukast works by blocking these receptors.

The drug is given as an additional medication when combined treatment with corticosteroids and bronchodilators does not give adequate control. It is usually given by mouth as tablets, and a chewable form is available for children.

Montelukast is not a bronchodilator, and cannot be used to treat an acute attack of asthma.

INFORMATION FOR USERS

Your drug prescription is tailored for you. Do not alter dosage without checking with your doctor.

How taken

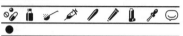

Tablets, chewable tablets.

Frequency and timing of doses
Once daily at bedtime.

Adult dosage range
10mg.

Onset of effect
2 hours.

Duration of action
24 hours.

Diet advice
None.

Storage
Keep in a closed container in a cool, dry place out of the reach of children. Protect from light.

Missed dose
Take as soon as you remember. If your next dose is due within 8 hours, take a single dose now and skip the next.

Stopping the drug
Do not stop the drug without consulting your doctor, symptoms may recur.

Exceeding the dose
An occasional unintentional extra dose is unlikely to be a cause for concern. But if you notice any unusual symptoms, or if a large overdose has been taken, notify your doctor.

SPECIAL PRECAUTIONS

Be sure to tell your doctor if:
▼ You have phenylketonuria.
▼ You are taking other medications.

Pregnancy
▼ Safety not established. Discuss with your doctor.

Breast-feeding
▼ Safety not established. Discuss with your doctor.

Infants and children
▼ Safety not established under 6 years. Reduced dose necessary.

Over 60
▼ No special problems.

Driving and hazardous work
▼ Avoid such activities until you have learned how montelukast affects you because the drug can cause dizziness.

Alcohol
▼ No special problems.

POSSIBLE ADVERSE EFFECTS

Severe *adverse effects* are rare with montelukast. There seems to be an increase in the incidence of chest infections among people taking this drug.

Symptom/effect	Frequency		Discuss with doctor		Stop taking drug now	Call doctor now
	Common	Rare	Only if severe	In all cases		
Abdominal pain	●		■			
Headache	●		■			
Diarrhoea		●	■			
Dizziness		●	■			
Weakness		●	■			
Fever		●			■	
Productive cough		●			■	

INTERACTIONS

None.

PROLONGED USE

No special problems.

MORPHINE/DIAMORPHINE

Brand names Diagesil, MST Continus, MXL, Oramorph, Oramorph SR, Sevredol
Used in the following combined preparations Cyclimorph, Omnopon

GENERAL INFORMATION

In use since the 19th century, morphine and diamorphine belong to a group of drugs called the *opioid* analgesics (see p.80). These drugs are derived from opium, which is obtained from the unripe seed capsules of the opium poppy.

The drugs are used to relieve severe pain that can be caused by heart attack, injury, surgery, or chronic diseases such as cancer. They are also sometimes given as *premedication* before surgery.

The drugs' painkilling effect wears off quickly, in contrast to some other opioid analgesics, and they may be given in a special slow-release (long-acting) form to relieve continuous severe pain.

These drugs are habit-forming, and dependence and addiction can occur. However, most patients who take them for pain relief over brief periods of time do not become dependent and are able to stop taking them without difficulty.

INFORMATION FOR USERS

Your drug prescription is tailored for you. Do not alter your dosage without checking with your doctor.

How taken

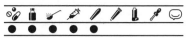

Tablets, SR-tablets, capsules, SR-capsules, liquid, SR-granules, injection, suppositories.

Frequency and timing of doses
Every 4 hours; every 12–24 hours (SR-preparations).

Adult dosage range
5–25mg per dose; however, some patients may need 75mg or more per dose. Doses vary considerably for each individual.

Onset of effect
Within 1 hour; within 4 hours (SR-preparations).

Duration of action
4 hours; up to 24 hours (SR-tablets).

Diet advice
None.

Storage
Keep in a closed container in a cool, dry place out of the reach of children.

Missed dose
Take as soon as you remember. Return to your normal dosing schedule as soon as possible.

Stopping the drug
If the reason for taking the drug no longer exists, you may stop the drug and notify your doctor.

OVERDOSE ACTION

Seek immediate medical advice in all cases. Take emergency action if symptoms such as slow or irregular breathing, severe drowsiness, or loss of consciousness occur.

See Drug poisoning emergency guide (p.494).

POSSIBLE ADVERSE EFFECTS

Nausea, vomiting, and constipation are common, especially with high doses.

Anti-nausea drugs or laxatives may be needed to counteract these symptoms.

Symptom/effect	Frequency		Discuss with doctor		Stop taking drug now	Call doctor now
	Common	Rare	Only if severe	In all cases		
Drowsiness	●		■			
Nausea/vomiting	●		■			
Constipation	●		■			
Dizziness	●			■		
Confusion		●		■		
Breathing difficulties		●		■	▲	■

INTERACTIONS

Sedatives Morphine and diamorphine increase the sedative effects of other sedating drugs including antidepressants, antipsychotics, sleeping drugs, and antihistamines.

Monoamine oxidase inhibitors (MAOIs) These drugs may produce a severe rise in blood pressure when taken with morphine and diamorphine.

SPECIAL PRECAUTIONS

Be sure to tell your doctor if:
▼ You have long-term liver or kidney problems.
▼ You have heart or circulatory problems.
▼ You have a lung disorder such as asthma or bronchitis.
▼ You have thyroid disease.
▼ You have a history of epileptic fits.
▼ You are taking other medications.

Pregnancy
▼ Not usually prescribed. May cause breathing difficulties in the newborn baby. Discuss with your doctor.

Breast-feeding
▼ The drug passes into the breast milk, but at low doses adverse effects on the baby are unlikely. Discuss with your doctor.

Infants and children
▼ Reduced dose necessary.

Over 60
▼ Increased likelihood of adverse effects. Reduced dose may therefore be necessary.

Driving and hazardous work
▼ People on morphine treatment are unlikely to be well enough to undertake such activities.

Alcohol
▼ Avoid. Alcohol may increase the sedative effects of these drugs.

PROLONGED USE

The effects of these drugs usually become weaker during prolonged use as the body adapts. Dependence may occur if they are taken for extended periods.

MOXONIDINE

Brand name Physiotens
Used in the following combined preparations None

GENERAL INFORMATION

Moxonidine is a new antihypertensive drug that is related to clonidine (p.243) but is more selective and may therefore have fewer *side effects*. It works by stimulating alpha-receptors within the central nervous system, reducing the signals that constrict the blood vessels. Moxonidine also reduces resistance to blood flow in the peripheral blood vessels. It also seems to have actions on the kidneys that result in more sodium and water being excreted.

The drug is less likely than clonidine to cause dry mouth, and, unlike clonidine, has no effect on blood fat levels or glucose. However, other side effects, such as headache and dizziness, may still occur.

QUICK REFERENCE

Drug group Antihypertensive drug (p.102)

Overdose danger rating Medium

Dependence rating Low

Prescription needed Yes

Available as generic No

INFORMATION FOR USERS

Your drug prescription is tailored for you. Do not alter dosage without checking with your doctor.

How taken

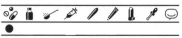

Tablets.

Frequency and timing of doses
Once daily in the morning (initially); 1–2 x daily.

Adult dosage range
200mcg daily initially; increasing after 3 weeks to 400mcg daily, if necessary; increasing again after a further 3 weeks to maximum of 600mcg daily in 2 divided doses if necessary.

Onset of effect
30–180 minutes.

Duration of action
12 hours.

Diet advice
None.

Storage
Keep in a closed container in a cool, dry place out of the reach of children.

Missed dose
Take as soon as you remember. If your next dose is due within 4 hours, take a single dose now and skip the next.

Stopping the drug
Do not stop taking the drug without consulting your doctor, who will supervise a gradual reduction in dosage over a period of 2 weeks.

Exceeding the dose
An occasional unintentional extra dose is unlikely to cause problems. Large overdoses may cause drowsiness and a fall in blood pressure.

SPECIAL PRECAUTIONS

Be sure to tell your doctor if:
▼ You have liver or kidney problems.
▼ You have heart problems.
▼ You have a history of angioedema.
▼ You have Raynaud's syndrome.
▼ You have epilepsy.
▼ You suffer from depression.
▼ You have Parkinson's disease.
▼ You have glaucoma.
▼ You are taking other medications.

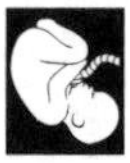

Pregnancy
▼ Safety not established. Discuss with your doctor.

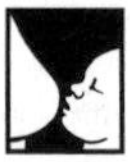

Breast-feeding
▼ Safety in breast-feeding not established. Discuss with your doctor.

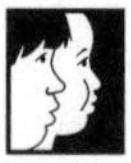

Infants and children
▼ Not recommended.

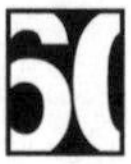

Over 60
▼ No special problems.

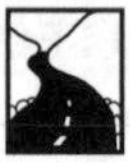

Driving and hazardous work
▼ Avoid such activities until you have learned how moxonidine affects you because the drug can cause drowsiness and dizziness.

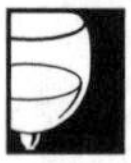

Alcohol
▼ Avoid. Alcohol may increase the sedative effects of this drug.

POSSIBLE ADVERSE EFFECTS

Side effects that appear at the start of treatment with moxonidine often decrease in frequency and intensity during the course of treatment.

Symptom/effect	Frequency		Discuss with doctor		Stop taking drug now	Call doctor now
	Common	Rare	Only if severe	In all cases		
Dry mouth	●		■			
Headache	●		■			
Weakness/fatigue	●		■			
Dizziness		●	■			
Nausea		●	■			
Sleep disturbance		●	■			
Sedation		●	■			

INTERACTIONS

Other antihypertensives, thymoxamine and muscle relaxants These drugs may increase the blood-pressure lowering effect of moxonidine.

Sedatives and hypnotics The effect of these drugs may be increased by moxonidine.

PROLONGED USE

No special problems.

NAFTIDROFURYL

Brand names Praxilene, Stimlor
Used in the following combined preparations None

GENERAL INFORMATION

Naftidrofuryl is a vasodilator drug used in the treatment of peripheral circulatory disorders such as Raynaud's syndrome or intermittent claudication (cramplike pain). Most of these conditions are caused by blockage of blood vessels due to spasms or sclerosis (hardening) of the vessel walls.

Naftidrofuryl may improve symptoms and mobility in these conditions, but it is not known if it has any influence on their progress. Lifestyle changes such as giving up smoking and taking exercise (and keeping warm in the case of Raynaud's) are often helpful.

Naftidrofuryl has also been used for treating night cramps, but it is not known how the drug works to reduce them. It has also been tried for circulatory disorders in the brain.

QUICK REFERENCE

Drug group Vasodilator (p.98)
Overdose danger rating Medium
Dependence rating Low
Prescription needed Yes
Available as generic Yes

INFORMATION FOR USERS

Your drug prescription is tailored for you. Do not alter dosage without checking with your doctor.

How taken

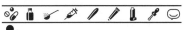

Capsules.

Frequency and timing of doses
3 x daily.

Adult dosage range
300–600mg daily.

Onset of effect
1 hour.

Duration of action
8 hours.

Diet advice
None.

Storage
Keep in a closed container in a cool, dry place out of the reach of children.

Missed dose
Take when you remember. If your next dose is due within 2 hours, take a single dose now and skip the next.

Stopping the drug
Do not stop taking the drug without consulting your doctor; symptoms may recur.

Exceeding the dose
An occasional unintentional extra dose is unlikely to cause problems. Large overdoses may cause heart problems and convulsions. Notify your doctor immediately.

SPECIAL PRECAUTIONS

Be sure to tell your doctor if:
▼ You have liver or kidney problems.
▼ You are taking other medications.

Pregnancy
▼ Safety not established. Discuss with your doctor.

Breast-feeding
▼ Safety not established. Discuss with your doctor.

Infants and children
▼ Not recommended.

Over 60
▼ No special problems.

Driving and hazardous work
▼ No special problems.

Alcohol
▼ No special problems.

POSSIBLE ADVERSE EFFECTS

Naftidrofuryl is generally well tolerated.

Symptom/effect	Frequency		Discuss with doctor		Stop taking drug now	Call doctor now
	Common	Rare	Only if severe	In all cases		
Nausea	●		■			
Chest pain		●		■		
Skin rash		●		■		
Jaundice		●		■	▲	
Convulsions		●		■	▲	

INTERACTIONS

None.

PROLONGED USE

Treatment should be reviewed after 3 months to see if the condition is improving, or if the drug should be stopped.

NAPROXEN

Brand names Arthrosin, Arthroxen, Laraflex, Naprosyn, Nycopren, Prosaid, Synflex, Timpron, Valrox
Used in the following combined preparations Condrotec, Napratec

GENERAL INFORMATION

Naproxen, one of the non-steroidal anti-inflammatory drugs (NSAIDs), is used to reduce pain, stiffness, and inflammation.

The drug relieves the symptoms of adult and juvenile rheumatoid arthritis, ankylosing spondylitis, and osteo-arthritis, although it does not cure the underlying disease.

Naproxen is also used to treat acute attacks of gout, and may sometimes be prescribed for the relief of migraine and pain following orthopaedic surgery, dental treatment, strains, and sprains. It is also effective for treating painful menstrual cramps.

Gastrointestinal *side effects* are fairly common, and there is an increased risk of bleeding. However, it is safer than aspirin, and in long-term use it needs to be taken only twice daily.

QUICK REFERENCE

Drug group Non-steroidal anti-inflammatory drug (p.116) and drug for gout (p.119)

Overdose danger rating Medium

Dependence rating Low

Prescription needed Yes

Available as generic Yes

INFORMATION FOR USERS

Your drug prescription is tailored for you. Do not alter dosage without checking with your doctor.

How taken

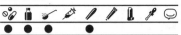

Tablets, liquid, granules, suppositories.

Frequency and timing of doses
Every 6–8 hours as required (general pain relief); 1–2 x daily (muscular pain and arthritis); every 8 hours (gout).
All doses should be taken with food.

Adult dosage range
Mild to moderate pain, menstrual cramps 500mg (starting dose), then 250mg every 6–8 hours as required. *Muscular pain and arthritis* 500–1,250mg daily. *Gout* 750mg (starting dose), then 250mg every 8 hours until attack has subsided.

Onset of effect
Pain relief begins within 1 hour. Full anti-inflammatory effect may take 2 weeks.

Duration of action
Up to 12 hours.

Diet advice
None.

Storage
Keep in a closed container in a cool, dry place out of the reach of children. Protect from light.

Missed dose
Take as soon as you remember. If your next dose is due within 4 hours, take a single dose now and skip the next.

Stopping the drug
When taken for short-term pain relief, naproxen can be safely stopped as soon as you no longer need it. If prescribed for long-term treatment, however, you should seek medical advice before stopping the drug.

Exceeding the dose
An occasional unintentional extra dose is unlikely to be a cause for concern. But if you notice any unusual symptoms, or if a large overdose has been taken, notify your doctor.

SPECIAL PRECAUTIONS

Be sure to tell your doctor if:
▼ You have long-term liver or kidney problems.
▼ You have heart problems.
▼ You have a bleeding disorder.
▼ You have high blood pressure.
▼ You have had a peptic ulcer, oesophagitis, or acid indigestion.
▼ You are allergic to aspirin.
▼ You suffer from asthma.
▼ You are taking other medications.

Pregnancy
▼ Not usually prescribed. When taken in the last three months of pregnancy, may increase the risk of adverse effects on the baby's heart and may prolong labour. Discuss with your doctor.

Breast-feeding
▼ The drug passes into the breast milk, but at normal doses adverse effects on the baby are unlikely. Discuss with your doctor.

Infants and children
▼ Prescribed only to treat juvenile arthritis. Reduced dose necessary.

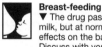

Over 60
▼ Increased likelihood of adverse effects. Reduced dose may therefore be necessary.

Driving and hazardous work
▼ Avoid such activities until you have learned how naproxen affects you because the drug may reduce your ability to concentrate.

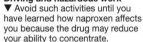

Alcohol
▼ Keep consumption low. Alcohol may increase the risk of stomach irritation with naproxen.

Surgery and general anaesthetics
▼ Naproxen may prolong bleeding. Discuss with your doctor or dentist before surgery.

POSSIBLE ADVERSE EFFECTS

Most adverse effects are not serious and may diminish with time. Black or bloodstained bowel movements should be reported to your doctor without delay.

Symptom/effect	Frequency		Discuss with doctor		Stop taking drug now	Call doctor now
	Common	Rare	Only if severe	In all cases		
Gastrointestinal disorders	●		■			
Headache		●	■			
Inability to concentrate		●	■			
Ringing in the ears		●		■		
Swollen feet/ankles		●		■		
Rash/itching		●		■	▲	
Wheezing/breathlessness		●		■	▲	▮
Black/bloodstained faeces		●		■	▲	▮

INTERACTIONS

General note Naproxen interacts with a wide range of drugs to increase the risk of bleeding and/or peptic ulcers. It may also alter the blood levels of lithium.

Antihypertensive drugs and diuretics The beneficial effects of these drugs may be reduced by naproxen.

PROLONGED USE

There is an increased risk of bleeding from peptic ulcers and in the bowel when naproxen is used long term.

NICORANDIL

Brand name Ikorel
Used in the following combined preparations None

GENERAL INFORMATION

Nicorandil, introduced in 1994 for the treatment of angina pectoris, is the first of a new group of drugs known as the potassium channel openers.

The symptoms of angina result from the failure of narrowed coronary blood vessels to deliver sufficient oxygen to the heart. Like the older drugs used to treat angina, nicorandil acts by widening blood vessels. However, this drug dilates them by a different mechanism and is notable because it widens both veins and arteries. As a result of this widening of the vessels, more oxygen-carrying blood reaches the heart muscle and, at the same time, the heart's work load is reduced since the resistance against which it has to pump is decreased.

Because nicorandil is a new drug, its precise role is still unclear and, at present, it is used mostly for treating angina that is resistant to older drugs.

QUICK REFERENCE

Drug group Anti-angina drug (p.101)

Overdose danger rating Medium

Dependence rating Low

Prescription needed Yes

Available as generic No

INFORMATION FOR USERS

Your drug prescription is tailored for you. Do not alter dosage without checking with your doctor.

How taken

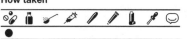

Tablets.

Frequency and timing of doses
2 x daily.

Adult dosage range
10–60mg daily.

Onset of effect
Within 1 hour.

Duration of action
Approximately 12 hours.

Diet advice
None.

Storage
Keep in a closed container in a cool, dry place out of the reach of children.

Missed dose
Take as soon as you remember. If your next dose is due within 4 hours, take a single dose now and skip the next.

Stopping the drug
Do not stop taking the drug without consulting your doctor; stopping the drug may lead to worsening of the underlying condition.

Exceeding the dose
An occasional unintentional extra dose is unlikely to cause problems. Large overdoses may cause unusual dizziness and dangerously low blood pressure. Notify your doctor.

SPECIAL PRECAUTIONS

Be sure to tell your doctor if:
▼ You are taking other medications.

Pregnancy
▼ Safety in pregnancy not established. Discuss with your doctor.

Breast-feeding
▼ Safety not established. Discuss with your doctor.

Infants and children
▼ Not recommended.

Over 60
▼ No special problems.

Driving and hazardous work
▼ Avoid such activities until you have learned how nicorandil affects you because the drug can cause dizziness as a result of lowered blood pressure.

Alcohol
▼ Avoid until you are accustomed to the effect of nicorandil. Alcohol may further reduce blood pressure, causing dizziness or other symptoms.

POSSIBLE ADVERSE EFFECTS

Adverse effects of nicorandil are generally minor. They usually wear off with continued treatment, but may necessitate a dose reduction in some cases.

Symptom/effect	Frequency		Discuss with doctor		Stop taking drug now	Call doctor now
	Common	Rare	Only if severe	In all cases		
Headache	●			■		
Flushing	●			■		
Nausea	●			■		
Dizziness		●	■			
Palpitations		●	■		▲	■

INTERACTIONS

Tricyclic antidepressant drugs may increase the effects of nicorandil on blood pressure, resulting in dizziness.

Antihypertensive drugs Nicorandil may increase the effects of these drugs.

PROLONGED USE

No problems expected.

NICOTINE

Brand names Boots Nicotine Gum, Boots NRT Patch, Nicorette, Nicotinell, NiQuitin CQ
Used in the following combined preparations None

GENERAL INFORMATION

Smoking is a difficult habit to stop due to the addiction to nicotine and the psychological attachment to cigarettes or a pipe. Taking nicotine in a different form can help the smoker deal with the two aspects of the habit separately.

Nicotine is available as chewing gum, nasal spray, and skin patches for the relief of withdrawal symptoms on giving up smoking.

The patches should be applied every 24 hours to unbroken, dry, and non-hairy skin on the trunk or the upper arm. Replacement patches should be placed on a different area, and the same area of application avoided for several days. The strength of the patch is gradually reduced, and abstinence is generally achieved within three months.

The chewing gum or nasal spray are used when the urge to smoke occurs. The gum is chewed slowly for up to 30 minutes, by which time all available nicotine has been released.

QUICK REFERENCE

Overdose danger rating Medium
Dependence rating Low
Prescription needed No
Available as generic No

INFORMATION FOR USERS

Follow instructions on the label. Call your doctor if symptoms worsen.

How taken

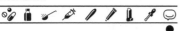

Skin patch, nasal spray, chewing gum.

Frequency and timing of doses
Every 24 hours, removing the patch after 16 hours (patches); when the urge to smoke is felt (gum or spray).

Adult dosage range
Will depend on your previous smoking habits. 7–22mg per day (patches); 1 x 2mg piece to 15 x 4mg pieces per day (gum); up to 64 x 0.5mg puffs (spray).

Onset of effect
A few hours (patches); within minutes (gum and spray).

Duration of action
Up to 24 hours (patches); 30 minutes (gum and spray).

Diet advice
None.

Storage
Keep in a cool, dry place out of the reach of children.

Missed dose
Change your patch as soon as you remember, and keep the new patch on for the required amount of time before removing it.

Stopping the drug
The dose of nicotine is normally reduced gradually.

Exceeding the dose
Application of several nicotine patches at the same time could result in serious overdosage. Seek immediate medical help. Overdosage with the gum or spray can occur only if many pieces are chewed simultaneously or if the spray is used more than 4 times an hour. Seek immediate medical help.

SPECIAL PRECAUTIONS

Be sure to consult your doctor or pharmacist before taking this drug if:
▼ You have long-term liver or kidney problems.
▼ You have diabetes mellitus.
▼ You have thyroid disease.
▼ You have circulation problems.
▼ You have heart problems.
▼ You have a peptic ulcer.
▼ You have phaeochromocytoma.
▼ You have any skin disorders.
▼ You are taking other medications.

Pregnancy
▼ Nicotine should not be used (in any form) during pregnancy.

Breast-feeding
▼ Nicotine should not be used (in any form) while breast-feeding.

Infants and children
▼ Nicotine products should not be administered to children.

Over 60
▼ No special problems.

Driving and hazardous work
▼ Usually no problems.

Alcohol
▼ No special problems.

POSSIBLE ADVERSE EFFECTS

Any skin reaction to patches will usually disappear in a couple of days. The chewing gum and nasal spray may cause local irritation of the throat or nose and increased salivation.

Symptom/effect	Frequency		Discuss with doctor		Stop taking drug now	Call doctor now
	Common	Rare	Only if severe	In all cases		
Local irritation	●			■		
Headache	●			■		
Dizziness		●		■		
Nausea		●		■		
Cold/flu-like symptoms		●		■		
Insomnia		●		■		
Indigestion		●		■		

PROLONGED USE

Nicotine should not normally be used for more than three months.

INTERACTIONS

General note Nicotine patches, chewing gum, and nasal spray should not be used with other nicotine-containing products, including cigarettes.

Stopping smoking may increase the blood levels of some drugs (such as warfarin and theophylline/aminophylline). Discuss with your doctor or pharmacist.

NIFEDIPINE

Brand names Adalat, Adipine, Angiopine, Cardilate MR, Coracten, Nifelease, Tensipine MR, and others
Used in the following combined preparations Beta-Adalat, Tenif

GENERAL INFORMATION

Nifedipine belongs to a group of drugs known as calcium channel blockers (p.101), which interfere with conduction of signals in the muscles of the heart and blood vessels.

Nifedipine is given for the treatment of angina, as a regular medication to help prevent attacks. The drug can be used safely by asthmatics, unlike some other anti-angina drugs (such as beta blockers).

Nifedipine is also widely used to reduce high blood pressure and is often helpful in improving circulation to the limbs in disorders such as Raynaud's disease.

In common with other drugs of its class, it may cause blood pressure to fall too low, and may occasionally cause disturbances of heart rhythm. In rare cases, angina worsens as a result of taking nifedipine, and another drug must be substituted.

INFORMATION FOR USERS

Your drug prescription is tailored for you. Do not alter dosage without checking with your doctor.

How taken

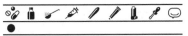

Tablets, capsules, SR-tablets, SR-capsules.

Frequency and timing of doses
3 x daily; 1–2 x daily (SR-preparations). For angina attacks, a capsule may be bitten and the liquid kept in the mouth or swallowed.

Adult dosage range
15–90mg daily.

Onset of effect
30–60 minutes. When capsules are bitten effects may be felt within minutes.

Duration of action
6–24 hours.

Diet advice
Nifedipine should not be taken with grapefruit juice.

Storage
Keep in a closed container in a cool, dry place out of the reach of children. Protect from light.

Missed dose
Take as soon as you remember, or when needed. If your next dose is due within 3 hours, take a single dose now and skip the next.

Stopping the drug
Do not stop the drug without consulting your doctor; symptoms may recur.

Exceeding the dose
An occasional unintentional extra dose is unlikely to cause problems. Large overdoses may cause dizziness. Notify your doctor.

SPECIAL PRECAUTIONS

Be sure to tell your doctor if:
▼ You have liver or kidney problems.
▼ You have heart failure.
▼ You have had a recent heart attack.
▼ You have aortic stenosis.
▼ You have diabetes.
▼ You are taking other medications.

 Pregnancy
▼ Not usually prescribed. The drug may cause abnormalities in the developing fetus and delay labour. Discuss with your doctor.

 Breast-feeding
▼ The drug passes into the breast milk and may affect the baby. Discuss with your doctor.

 Infants and children
▼ Not recommended.

 Over 60
▼ Increased likelihood of adverse effects. Reduced dose may therefore be necessary.

 Driving and hazardous work
▼ Avoid such activities until you have learned how nifedipine affects you because the drug can cause dizziness as a result of lowered blood pressure.

Alcohol
▼ Avoid. Alcohol may further reduce blood pressure, causing dizziness or other symptoms.

POSSIBLE ADVERSE EFFECTS

Nifedipine can cause a variety of minor *adverse effects*. Dizziness, especially on rising, may be caused by an excessive reduction in blood pressure. Patients with angina may notice an increase in the severity or frequency of attacks after starting nifedipine treatment. This should always be reported to your doctor. Sometimes an adjustment in dosage or a change of drug may be necessary.

Symptom/effect	Frequency		Discuss with doctor		Stop taking drug now	Call doctor now
	Common	Rare	Only if severe	In all cases		
Headache	●		■			
Dizziness/fatigue	●		■			
Flushing	●		■			
Ankle swelling	●		■			
Frequency in passing urine		●		■		
Increased angina		●			■	▲

PROLONGED USE

No problems expected.

INTERACTIONS

Antihypertensive drugs Nifedipine may increase the effects of these drugs.

Phenytoin Nifedipine may increase the effects of phenytoin.

Digoxin Nifedipine may increase the effects and *toxicity* of digoxin.

Rifampicin This drug may decrease the effects of nifedipine.

Grapefruit juice This may block the breakdown of nifedipine, increasing its effects.

NORETHISTERONE

Brand names Micronor, Noriday, Noristerat, Primolut N, Utovlan, and others
Used in the following combined preparations Brevinor, Loestrin, Norinyl, Synphase, TriNovum, and others

GENERAL INFORMATION

Norethisterone is a progestogen, a synthetic hormone similar to a natural female sex hormone, progesterone. It has a wide variety of uses including the postponement of menstruation and the treatment of menstrual disorders such as endometriosis (p.160). When used for these disorders, it is only taken on certain days during the menstrual cycle. It is also prescribed in the treatment of certain types of breast cancer.

One of the major uses for norethisterone is as an ingredient of oral contraceptive preparations, either on its own or with an oestrogen drug. The drug is also available in an injectable contraceptive preparation, which is used in special circumstances.

Adverse effects from this drug are rare, but contraceptive preparations containing this drug may cause "breakthrough" bleeding (see p.161).

INFORMATION FOR USERS

Your drug prescription is tailored for you. Do not alter dosage without checking with your doctor.

How taken

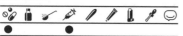

Tablets, injection.

Frequency and timing of doses
1–3 x daily (tablets); once every 8 weeks (injection).

Adult dosage range
10–15mg daily (menstrual disorders); 15mg daily (postponement of menstruation); 350 mcg daily (progestogen-only contraceptives); 30–60mg daily (cancer).

Onset of effect
The drug starts to act within a few hours.

Duration of action
24 hours.

Diet advice
None.

Storage
Keep in a closed container in a cool, dry place out of the reach of children. Protect from light.

Missed dose
Take as soon as you remember. If you are taking the drug for contraception, see What to do if you miss a pill (p.163).

Stopping the drug
The drug can be safely stopped as soon as contraceptive protection is no longer required. If prescribed for an underlying disorder, do not stop taking the drug without consulting your doctor.

Exceeding the dose
An occasional unintentional extra dose is unlikely to be a cause for concern. But if you notice any unusual symptoms, or if a large overdose has been taken, notify your doctor.

SPECIAL PRECAUTIONS

Be sure to tell your doctor if:
▼ You have liver or kidney problems.
▼ You have diabetes.
▼ You have had epileptic fits.
▼ You suffer from migraines.
▼ You have acute porphyria.
▼ You have heart or circulatory problems.
▼ You are taking other medications.

Pregnancy
▼ Not usually prescribed. May cause defects in the baby. Discuss with your doctor.

Breast-feeding
▼ The drug passes into the breast milk, but at normal doses adverse effects on the baby are unlikely. Discuss with your doctor.

Infants and children
▼ Not prescribed.

Over 60
▼ Not usually prescribed.

Driving and hazardous work
▼ No special problems.

Alcohol
▼ No special problems.

POSSIBLE ADVERSE EFFECTS

Adverse effects of norethisterone are rarely troublesome and are generally typical of drugs of this type. Prolonged treatment may cause *jaundice* due to liver damage.

Symptom/effect	Frequency		Discuss with doctor		Stop taking drug now	Call doctor now
	Common	Rare	Only if severe	In all cases		
Breakthrough bleeding	●			■		
Swollen feet/ankles		●	■			
Weight gain		●	■			
Depression/headache		●		■		
Jaundice		●		■	▲	

INTERACTIONS

General note Norethisterone may interfere with the beneficial effects of many drugs, including oral anticoagulants, anticonvulsants, antihypertensives, and antidiabetic drugs. Many other drugs may reduce the contraceptive effect of norethisterone-containing pills. These include anticonvulsants, antituberculous drugs, and antibiotics. Be sure to inform your doctor that you are taking norethisterone before taking additional prescribed medication.

Cyclosporin Levels of cyclosporin may be raised by norethisterone.

PROLONGED USE

Prolonged use may in rare cases cause liver damage.

Monitoring Blood tests to check liver function may be carried out.

NYSTATIN

Brand names Nystamont, Nystan
Used in the following combined preparations Dermovate-NN, Nystaform, Timodine, Tinaderm-M, and others

GENERAL INFORMATION

Nystatin is an antifungal drug named after the New York State Institute of Health, where it was developed in the early 1950s.

The drug has been used effectively against candidiasis (thrush), an infection caused by the *Candida* yeast. Available in a variety of dosage forms, it is used to treat infections of the skin, mouth, throat, intestinal tract, oesophagus, and vagina. As the drug is poorly absorbed into the bloodstream from the digestive tract, it is of little use against *systemic* infections. It is not given by injection.

Nystatin rarely causes *adverse effects* and can be used during pregnancy to treat vaginal candidiasis.

QUICK REFERENCE

Drug group Antifungal drug (p.138)
Overdose danger rating Low
Dependence rating Low
Prescription needed Yes
Available as generic Yes

INFORMATION FOR USERS

Your drug prescription is tailored for you. Do not alter dosage without checking with your doctor.

How taken

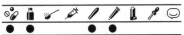

Tablets, pastilles, liquid, pessaries, cream, ointment, gel.

Frequency and timing of doses
Mouth or throat infections 4 x daily. Liquid should be held in the mouth for several minutes before swallowing.
Intestinal infections 4 x daily.
Skin infections 2–4 x daily.
Vaginal infections Once daily for 2 weeks.

Adult dosage range
2–4 million units daily (by mouth); 100,000–200,000 units at night (pessaries); 1–2 applicatorfuls (vaginal cream); as directed (skin preparations).

Onset of effect
Full beneficial effect may not be felt for 7–14 days.

Duration of action
Up to 6 hours.

Diet advice
None.

Storage
Keep in a closed container in a cool, dry place out of the reach of children. Protect from light.

Missed dose
Take as soon as you remember. Take your next dose as usual.

Stopping the drug
Take the full course. Even if the affected area seems to be cured, the original infection may still be present, and symptoms may recur if treatment is stopped too soon.

Exceeding the dose
An occasional unintentional extra dose is unlikely to be a cause for concern. But if you notice any unusual symptoms, or if a large overdose has been taken, notify your doctor.

SPECIAL PRECAUTIONS

Be sure to tell your doctor if:
▼ You are taking other medications.

Pregnancy
▼ No evidence of risk to developing fetus.

Breast-feeding
▼ No evidence of risk.

Infants and children
▼ Reduced dose necessary.

Over 60
▼ No special problems.

Driving and hazardous work
▼ No known problems.

Alcohol
▼ No known problems.

POSSIBLE ADVERSE EFFECTS

Adverse effects are uncommon, and are usually mild and transient. Nausea and vomiting may occur when high doses of the drug are taken by mouth.

Symptom/effect	Frequency		Discuss with doctor		Stop taking drug now	Call doctor now
	Common	Rare	Only if severe	In all cases		
Diarrhoea		●	■			
Nausea/vomiting		●	■			
Rash		●		■		

INTERACTIONS

None.

PROLONGED USE

No problems expected. Usually given as a course of treatment until the infection is cured.

OLANZAPINE

Brand name Zyprexa
Used in the following combined preparations None

GENERAL INFORMATION

Olanzapine is a benzodiazepine antipsychotic drug prescribed for the treatment of schizophrenia. It works by blocking several different receptors, including dopamine, histamine, and serotonin receptors.

The drug is effective in maintaining control of the condition in people who have responded to initial treatment. It can be used to treat both "positive"

symptoms (delusions, hallucinations, and thought disorders) and "negative" symptoms (blunted affect, emotional and social withdrawal).

The drug stays in the body longer in women, non-smokers, and the elderly than in younger men and smokers. As a result, women, non-smokers, and older people may need a lower starting dose and lower maintenance doses.

INFORMATION FOR USERS

Your drug prescription is tailored for you. Do not alter dosage without checking with your doctor.

How taken

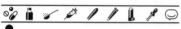

Tablets.

Frequency and timing of doses
Once daily.

Adult dosage range
10mg daily (starting dose), then 5–20mg daily. Doses greater than 15mg are prescribed only after clinical reassessment.

Onset of effect
4–8 hours.

Duration of action
30–38 hours, but longer in women than in men, and longer in the elderly.

Diet advice
None.

Storage
Keep in a closed container in a cool, dry place out of the reach of children. Protect from light.

Missed dose
Take as soon as you remember. If your next dose is due within 8 hours take a single dose now and skip the next.

Stopping the drug
Do not stop the drug without consulting your doctor; symptoms may recur.

Exceeding the dose
An occasional unintentional extra dose is unlikely to cause problems. Large overdoses may cause unusual drowsiness, depressed breathing, and low blood pressure. Notify your doctor.

SPECIAL PRECAUTIONS

Be sure to tell your doctor if:
▼ You have an enlarged prostate.
▼ You have glaucoma.
▼ You are taking other medications.

Pregnancy
▼ Safety not established. Discuss with your doctor.

Breast-feeding
▼ Safety not established. Discuss with your doctor.

Infants and children
▼ Not recommended.

Over 60
▼ Reduced dose necessary.

Driving and hazardous work
▼ Avoid. Olanzapine can cause unusual drowsiness.

Alcohol
▼ Avoid. Alcohol increases the sedative effects of this drug.

POSSIBLE ADVERSE EFFECTS

Unusual drowsiness and weight gain are the most common *adverse effects* of olanzapine.

Symptom/effect	Frequency		Discuss with doctor		Stop taking drug now	Call doctor now
	Common	Rare	Only if severe	In all cases		
Unusual drowsiness	●		■			
Weight gain	●		■			
Dizziness/fainting	●				■	
Parkinsonism	●				■	
Persistent sore throat		●			■	

PROLONGED USE

Prolonged use of olanzapine may, rarely, cause *tardive dyskinesia*, in which there are involuntary movements of the tongue and face.

INTERACTIONS

Sedatives All drugs that have a *sedative* effect on the central nervous system may increase the sedative effects of olanzapine.

Anticonvulsant drugs Olanzapine opposes the effect of these drugs. Carbamazepine decreases the effect of olanzapine.

Anti-arrhythmics There is an increased risk of arrhythmias when certain of these drugs are used with olanzapine.

OMEPRAZOLE

Brand name Losec
Used in the following combined preparations None

GENERAL INFORMATION

Omeprazole is an anti-ulcer drug that was introduced in 1989. It is used to treat stomach and duodenal ulcers as well as reflux oesophagitis, a condition in which acid from the stomach rises into the oesophagus. It reduces (by about 70 per cent) the amount of acid produced by the stomach and works in a different way from other anti-ulcer drugs that reduce acid secretion.

Treatment is usually given for four to eight weeks, depending on where the ulcer is situated. Omeprazole may also be given with antibiotics to eradicate the *Helicobacter pylori* bacteria that cause

many gastric ulcers. Reflux oesophagitis may be treated for four to twelve weeks.

Omeprazole causes few serious *side effects*. However, because the drug may affect the actions of enzymes in the liver, where many drugs are broken down, it may increase the effects of cyclosporin, warfarin, and phenytoin, and these drugs require more careful monitoring when used with omeprazole. As with other anti-ulcer drugs, it may mask signs of stomach cancer, so it is used only when the possibility of this disease has been ruled out.

QUICK REFERENCE

Drug group Anti-ulcer drug (p.109)
Overdose danger rating Low
Dependence rating Low
Prescription needed Yes
Available as generic No

INFORMATION FOR USERS

Your drug prescription is tailored for you. Do not alter dosage without checking with your doctor.

How taken

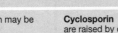

Capsules.

Frequency and timing of doses
1–2 x daily.

Adult dosage range
10–40mg daily and sometimes up to 120mg daily.

Onset of effect
2–5 hours.

Duration of action
24 hours.

Diet advice
None, although spicy foods and alcohol may exacerbate the underlying condition.

Storage
Keep in a closed container in a cool, dry place out of the reach of children. Omeprazole is very sensitive to moisture. It must not be transferred to another container and must be used within 3 months of opening.

Missed dose
Take as soon as you remember. If your next dose is due within 8 hours, take a single dose now and skip the next.

Stopping the drug
Do not stop the drug without consulting your doctor; symptoms may recur.

Exceeding the dose
An occasional unintentional extra dose is unlikely to be a cause for concern. But if you notice any unusual symptoms, or if a large overdose has been taken, notify your doctor.

SPECIAL PRECAUTIONS

Be sure to tell your doctor if:
▼ You have a long-term liver problem.
▼ You are taking other medications.

Pregnancy
▼ Safety in pregnancy not established. Discuss with your doctor.

Breast-feeding
▼ The drug may pass into the breast milk. Safety in breast-feeding not established. Discuss with your doctor.

Infants and children
▼ Not recommended.

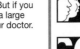
Over 60
▼ No special problems.

Driving and hazardous work
▼ No special problems.

Alcohol
▼ Avoid. Alcohol may aggravate your underlying condition and reduce the beneficial effects of this drug.

POSSIBLE ADVERSE EFFECTS

Adverse effects such as headache and diarrhoea are usually mild, and often diminish with continued use of the drug. If you develop a rash, however, you should notify your doctor.

Symptom/effect	Frequency		Discuss with doctor		Stop taking drug now	Call doctor now
	Common	Rare	Only if severe	In all cases		
Nausea		●	■			
Headache	●		■			
Diarrhoea	●		■			
Constipation		●	■			
Rash		●		■	▲	

INTERACTIONS

Warfarin The effects of warfarin may be increased by omeprazole.

Phenytoin The effects of phenytoin may be increased by omeprazole.

Cyclosporin Blood levels of cyclosporin are raised by omeprazole.

PROLONGED USE

No problems expected.

ONDANSETRON

Brand name Zofran
Used in the following combined preparations None

GENERAL INFORMATION

Ondansetron, an anti-emetic, is used especially for treating the nausea and vomiting associated with radiotherapy and anticancer drugs such as cisplatin. It may also be prescribed for the nausea and vomiting that occur after surgery.

The dose given and the frequency will depend on which anti-cancer drug you are having and the dose of that drug. In most instances, you will receive a dose of ondansetron, either by mouth or injection, before infusion of the anti-cancer agent, then tablets for up to five days after the treatment has finished. The activity of ondansetron against the delayed nausea and vomiting that occur several days after chemotherapy is much less than its activity against the symptoms that occur soon after anticancer treatment.

To enhance the effectiveness of ondansetron, it is usually taken with other drugs, such as dexamethasone. Serious *adverse effects* are unlikely to occur.

INFORMATION FOR USERS

Your drug prescription is tailored for you. Do not alter dosage without checking with your doctor.

How taken

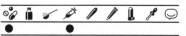

Tablets, injection.

Frequency and timing of doses
Normally 2 x daily but the frequency will depend on the reason for which it is being used.

Adult dosage range
4–32mg daily depending on the reason for which it is being used.

Onset of effect
Within 1 hour.

Duration of action
Approximately 12 hours.

Diet advice
None.

Storage
Keep in a closed container in a cool, dry place out of the reach of children. Protect from light.

Missed dose
Take as soon as you remember. If your next dose is due within 2 hours, take a single dose now and skip the next.

Stopping the drug
Can be safely stopped as soon as you no longer need it.

Exceeding the dose
An occasional unintentional extra dose is unlikely to be a cause for concern. But if you notice any unusual symptoms, or if a large overdose has been taken, notify your doctor.

SPECIAL PRECAUTIONS

Be sure to tell your doctor if:
▼ You have a long-term liver problem.
▼ You are taking other medications.

 Pregnancy
▼ Safety in pregnancy not established. Discuss with your doctor.

 Breast-feeding
▼ The drug passes into the breast milk. Discuss with your doctor.

 Infants and children
▼ Reduced dose necessary.

 Over 60
▼ No special problems.

 Driving and hazardous work
▼ No problems expected.

Alcohol
▼ No known problems.

POSSIBLE ADVERSE EFFECTS

Ondansetron is considered to be safe and is generally well tolerated. It does not cause sedation and movement disorders – adverse effects of some of the other anti-emetics.

Symptom/effect	Frequency		Discuss with doctor		Stop taking drug now	Call doctor now
	Common	Rare	Only if severe	In all cases		
Constipation	●		■			
Headache	●		■			
Warm feeling in head/stomach		●	■			

INTERACTIONS

None.

PROLONGED USE

Not generally prescribed for long-term treatment.

ORLISTAT

Brand name Xenical
Used in the following combined preparations None

GENERAL INFORMATION

Orlistat blocks the action of stomach and pancreatic enzymes (lipases) that digest fats. This means that the fats are not absorbed into the body but pass through and are excreted in the faeces. As a result, the body must burn stored fat from the tissues to provide energy, which should gradually reduce the fat stores and produce weight loss. The effectiveness of orlistat varies from person to person.

Because of the way orlistat works, the faeces become oily and this can cause flatulence. Part of the drug's effect may be due to people reducing their fat intake in order to avoid the unpleasantness of these *side effects*.

As fat absorption is greatly reduced, there is a danger that fat soluble vitamins might be lost to the body. Vitamin supplements may be prescribed to compensate for this. The vitamins should be taken at a different time from the orlistat; bedtime might be best, or at least 2 hours apart from any orlistat dose.

INFORMATION FOR USERS

Your drug prescription is tailored for you. Do not alter dosage without checking with your doctor.

How taken

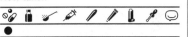

Capsules.

Frequency and timing of doses
Just before, during, or up to 1 hour after each main meal (up to 3 x daily). If a meal is omitted or contains no fat, do not take the dose of orlistat.

Adult dosage range
120–360mg daily.

Onset of effect
30 minutes; excretion of excess faecal fat begins about 24–48 hours after the first dose.

Duration of action
Orlistat is not absorbed from the gut, and potentially continues to work as it passes through the intestines. If you stop taking the drug, faecal fat returns to normal in 48–72 hours.

Diet advice
Eat a nutritionally balanced diet that does not contain quite enough calories, and that provides about 30 percent of the calories as fat. Eat lots of fruit and vegetables. The intake of fat, carbohydrate and protein should be distributed over the three main meals.

Storage
Keep in a closed container in a cool dry place. Keep out of the reach of children.

Missed dose
No cause for concern. Take the next dose with the next meal.

Stopping the drug
The drug can be safely stopped as soon as it is no longer needed, but notify your doctor.

SPECIAL PRECAUTIONS

Be sure to tell your doctor if:
▼ You have diabetes.
▼ You have chronic malabsorption syndrome.
▼ You have gallbladder or liver problems.
▼ You are taking lipid-lowering drugs.
▼ You are taking other medications.

Pregnancy
▼ Safety not established. Discuss with your doctor.

Breast-feeding
▼ Safety not established. Discuss with your doctor.

Infants and children
▼ Not prescribed.

Over 60
▼ No known problems.

Driving and hazardous work
▼ No special problems.

Alcohol
▼ No special problems.

POSSIBLE ADVERSE EFFECTS

Most of the *side effects* depend on how much fat is eaten, as well as the dose of orlistat.

Symptom/effect	Frequency		Discuss with doctor		Stop taking drug now	Call doctor now
	Common	Rare	Only if severe	In all cases		
Liquid, oily stools	●		■			
Faecal urgency	●		■			
Flatulence	●		■			
Abdominal/rectal pain	●		■			
Headache		●	■			
Menstrual irregularities		●	■			
Anxiety/fatigue/nausea		●	■			

INTERACTIONS

Lipid lowering drugs Orlistat increases blood levels and *toxicity* of pravastatin.

PROLONGED USE

Orlistat treatment should be stopped after 12 weeks if you have not lost 5 percent of your body weight since the start of treatment. If you have, then the drug may be continued, for up to a maximum of 2 years, until your target weight is approached.

ORPHENADRINE

Brand names Biorphen, Disipal
Used in the following combined preparations None

GENERAL INFORMATION

Orphenadrine is an *anticholinergic* drug that is prescribed to treat all forms of Parkinson's disease. Although it is less effective than other drugs used in the treatment of this disorder, it is often preferred because its *adverse effects* tend to be less severe. Orphenadrine is particularly valuable for relieving the muscle rigidity that often occurs with Parkinson's disease; it is less helpful for improving slowing of movement that also commonly affects sufferers.

Orphenadrine possesses significant muscle-relaxant properties. It produces this effect by blocking nerve pathways responsible for muscle rigidity and spasm. Consequently, it is prescribed for the relief of muscle spasm caused by muscle injury, prolapsed ("slipped") disc, and whiplash injuries.

INFORMATION FOR USERS

Your drug prescription is tailored for you. Do not alter dosage without checking with your doctor.

How taken

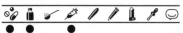

Tablets, liquid, injection.

Frequency and timing of doses
2–3 x daily.

Adult dosage range
150–400mg daily.

Onset of effect
Within 60 minutes (by mouth); within 5 minutes (by injection).

Duration of action
8–12 hours.

Diet advice
None.

Storage
Keep in a closed container in a cool, dry place out of the reach of children. Protect from light.

Missed dose
Take as soon as you remember. If your next dose is due within 2 hours, take a single dose now and skip the next.

Stopping the drug
Do not stop the drug without consulting your doctor; symptoms may recur.

OVERDOSE ACTION

 Seek immediate medical advice in all cases. Take emergency action if palpitations, fits, or loss of consciousness occur.

See Drug poisoning emergency guide (p.494).

SPECIAL PRECAUTIONS

Be sure to tell your doctor if:
▼ You have long-term liver or kidney problems.
▼ You have heart problems.
▼ You have had glaucoma.
▼ You have difficulty in passing urine.
▼ You have myasthenia gravis.
▼ You are taking other medications.

 Pregnancy
▼ Safety in pregnancy not established. Discuss with your doctor.

 Breast-feeding
▼ The drug passes into the breast milk, but at normal doses adverse effects on the baby are unlikely. Discuss with your doctor.

 Infants and children
▼ Not usually prescribed.

 Over 60
▼ Increased likelihood of adverse effects. Reduced dose may therefore be necessary.

 Driving and hazardous work
▼ Avoid such activities until you have learned how orphenadrine affects you because the drug can cause dizziness, lightheadedness, and blurred vision.

Alcohol
▼ Avoid. Alcohol may increase the sedative effects of this drug.

PROLONGED USE

No problems expected. Effectiveness in treating Parkinson's disease may diminish with time.

POSSIBLE ADVERSE EFFECTS

The adverse effects of orphenadrine are similar to those of other anticholinergic drugs. The more common symptoms, such as dryness of the mouth and blurred vision, can often be overcome by an adjustment in dosage.

Symptom/effect	Frequency		Discuss with doctor		Stop taking drug now	Call doctor now
	Common	Rare	Only if severe	In all cases		
Dry mouth/skin	●		■			
Difficulty in passing urine	●		■			
Constipation	●		■			
Dizziness	●		■			
Blurred vision	●			■		
Confusion/agitation		●		■		
Rash/itching		●		■	▲	
Palpitations		●		■	▲	■

INTERACTIONS

Anticholinergic drugs The anticholinergic effects of orphenadrine are likely to be increased by these drugs.

Dextropropoxyphene/co-proxamol Confusion, anxiety, and tremors may occur if these drugs are taken with orphenadrine.

Sedatives The effects of all drugs that have a sedative effect on the central nervous system are likely to be increased with orphenadrine.

OXYBUTYNIN

Brand names Contimin, Cystrin, Ditropan
Used in the following combined preparations None

GENERAL INFORMATION

Oxybutynin is an *anticholinergic* and *antispasmodic* drug used to treat urinary incontinence and frequency in adults and bedwetting in children. It works by reducing bladder contraction, allowing the bladder to hold more urine. The drug stops bladder spasms and delays the desire to empty the bladder. It also has some local *anaesthetic* effect.

The drug's usefulness is limited to some extent by its *side effects*, especially in children and the elderly. It can aggravate conditions such as an enlarged prostate or coronary heart disease in the elderly. Children are more susceptible to effects on the central nervous system (CNS), such as restlessness, disorientation, hallucinations, and convulsions.

QUICK REFERENCE

Drug group Drug for urinary disorder (p.166)

Overdose danger rating Medium

Dependence rating Low

Prescription needed Yes

Available as generic Yes

INFORMATION FOR USERS

Your drug prescription is tailored for you. Do not alter dosage without checking with your doctor.

How taken

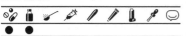

Tablets, liquid.

Frequency and timing of doses
2–4 x daily.

Adult dosage range
10–20mg daily.

Onset of effect
1 hour.

Duration of action
Up to 10 hours.

Diet advice
None.

Storage
Keep in a closed container in a cool, dry place out of the reach of children. Protect liquid from light.

Missed dose
Take as soon as you remember. If your next dose is due within 2 hours, take a single dose now and skip the next.

Stopping the drug
Do not stop taking the drug without consulting your doctor; symptoms may recur.

Exceeding the dose
An occasional unintentional extra dose is unlikely to cause problems. Larger overdoses may cause restlessness or psychotic behaviour, fall in blood pressure, breathing difficulties, paralysis, or coma. Notify your doctor immediately.

SPECIAL PRECAUTIONS

Be sure to tell your doctor if:
▼ You have liver or kidney problems.
▼ You have hyperthyroidism.
▼ You have heart problems.
▼ You have an enlarged prostate.
▼ You have porphyria.
▼ You have hiatus hernia.
▼ You have ulcerative colitis.
▼ You have glaucoma.
▼ You have myasthenia gravis.
▼ You are taking other medications.

Pregnancy
▼ Safety not established. May harm the unborn baby. Discuss with your doctor.

Breast-feeding
▼ Safety not established. Discuss with your doctor.

Infants and children
▼ Not recommended under 5 years. Reduced dose necessary in older children.

Over 60
▼ Reduced dose necessary.

Driving and hazardous work
▼ Avoid such activities until you have learned how oxybutynin affects you because the drug can cause drowsiness, disorientation, and blurred vision.

Alcohol
▼ Avoid. Alcohol increases the sedative effects of oxybutynin.

POSSIBLE ADVERSE EFFECTS

An adjustment in dosage is necessary in children and the elderly to minimize oxybutynin's adverse effects. The drug can also precipitate glaucoma.

Symptom/effect	Frequency		Discuss with doctor		Stop taking drug now	Call doctor now
	Common	Rare	Only if severe	In all cases		
Dry mouth	●		■			
Blurred vision/eye pain		●	■			
Constipation	●		■			
Nausea	●		■			
Facial flushing	●		■			
Difficulty in passing urine	●		■			
Headache/confusion		●	■			
Dry skin/rash		●		■		

INTERACTIONS

General note If oxybutynin is taken with other drugs that have anticholinergic effects, the risk of accumulated side effects is increased.

PROLONGED USE

No special problems.

PARACETAMOL

Brand names Alvedon, Calpol, Disprol, Hedex, Panadol, Panaleve, and many others
Used in the following combined preparations Anadin Extra, Migraleve, Panadeine, Paradote, Tylex, and others

GENERAL INFORMATION

Although paracetamol has been known since the early 1900s, it was not widely used as an analgesic until the 1950s. One of a group of drugs known as the non-*opioid* analgesics, it is kept in the home to relieve occasional bouts of mild pain and to reduce fever. It is suitable for children as well as adults.

One of the primary advantages of paracetamol is that it does not cause stomach upset or bleeding problems. This makes it a particularly useful

alternative for people who suffer from peptic ulcers or those who cannot tolerate aspirin. The drug is also safe for occasional use by those who are being treated with anticoagulants.

Although safe when used as directed, paracetamol is dangerous when it is taken in overdose, and it is capable of causing serious damage to the liver and kidneys. Large doses of paracetamol may also be *toxic* if you regularly drink even moderate amounts of alcohol.

QUICK REFERENCE

Drug group Non-opioid analgesic (p.80)

Overdose danger rating High

Dependence rating Low

Prescription needed No

Available as generic Yes

INFORMATION FOR USERS

Follow instructions on the label. Call your doctor if symptoms worsen.

How taken

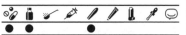

Tablets, capsules, liquid, suppositories.

Frequency and timing of doses
Every 4–6 hours as necessary, but not more than 4 doses per 24 hours in children.

Dosage range
Adults 500mg–1g per dose up to 4g daily.
Children 60–120mg per dose (3 months–1 year); 120–250mg per dose (1–5 years); 250–500mg per dose (6–12 years).

Onset of effect
Within 15–60 minutes.

Duration of action
Up to 6 hours.

Diet advice
None.

Storage
Keep in a closed container in a cool, dry place out of the reach of children.

Missed dose
Take as soon as you remember if required to relieve pain. Otherwise do not take the missed dose, and take a further dose only when you are in pain.

Stopping the drug
Can be safely stopped as soon as you no longer need it.

OVERDOSE ACTION

 Seek immediate medical advice in all cases. Take emergency action if nausea, vomiting, or stomach pain occur.

See Drug poisoning emergency guide (p.494).

SPECIAL PRECAUTIONS

Be sure to consult your doctor or pharmacist before using this drug if:
▼ You have long-term liver or kidney problems.
▼ You are taking other medications.

Pregnancy
▼ No evidence of risk with occasional use.

Breast-feeding
▼ No evidence of risk.

Infants and children
▼ Infants under 3 months on doctor's advice only. Reduced dose necessary up to 12 years.

 Over 60
▼ No special problems.

 Driving and hazardous work
▼ No special problems.

 Alcohol
▼ Prolonged heavy intake of alcohol in combination with excess paracetamol may substantially increase the risk of injury to the liver.

POSSIBLE ADVERSE EFFECTS

Paracetamol has rarely been found to produce any side effects when taken as recommended.

The drug should be stopped and your doctor notified if a rash occurs.

Symptom/effect	Frequency		Discuss with doctor		Stop taking drug now	Call doctor now
	Common	Rare	Only if severe	In all cases		
Nausea		●	■			
Rash		●		■	▲	

PROLONGED USE

You should not normally take this drug for longer than 48 hours except on the advice of your doctor. However, there is no evidence of harm from long-term use.

INTERACTIONS

Anticoagulants such as warfarin may need dosage adjustment if paracetamol is taken regularly in high doses.

Cholestyramine reduces the absorption of paracetamol and may reduce its effectiveness.

PAROXETINE

Brand name Seroxat
Used in the following combined preparations None

GENERAL INFORMATION

Paroxetine is one of the group known as selective serotonin re-uptake inhibitors (SSRIs). It is used in the treatment of mild to moderate depression. It helps control the anxiety often accompanying depression. It is also used to treat panic and obsessive-compulsive disorders.

Compared with the older tricyclic antidepressants, paroxetine and other other SSRIs are less likely to cause *anticholinergic side effects* such as dry mouth, blurred vision, and difficulty in passing urine. They are also much less dangerous if taken in overdose.

The most common *adverse effects* of paroxetine include nausea, drowsiness, sweating, tremor, weakness, insomnia, and sexual dysfunction.

INFORMATION FOR USERS

Your drug prescription is tailored for you. Do not alter dosage without checking with your doctor.

How taken

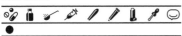

Tablets.

Frequency and timing of doses
Once daily, in the morning.

Dosage range
20–60mg daily.

Onset of effect
The onset of therapeutic response usually occurs within 7–14 days of starting treatment, but full antidepressant effect may not be felt for 3–4 weeks.

Duration of action
Up to 24 hours.

Diet advice
None.

Storage
Keep in a closed container in a cool, dry place out of the reach of children.

Missed dose
Take as soon as you remember.

Stopping the drug
Do not stop the drug without consulting your doctor. Stopping abruptly can cause withdrawal symptoms.

Exceeding the dose
An occasional unintentional extra dose is unlikely to be a cause for concern. Large doses may cause unusual drowsiness. Notify your doctor immediately.

SPECIAL PRECAUTIONS

Be sure to tell your doctor if:
▼ You have long-term liver or kidney problems.
▼ You have a heart problem.
▼ You have a history or a family history of fits.
▼ You are taking other medications.

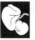 **Pregnancy**
▼ Safety in pregnancy not established. Discuss with your doctor.

 Breast-feeding
▼ The drug passes into the breast milk. Discuss with your doctor.

 Infants and children
▼ Not recommended under 18 years.

 Over 60
▼ No special problems.

 Driving and hazardous work
▼ Avoid such activities until you have learned how paroxetine affects you because the drug can cause drowsiness.

 Alcohol
▼ Avoid. Alcohol may increase the sedative effects of this drug.

POSSIBLE ADVERSE EFFECTS

The most commonly observed adverse effects are nausea, drowsiness, sweating, tremor, weakness, insomnia, and sexual dysfunction (lack of orgasm, male ejaculation problems).

Symptom/effect	Frequency		Discuss with doctor		Stop taking drug now	Call doctor now
	Common	Rare	Only if severe	In all cases		
Nausea	●			■		
Sweating	●			■		
Drowsiness/dizziness	●			■		
Sexual dysfunction (both sexes)	●			■		
Nervousness/anxiety/agitation		●		■		
Rash/itching/hives/joint pain		●		■	▲	■
Poor appetite/weight loss		●		■		
Convulsions		●		■		■

PROLONGED USE

No problems expected. However, mild withdrawal symptoms may occur if the drug is not stopped gradually.

INTERACTIONS

General note Any drug that affects the breakdown of others in the liver may alter blood levels of paroxetine or vice versa.

Anticoagulants Paroxetine may increase the effects of these drugs.

Sedatives All sedatives are likely to increase the sedative effects of paroxetine.

Tricyclic antidepressants Paroxetine may increase the *toxicity* of these drugs.

Monoamine oxidase inhibitors (MAOIs) Paroxetine should not be taken during or within 14 days of MAOI treatment because serious reactions may occur.

PERMETHRIN

Brand name Lyclear
Used in the following combined preparations None

GENERAL INFORMATION

Permethrin is an insecticide related to the natural substance, pyrethrum, which is obtained from the flower of the same name. The drug is used to treat head lice and scabies infestations. It works by interfering with the nervous system function of the parasites, causing paralysis and death. Permethrin has the advantage of being less *toxic* than some other types of insecticide.

Permethrin is applied *topically* as a liquid to treat head lice and a cream for scabies infestations. In children, the entire body surface, including the face, scalp, neck, and ears, is covered; adults are treated from the neck downwards.

For both head lice and scabies, all family members should be treated at the same time, to prevent recontamination, and the process repeated after a week.

There are signs that the parasites are developing resistance to permethrin. If the drug does not work for you, your pharmacist should be able to suggest an alternative treatment.

INFORMATION FOR USERS

Follow instructions on the label. Call your doctor if symptoms worsen.

How taken

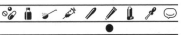

Cream, topical liquid.

Frequency and timing of doses
Once only, repeating after 7 days. Avoid contact with eyes and broken or infected skin.

Adult dosage range
As directed.

Onset of effect
Liquid should be rinsed off after 10 minutes (head lice); cream should be washed off after 8–12 hours (scabies).

Duration of action
Until washed off.

Diet advice
None.

Storage
Keep in a closed container in a cool, dry place out of the reach of children. Protect from light.

Missed dose
Timing of the second application is not rigid; use as soon as you remember.

Stopping the drug
Not applicable

Exceeding the dose
An occasional extra application is unlikely to cause problems. If the drug is accidentally swallowed, take emergency action.

POSSIBLE ADVERSE EFFECTS

In general, permethrin is well tolerated on the skin, although mild skin irritation is common.

Symptom/effect	Frequency		Discuss with doctor		Stop taking drug now	Call doctor now
	Common	Rare	Only if severe	In all cases		
Itching	●		■			
Reddened skin/stinging	●		■			
Rash		●	■			

INTERACTIONS

None.

SPECIAL PRECAUTIONS

Be sure to consult your doctor or pharmacist before taking this drug if:
▼ You are taking other medications.

Pregnancy
▼ Safety not established. Discuss with your doctor.

Breast-feeding
▼ Safety not established. Discuss with your doctor.

Infants and children
▼ No special problems.

Over 60
▼ No special problems.

Driving and hazardous work
▼ No special problems.

Alcohol
▼ No special problems.

PROLONGED USE

Permethrin should not be used for prolonged periods; it is intended for intermittent use only.

PHENOBARBITAL

Brand name Gardenal
Used in the following combined preparations None

GENERAL INFORMATION

Phenobarbital, introduced more than 70 years ago, belongs to the group of drugs known as barbiturates. It is used mainly in the treatment of epilepsy, but it was also used as a sleeping drug and sedative before the development of safer drugs.

In the treatment of epilepsy, the drug is usually given together with another anticonvulsant drug such as phenytoin.

The main disadvantage of the drug is that it often causes unwanted sedation. However, tolerance develops within a week or two, and most patients have no problem in long-term use. In children and the elderly, it may occasionally cause excessive excitement.

Because of their sedative effects, phenobarbital and other barbiturates are sometimes abused.

INFORMATION FOR USERS

Your drug prescription is tailored for you. Do not alter dosage without checking with your doctor.

How taken

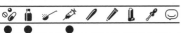

Tablets, liquid, injection.

Frequency and timing of doses
1–3 x daily.

Dosage range
Adults 60–180mg daily.

Onset of effect
30–60 minutes (by mouth).

Duration of action
24–48 hours (some effect may persist for up to 6 days).

Diet advice
None.

Storage
Keep in a closed container in a cool, dry place out of the reach of children.

Missed dose
Take as soon as you remember. If you take once daily and the next dose is due within 10 hours, take a single dose now and skip the next. If you take 2–3 times daily and the next dose is due within 2 hours, take a single dose now and skip the next.

Stopping the drug
Do not stop taking the drug without consulting your doctor, who may supervise a gradual reduction in dosage. Abrupt cessation may cause fits or lead to restlessness, trembling, and insomnia.

OVERDOSE ACTION

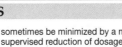

Seek immediate medical advice in all cases. Take emergency action if unsteadiness, severe weakness, confusion, or loss of consciousness occur.

See Drug poisoning emergency guide (p.494).

POSSIBLE ADVERSE EFFECTS

Most of the adverse effects of phenobarbital are the result of its sedative effect. They can sometimes be minimized by a medically supervised reduction of dosage.

Symptom/effect	Frequency		Discuss with doctor		Stop taking drug now	Call doctor now
	Common	Rare	Only if severe	In all cases		
Drowsiness	●		■			
Clumsiness/unsteadiness	●		■			
Dizziness/faintness	●		■			
Confusion		●		■		
Rash/localized swellings		●		■	▲	▮

INTERACTIONS

Corticosteroids Phenobarbital may reduce the effect of corticosteroid drugs.

Antipsychotics and antidepressants may reduce the anticonvulsant effect of phenobarbital.

Anticoagulants The effect of these drugs may be reduced when they are taken with phenobarbital.

Oral contraceptives Phenobarbital may reduce the effectiveness of oral contraceptives. Discuss with your doctor.

Sedatives All drugs that have a sedative effect on the central nervous system are likely to increase the sedative properties of phenobarbital.

SPECIAL PRECAUTIONS

Be sure to tell your doctor if:
▼ You have long-term liver or kidney problems.
▼ You have heart problems.
▼ You have poor circulation.
▼ You have porphyria.
▼ You have breathing problems.
▼ You are taking other medications.

 Pregnancy
▼ The drug may affect the fetus and increase the tendency of bleeding in the newborn. Discuss with your doctor.

 Breast-feeding
▼ The drug passes into the breast milk and could cause drowsiness in the baby. Discuss with your doctor.

 Infants and children
▼ Reduced dose necessary.

 Over 60
▼ Increased likelihood of confusion. Reduced dose may therefore be necessary.

 Driving and hazardous work
▼ Your underlying condition, in addition to the possibility of reduced alertness while taking phenobarbital, may make such activities inadvisable. Discuss with your doctor.

 Alcohol
▼ Never drink while under treatment with phenobarbital. Alcohol may interact dangerously with this drug.

PROLONGED USE

The sedative effect of phenobarbital can build up after starting use of the drug, causing excessive drowsiness and lethargy. However, *tolerance* may develop, so reducing these effects. Withdrawal symptoms may occur if the drug is stopped suddenly.

Monitoring Blood samples may be taken periodically to test blood levels of the drug.

PHENOXYMETHYLPENICILLIN

Brand names Apsin, Tenkicin
Used in the following combined preparations None

GENERAL INFORMATION

Phenoxymethylpenicillin, also known as Penicillin V, is a synthetic penicillin-type antibiotic that is prescribed for a wide range of infections.

Various commonly occurring respiratory tract infections, such as some types of tonsillitis and pharyngitis, as well as ear infections, often respond well to this drug. It is also effective for the treatment of the gum disease, Vincent's gingivitis.

Phenoxymethylpenicillin is also used to treat less common infections caused by the *Streptococcus* bacterium, such as scarlet fever and erysipelas (a skin infection). It is also prescribed long term to prevent the recurrence of rheumatic fever, a rare, although potentially serious condition. It is also used long term to prevent infections following removal of the spleen or in sickle cell disease.

As with other penicillin antibiotics, the most serious *adverse effect* that may rarely occur is an allergic reaction that may cause collapse, wheezing, and a rash in susceptible people.

QUICK REFERENCE

Drug group Penicillin antibiotic (p.128)

Overdose danger rating Low

Dependence rating Low

Prescription needed Yes

Available as generic Yes

INFORMATION FOR USERS

Your drug prescription is tailored for you. Do not alter dosage without checking with your doctor.

How taken

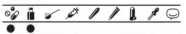

Tablets, liquid.

Frequency and timing of doses
2–4 x daily, at least 30 minutes before food.

Dosage range
Adults 2–3g daily.
Children Reduced dose according to age.

Onset of effect
1–2 days.

Duration of action
Up to 12 hours.

Diet advice
None.

Storage
Keep in a closed container in a cool, dry place out of the reach of children.

Missed dose
Take as soon as you remember. If your next dose is due within 2 hours, take a single dose now and skip the next.

Stopping the drug
Take the full course. Even if you feel better, the original infection may still be present and may recur if the treatment is stopped too soon.

Exceeding the dose
An occasional unintentional extra dose is unlikely to be a cause for concern. But if you notice any unusual symptoms, or if a large overdose has been taken, notify your doctor.

SPECIAL PRECAUTIONS

Be sure to tell your doctor if:
▼ You have a long-term kidney problem.
▼ You have had a previous allergic reaction to a penicillin or cephalosporin antibiotic.
▼ You have an allergic disorder such as asthma or urticaria.
▼ You are taking other medications.

Pregnancy
▼ No evidence of risk.

Breast-feeding
▼ The drug passes into the breast milk, but at normal doses adverse effects on the baby are unlikely. Discuss with your doctor.

Infants and children
▼ Reduced dose necessary.

Over 60
▼ No special problems.

Driving and hazardous work
▼ No known problems.

Alcohol
▼ No known problems.

POSSIBLE ADVERSE EFFECTS

Most people do not experience any serious adverse effects when taking phenoxymethyl-penicillin. However, this drug may provoke an allergic reaction in susceptible people.

Symptom/effect	Frequency		Discuss with doctor		Stop taking drug now	Call doctor now
	Common	Rare	Only if severe	In all cases		
Nausea/vomiting	●		■			
Diarrhoea		●	■			
Rash/itching		●		■	▲	▮
Breathing difficulties		●		■	▲	▮

INTERACTIONS

Oral contraceptives Phenoxymethyl-penicillin may reduce the contraceptive effect of these drugs. Discuss with your doctor.

Probenecid increases the level of phenoxymethylpenicillin in the blood.

PROLONGED USE

Prolonged use may increase the risk of *Candida* infections and diarrhoea.

PHENYLPROPANOLAMINE

Used in the following combined preparations Contac 400, Day Nurse Capsules, Dimotapp, Eskornade, Mucron, Sinutab, Triogesic, Triominic, Vicks Coldcare, and others.

GENERAL INFORMATION

Phenylpropanolamine belongs to the *sympathomimetic* group of drugs. It is used as a decongestant in many over-the-counter cold relief preparations. By reducing inflammation and swelling of blood vessels in the lining of the nose, the drug relieves the nasal congestion in head colds, hay fever, and sinusitis.

Phenylpropanolamine mimics some of the actions of the sympathetic nervous system (p.75), and as a consequence it can produce undesirable stimulant *side effects*. The drug may raise the heart rate and severely elevate blood pressure. It can also cause palpitations and wakefulness.

QUICK REFERENCE

Drug group Decongestant (p.93)

Overdose danger rating High

Dependence rating Low

Prescription needed No

Available as generic No

INFORMATION FOR USERS

Follow instructions on the label. Call your doctor if symptoms worsen.

How taken

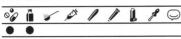

Tablets, SR-tablets, capsules, liquid.

Frequency and timing of doses
3–4 x daily; 2 x daily (SR-tablets).

Dosage range
75–100mg daily.

Onset of effect
Within 30 minutes.

Duration of action
4–6 hours. Up to 12 hours (SR-tablets).

Diet advice
None.

Storage
Keep in a closed container in a cool, dry place out of the reach of children. Protect from light.

Missed dose
Take as soon as you remember if needed. If you take the medication twice daily, and your next dose is due within 12 hours, take a single dose now and skip the next. If you take it 3–4 times daily and your next dose is due within 2 hours, take a single dose now and skip the next.

Stopping the drug
Can be safely stopped as soon as you no longer need it.

OVERDOSE ACTION

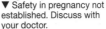

Seek immediate medical advice in all cases. Take emergency action if delirium, convulsions, or loss of consciousness occur.

See Drug poisoning emergency guide (p.494).

SPECIAL PRECAUTIONS

Be sure to consult your doctor or pharmacist before taking this drug if:
▼ You have high blood pressure.
▼ You have heart problems.
▼ You have had glaucoma.
▼ You have an overactive thyroid gland.
▼ You have diabetes.
▼ You have urinary difficulties.
▼ You are taking other medications.

Pregnancy
▼ Safety in pregnancy not established. Discuss with your doctor.

Breast-feeding
▼ The drug passes into the breast milk and may affect the baby. Discuss with your doctor.

Infants and children
▼ Not recommended under 8 years.

Over 60
▼ Increased likelihood of adverse effects. Reduced dose may therefore be necessary.

Driving and hazardous work
▼ Do not undertake such activities until you know how phenylpropanolamine affects you because the drug can cause dizziness.

Alcohol
▼ No known problems.

POSSIBLE ADVERSE EFFECTS

High doses may be associated with anxiety, nausea, dizziness, and, rarely, with a marked rise in blood pressure, causing palpitations, headache, and breathlessness.

Symptom/effect	Frequency		Discuss with doctor		Stop taking drug now	Call doctor now
	Common	Rare	Only if severe	In all cases		
Nausea/vomiting		●	■			
Dizziness/lightheadedness		●	■			
Nervousness/insomnia		●	■			
Confusion		●		■		
Rash		●		■	▲	
Palpitations/breathlessness		●		■	▲	▌
Headache		●		■		▌

INTERACTIONS

Other sympathomimetics increase the risk of adverse effects with this drug.

Beta blockers A severe rise in blood pressure can occur if beta blockers are taken with phenylpropanolamine.

Tricyclic antidepressants and digoxin There is an increased risk of abnormal heart rhythms if these drugs are taken with phenylpropanolamine.

Monoamine oxidase inhibitors (MAOIs) dangerously increase the risk of high blood pressure with phenylpropanolamine. It should not be taken during or within 14 days of MAOI treatment.

PROLONGED USE

Phenylpropanolamine should not be taken for long periods without medical supervision because it may raise the blood pressure and put a strain on the heart.

PHENYTOIN/FOSPHENYTOIN

Brand names Epanutin, Pentran
Used in the following combined preparations None

GENERAL INFORMATION

Phenytoin decreases the likelihood of convulsions by reducing abnormal electrical discharges within the brain. Introduced in the 1930s, it is prescribed for the treatment of epilepsy, including grand mal and temporal lobe epilepsy. Fosphenytoin is a new type of phenytoin given by injection for severe fits.

Over the years, various other uses have been found for the drug. It has been given for migraine, trigeminal neuralgia, and the correction of certain abnormal heart rhythms.

Some *adverse effects* of phenytoin (such as overgrowth of the gums) are more pronounced in children, so it is prescribed for children only when other drugs are unsuitable. Phenytoin is also avoided, if possible, in young women as it can affect the developing fetus.

QUICK REFERENCE

Drug group Anticonvulsant drug (p.86)

Overdose danger rating Medium

Dependence rating Low

Prescription needed Yes

Available as generic Yes

INFORMATION FOR USERS

Your drug prescription is tailored for you. Do not alter dosage without checking with your doctor.

How taken

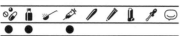

Tablets, capsules, liquid, injection.

Frequency and timing of doses
1–3 x daily with food or plenty of water.

Dosage range
Adults 200–500mg daily.
Children According to age and weight.

Onset of effect
Full anticonvulsant effect may not be felt for 7–10 days.

Duration of action
24 hours.

Diet advice
Folic acid and vitamin D deficiency may occasionally occur while taking this drug. Make sure you eat a balanced diet containing fresh, green vegetables.

Storage
Keep in a tightly closed container in a cool, dry place out of the reach of children.

Missed dose
Take as soon as you remember.

Stopping the drug
Do not stop the drug without consulting your doctor; symptoms may recur.

Exceeding the dose
An occasional, unintentional extra dose is unlikely to cause problems. However, if you notice unusual drowsiness, slurred speech, or confusion, notify your doctor.

SPECIAL PRECAUTIONS

Be sure to tell your doctor if:
▼ You have long-term liver or kidney problems.
▼ You have diabetes.
▼ You have porphyria.
▼ You are taking other medications.

 Pregnancy
▼ The drug may be associated with malformation and a tendency to bleeding in the newborn baby. Folic acid supplements should be taken by the mother. Discuss with your doctor.

 Breast-feeding
▼ The drug passes into the breast milk, but at normal doses adverse effects on the baby are unlikely. Discuss with your doctor.

 Infants and children
▼ Reduced dose necessary. Increased likelihood of overgrowth of the gums and excessive growth of body hair.

 Over 60
▼ Reduced dose may be necessary.

 Driving and hazardous work
▼ Your underlying condition, as well as the effects of phenytoin, may make such activities inadvisable. Discuss with your doctor.

 Alcohol
▼ Avoid. Alcohol increases the sedative effects of this drug.

POSSIBLE ADVERSE EFFECTS

Phenytoin has a number of adverse effects, many of which appear only after prolonged use. If they become severe, your doctor may prescribe a different anticonvulsant.

Symptom/effect	Frequency		Discuss with doctor		Stop taking drug now	Call doctor now
	Common	Rare	Only if severe	In all cases		
Dizziness/headache	●		■			
Confusion	●		■			
Nausea/vomiting	●		■			
Insomnia	●		■			
Increased body hair		●	■			
Overgrowth of gums		●		■		
Rash		●		■		
Fever/sore throat/mouth ulcers		●		■		

INTERACTIONS

General note Many drugs may interact with phenytoin, causing either an increase or a reduction in the phenytoin blood level. The dosage of phenytoin may need to be adjusted. Consult your doctor.

Cyclosporin Blood levels of cyclosporin may be reduced with phenytoin.

Antidepressants/antipsychotics These drugs may reduce the effect of phenytoin.

Warfarin The anticoagulant effect of this drug may be altered. An adjustment in its dosage may be necessary.

Oral contraceptives Phenytoin may reduce their effectiveness.

PROLONGED USE

There is a slight risk that blood abnormalities may occur. Prolonged use may also lead to adverse effects on skin, gums, and bones. It may also disrupt control of diabetes.

Monitoring Periodic blood tests may be performed to monitor levels of the drug in the body and composition of the blood cells and blood chemistry.

PILOCARPINE

Brand names Minims Pilocarpine, Ocusert Pilo, Salagen, Sno Pilo
Used in the following combined preparation Isopto Carpine

GENERAL INFORMATION

Pilocarpine, in use since 1875, is a *miotic* drug used to treat chronic glaucoma and, less often, severe glaucoma prior to surgery.

It is prescribed most frequently as eye drops. These are quick-acting but have to be re-applied every four to eight hours in chronic glaucoma. A slow-release formulation inserted once a week under the eyelid (Ocusert) may be more convenient for long-term use.

Pilocarpine, like other similar drugs, frequently causes blurred vision; and excessive spasm of the eye muscles may cause headaches, particularly at the start of treatment. However, serious *adverse effects* are rare.

Pilocarpine tablets are used to treat dry mouth following radiotherapy to the head and neck.

QUICK REFERENCE

Drug group Miotic drug for glaucoma (p.168)

Overdose danger rating Medium

Dependence rating Low

Prescription needed Yes

Available as generic Yes

INFORMATION FOR USERS

Your drug prescription is tailored for you. Do not alter dosage without checking with your doctor.

How taken

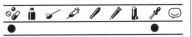

Tablets, eye drops, SR-inserts (Ocuserts).

Frequency and timing of doses
Eye drops 3–6 x daily (chronic glaucoma). In acute glaucoma, pilocarpine is given at 5-minute intervals until the condition is controlled.
Ocusert Once every 7 days at bedtime.
Tablets 3 x daily after food with plenty of water.

Dosage range
According to formulation and condition. In general, 1–2 eye drops are used per application.
Tablets 15–30 mg daily.

Onset of effect
15–30 minutes.

Duration of action
4–8 weeks for maximum effect (tablets); 3–8 hours (eye drops); about 7 days (Ocuserts).

Diet advice
None.

Storage
Keep in a closed container in a cool, dry place out of the reach of children (tablets/eye drops). Discard eye drops 1 month after opening.

Missed dose
Use as soon as you remember. If not remembered until 2 hours before your next dose, skip the missed dose and take the next dose now.

Stopping the drug
Do not stop the drug without consulting your doctor; symptoms may recur.

Exceeding the dose
An occasional unintentional extra application is unlikely to cause problems. Excessive use may cause facial flushing, an increase in the flow of saliva, and sweating. If accidentally swallowed, seek medical attention immediately.

SPECIAL PRECAUTIONS

Be sure to tell your doctor if:
▼ You have asthma.
▼ You have inflamed eyes.
▼ You wear contact lenses.
▼ You have heart, liver, or gastrointestinal problems.
▼ You are taking other medications.

Pregnancy
▼ No evidence of risk at the doses used for chronic glaucoma.

Breast-feeding
▼ The drug passes into the breast milk, but at normal doses adverse effects on the baby are unlikely. Discuss with your doctor.

Infants and children
▼ Not usually prescribed.

Over 60
▼ Reduced night vision is particularly noticeable.

Driving and hazardous work
▼ Avoid such activities, especially in poor light, until you have learned how pilocarpine affects you because it may cause short sight and poor night vision.

Alcohol
▼ No known problems.

PROLONGED USE

The effect of the drug may occasionally wear off with prolonged use as the body adapts, but may be restored by changing temporarily to another antiglaucoma drug.

POSSIBLE ADVERSE EFFECTS

Alteration in vision is common. Ocuserts may cause irritation if they move out of position. Brow ache and eye pain are common at the start of treatment, but usually wear off after a few days.

Symptom/effect	Frequency		Discuss with doctor		Stop taking drug now	Call doctor now
	Common	Rare	Only if severe	In all cases		
Blurred vision	●		■			
Poor night vision	●		■			
Headache/brow ache	●		■			
Sweating/chills	●		■			
Eye pain/irritation	●				■	■
Twitching eyelids		●			■	
Red, watery eyes		●	■			

INTERACTIONS

General note A wide range of drugs (including aminoglycoside antibiotics, clindamycin, colistin, chloroquine, quinine, quinidine, lithium, and procainamide) may antagonize pilocarpine.

Beta blockers These drugs may reduce the effects of pilocarpine.

Calcium channel blockers These drugs may increase pilocarpine's *systemic* effects.

PIROXICAM

Brand names Feldene, Flamatrol, Kentene, Larapram, Piroflam, Pirozip
Used in the following combined preparations None

GENERAL INFORMATION

Piroxicam, introduced in 1980, is a non-steroidal anti-inflammatory drug (NSAID) that, like others in this group, reduces pain, stiffness, and inflammation. Blood levels of the drug remain high for many hours after a dose, so it needs to be taken only once daily.

Piroxicam is used for osteoarthritis, rheumatoid arthritis, acute attacks of gout, and ankylosing spondylitis. It gives relief of the symptoms of arthritis, although it does not cure the disease. It is sometimes prescribed in conjunction with slow-acting drugs in rheumatoid arthritis to relieve pain and inflammation while these drugs take effect. The drug may also be given for pain relief after sports injuries, for conditions such as tendinitis and bursitis, and following minor surgery.

This drug is less likely than aspirin to cause stomach ulcers.

QUICK REFERENCE

Drug group Non-steroidal anti-inflammatory drug (p.116) and drug for gout (p.119)

Overdose danger rating Medium

Dependence rating Low

Prescription needed Yes

Available as generic Yes

INFORMATION FOR USERS

Your drug prescription is tailored for you. Do not alter dosage without checking with your doctor.

How taken

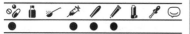

Tablets, dispersible tablets, capsules, injection, suppositories, gel.

Frequency and timing of doses
1–3 x daily with food or plenty of water.

Adult dosage range
10–40mg daily.

Onset of effect
Pain relief begins in 3–4 hours. Used for arthritis, the full anti-inflammatory effect develops over 2–4 weeks. Used for gout, this effect develops over 4–5 days.

Duration of action
Up to 2 days. Some effect may last for 7–10 days after treatment has been stopped.

Diet advice
None.

Storage
Keep in a closed container in a cool, dry place out of the reach of children. Protect from light.

Missed dose
Take as soon as you remember. If your next dose is due within 4 hours, take a single dose now and skip the next.

Stopping the drug
When taken for short-term pain relief, the drug can be safely stopped as soon as you no longer need it. If prescribed for the long-term treatment of arthritis, however, you should seek medical advice before stopping the drug.

Exceeding the dose
An occasional unintentional extra dose is unlikely to be a cause for concern. Large overdoses may cause nausea and vomiting. Notify your doctor.

SPECIAL PRECAUTIONS

Be sure to tell your doctor if:
▼ You have liver or kidney problems.
▼ You have heart problems or high blood pressure
▼ You have had a peptic ulcer, oesophagitis, or acid indigestion.
▼ You have porphyria.
▼ You have asthma.
▼ You are allergic to aspirin.
▼ You are taking other medications.

Pregnancy
▼ Not usually prescribed. When taken in the last three months of pregnancy, the drug increase the risk of adverse effects on the baby's heart and may prolong labour. Discuss with your doctor.

Breast-feeding
▼ The drug passes into the breast milk but at normal doses adverse effects are unlikely. Discuss with your doctor.

Infants and children
▼ Not recommended under 6 years. Reduced dose necessary.

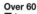

Over 60
▼ Increased likelihood of adverse effects. Reduced dose may therefore be necessary.

Driving and hazardous work
▼ Avoid such activities until you have learned how piroxicam affects you because the drug can cause dizziness.

Alcohol
▼ Avoid. Alcohol may increase the risk of stomach disorders with piroxicam.

Surgery and general anaesthetics
▼ Piroxicam may prolong bleeding. Discuss with your doctor or dentist before any surgery.

POSSIBLE ADVERSE EFFECTS

Gastrointestinal *side effects*, dizziness, and headache are not generally serious. Black or bloodstained bowel movements should be reported to your doctor immediately.

Symptom/effect	Frequency		Discuss with doctor		Stop taking drug now	Call doctor now
	Common	Rare	Only if severe	In all cases		
Nausea/indigestion	●		■			
Abdominal pain	●			■		
Dizziness/headache		●	■			
Swollen feet/ankles		●		■		
Rash/itching		●		■	▲	
Wheezing/breathlessness		●		■	▲	▮
Bruising or bleeding		●		■	▲	▮

INTERACTIONS

General note Piroxicam interacts with many drugs, including other NSAIDs, corticosteroids, and oral anticoagulant drugs, to increase the risk of bleeding and/or peptic ulcers.

Lithium Piroxicam may raise blood levels of lithium.

Antihypertensive drugs and diuretics The beneficial effects of these drugs may be reduced by piroxicam.

Ciprofloxacin, norfloxacin, and ofloxacin Piroxicam may increase the risk of convulsions when taken with these drugs.

PROLONGED USE

There is an increased risk of bleeding from peptic ulcers and in the bowel.

Monitoring Periodic blood counts and liver function tests may be performed.

PIZOTIFEN

Brand name Sanomigran
Used in the following combined preparations None

GENERAL INFORMATION

Pizotifen is an antihistamine drug with a chemical structure similar to that of the tricyclic antidepressants (p.84); it also has similar *anticholinergic* effects. This drug is prescribed for the prevention of migraine headaches in people who suffer frequent, disabling attacks. The drug is thought to work by blocking the chemicals (histamine and serotonin) that act on blood vessels in the brain.

Pizotifen has also been prescribed to relieve the symptoms of carcinoid syndrome, a disorder in which excess production of serotonin causes attacks of flushing and diarrhoea.

The main disadvantage of prolonged use of pizotifen is that it stimulates the appetite and, as a result, often causes weight gain. It is usually prescribed only for people in whom other measures for migraine prevention – for example, avoidance of stress and foods that trigger attacks – have failed.

The sweetener used in the liquid medicine may affect blood sugar levels.

QUICK REFERENCE

Drug group Drug for migraine (p.89)

Overdose danger rating Medium

Dependence rating Low

Prescription needed Yes

Available as generic No

INFORMATION FOR USERS

Your drug prescription is tailored for you. Do not alter dosage without checking with your doctor.

How taken

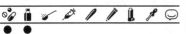

Tablets, liquid.

Frequency and timing of doses
Once a day (at night) or 3 x daily.

Adult dosage range
1.5–4.5mg daily. Maximum single dose 3mg.

Onset of effect
Full beneficial effects may not be felt for several days.

Duration of action
Effects of this drug may last for several weeks.

Diet advice
Migraine sufferers may be advised to avoid foods that trigger headaches in their case.

Storage
Keep in a closed container in a cool, dry place out of the reach of children. Protect from light.

Missed dose
Take as soon as you remember. If your next dose is due within 4 hours, take a single dose now and skip the next.

Stopping the drug
Do not stop the drug without consulting your doctor; symptoms may recur.

Exceeding the dose
An occasional unintentional extra dose is unlikely to cause problems. Large overdoses may cause drowsiness, nausea, palpitations, and fits. Notify your doctor.

SPECIAL PRECAUTIONS

Be sure to tell your doctor if:
▼ You have a long-term kidney problem.
▼ You have glaucoma.
▼ You have prostate trouble.
▼ You are taking other medications.

Pregnancy
▼ Safety in pregnancy not established. Discuss with your doctor.

Breast-feeding
▼ The drug passes into the breast milk, but at normal doses adverse effects on the baby are unlikely. Discuss with your doctor.

Infants and children
▼ Reduced dose usually necessary.

Over 60
▼ No special problems.

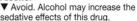
Driving and hazardous work
▼ Avoid such activities until you have learned how pizotifen affects you because the drug can cause drowsiness.

Alcohol
▼ Avoid. Alcohol may increase the sedative effects of this drug.

POSSIBLE ADVERSE EFFECTS

Drowsiness is a common *adverse effect* that can often be minimized by starting treatment with a low dose that is gradually increased.

Symptom/effect	Frequency		Discuss with doctor		Stop taking drug now	Call doctor now
	Common	Rare	Only if severe	In all cases		
Weight gain/increased appetite	●		■			
Drowsiness	●		■			
Nausea/dizziness		●	■			
Muscle pains		●	■			
Dry mouth		●	■			
Blurred vision		●	■			
Depression		●		■		

PROLONGED USE

Pizotifen often causes weight gain during long-term use. Treatment is usually reviewed every 6 months.

INTERACTIONS

Anticholinergic drugs The weak anticholinergic effects of pizotifen may be increased by other anticholinergic drugs, including tricyclic antidepressants.

Monoamine oxidase inhibitors (MAOIs) A dangerous rise in blood pressure may occur if pizotifen is taken with these drugs.

Sedatives All drugs that have a sedative effect on the central nervous system are likely to increase the sedative properties of pizotifen. These include sleeping drugs, anti-anxiety drugs, *opioid* analgesics, and antihistamines.

PRAVASTATIN

Brand name Lipostat
Used in the following combined preparations None

GENERAL INFORMATION

Pravastatin belongs to the statin group of lipid-lowering drugs. It is prescribed for people with hypercholesterolaemia (high levels of cholesterol in the blood) who have not responded to other treatments, such as a special diet, and who are at risk of developing heart disease. The drug works by blocking the action of an enzyme that is needed for the manufacture of cholesterol, mainly in the liver. As a result, blood levels of cholesterol are lowered, which can help to prevent heart disease.

Rarely, statins can cause muscle pain, inflammation, and damage. This seems to be more likely if another kind of lipid-lowering drug called a fibrate is given with the statin.

INFORMATION FOR USERS

Your drug prescription is tailored for you. Do not alter dosage without checking with your doctor.

How taken

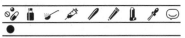

Tablets.

Frequency and timing of doses
Once daily at night.

Adult dosage range
10–40mg daily, changed after intervals of at least 4 weeks.

Onset of effect
Within 2 weeks. Full beneficial effect may be felt within 4 weeks.

Duration of action
24 hours.

Diet advice
A low fat diet is usually recommended.

Storage
Keep in a closed container in a cool, dry place out of the reach of children. Protect from light.

Missed dose
Take as soon as you remember. If your next dose is due within 8 hours, do not take the missed dose, but take the next dose as usual.

Stopping the drug
Do not stop taking the drug without consulting your doctor; stopping the drug may lead to worsening of the underlying condition.

Exceeding the dose
An occasional unintentional extra dose is unlikely to cause problems. Large overdoses may cause liver problems. Notify your doctor.

SPECIAL PRECAUTIONS

Be sure to tell your doctor if:
▼ You have had liver problems.
▼ You are taking other medications.

 Pregnancy
▼ Not usually prescribed. Safety not established. Discuss with your doctor.

 Breast-feeding
▼ Safety not established. Discuss with your doctor.

 Infants and children
▼ Not recommended.

 Over 60
▼ No special problems.

 Driving and hazardous work
▼ No special problems.

Alcohol
▼ Avoid excessive amounts. Alcohol may increase the risk of developing liver problems with this drug.

POSSIBLE ADVERSE EFFECTS

Most *adverse effects* are mild and usually disappear with time. You should report any muscle pains to your doctor straight away.

Symptom/effect	Frequency		Discuss with doctor		Stop taking drug now	Call doctor now
	Common	Rare	Only if severe	In all cases		
Headache	●		■			
Nausea	●		■			
Fatigue		●	■			
Chest pain		●	■			
Jaundice/abdominal pain		●		■		
Rash		●		■	▲	
Muscle pain/weakness		●		■	▲	■

INTERACTIONS

Anticoagulants Pravastatin may increase the effect of these drugs.

Antifungal drugs Taken with pravastatin, itraconazole, ketoconazole, and possibly other antifungal drugs, may increase the risk of muscle damage.

Orlistat This drug increases blood levels and *toxicity* of pravastatin.

Other lipid-lowering drugs (fibrates)
Taken with pravastatin, these drugs may increase the risk of muscle damage.

Cyclosporin and other immuno-suppressant drugs There is an increased risk of muscle damage if pravastatin is taken with these drugs. They are not usually prescribed together.

PROLONGED USE

Long-term use of pravastatin can affect liver function.

Monitoring Regular blood tests to check liver and muscle function are usually required.

PREDNISOLONE

Brand names Deltacortril, Deltastab, Minims prednisolone, Precortisyl, Predenema, Predfoam, Pred Forte, Predsol, and others
Used in the following combined preparations Predsol-N, Scheriproct

GENERAL INFORMATION

Prednisolone, a powerful corticosteroid, is used for a wide range of conditions, including some skin diseases, rheumatic disorders, allergic states, and certain blood disorders. It is used in the form of eye drops to reduce inflammation in conjunctivitis or iritis and may be given as an enema to treat inflammatory bowel disease. The drug can also be injected into joints to relieve rheumatoid and other forms of arthritis. Prednisolone is also prescribed with fludrocortisone for pituitary or adrenal gland disorders.

Low doses taken short term either by mouth or *topically* rarely cause serious *side effects*. However, long-term treatment with large doses can cause fluid retention, indigestion, diabetes, hypertension, and acne. *Enteric*-coated tablets reduce the local effects of the drug on the stomach but not the *systemic* effects .

INFORMATION FOR USERS

Your drug prescription is tailored for you. Do not alter dosage without checking with your doctor.

How taken

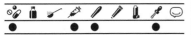

Tablets, injection, suppositories, enema, foam, eye and ear drops.

Frequency and timing of doses
1–2 x daily or on alternate days with food (tablets/injection); 2–4 x daily, more frequently initially (eye/ear drops).

Adult dosage range
Considerable variation. Follow your doctor's instructions.

Onset of effect
2–4 days.

Duration of action
12–72 hours.

Diet advice
A low-sodium and high-potassium diet is recommended when the oral or injected form of the drug is prescribed for extended periods. Follow the advice of your doctor.

Storage
Keep in a closed container in a cool, dry place out of the reach of children. Protect from light.

Missed dose
Take as soon as you remember. If your next dose is due within 6 hours, take a single dose now and skip the next.

Stopping the drug
Do not stop the drug without consulting your doctor. Abrupt cessation of long-term treatment by mouth or injection may be dangerous.

Exceeding the dose
An occasional unintentional extra dose is unlikely to be a cause for concern. But if you notice any unusual symptoms, or if a large overdose has been taken, notify your doctor.

SPECIAL PRECAUTIONS

Be sure to tell your doctor if:
▼ You have had a peptic ulcer.
▼ You have glaucoma.
▼ You have had tuberculosis.
▼ You suffer from depression.
▼ You have any infection.
▼ You have diabetes.
▼ You have osteoporosis.
▼ You are taking other medications.

Avoid exposure to chickenpox, shingles, or measles if you are on systemic treatment.

Pregnancy
▼ No evidence of risk with drops or joint injections. Taken as tablets in low doses, harm to the fetus is unlikely. Discuss with your doctor.

Breast-feeding
▼ No evidence of risk with drops or injections. Taken by mouth, it passes into the breast milk, but at low doses adverse effects on the baby are unlikely. Discuss with your doctor.

Infants and children
▼ Only given when essential. Reduced dose may be necessary.

Over 60
▼ Increased likelihood of adverse effects. Reduced dose may therefore be necessary.

Driving and hazardous work
▼ No known problems.

Alcohol
▼ Keep consumption low. Alcohol may increase the risk of peptic ulcers with prednisolone taken by mouth or injection.

POSSIBLE ADVERSE EFFECTS

The rare but more serious adverse effects occur only when high doses are taken by mouth or injection or for long periods. If taking oral forms, you should avoid close personal contact with chickenpox or herpes zoster, and seek urgent medical attention if exposed.

Symptom/effect	Frequency		Discuss with doctor		Stop taking drug now	Call doctor now
	Common	Rare	Only if severe	In all cases		
Indigestion	●			■		
Acne	●			■		
Weight gain		●	■			
Muscle weakness		●		■		
Mood changes/depression		●		■		
Black/bloodstained faeces		●		■	▲	■

INTERACTIONS

Anticonvulsant drugs Carbamazepine, phenytoin, and phenobarbital can reduce the effects of prednisolone.

Anticoagulant drugs Prednisolone may affect the response to these drugs.

Diuretics Prednisolone may increase the adverse effects of these drugs.

Antihypertensive and antidiabetic drugs and insulin Prednisolone may reduce the effects of these drugs.

Vaccines Serious reactions can occur when vaccinations are given with this drug. Discuss with your doctor.

PROLONGED USE

Prolonged systemic use can lead to such adverse effects as diabetes, glaucoma, cataracts, and fragile bones, and may retard growth in children. Dosages are usually tailored to minimize these effects. People on long-term treatment are advised to carry a treatment card.

PRIMIDONE

Brand name Mysoline
Used in the following combined preparations None

GENERAL INFORMATION

Introduced in the 1950s, primidone is in the anticonvulsant group of drugs. It is chemically related to the barbiturates (see Sleeping drugs, p.82) and is partially converted to phenobarbital in the body. Primidone is used mainly for its effect in suppressing epileptic fits. However, the drug is also occasionally prescribed to treat people who suffer from certain types of tremor.

Although this drug may be prescribed on its own, it is more frequently taken with another anticonvulsant. Its major *adverse effects* are due to its sedative action on the central nervous system.

QUICK REFERENCE

Drug group Anticonvulsant (p.86)
Overdose danger rating High
Dependence rating Medium
Prescription needed Yes
Available as generic No

INFORMATION FOR USERS

Your drug prescription is tailored for you. Do not alter dosage without checking with your doctor.

How taken

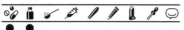

Tablets, liquid.

Frequency and timing of doses
1–3 x daily, usually 2 x daily.

Adult dosage range
Initially 125mg, increased gradually to a maximum of 1.5g daily (1g daily in children).

Onset of effect
Within 1 hour.

Duration of action
Up to 24 hours.

Diet advice
None.

Storage
Keep in a closed container in a cool, dry place out of the reach of children.

Missed dose
Take as soon as you remember. If you normally take once daily, and your next dose is due within 8 hours, take a single dose now and skip the next. If you normally take 2–3 times daily, and your next dose is due within 2 hours, take a single dose now and skip the next.

Stopping the drug
Do not stop the drug without consulting your doctor; symptoms may recur and *withdrawal* reactions can result.

OVERDOSE ACTION

Seek immediate medical advice in all cases. Take emergency action if loss of consciousness occurs.

See Drug poisoning emergency guide (p.494).

POSSIBLE ADVERSE EFFECTS

Most people experience very few adverse effects with this drug, but when blood levels get too high, adverse effects are common and the dose may need to be reduced.

Symptom/effect	Frequency		Discuss with doctor		Stop taking drug now	Call doctor now
	Common	Rare	Only if severe	In all cases		
Drowsiness	●		■			
Clumsiness/unsteadiness	●		■			
Dizziness/lightheadedness	●		■			
Headache		●	■			
Nausea/vomiting		●	■			
Rash		●		■		

INTERACTIONS

Sedatives All drugs that have a sedative effect are likely to increase the sedative properties of primidone. Such drugs include sleeping drugs, antihistamines, *opioid* analgesics, antipsychotic drugs, and antidepressant drugs.

Anticoagulants Primidone may reduce the effect of anticoagulant drugs.

Oral contraceptives Primidone may reduce the effectiveness of oral contraceptives. An alternative form of contraception may be necessary. Discuss with your doctor.

Corticosteroids Primidone may reduce the effect of some of these drugs.

SPECIAL PRECAUTIONS

Be sure to tell your doctor if:
▼ You have long-term liver or kidney problems.
▼ You have heart problems.
▼ You have poor circulation.
▼ You have a lung disorder such as asthma or bronchitis.
▼ You have porphyria.
▼ You are taking other medications.

Pregnancy
▼ Not usually prescribed. May cause abnormalities in the fetus. Discuss with your doctor.

Breast-feeding
▼ The drug passes into the breast milk and may affect the baby. Discuss with your doctor.

Infants and children
▼ Reduced dose necessary, depending on weight.

Over 60
▼ Reduced dose may be necessary.

Driving and hazardous work
▼ Your underlying condition, as well as the possibility of reduced alertness while taking primidone, may make such activities inadvisable. Discuss with your doctor.

Alcohol
▼ Avoid. Alcohol may dangerously increase the sedative effects of this drug.

PROLONGED USE

Continued use of this drug may sometimes lead to dependence.

In rare cases, joint pain may occur.

Monitoring Regular blood tests may be performed to measure blood levels and to check the blood cells.

PROCHLORPERAZINE

Brand names Buccastem, Prozière, Stemetil
Used in the following combined preparations None

GENERAL INFORMATION

Prochlorperazine was introduced in the late 1950s and belongs to a group of drugs called the phenothiazines, which act on the central nervous system.

In small doses, the drug controls nausea and vomiting, especially when they occur as the *side effects* of medical treatment by drugs or radiation, or of anaesthesia. Prochlorperazine is also used to treat the nausea that occurs with inner-ear disorders, for example, vertigo. In large doses, it is used as an antipsychotic to tranquillize, reduce aggressiveness, and suppress abnormal behaviour (see p.85). It thus minimizes and controls the abnormal behaviour of schizophrenia, mania, and other mental disorders. Prochlorperazine does not cure any of these diseases, but it helps to relieve symptoms.

QUICK REFERENCE

Drug group Phenothiazine antipsychotic drug (p.85) and anti-emetic (p.90)

Overdose danger rating Medium

Dependence rating Low

Prescription needed Yes

Available as generic Yes

INFORMATION FOR USERS

Your drug prescription is tailored for you. Do not alter the dosage without checking with your doctor.

How taken

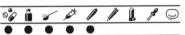

Tablets, capsules, SR-capsules, liquid, powder, injection, suppositories.

Frequency and timing of doses
2–3 x daily (tablets); 2–3 x daily (suppositories); 1–2 x daily (SR-capsules); 2–3 x daily (injection).

Adult dosage range
Nausea and vomiting 20mg initially, then 5–10mg per dose (tablets); 5–25mg per dose (suppositories); 10–15mg per dose (SR-capsules). *Mental illness* 15–40mg daily. Larger doses may be given.

Onset of effect
Within 60 minutes (by mouth or suppository); 10–20 minutes (by injection).

Duration of action
3–6 hours (up to 12 hours SR-preparations).

Diet advice
None.

Storage
Keep in a closed container in a cool, dry place out of the reach of children. Protect from light.

Missed dose
Take as soon as you remember. If your next dose is due within 2 hours, take a single dose now and skip the next.

Stopping the drug
Do not stop the drug without consulting your doctor; symptoms may recur.

Exceeding the dose
An occasional unintentional extra dose is unlikely to be a cause for concern. Large overdoses may cause unusual drowsiness and may affect the heart. Notify your doctor.

SPECIAL PRECAUTIONS

Be sure to tell your doctor if:
▼ You have heart problems.
▼ You have liver or kidney problems.
▼ You have had epileptic fits.
▼ You have Parkinson's disease.
▼ You have an underactive thyroid gland.
▼ You have prostate problems.
▼ You have glaucoma.
▼ You are taking other medications.

Pregnancy
▼ Safety in pregnancy not established. Discuss with your doctor.

Breast-feeding
▼ The drug passes into the breast milk and may affect the baby. Discuss with your doctor.

Infants and children
▼ Not recommended in infants weighing less than 10kg and young children. Reduced dose necessary in older children due to increased risk of adverse effects.

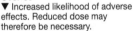

Over 60
▼ Increased likelihood of adverse effects. Reduced dose may therefore be necessary.

Driving and hazardous work
▼ Avoid such activities until you have learned how prochlorperazine affects you because it can cause drowsiness and reduced alertness.

Alcohol
▼ Avoid. Alcohol may increase and prolong the sedative effects of this drug.

POSSIBLE ADVERSE EFFECTS

Prochlorperazine has a strong *anticholinergic* effect, which can cause a variety of minor symptoms that often become less marked with time. The most significant adverse effect with high doses is abnormal movements of the face and limbs (*parkinsonism*) caused by changes in the balance of brain chemicals.

Symptom/effect	Frequency		Discuss with doctor		Stop taking drug now	Call doctor now
	Common	Rare	Only if severe	In all cases		
Drowsiness/lethargy	●		■			
Dry mouth	●		■			
Dizziness/fainting	●			■		
Parkinsonism	●			■		
Rash		●		■	▲	
Jaundice/fever		●		■		■
Tensing of muscles		●		■		

INTERACTIONS

Sedatives All drugs with a sedative effect are likely to increase the sedative effects of prochlorperazine.

Drugs for parkinsonism Prochlorperazine may block the beneficial effect of these.

Terfenadine and cisapride When taken with prochlorperazine, these drugs increase the risk of abnormal heart rhythms.

Anticholinergic drugs Prochlorperazine may increase the side effects of these drugs.

PROLONGED USE

Use of this drug for more than a few months may lead to the development of involuntary, potentially irreversible, eye mouth, and tongue, movements (*tardive dyskinesia*). Occasionally, *jaundice* may occur.

Monitoring Periodic blood tests may be performed.

PROCYCLIDINE

Brand names Arpicolin, Kemadrin
Used in the following combined preparations None

GENERAL INFORMATION

Introduced in the 1950s, procyclidine is an *anticholinergic* drug that is used to treat Parkinson's disease. It is especially helpful in the early stages of the disorder for treating muscle rigidity. It also helps to reduce excess salivation. However, the drug has little effect on the shuffling gait and slow muscular movements that characterize Parkinson's disease.

Procyclidine is also often used to treat *parkinsonism* resulting from treatment with antipsychotic drugs.
The drug may cause various minor *adverse effects* (see below), but these are rarely serious enough to warrant stopping treatment.

INFORMATION FOR USERS

Your drug prescription is tailored for you. Do not alter dosage without checking with your doctor.

How taken

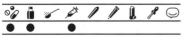

Tablets, liquid, injection.

Frequency and timing of doses
2–3 x daily.

Adult dosage range
7.5–30mg daily, exceptionally up to 60mg daily. Dosage is determined individually in order to find the best balance between effective relief of symptoms and the occurrence of adverse effects.

Onset of effect
Within 30 minutes.

Duration of action
8–12 hours.

Diet advice
None.

Storage
Keep in a closed container in a cool, dry place out of the reach of children.

Missed dose
Take as soon as you remember. If your next dose is due within 2 hours, take a single dose now and skip the next.

Stopping the drug
Do not stop the drug without consulting your doctor; symptoms may recur.

OVERDOSE ACTION

 Seek immediate medical advice in all cases. Take emergency action if palpitations, fits, or unconsciousness occur.

See Drug poisoning emergency guide (p.494).

POSSIBLE ADVERSE EFFECTS

The possible adverse effects of procyclidine are mainly the result of its anticholinergic action. Some of the more common symptoms, such as dry mouth, constipation, and blurred vision, may be overcome by adjustment in dosage. Nausea and vomiting, nervousness, and rash have occasionally been reported.

Symptom/effect	Frequency		Discuss with doctor		Stop taking drug now	Call doctor now
	Common	Rare	Only if severe	In all cases		
Dry mouth	●		■			
Constipation	●		■			
Nervousness	●		■			
Drowsiness/dizziness	●		■			
Blurred vision	●			■		
Confusion		●		■		
Difficulty in passing urine		●		■		▮
Palpitations		●		■	▲	▮

INTERACTIONS

Anticholinergic and antihistamine drugs These drugs may increase the adverse effects of procyclidine.

Antidepressant drugs may increase the *side effects* of procyclidine.

Glyceryl trinitrate may be less effective in relief of heart pain, since dry mouth may prevent its dissolution under the tongue.

SPECIAL PRECAUTIONS

Be sure to tell your doctor if:
▼ You have long-term liver or kidney problems.
▼ You suffer from or have a family history of glaucoma.
▼ You have high blood pressure.
▼ You suffer from constipation.
▼ You have prostate trouble.
▼ You are taking other medications.

 Pregnancy
▼ Safety in pregnancy not established. Discuss with your doctor.

 Breast-feeding
▼ The drug passes into the breast milk and may affect the baby. Discuss with your doctor.

 Infants and children
▼ Not recommended.

Over 60
▼ Reduced dose may be necessary.

Driving and hazardous work
▼ Avoid such activities until you have learned how procyclidine affects you because the drug can cause drowsiness, blurred vision, and mild confusion.

Alcohol
▼ Avoid. Alcohol may increase the sedative effect of this drug.

PROLONGED USE

Prolonged use of this drug may provoke the onset of glaucoma.

Monitoring Periodic eye examinations are usually advised.

PROGUANIL

Brand name Paludrine
Used in the following combined preparations None

GENERAL INFORMATION

Proguanil is an antimalarial drug that has been used for over 30 years. It is given to prevent the development of malaria in people visiting parts of the world where the disease is prevalent. Treatment with the drug needs to be started one week before travel and should be continued for four weeks after your return. In some parts of the world the malaria parasite is resistant to proguanil, so another drug such as chloroquine may be needed as well to ensure adequate protection. Always seek expert advice on the prevention of malaria well ahead of travelling. The drug must be taken regularly in order to be effective. See your doctor at once if you become ill within three months of returning. *Adverse effects* from this drug are rare and usually subside with continued treatment.

Preventative drug treatment should be combined with personal protection against being bitten, such as keeping well covered and using mosquito nets and repellents.

INFORMATION FOR USERS

Follow instructions on the label.

How taken

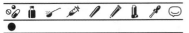

Tablets.

Frequency and timing of doses
Once daily with water after food.

Adult dosage range
200mg (2 tablets) daily.

Onset of effect
After 24 hours.

Duration of action
24–48 hours.

Diet advice
None.

Storage
Keep in a closed container in a cool, dry place out of the reach of children.

Missed dose
Take as soon as you remember. If your next dose is due at this time, take both doses together.

Stopping the drug
Do not stop taking the drug for 4 weeks after leaving a malaria-infected area, otherwise there is a risk that you may develop the disease.

Exceeding the dose
An occasional unintentional extra dose is unlikely to cause problems. Large overdoses may cause abdominal pain and vomiting. Notify your doctor.

POSSIBLE ADVERSE EFFECTS

Adverse effects from proguanil are rare. Stomach irritation is the most common problem, but this usually settles as the treatment continues.

Symptom/effect	Frequency		Discuss with doctor		Stop taking drug now	Call doctor now
	Common	Rare	Only if severe	In all cases		
Nausea/vomiting		●	■			
Abdominal pain/indigestion		●	■			
Mouth ulcers		●	■			
Hair loss		●		■		

INTERACTIONS

Warfarin The effects of warfarin may be enhanced by proguanil.

Antacids The absorption of proguanil may be reduced by antacids.

SPECIAL PRECAUTIONS

Be sure to tell your doctor if:
▼ You have a long-term kidney problem.
▼ You are taking other medications.

Pregnancy
▼ Safety in pregnancy not established, although benefits are generally considered to outweigh risks. Folic acid supplements must be taken. Discuss with your doctor.

Breast-feeding
▼ The drug passes into the breast milk, but at normal doses adverse effects on the baby are unlikely. Breast-feeding while you are taking proguanil will not protect your baby from malaria. Discuss with your doctor.

Infants and children
▼ Reduced dose necessary.

Over 60
▼ No known problems.

Driving and hazardous work
▼ No known problems.

Alcohol
▼ No special problems.

PROLONGED USE

No known problems.

PROMAZINE

Brand name Sparine
Used in the following combined preparations None

GENERAL INFORMATION

Promazine, introduced in the late 1950s, is a member of a group of drugs called phenothiazines, which act on the brain to regulate abnormal behaviour (see Antipsychotics, p.85).

Its main use is to calm agitated and restless behaviour. It is also given as a sedative for the short-term treatment of severe anxiety, especially in the elderly and during terminal illness.

In theory, promazine may cause the unpleasant *side effects* experienced with most of the other phenothiazine drugs – in particular, the abnormal movements and shaking of the arms and legs (*parkinsonism*). However, in practice the drug is rarely used for periods that are long enough to produce these problems.

INFORMATION FOR USERS

Your drug prescription is tailored for you. Do not alter dosage without checking with your doctor.

How taken

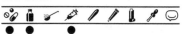

Tablets, liquid, injection.

Frequency and timing of doses
4 x daily.

Adult dosage range
100–800mg daily (tablets).

Onset of effect
30 minutes–1 hour.

Duration of action
4–6 hours.

Diet advice
None.

Storage
Keep in a closed container in a cool, dry place out of the reach of children. Protect from light.

Missed dose
Take as soon as you remember. If your next dose is due within 2 hours, take a single dose now and skip the next.

Stopping the drug
Do not stop the drug without consulting your doctor; symptoms may recur.

Exceeding the dose
An occasional unintentional extra dose is unlikely to be a cause for concern. Large overdoses may cause drowsiness, dizziness, unsteadiness, fits, and coma. Notify your doctor.

SPECIAL PRECAUTIONS

Be sure to tell your doctor if:
▼ You have heart problems.
▼ You have long-term liver or kidney problems.
▼ You have myasthenia gravis or phaeochromocytoma.
▼ You have had epileptic fits.
▼ You have breathing problems.
▼ You have prostate problems.
▼ You have glaucoma.
▼ You have Parkinson's disease.
▼ You are diabetic.
▼ You are taking other medications.

Pregnancy
▼ Safety in early pregnancy not established. The drug is sometimes injected during labour. Discuss with your doctor.

Breast-feeding
▼ The drug passes into the breast milk, but at normal doses adverse effects on the baby are unlikely. Discuss with your doctor.

Infants and children
▼ Not recommended.

Over 60
▼ Increased likelihood of adverse effects. Reduced dose may therefore be necessary.

Driving and hazardous work
▼ Avoid such activities until you have learned how promazine affects you because the drug can cause drowsiness and reduced alertness.

Alcohol
▼ Avoid. Alcohol may increase the sedative effect of this drug.

POSSIBLE ADVERSE EFFECTS

The more common adverse effects of promazine, such as drowsiness, dry mouth, and blurred vision, may be helped by an adjustment of dosage. Promazine may affect the body's ability to regulate temperature (especially in the elderly). Parkinsonism is rare.

Symptom/effect	Frequency		Discuss with doctor		Stop taking drug now	Call doctor now
	Common	Rare	Only if severe	In all cases		
Drowsiness/lethargy	●		■			
Dry mouth	●		■			
Constipation	●		■			
Blurred vision	●			■		
Parkinsonism		●		■		
Jaundice		●		■		▮
Rash		●		■	▲	
Photosensitivity		●		■		

INTERACTIONS

Sedatives All drugs that have a sedative effect are likely to increase the sedative properties of promazine.

Antihistamines There may be an increased risk of abnormal heart rhythms occurring with terfenadine.

Anticonvulsants Promazine may reduce the effectiveness of anticonvulsants.

Drugs for parkinsonism Promazine may reduce the effectiveness of these drugs.

Antiemetics There is an increased risk of parkinsonism if antiemetic drugs such as metoclopramide are taken with promazine.

PROLONGED USE

Use of this drug for more than a few months may be associated with *jaundice* and abnormal movements. Sometimes a reduction in dose may be recommended.

Monitoring Periodic blood tests and eye examinations may be performed.

PROMETHAZINE

Brand names Avomine, Phenergan, Sominex
Used in the following combined preparations Medised, Night Nurse, Pamergan P100, Phensedyl Plus, Tixylix Night-time

GENERAL INFORMATION

Promethazine is one of a class of drugs known as the phenothiazines, which were developed in the 1950s for their beneficial effect on abnormal behaviour arising from mental illnesses (see Antipsychotics, p.85). Promethazine was found, however, to have effects more like the antihistamines used to treat allergies (see p.124) and some types of nausea and vomiting (see Anti-emetics, p.90). The drug is widely used to reduce itching in a variety of skin conditions including urticaria (hives), chickenpox, and eczema. It can also relieve the nausea and vomiting caused by inner ear disturbances such as Ménière's disease and motion sickness. Because of its sedative effect, promethazine is sometimes used for short periods as a sleeping medicine, and is also given as *premedication* before surgery.

Promethazine is used in combined preparations together with *opioid* cough suppressants for the relief of coughs and nasal congestion, and it is given at night for its sedative effect.

INFORMATION FOR USERS

Follow instructions on the label. Call your doctor if symptoms worsen.

How taken

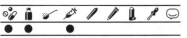

Tablets, liquid, injection.

Frequency and timing of doses
Allergic symptoms 1–3 x daily or as a single dose at night.
Motion sickness Bedtime on night before travelling, repeating following morning if necessary, then every 6–8 hours as necessary.
Nausea and vomiting Every 4–6 hours as necessary.

Dosage range (promethazine hydrochloride)
Adults 20–75mg per dose.
Children Reduced dose according to age.

Onset of effect
Within 1 hour. If dose is taken after nausea has started, the onset of effect is delayed.

Duration of action
8–16 hours.

Diet advice
None.

Storage
Keep in a closed container in a cool, dry place out of the reach of children. Protect from light.

Missed dose
No cause for concern, but take as soon as you remember. Adjust the timing of your next dose accordingly.

Stopping the drug
Can be safely stopped as soon as symptoms disappear.

Exceeding the dose
An occasional unintentional extra dose is unlikely to cause problems. Large overdoses may cause drowsiness or agitation, fits, unsteadiness, and coma. Notify your doctor.

SPECIAL PRECAUTIONS

Be sure to consult your doctor or pharmacist before taking this drug if:
▼ You have liver or kidney problems.
▼ You have had epileptic fits.
▼ You have heart disease.
▼ You have glaucoma.
▼ You suffer from asthma.
▼ You have Parkinson's disease.
▼ You have urinary difficulties.
▼ You are taking other medications.

 Pregnancy
▼ Safety in pregnancy not established. Discuss with your doctor.

 Breast-feeding
▼ The drug passes into the breast milk, but at normal doses adverse effects on the baby are unlikely. Discuss with your doctor.

 Infants and children
▼ Not recommended for infants under two years. Reduced dose necessary for older children.

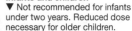 **Over 60**
▼ No special problems.

 Driving and hazardous work
▼ Avoid such activities until you have learned how promethazine affects you because the drug can cause drowsiness.

 Alcohol
▼ Avoid. Alcohol may increase the sedative effects of this drug.

Sunlight
▼ Avoid exposure to strong sunlight.

POSSIBLE ADVERSE EFFECTS

Promethazine usually causes only minor *anticholinergic* effects. More serious *adverse effects* generally occur only during long-term use or with abnormally high doses.

Symptom/effect	Frequency		Discuss with doctor		Stop taking drug now	Call doctor now
	Common	Rare	Only if severe	In all cases		
Drowsiness/lethargy	●		■			
Dry mouth	●		■			
Blurred vision	●		■			
Light-sensitive rash		●		■		▲

INTERACTIONS

Monamine oxidase inhibitors (MAOIs) These drugs may cause a severe reaction if taken with promethazine. Avoid taking promethazine if MAOIs have been taken in the last 14 days.

Antihistamines There may be an increased risk of abnormal heart rhythms occurring with terfenadine.

Sedatives All drugs that have a sedative effect are likely to increase the sedative properties of promethazine. Such drugs include other antihistamines, sleeping drugs, and antipsychotics.

PROLONGED USE

Use of this drug for long periods is rarely necessary, but may sometimes cause abnormal movements of the face and limbs (*parkinsonism*). The problem normally disappears when the drug is stopped.

PROPRANOLOL

Brand names Angilol, Apsolol, Berkolol, Beta-Prograne, Cardinol, Inderal, Inderal-LA, Propanix, and others
Used in the following combined preparations Inderetic, Inderex

GENERAL INFORMATION

Propranolol, introduced in 1965, was the first widely available beta blocker in the United Kingdom. It is most often used to treat hypertension, angina, and abnormal heart rhythms but is also helpful in controlling the fast heart rate and other symptoms of an overactive thyroid gland. Propranolol also helps to reduce the palpitations, sweating, and tremor of severe anxiety and is also used to prevent migraine headaches.

Propranolol is not prescribed to people with asthma, chronic bronchitis, or emphysema because it can cause breathing difficulties. The drug should be used with caution by diabetics, because, like all beta blockers, it affects the body's response to low blood sugar.

QUICK REFERENCE

Drug group Beta blocker (p.97) and anti-anxiety drug (p.83)

Overdose danger rating High

Dependence rating Low

Prescription needed Yes

Available as generic Yes

INFORMATION FOR USERS

Your drug prescription is tailored for you. Do not alter dosage without checking with your doctor.

How taken

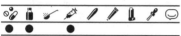

Tablets, SR-capsules, liquid, injection.

Frequency and timing of doses
2–4 x daily. Once daily (SR-capsules).

Adult dosage range
Abnormal heart rhythms 30–160mg daily.
Angina 80–240mg daily.
Hypertension 160–320mg daily.
Migraine prevention and anxiety 40–160mg daily.

Onset of effect
1–2 hours (tablets); after 4 hours (SR-capsules). In hypertension and migraine, it may be several weeks before full benefits of this drug are felt.

Duration of action
6–12 hours (tablets); 24–30 hours (SR-capsules).

Diet advice
None.

Storage
Keep in a closed container in a cool, dry place out of the reach of children. Protect from light.

Missed dose
Take as soon as you remember. If your next dose is due within 2 hours (tablets) or 12 hours (SR-capsules), take a single dose now and skip the next.

Stopping the drug
Do not stop the drug without consulting your doctor. Abrupt cessation may lead to worsening of the underlying condition.

OVERDOSE ACTION

Seek immediate medical advice in all cases. Take emergency action if breathing difficulties, collapse, or loss of consciousness occur.

See Drug poisoning emergency guide (p.494).

SPECIAL PRECAUTIONS

Be sure to tell your doctor if:
▼ You have long-term liver or kidney problems.
▼ You have a breathing disorder such as asthma, bronchitis, or emphysema.
▼ You have heart failure.
▼ You have diabetes.
▼ You have poor circulation in the legs.
▼ You are taking other medications.

 Pregnancy
▼ May affect the baby. Discuss with your doctor.

 Breast-feeding
▼ The drug passes into the breast milk, but at normal doses adverse effects on the baby are unlikely. Discuss with your doctor.

 Infants and children
▼ Reduced dose necessary.

 Over 60
▼ Increased risk of adverse effects.

 Driving and hazardous work
▼ No special problems.

 Alcohol
▼ No special problems.

Surgery and general anaesthetics
▼ Propranolol may need to be stopped before you have a general anaesthetic. Discuss this with your doctor or dentist before any surgery.

POSSIBLE ADVERSE EFFECTS

Propranolol has *adverse effects* that are common to most beta blockers. Symptoms such as fatigue and nausea are usually temporary and diminish with long-term use. Fainting may be a sign that the drug has slowed the heart beat excessively.

Symptom/effect	Frequency		Discuss with doctor		Stop taking drug now	Call doctor now
	Common	Rare	Only if severe	In all cases		
Lethargy/fatigue	●		■			
Cold hands and feet	●		■			
Nausea		●	■			
Nightmares/vivid dreams		●		■		
Dry eyes		●		■		
Fainting/breathlessness		●		■		■
Visual disturbances		●		■		

PROLONGED USE

No problems expected.

INTERACTIONS

Antihypertensive drugs Propranolol may enhance the blood pressure lowering effect.

Diltiazem and verapamil Combining either of these drugs with propranolol may have adverse effects on heart function.

Cimetidine and hydralazine These drugs may increase the effects of propranolol.

Non-steroidal anti-inflammatory drugs (NSAIDs) e.g., indomethacin may reduce the antihypertensive effect of propranolol.

PROPYLTHIOURACIL

Brand names None
Used in the following combined preparations None

GENERAL INFORMATION

Propylthiouracil is an antithyroid drug used to manage an overactive thyroid gland (hyperthyroidism). In some people, particularly those with Graves' disease (the most common form of the disorder), drug treatment alone may bring on a remission. Propylthiouracil may also be prescribed for long-term treatment of the disease in people who may be at special risk from surgery, such as children and pregnant women.

The drug is also used to restore the normal functioning of the thyroid gland before its partial removal by surgery. It is sometimes given with thyroxine in order to prevent the development of hypothyroidism (low thyroid hormone levels). Propylthiouracil is preferred to other antithyroid drugs when treatment is essential during pregnancy.

The most important *adverse effect* that sometimes occurs is a reduction in white blood cells, leading to the risk of infection. If you develop a sore throat or mouth ulceration, see your doctor immediately; this might be a sign that your blood is being affected.

INFORMATION FOR USERS

Your drug prescription is tailored for you. Do not alter dosage without consulting your doctor.

How taken

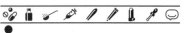

Tablets.

Frequency and timing of doses
1–3 x daily.

Dosage range
Initially 300–600mg daily. Usually the dose can be reduced to 50–150mg daily.

Onset of effect
10–20 days. Full beneficial effects may not be felt for 6–10 weeks.

Duration of action
24–36 hours.

Diet advice
Your doctor may advise you to avoid foods that are high in iodine (see p.441).

Storage
Keep in a closed container in a cool, dry place out of the reach of children. Protect from light.

Missed dose
Take as soon as you remember. If your next dose is due within 3 hours, take a single dose now and skip the next.

Stopping the drug
Do not stop the drug without consulting your doctor; stopping the drug may lead to a recurrence of hyperthyroidism.

Exceeding the dose
An occasional unintentional extra dose is unlikely to cause problems. Large overdoses may cause nausea, vomiting, and headache. Notify your doctor.

POSSIBLE ADVERSE EFFECTS

Serious side effects are rare with this drug. Skin rashes and itching are fairly common. A sore throat or fever may indicate adverse effects on the blood. If these occur, inform your doctor immediately.

Symptom/effect	Frequency		Discuss with doctor		Stop taking drug now	Call doctor now
	Common	Rare	Only if severe	In all cases		
Nausea/vomiting	●		■			
Joint pain	●			■		
Headache	●			■		
Rash/itching	●			■		
Jaundice		●		■	▲	▌
Sore throat/fever		●		■	▲	▌

INTERACTIONS

Anticoagulants Propylthiouracil may increase the effects of these drugs, making an adjustment in dosage necessary.

SPECIAL PRECAUTIONS

Be sure to tell your doctor if:
▼ You have long-term liver or kidney problems.
▼ You are taking other medications.

Pregnancy
▼ Prescribed with caution. Risk of goitre and thyroid hormone deficiency (hypothyroidism) in the newborn infant if too high a dose is used. Discuss with your doctor.

Breast-feeding
▼ The drug passes into the breast milk and may affect the baby. Discuss with your doctor.

Infants and children
▼ Reduced dose necessary.

Over 60
▼ No special problems.

Driving and hazardous work
▼ No problems expected.

Alcohol
▼ No known problems.

PROLONGED USE

High doses of propylthiouracil over a prolonged period may reduce the number of white blood cells.

Monitoring Periodic tests of thyroid function are usually required, and blood cell counts may also be carried out.

PYRIDOSTIGMINE

Brand name Mestinon
Used in the following combined preparations None

GENERAL INFORMATION

Pyridostigmine is used to treat a rare autoimmune condition involving the faulty transmission of nerve impulses to the muscles, known as myasthenia gravis (p.121). Pyridostigmine improves muscle strength by prolonging nerve signals, although it does not cure the disease. In severe cases, the drug may be prescribed with corticosteroids or other drugs. Pyridostigmine may also be given to reverse temporary paralysis of the bowel and urinary retention following operations.

Side effects, including abdominal cramps, nausea, and diarrhoea, usually disappear as a result of reducing the dosage of pyridostigmine.

QUICK REFERENCE

Drug group Drug for myasthenia gravis (p.121)

Overdose danger rating High

Dependence rating Low

Prescription needed Yes

Available as generic No

INFORMATION FOR USERS

Your drug prescription is tailored for you. Do not alter dosage without checking with your doctor.

How taken

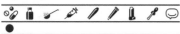

Tablets.

Frequency and timing of doses
Every 3–4 hours initially. Thereafter, according to the needs of the individual.

Dosage range
Adults 150mg–1.2g daily (by mouth) according to response and side effects.
Children Reduced dose necessary according to age and weight.

Onset of effect
30–60 minutes.

Duration of action
3–6 hours.

Diet advice
None.

Storage
Keep in a closed container in a cool, dry place out of the reach of children. Protect from light.

Missed dose
Take as soon as you remember. If your next dose is due within 2 hours, take a single dose now and skip the next.

Stopping the drug
Do not stop the drug without consulting your doctor; symptoms may recur.

OVERDOSE ACTION

 Seek immediate medical advice in all cases. You may experience severe abdominal cramps, vomiting, weakness, and tremor. Take emergency action if troubled breathing, unusually slow heart beat, fits, or loss of consciousness occur.

See Drug poisoning emergency guide (p.494).

SPECIAL PRECAUTIONS

Be sure to tell your doctor if:
▼ You have a long-term kidney problem.
▼ You have heart problems.
▼ You have had epileptic fits.
▼ You have asthma.
▼ You have difficulty in passing urine.
▼ You have a peptic ulcer.
▼ You have Parkinson's disease.
▼ You are taking other medications.

 Pregnancy
▼ No evidence of risk to the developing fetus in the first 6 months. Large doses near the time of delivery may cause premature labour and temporary muscle weakness in the baby. Discuss with your doctor.

 Breast-feeding
▼ No evidence of risk, but the baby should be monitored for signs of muscle weakness.

 Infants and children
▼ Reduced dose necessary, calculated according to age and weight.

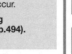 **Over 60**
▼ Reduced dose is usually given. Increased likelihood of adverse effects.

 Driving and hazardous work
▼ Your underlying condition may make such activities inadvisable. Discuss with your doctor.

 Alcohol
▼ No special problems.

Surgery and general anaesthetics
▼ Pyridostigmine interacts with some anaesthetic agents. Make sure your treatment is known to your doctor, dentist, and anaesthetist before any surgery.

POSSIBLE ADVERSE EFFECTS

Adverse effects of pyridostigmine are usually dose-related and can be avoided by adjusting the dose. In rare cases, hypersensitivity may occur leading to an allergic skin rash.

Symptom/effect	Frequency		Discuss with doctor		Stop taking drug now	Call doctor now
	Common	Rare	Only if severe	In all cases		
Nausea/vomiting	●		■			
Increased salivation	●		■			
Sweating	●		■			
Abdominal cramps/diarrhoea	●			■		
Watering eyes/small pupils		●		■		
Headache		●		■		
Rash		●		■		

INTERACTIONS

General note Drugs that suppress the transmission of nerve signals may oppose the effect of pyridostigmine. Such drugs include aminoglycoside antibiotics, digoxin, procainamide, quinidine, lithium, and chloroquine.

Propranolol antagonizes the effect of pyridostigmine.

PROLONGED USE

No problems expected.

PYRIMETHAMINE

Brand name Daraprim
Used in the following combined preparations Fansidar, Maloprim

GENERAL INFORMATION

Pyrimethamine is an antimalarial drug now reserved for use against types of malaria resistant to other drugs. Since the malaria parasites can readily develop resistance to pyrimethamine, the drug is now usually given combined with the antibacterial drug sulfadoxine (Fansidar) or with dapsone (Maloprim). The activity of these combinations greatly exceeds that of either drug alone. Fansidar is used to suppress the symptoms of malaria during treatment with quinine. Maloprim is now used with chloroquine only to protect against malaria in areas with a high risk of chloroquine-resistant malaria.

Pyrimethamine and sulfadiazine are given together to treat toxoplasmosis in immunocompromised patients.

Because blood disorders can arise during prolonged use, blood counts are monitored regularly and vitamin supplements are given.

QUICK REFERENCE

Drug group Antimalarial drug (p.137)

Overdose danger rating Medium

Dependence rating Low

Prescription needed Yes

Available as generic No

INFORMATION FOR USERS

Your drug prescription is tailored for you. Do not alter dosage without checking with your doctor.

How taken

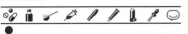

Tablets.

Frequency and timing of doses
Prevention of malaria Once weekly starting 1 week before travel and continuing for at least 4 weeks after leaving malarial area.

Dosage range
Adults 25mg per dose (prevention of malaria).
Children Reduced dose necessary according to age.

Onset of effect
24 hours.

Duration of action
Up to 1 week.

Diet advice
None.

Storage
Keep in a closed container in a cool, dry place out of the reach of children. Protect from light.

Missed dose
Take as soon as you remember. If your next dose is due within 24 hours, take a single dose now and alter the dosing day so that your next dose is one week later.

Stopping the drug
Do not stop taking the drug until 4 weeks after leaving a malaria-infected area, otherwise there is a risk that you may develop the disease.

Exceeding the dose
An occasional unintentional extra dose is unlikely to cause problems. Large overdoses may cause trembling, breathing difficulty, fits, and blood disorders. Notify your doctor.

SPECIAL PRECAUTIONS

Be sure to tell your doctor if:
▼ You have long-term liver or kidney problems.
▼ You have had epileptic fits.
▼ You have anaemia.
▼ You are allergic to sulphonamides.
▼ You have glucose-6-phosphate dehydrogenase (G6PD) deficiency.
▼ You are taking other medications.

Pregnancy
▼ Pyrimethamine may cause folic acid deficiency in the unborn fetus. Pregnant women receiving this drug should take a folic acid supplement. Discuss with your doctor.

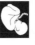

Breast-feeding
▼ The drug passes into the breast milk, but at normal doses adverse effects on the baby are unlikely. Discuss with your doctor.

Infants and children
▼ Reduced dose necessary.

Over 60
▼ No special problems.

Driving and hazardous work
▼ No special problems.

Alcohol
▼ No known problems.

POSSIBLE ADVERSE EFFECTS

Side effects of pyrimethamine occur only rarely with the low doses that are given for the prevention of malaria. Unusual tiredness, weakness, bleeding, bruising, and sore throat may be signs of a blood disorder. Notify your doctor promptly if they occur. Breathing difficulties or signs of chest infection should be reported to your doctor.

Symptom/effect	Frequency		Discuss with doctor		Stop taking drug now	Call doctor now
	Common	Rare	Only if severe	In all cases		
Loss of appetite	●			■		
Insomnia	●			■		
Gastric irritation	●			■		
Rash	●			■		▮
Unusual bleeding/bruising	●			■		▮
Sore throat/fever	●			■		▮
Breathing problems	●			■		▮

INTERACTIONS

General note Drugs that suppress the bone marrow or cause folic acid deficiency may increase the risk of serious blood disorders when taken with pyrimethamine. Such drugs include anticancer and antirheumatic drugs, phenylbutazone, sulfasalazine, co-trimoxazole, trimethoprim, and phenytoin.

PROLONGED USE

Prolonged use of this drug may cause folic acid deficiency, leading to serious blood disorders. Supplements of folic acid may be recommended (in the form of folinic acid).

Monitoring Regular blood cell counts are required during high-dose or long-term treatment.

QUETIAPINE

Brand name Seroquel
Used in the following combined preparations None

GENERAL INFORMATION

Quetiapine is an antipsychotic drug that is prescribed for the treatment of schizophrenia. It can be used to treat "positive" symptoms (thought disorders, delusions, and hallucinations) and "negative" symptoms (blunted affect and emotional and social withdrawal). The drug may be more effective when used for positive symptoms, however.

Unlike the similar drug olanzapine, quetiapine stays in the body for the same length of time in men and women. Elderly people excrete the drug up to 50 percent more slowly than the usual adult rate. They therefore require much lower doses in order to avoid *adverse effects*.

Parkinsonism is a common adverse effect of this and many other antipsychotic drugs.

INFORMATION FOR USERS

Your drug prescription is tailored for you. Do not alter dosage without checking with your doctor.

How taken

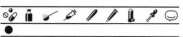

Tablets.

Frequency and timing of doses
2 x daily.

Adult dosage range
50mg daily (day 1), 100mg daily (day 2), 200mg daily (day 3), 300mg daily (day 4), then changing according to response. Usual range is 300-450mg daily, maximum 750mg daily.

Onset of effect
1 hour.

Duration of action
Up to 12 hours.

Diet advice
None.

Storage
Keep in a closed container in a cool, dry place out of the reach of children.

Missed dose
Take as soon as you remember. If your next dose is due within 4 hours take a single dose now and skip the next.

Stopping the drug
Do not stop the drug without consulting your doctor; symptoms may recur.

Exceeding the dose
An occasional unintentional extra dose is unlikely to cause problems. Large overdoses may cause unusual drowsiness, palpitations, and low blood pressure. Notify your doctor.

POSSIBLE ADVERSE EFFECTS

Unusual drowsiness and weight gain are common adverse effects of quetiapine.

Symptom/effect	Frequency		Discuss with doctor		Stop taking drug now	Call doctor now
	Common	Rare	Only if severe	In all cases		
Unusual drowsiness	●			■		
Weight gain	●			■		
Digestive upset	●			■		
Parkinsonism	●		■			
Dizziness/fainting		●	■			
Persistent sore throat		●	■			
Palpitations		●	■			▮

INTERACTIONS

Sedatives All drugs that have a sedative effect on the central nervous system are likely to increase the sedative properties of quetiapine.

Anticonvulsants Quetiapine opposes the effect of these drugs. Phenytoin decreases the effect of quetiapine.

SPECIAL PRECAUTIONS

Be sure to tell your doctor if:
▼ You have epilepsy.
▼ You have Parkinson's disease.
▼ You have liver or kidney problems.
▼ You have heart problems.
▼ You have blood problems.
▼ You are taking other medications.

Pregnancy
▼ Safety not established. Discuss with your doctor.

Breast-feeding
▼ Safety not established. Discuss with your doctor.

Infants and children
▼ Not recommended.

Over 60
▼ Reduced doses necessary. The elderly eliminate quetiapine much more slowly than younger adults.

Driving and hazardous work
▼ Avoid. Quetiapine can cause drowsiness.

Alcohol
▼ Avoid. Alcohol increases the sedative effects of this drug.

PROLONGED USE

Prolonged use of quetiapine has been reported to produce *tardive dyskinesia* (in which there are involuntary movements of the tongue and face).

QUININE

Brand names None
Used in the following combined preparations None

GENERAL INFORMATION

Quinine, obtained from the bark of the cinchona tree, was introduced in the last century and is the earliest antimalarial drug. It often causes *side effects*, but is still given for malaria resistant to safer treatments. Owing to malaria parasite resistance to chloroquine and some of the more modern antimalarials, quinine remains the mainstay of treatment, but it is not used as a preventative.

At the high doses used to treat malaria, quinine may cause ringing in the ears, headaches, nausea, hearing loss, and blurred vision: a group of symptoms known as cinchonism. In rare cases, it may cause bleeding into the skin due to reduced blood platelets.

In many countries quinine is often used, in small doses, to prevent painful night-time leg cramps.

QUICK REFERENCE

Drug group Antimalarial drug (p.137) and muscle relaxant (p.120)

Overdose danger rating High

Dependence rating Low

Prescription needed Yes

Available as generic Yes

INFORMATION FOR USERS

Your drug prescription is tailored for you. Do not alter dosage without checking with your doctor.

How taken

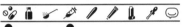

Tablets, injection.

Frequency and timing of doses
Malaria Every 8 hours.
Muscle cramps Once daily at bedtime.

Adult dosage range
1.8g daily (malaria);
200–300mg daily (cramps).

Onset of effect
1–2 days (malaria); 2–3 hours (cramps).

Duration of action
Up to 24 hours.

Diet advice
None.

Storage
Keep in a closed container in a cool, dry place out of the reach of children. Protect from light.

Missed dose
Take as soon as you remember. If your next dose is due within 4 hours, skip the missed one and return to your normal dosing schedule thereafter.

Stopping the drug
If prescribed for malaria, take the full course. Even if you feel better, the original infection may still be present and may recur if treatment is stopped too soon. If taken for muscle cramps, the drug can safely be stopped as soon as you no longer need it.

OVERDOSE ACTION

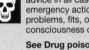

Seek immediate medical advice in all cases. Take emergency action if breathing problems, fits, or loss of consciousness occur.

See Drug poisoning emergency guide (p.494).

SPECIAL PRECAUTIONS

Be sure to consult your doctor if:
▼ You have a long-term kidney problem.
▼ You have tinnitus (ringing in the ears).
▼ You have optic neuritis.
▼ You have myasthenia gravis.
▼ You have glucose-6-phosphate dehydrogenase (G6PD) deficiency.
▼ You have heart problems.
▼ You are taking other medications.

Pregnancy
▼ Not usually prescribed. May cause defects in the unborn baby. Discuss with your doctor.

Breast-feeding
▼ The drug passes into the breast milk, but at normal doses adverse effects on the baby are unlikely. Discuss with your doctor.

Infants and children
▼ Reduced dose necessary.

Over 60
▼ No special problems.

Driving and hazardous work
▼ Avoid these activities until you know how quinine affects you because the drug's side effects may distract you.

Alcohol
▼ No known problems.

POSSIBLE ADVERSE EFFECTS

Adverse effects are unlikely with low doses. At antimalarial doses, hearing disturbances, headache, and blurred vision are more common. Nausea and diarrhoea may occur.

Symptom/effect	Frequency		Discuss with doctor		Stop taking drug now	Call doctor now
	Common	Rare	Only if severe	In all cases		
Nausea/vomiting/diarrhoea		●		■		
Headache		●		■		
Ringing in ears/giddiness		●		■		
Rash/itching		●		■	▲	▌
Loss of hearing		●		■	▲	▌
Blurred vision		●		■	▲	▌

PROLONGED USE

No problems expected with low doses used to control night-time leg cramps.

INTERACTIONS

Antihistamines There is an increased risk of adverse effects on the heart if quinine is taken with antihistamines such as terfenadine.

Cimetidine This drug increases the blood levels of quinine.

Digoxin Quinine increases the blood levels of digoxin, and so the dose of digoxin should be reduced. Discuss with your doctor.

RALOXIFENE

Brand name Evista
Used in the following combined preparations None

GENERAL INFORMATION

Raloxifene is a non-steroidal anti-oestrogen drug (oestrogen is a naturally occurring female sex hormone, see p.147) that is related to clomifene and tamoxifen. It is prescribed to prevent vertebral fractures in postmenopausal women who are at increased risk of osteoporosis. There is some evidence that the drug would also be useful for preventing fractures of the hip, but its use in the prevention of other bone fractures is uncertain.

Raloxifene has no beneficial effect on other menopausal problems such as hot flushes. It is not prescribed to women who might become pregnant because it may harm the unborn baby, and it is not prescribed to men.

There is an increased risk of a thrombosis (blood clot) developing in a vein in the leg, but the risk is similar to that due to HRT (see p.147). However, because of this risk, raloxifene is usually stopped if the woman taking it becomes immobile or bedbound, when clots are more likely to form. Treatment is restarted when full activity is resumed.

INFORMATION FOR USERS

Your drug prescription is tailored for you. Do not alter dosage without checking with your doctor.

How taken

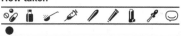
●

Tablets.

Frequency and timing of doses
Once daily.

Adult dosage range
60mg daily.

Onset of effect
1–4 hours.

Duration of action
24–48 hours.

Diet advice
Calcium supplements are recommended if dietary calcium is low.

Storage
Keep in a closed container in a cool, dry place out of the reach of children. Protect from light.

Missed dose
Take as soon as you remember. If your next dose is due within 8 hours, take a single dose now and skip the next.

Stopping the drug
Do not stop the drug without consulting your doctor except under conditions specified in advance, such as immobility, which increases the risk of blood clots forming.

Exceeding the dose
An occasional unintentional extra dose is unlikely to be a cause for concern. But if you notice any unusual symptoms, or if a large overdose has been taken, notify your doctor.

SPECIAL PRECAUTIONS

Be sure to tell your doctor if:
▼ You have had a blood clot in a vein.
▼ You have uterine bleeding.
▼ You have liver or kidney problems.
▼ You are taking other medications.

 Pregnancy
▼ Not prescribed to premenopausal women.

 Breast-feeding
▼ Not prescribed to premenopausal women.

 Infants and children
▼ Not prescribed.

 Over 60
▼ No special problems.

 Driving and hazardous work
▼ No special problems.

 Alcohol
▼ No special problems.

POSSIBLE ADVERSE EFFECTS

Some adverse effects of raloxifene are indications of a thrombosis (blood clot) in a vein in the leg. If a clot occurs somewhere else in the body, there might not be any obvious symptoms.

Symptom/effect	Frequency		Discuss with doctor		Stop taking drug now	Call doctor now
	Common	Rare	Only if severe	In all cases		
Hot flushes	●		■			
Leg cramps	●		■			
Swollen ankles/feet	●		■			
Leg pain/tenderness		●		■	▲	❙
Leg swelling		●		■	▲	❙
Leg discoloration/ulceration		●		■	▲	❙
Inflammation of capillaries		●		■	▲	❙

PROLONGED USE

No special problems. Raloxifene is normally used long term.

Monitoring Liver function tests may be performed periodically.

INTERACTIONS

Anticoagulants Raloxifene reduces the effect of warfarin and acenocoumarol (nicoumalone).

Cholestyramine This drug reduces the absorption of raloxifene by the body.

RAMIPRIL

Brand name Tritace
Used in the following combined preparations None

GENERAL INFORMATION

Ramipril belongs to a group of drugs known as ACE (angiotensin converting enzyme) inhibitors. It works by dilating the blood vessels, which enables the blood to circulate more easily. The drug is used to treat high blood pressure (p.102) and to reduce the strain on the heart in patients with heart failure after a heart attack. The first dose of an ACE inhibitor can cause the blood pressure to drop very suddenly, so a few hours' bed rest afterwards may be advised. You may need to stay in hospital until you are stabilized on the treatment.

Side effects such as headache, nausea, and dizziness are usually mild. Like all ACE inhibitors, however, ramipril causes the body to retain potassium, an excess of which can cause a number of *adverse effects*.

QUICK REFERENCE

Drug group ACE inhibitor (p.98) and drug for hypertension (p.102)

Overdose danger rating Medium

Dependence rating Low

Prescription needed Yes

Available as generic No

INFORMATION FOR USERS

Your drug prescription is tailored for you. Do not alter dosage without checking with your doctor.

How taken

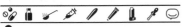

Capsules.

Frequency and timing of doses
With water, with or after food.
High blood pressure Usually once daily.
Heart failure after a heart attack 2 x daily.

Adult dosage range
High blood pressure 1.25–10mg daily.
Heart failure after heart attack 5–10mg daily.

Onset of effect
Within 2 hours.

Duration of action
Up to 24 hours.

Diet advice
Your doctor may advise you to decrease your salt intake to help control your blood pressure.

Storage
Keep in a closed container in a cool, dry place out of the reach of children.

Missed dose
Take as soon as you remember. If your next dose is due within 6 hours, take a single dose now and skip the next. Subsequently, continue with your usual routine.

Stopping the drug
Do not stop taking the drug without consulting your doctor. Treatment of hypertension and heart failure is normally lifelong, it may be necessary to substitute alternative therapy.

Exceeding the dose
If you notice any unusual symptoms or if a large overdose has been taken, notify your doctor.

SPECIAL PRECAUTIONS

Be sure to tell your doctor if:
▼ You have long-term liver or kidney problems.
▼ You have ever suffered from severe allergies.
▼ You have peripheral vascular disease.
▼ You suffer from systemic lupus erythematosus or scleroderma.
▼ You are taking other medications.

Pregnancy
▼ Not usually prescribed. May cause defects in the unborn baby. Discuss with your doctor.

Breast-feeding
▼ The drug passes into the breast milk and may affect the baby adversely. Discuss with your doctor.

Infants and children
▼ Not recommended.

Over 60s
▼ Reduced dose may be necessary.

Driving and hazardous work
▼ Avoid such activities until you have learned how ramipril affects you because the drug may cause dizziness due to low blood pressure.

Alcohol
▼ Avoid. Alcohol may reduce blood pressure further at first dose or dosage adjustment.

Surgery and general anaesthetics
▼ Notify your doctor or dentist that you are taking ramipril.

POSSIBLE ADVERSE EFFECTS

Nausea, dizziness, and headache are common but are usually mild and transient. An irritating dry cough may necessitate withdrawal of the drug. High potassium levels may occur. Rarely, ramipril may cause deterioration of kidney function, digestive tract disturbance, severe rash, or severe swelling of the face accompanied by breathing difficulties.

Symptom/effect	Frequency		Discuss with doctor		Stop taking drug now	Call doctor now
	Common	Rare	Only if severe	In all cases		
Nausea	●		■			
Dizziness/headache	●		■			
Cough	●		■			
Dry mouth/taste disturbance	●		■			
Rash/itching		●		■		▌
Swelling of face/mouth		●		■	▲	▌
Difficulty in breathing		●		■	▲	▌

INTERACTIONS

Non-steroidal anti-inflammatory drugs (NSAIDs) (e.g., ibuprofen) may reduce the antihypertensive effect of ramipril and increase the risk of kidney damage.

Cyclosporin increases the risk of high potassium.

Potassium supplements and potassium-sparing diuretics may cause excess levels of potassium in the body.

Lithium Like other ACE inhibitors, ramipril may cause raised blood lithium levels and *toxicity*.

PROLONGED USE

No problems expected.

RANITIDINE

Brand name Zantac
Used in the following combined preparations None

GENERAL INFORMATION

Ranitidine is prescribed in the treatment of stomach and duodenal ulcers. In combination with antibiotics, the drug is used for ulcers caused by *Helicobacter pylori* infection. It is also used to protect against duodenal (but not stomach) ulcers in people taking NSAIDs (p.116), who may be prone to ulcers. This drug reduces the discomfort and ulceration of reflux oesophagitis, and may prevent stress ulceration and gastric bleeding in severely ill patients. Ranitidine reduces the amount of stomach acid produced, allowing ulcers to heal. It is usually given in courses lasting four to eight weeks, with further courses if symptoms recur.

Ranitidine does not affect the actions of *enzymes* in the liver, where many drugs are broken down. Consequently, unlike the similar drug cimetidine, ranitidine does not increase blood levels of other drugs such as anticoagulants and anti-convulsants, which might reduce the effectiveness of treatment.

Most people experience no serious effects during ranitidine treatment. As it promotes healing of the stomach lining, there is a risk that ranitidine may mask stomach cancer, delaying diagnosis. It is therefore usually prescribed only when the possibility of stomach cancer has been ruled out.

QUICK REFERENCE

Drug group Anti-ulcer drug (p.109)
Overdose danger rating Low
Dependence rating Low
Prescription needed No (tablets in limited quantities); Yes (other preparations)
Available as generic Yes

INFORMATION FOR USERS

Your drug prescription is tailored for you. Do not alter dosage without checking with your doctor.

How taken

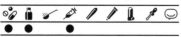

Tablets, capsules, oral liquid, injection.

Frequency and timing of doses
Once daily at bedtime or 2–3 x daily.

Adult dosage range
150mg–6g daily, depending on the condition being treated. Usual dose is 150mg twice daily.

Onset of effect
Within 1 hour.

Duration of action
12 hours.

Diet advice
None.

Storage
Keep in a closed container in a cool, dry place out of the reach of children. Protect from light.

Missed dose
Take as soon as you remember. If your next dose is due within 3 hours, take a single dose now and skip the next.

Stopping the drug
Do not stop the drug without consulting your doctor; symptoms may recur.

Exceeding the dose
An occasional unintentional extra dose is unlikely to be a cause for concern. But if you notice any unusual symptoms, or if a large overdose has been taken, notify your doctor.

SPECIAL PRECAUTIONS

Be sure to tell your doctor if:
▼ You have long-term liver or kidney problems.
▼ You are taking other medications.

 Pregnancy
▼ Safety in pregnancy not established. Discuss with your doctor.

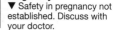

 Breast-feeding
▼ The drug passes into the breast milk and may affect the baby. Discuss with your doctor.

 Infants and children
▼ Reduced dose necessary.

 Over 60
▼ No special problems.

 Driving and hazardous work
▼ No known problems. Dizziness can occur in a very small proportion of patients.

 Alcohol
▼ Avoid. Alcohol may aggravate your underlying condition and reduce the beneficial effects of this drug.

POSSIBLE ADVERSE EFFECTS

The *adverse effects* of ranitidine, of which headache is the most common, are usually related to dosage level and almost always disappear when treatment finishes.

Symptom/effect	Frequency		Discuss with doctor		Stop taking drug now	Call doctor now
	Common	Rare	Only if severe	In all cases		
Headache/dizziness	●		■			
Nausea/vomiting		●	■			
Constipation		●	■			
Diarrhoea		●	■			

PROLONGED USE

No problems expected.

INTERACTIONS

Ketoconazole Ranitidine may reduce the absorption of ketoconazole. Ranitidine should be taken at least 2 hours after ketoconazole.

Cisapride Peak levels of ranitidine in the blood may be reached more rapidly when it is taken with cisapride.

Sucralfate High doses (2g) of sucralfate may reduce the absorption of ranitidine. Sucralfate should be taken at least 2 hours after ranitidine.

REPAGLINIDE

Brand name NovoNorm
Used in the following combined preparations None

GENERAL INFORMATION

Repaglinide is a drug used to treat non-insulin dependent diabetes that cannot be adequately controlled by diet and exercise alone. It acts in a similar manner to sulphonylurea drugs by stimulating the release of insulin from the pancreas. Therefore, some of the pancreatic cells need to be functioning in order for it to be effective.

Repaglinide is quick acting, but its effects last for only about four hours. The drug is sometimes given with metformin if that drug is not providing adequate diabetic control.

Repaglinide is best taken just before a meal in order for the insulin that is released to cope with the food. If a meal is likely to be missed, the dose of repaglinide should not be taken. If a tablet has been taken and a meal is not forthcoming, some carbohydrate (as specified by your doctor or dietitian) should be eaten as soon as possible.

INFORMATION FOR USERS

Your drug prescription is tailored for you. Do not alter dosage without checking with your doctor.

How taken

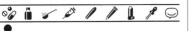

Tablets.

Frequency and timing of doses
1–4 x daily (up to 30 minutes before a meal, and up to 4 meals a day). If you are going to miss a meal, do not take the tablet.

Adult dosage range
500mcg (starting dose), increased at intervals of 1–2 weeks according to response; 4–16mg daily (maintenance dose).

Onset of effect
30 minutes.

Duration of action
4 hours.

Diet advice
Follow the diet advised by your doctor or dietitian.

Storage
Keep in a closed container in a cool, dry place out of the reach of children.

Missed dose
Do not take tablets between meals. Discuss with your doctor.

Stopping the drug
Do not stop taking the drug without consulting your doctor.

Exceeding the dose
An overdose will cause hypoglycaemia with dizziness, sweating, trembling, confusion, and headache. Notify your doctor.

SPECIAL PRECAUTIONS

Be sure to tell your doctor if:
▼ You have liver or kidney problems.
▼ You are taking other medications.

 Pregnancy
▼ Safety not established. Discuss with your doctor.

 Breast-feeding
▼ Safety not established. Discuss with your doctor.

 Infants and children
▼ Not recommended.

 Over 60
▼ No special problems, but safety not established over 75 years.

 Driving and hazardous work
▼ Avoid if low blood sugar without warning signs is likely.

 Alcohol
▼ Avoid. Alcohol may upset diabetic control and may increase and prolong the effects of repaglinide.

POSSIBLE ADVERSE EFFECTS

Intestinal problems are common at the start of treatment with repaglinide. However, such *adverse effects* tend to become less troublesome as treatment continues.

Symptom/effect	Frequency		Discuss with doctor		Stop taking drug now	Call doctor now
	Common	Rare	Only if severe	In all cases		
Nausea/vomiting	●		■			
Abdominal pain	●		■			
Diarrhoea/constipation	●		■			
Rash/itching		●			■	

PROLONGED USE

Repaglinide is usually prescribed indefinitely. No special problems.

INTERACTIONS

Monoamine oxidase inhibitors (MAOIs), beta-blockers, ACE inhibitors, and NSAIDs These drugs may increase the effect of repaglinide.

Oral contraceptives, thiazide diuretics, corticosteroids, danazol, thyroid hormones and sympathomimetics These drugs may decrease the effect of repaglinide.

RIFAMPICIN

Brand names Rifadin, Rimactane
Used in the following combined preparations Rifater, Rifinah, Rimactazid

GENERAL INFORMATION

Rifampicin is an antibacterial drug that is highly effective in the treatment of tuberculosis. Taken by mouth, the drug is well absorbed in the intestine and widely distributed throughout the body, including the brain. As a result, it is particularly useful in the treatment of tuberculous meningitis.

The drug is also used to treat leprosy and other serious infections, including Legionnaires' disease and infections of the bone (osteomyelitis). Additionally, it is given to anyone in close contact with meningococcal meningitis in order to prevent infection. Rifampicin is always prescribed with antibiotics or other antituberculous drugs because of rapid resistance in some bacteria.

A harmless red-orange coloration may be imparted to the urine, saliva, and tears, and soft contact lenses may become permanently stained.

QUICK REFERENCE

Drug group Antituberculous drug (p.132)

Overdose danger rating Medium

Dependence rating Low

Prescription needed Yes

Available as generic Yes

INFORMATION FOR USERS

Your drug prescription is tailored for you. Do not alter dosage without checking with your doctor.

How taken

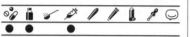

Tablets, capsules, liquid, injection.

Frequency and timing of doses
1 x daily, 30 minutes before breakfast (leprosy, tuberculosis) or once a month (leprosy); 2 x daily (prevention of meningococcal meningitis); 2–4 x daily, 30 minutes before or 2 hours after meals (other serious infections).

Adult dosage range
According to weight; usually 450–600mg daily (tuberculosis, leprosy) or 600mg once a month (leprosy); 600mg–1.2g daily (other serious infections); 1.2g daily for 2 days (meningococcal meningitis).

Onset of effect
Over several days.

Duration of action
Up to 24 hours.

Diet advice
None.

Storage
Keep in a closed container in a cool, dry place out of the reach of children. Protect from light.

Missed dose
Take as soon as you remember. If your next dose is due within 6 hours, take a single dose now, then return to normal dosing schedule.

Stopping the drug
Take the full course. Even if you feel better, the original infection may still be present and symptoms may recur if treatment is stopped too soon. In rare cases stopping the drug suddenly after high-dose treatment can lead to a severe flu-like illness.

Exceeding the dose
An occasional unintentional extra dose is unlikely to cause problems. Large overdoses may cause liver damage, nausea, vomiting, and lethargy. Notify your doctor immediately.

SPECIAL PRECAUTIONS

Be sure to tell your doctor if:
▼ You have a long-term liver problem.
▼ You wear contact lenses.
▼ You are taking other medications.

Pregnancy
▼ Safety in pregnancy not established. Discuss with your doctor.

Breast-feeding
▼ The drug passes into the breast milk, but at normal doses adverse effects on the baby are unlikely. Discuss with your doctor.

Infants and children
▼ Reduced dose necessary.

Over 60
▼ Increased risk of adverse effects. Reduced dose may therefore be necessary.

Driving and hazardous work
▼ No problems expected.

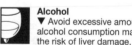

Alcohol
▼ Avoid excessive amounts. Heavy alcohol consumption may increase the risk of liver damage.

POSSIBLE ADVERSE EFFECTS

A harmless red-orange discoloration of body fluids normally occurs. Serious adverse effects are rare. *Jaundice* usually improves during treatment but should be reported to your doctor. Headache and breathing difficulties may occur after stopping high-dose treatment.

Symptom/effect	Frequency		Discuss with doctor		Stop taking drug now	Call doctor now
	Common	Rare	Only if severe	In all cases		
Muscle cramps/aches		●		■		
Nausea/vomiting/diarrhoea		●	■			
Jaundice		●		■	▲	▌
Flu-like illness		●		■	▲	▌
Rash/itching		●		■		

PROLONGED USE

Prolonged use of rifampicin may cause liver damage.

Monitoring Periodic blood tests may be performed to monitor liver function.

INTERACTIONS

General note Rifampicin may reduce the effectiveness of a wide variety of drugs, such as oral contraceptives (in which case alternative contraceptive methods may be necessary), phenytoin, corticosteroids, oral antidiabetics, disopyramide, and oral anticoagulants. Dosage adjustment of these drugs may be necessary at the start or end of treatment with rifampicin. Consult your doctor or pharmacist for advice.

RISPERIDONE

Brand name Risperdal
Used in the following combined preparations None

GENERAL INFORMATION

Risperidone is used to treat patients with acute psychiatric disorders and long-term psychotic illness such as schizophrenia. Although it does not cure the underlying disorder, the drug helps to alleviate the distressing symptoms. It is effective for relieving both "positive" symptoms (for example, hallucinations, thought disturbances, and hostility) and "negative" symptoms (for example, emotional and social withdrawal). The drug may also help with various other symptoms that are often associated with schizophrenia, such as depression and anxiety. Risperidone has less of a sedative effect and is also less likely to cause movement disorders as a *side effect* than some other antipsychotics.

INFORMATION FOR USERS

Your drug prescription is tailored for you. Do not alter dosage without checking with your doctor.

How taken

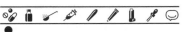

Tablets.

Frequency and timing of doses
1–2 x daily.

Adult dosage range
2mg daily (starting dose) increasing to 6–10mg, sometimes up to 16mg, daily (maintenance dose).

Onset of effect
Within 2–3 days, but may take up to 4 weeks before maximum effect is seen.

Duration of action
Approximately 2 days.

Diet advice
None.

Storage
Keep in a closed container in a cool, dry place out of the reach of children. Protect from light.

Missed dose
Take as soon as you remember. If your next dose is due within 3 hours, take a single dose now and skip the next.

Stopping the drug
Do not stop taking the drug without consulting your doctor; symptoms may recur.

Exceeding the dose
An occasional unintentional extra dose is unlikely to cause problems. If larger doses have been taken, notify your doctor.

SPECIAL PRECAUTIONS

Be sure to tell your doctor if:
▼ You have liver or kidney problems.
▼ You have heart or circulation problems.
▼ You have had epileptic fits.
▼ You have Parkinson's disease.
▼ You are taking other medications.

Pregnancy
▼ Safety in pregnancy not established. Discuss with your doctor.

Breast-feeding
▼ The drug probably passes into breast milk. Discuss with your doctor.

Infants and children
▼ Not recommended under 15 years.

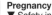

Over 60
▼ Reduced dose necessary.

Driving and hazardous work
▼ Avoid such activities until you have learned how risperidone affects you because the drug may cause difficulty in concentration and slowed reactions.

Alcohol
▼ Avoid. Alcohol may increase the sedative effects of this drug.

Surgery and general anaesthetics
▼ Risperidone treatment may need to be stopped before you have a general anaesthetic. Discuss this with your doctor or dentist before any operation.

POSSIBLE ADVERSE EFFECTS

Risperidone is generally well tolerated with a low incidence of movement disorders. This drug is less sedating than some of the other antipsychotics.

Symptom/effect	Frequency		Discuss with doctor		Stop taking drug now	Call doctor now
	Common	Rare	Only if severe	In all cases		
Insomnia/anxiety/agitation	●			■		
Headache	●			■		
Difficulty in concentration	●			■		
Dizziness/drowsiness		●		■		
Shakiness/tremor		●		■		
Rash		●		■		
High fever/rigid muscles		●		■	▲	■
Unusual thirst		●		■		
Weight gain	●			■		

INTERACTIONS

Drugs for parkinsonism Risperidone may reduce the effect of these drugs.

Carbamazepine This drug reduces the effects of risperidone.

Sedatives All drugs that have a sedative effect on the central nervous system are likely to increase any sedative effect of risperidone.

PROLONGED USE

If used long term, permanent movement disorders (*tardive dyskinesia*) may occur, although they are less likely than with many other antipsychotic drugs.

RIVASTIGMINE

Brand name Exelon
Used in the following combined preparations None

GENERAL INFORMATION

Rivastigmine is an anticholinesterase drug (an inhibitor of the enzyme acetyl-cholinesterase). The enzyme usually breaks down the *neurotransmitter* acetylcholine from the blood, thus limiting its effects. Blocking the enzyme increases and prolongs the effect of acetylcholine. Rivastigmine has been found to improve the symptoms of dementia due to Alzheimer's disease, and is used to slow the rate of deterioration in that disease. The drug has no effect on dementia due to other causes. It is usual to assess anyone being treated with rivastigmine after about three months to decide whether the drug is helping and whether it is worth continuing treatment. As the disease progresses, the benefit obtained may diminish.

Side effects may include agitation, confusion and depression, which could be thought due to Alzheimer's disease. Weight loss should be watched for.

INFORMATION FOR USERS

Your drug prescription is tailored for you. Do not alter dosage without checking with your doctor.

How taken

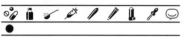

Capsules.

Frequency and timing of doses
2 x daily.

Adult dosage range
3mg daily (starting dose); 6–12mg daily (maintenance dose).

Onset of effect
30–60 minutes.

Duration of action
9–12 hours.

Diet advice
None.

Storage
Keep in a closed container in a cool, dry place out of the reach of children.

Missed dose
Take as soon as you remember. If your next dose is due within 4 hours, take a single dose now and skip the next. A carer should be overseeing the taking of tablets.

Stopping the drug
Do not stop the drug without consulting your doctor; symptoms may recur.

Exceeding the dose
An occasional unintentional extra dose is unlikely to be a problem. Large overdoses may cause nausea, vomiting and diarrhoea. Notify your doctor.

SPECIAL PRECAUTIONS

Be sure to tell your doctor if:
▼ You have a heart problem.
▼ You have liver or kidney problems.
▼ You have asthma or respiratory problems.
▼ You have had a peptic ulcer.
▼ You are taking an NSAID regularly.
▼ You are taking other medications.

Pregnancy
▼ Not usually prescribed. Safety not established.

Breast-feeding
▼ Not usually prescribed. Safety not established.

Infants and children
▼ Not usually prescribed.

Over 60
▼ No special problems.

Driving and hazardous work
▼ Your underlying condition may make such activities inadvisable. Discuss with your doctor.

Alcohol
▼ Avoid. Alcohol increases the sedative effects of rivastigmine.

Surgery and general anaesthetics
▼ Treatment with rivastigmine may need to be stopped before you have a general anaesthetic. Discuss this with your doctor or dentist before any operation.

POSSIBLE ADVERSE EFFECTS

Adverse effects include mental changes and intestinal problems. Though common, these effects are usually quite mild.

Symptom/effect	Frequency		Discuss with doctor		Stop taking drug now	Call doctor now
	Common	Rare	Only if severe	In all cases		
Reduced appetite/weight loss	●			■		
Nausea/abdominal pain	●			■		
Agitation/confusion/depression	●			■		
Drowsiness/dizziness	●		■			
Weakness/trembling	●		■			
Headache/insomnia	●		■			
Sweating/malaise	●		■			
Difficulty in passing urine		●			■	
Convulsions		●			■	

INTERACTIONS

Aminoglycoside antibiotics, clindamycin, and colistin These antibiotics block the effect of rivastigmine.

Antimalarials and anti-arrhythmics Certain drugs from these groups may block the effects of rivastigmine.

Muscle relaxants used in surgery Rivastigmine may increase the effects of some muscle relaxants, but it may also block the effects of some others.

PROLONGED USE

May be continued for as long as there is benefit. Stopping the drug leads to a gradual loss of the improvements.

Monitoring Periodic checks may be performed to test whether the drug is still providing some benefit.

SALBUTAMOL

Brand names Aerolin, Airomir, Asmasal, Asmaven, Maxivent, Salamol, Salbulin, Ventodisks, Ventolin, Volmax
Used in the following combined preparations Aerocrom, Combivent, Ventide

GENERAL INFORMATION

Salbutamol is a *sympathomimetic bronchodilator* that relaxes the muscle surrounding the bronchioles (airways in the lungs).

This drug is used to relieve symptoms of asthma, chronic bronchitis, and emphysema. Although it can be taken by mouth, inhalation is considered more effective because the drug is delivered directly to the bronchioles, thus giving rapid relief, allowing smaller doses, and causing fewer *side effects*.

Compared with some similar drugs, it has little stimulant effect on the heart rate and blood pressure, making it safer for people with heart problems or high blood pressure. Because salbutamol relaxes the muscles of the uterus, it is also used to prevent premature labour.

The most common side effect of salbutamol is fine tremor of the hands, which may interfere with precise manual work. Anxiety, tension, and restlessness may also occur.

QUICK REFERENCE

Drug group Bronchodilator (p.92) and drug used in premature labour (p.165)

Overdose danger rating Low

Dependence rating Low

Prescription needed Yes

Available as generic Yes

INFORMATION FOR USERS

Your drug prescription is tailored for you. Do not alter dosage without checking with your doctor.

How taken

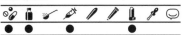

Tablets, SR-tablets, liquid, injection, inhaler, powder for inhalation.

Frequency and timing of doses
1–2 inhalations 3–4 x daily (inhaler); 3–4 x daily (tablets/liquid); 2 x daily (SR-tablets).

Dosage range
400–800mcg daily (inhaler); 8–32mg daily (by mouth).

Onset of effect
Within 5–15 minutes (inhaler); within 30–60 minutes (by mouth).

Duration of action
Up to 6 hours (inhaler); up to 8 hours (by mouth).

Diet advice
None.

Storage
Keep in a closed container in a cool, dry place out of the reach of children. Protect from light. Do not puncture or burn inhalers.

Missed dose
Take as soon as you remember if you need it. If your next dose is due within 2 hours, take a single dose now and skip the next.

Stopping the drug
Do not stop the drug without consulting your doctor; symptoms may recur.

Exceeding the dose
An occasional unintentional extra dose is unlikely to be a cause for concern. But if you notice any unusual symptoms, or if a large overdose has been taken, notify your doctor.

SPECIAL PRECAUTIONS

Be sure to tell your doctor if:
▼ You have heart problems.
▼ You have high blood pressure.
▼ You have an overactive thyroid gland.
▼ You have diabetes.
▼ You are taking other medications.

Pregnancy
▼ No evidence of risk when used to treat asthma, or to treat or prevent premature labour. Discuss with your doctor.

Breast-feeding
▼ The drug passes into the breast milk, but at normal doses adverse effects on the baby are unlikely. Discuss with your doctor.

Infants and children
▼ Reduced dose necessary.

Over 60
▼ Increased likelihood of adverse effects. Reduced dose may therefore be necessary.

Driving and hazardous work
▼ Avoid such activities until you have learned how salbutamol affects you because the drug can cause tremors.

Alcohol
▼ No known problems.

POSSIBLE ADVERSE EFFECTS

Muscle tremor, which particularly affects the hands, anxiety, and restlessness are the most common adverse effects. Palpitations and headache are rare.

Symptom/effect	Frequency		Discuss with doctor		Stop taking drug now	Call doctor now
	Common	Rare	Only if severe	In all cases		
Anxiety/nervous tension	●		■			
Tremor	●		■			
Restlessness	●		■			
Headache		●		■		
Palpitations		●		■	▲	
Muscle cramps		●		■		

INTERACTIONS

Theophylline There is a risk of low potassium levels in blood occurring if this drug is taken with salbutamol.

Monoamine oxidase inhibitors (MAOIs) can interact with salbutamol to produce a dangerous rise in blood pressure.

Other sympathomimetic drugs may increase the effects of salbutamol, thereby also increasing the risk of adverse effects.

Beta blockers Drugs in this group may reduce the action of salbutamol.

PROLONGED USE

No problems expected. However, you should contact your doctor if you find you are needing to use your salbutamol inhaler more than usual (more than 8 puffs in 24 hours). Failure to respond to the drug may be a result of worsening asthma that requires urgent medical attention.

SALMETEROL

Brand name Serevent
Used in the following combined preparation Seretide

GENERAL INFORMATION

Salmeterol is a *sympathomimetic* bronchodilator used to treat conditions, such as asthma and bronchospasm, in which the airways become constricted. Its advantage over salbutamol (p.399) is that it is longer acting.

Salmeterol relaxes the muscle surrounding the airways in the lungs but, because of its slow onset of effect,

it is not used to relieve symptoms of asthma. It is prescribed to prevent attacks, however, and can be helpful in preventing night-time asthma.

Taken by inhalation, salmeterol is delivered directly to the airways. This allows smaller doses to be taken and reduces the risk of *adverse effects*.

INFORMATION FOR USERS

Your drug prescription is tailored for you. Do not alter dosage without checking with your doctor.

How taken

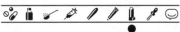

Inhaler, powder for inhalation.

Frequency and timing of doses
2 x daily.

Adult dosage range
100–200 mcg daily.

Onset of effect
10–20 minutes.

Duration of action
12 hours.

Diet advice
None.

Storage
Keep in a cool, dry place out of the reach of children.

Missed dose
Take as soon as you remember. If your next dose is due within 4 hours, take a single dose now and skip the next.

Stopping the drug
Do not stop the drug without consulting your doctor; symptoms may recur.

Exceeding the dose
An occasional unintentional extra dose is unlikely to be a cause for concern. But if you notice any unusual symptoms, or if a large overdose has been taken, notify your doctor.

SPECIAL PRECAUTIONS

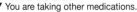

Be sure to tell your doctor if:
▼ You have heart problems.
▼ You have high blood pressure.
▼ You have an overactive thyroid.
▼ You have diabetes.
▼ You are taking other medications.

Pregnancy
▼ No evidence of risk when used to treat asthma. Discuss with your doctor.

Breast-feeding
▼ The drug passes into the breast milk, but at normal doses adverse effects on the baby are unlikely. Discuss with your doctor.

Infants and children
▼ Reduced dose necessary. Not recommended for children under 4 years.

Over 60
▼ No special problems.

Driving and hazardous work
▼ No special problems.

Alcohol
▼ No known problems.

POSSIBLE ADVERSE EFFECTS

Side effects are usually mild. If wheezing and breathlessness (paradoxical bronchospasm)

occur, stop taking the drug and notify your doctor immediately.

Symptom/effect	Frequency		Discuss with doctor		Stop taking drug now	Call doctor now
	Common	Rare	Only if severe	In all cases		
Tremor	●		■			
Palpitations		●		■		
Headache		●		■		
Sudden breathlessness		●		■	▲	▮

INTERACTIONS

Corticosteroids, theophylline, and diuretics There is an increased risk of low blood potassium levels when high doses of salmeterol are taken with these drugs.

PROLONGED USE

Salmeterol is intended to be used long term. The main problem comes from using combinations of anti-asthma drugs, leading to low blood potassium levels.

Monitoring
Periodic blood tests are usually carried out to monitor potassium levels.

SILDENAFIL

Brand name Viagra
Used in the following combined preparations None

GENERAL INFORMATION

Sildenafil is a new type of drug that is used to treat impotence. It does not cause an erection directly, but it produces a chemical change that prevents the muscle walls of the blood-filled chambers in the penis from relaxing.

Sildenafil does not need to be taken regularly; it is only used to produce an erection and only needs to be taken before sexual activity is undertaken.

Because it is a vasodilator, sildenafil can cause a small fall in blood pressure while it is active, and it may increase the effect of anti-hypertensive drugs. The drug is not usually prescribed with nitrates (see p.98) because it greatly increases their effects.

INFORMATION FOR USERS

Your drug prescription is tailored for you. Do not alter dosage without checking with your doctor.

How taken

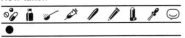

Tablets.

Frequency and timing of doses
Maximum once daily, 1 hour before sexual activity.

Adult dosage range
25–100mg.

Onset of effect
30 minutes.

Duration of action
4 hours.

Diet advice
None, although sildenafil will take longer to work after a meal, especially a high fat meal. It is absorbed faster on an empty stomach.

Storage
Keep in a closed container in a cool, dry place out of the reach of children.

Missed dose
Take the next dose when you need to. Do not use more than one dose in a 24-hour period.

Stopping the drug
Can be safely stopped as soon as you no longer need it.

Exceeding the dose
An occasional unintentional extra dose is unlikely to cause problems. Large overdoses may cause headache, dizziness, flushing, altered vision, and nasal congestion. Notify your doctor.

SPECIAL PRECAUTIONS

Be sure to tell your doctor if:
▼ You have heart problems.
▼ You have had a stroke or heart attack.
▼ You have sickle cell anaemia.
▼ You have multiple myeloma.
▼ You have leukaemia.
▼ You have liver or kidney problems.
▼ You have an inherited eye problem.
▼ You have an abnormality of the penis.
▼ You are taking a nitrate drug.
▼ You are taking other medications.

 Pregnancy
▼ Not prescribed.

 **Breast-feeding**
▼ Not prescribed.

 Infants and children
▼ Not prescribed under 18 years.

 Over 60
▼ Reduced dose may be necessary.

 Driving and hazardous work
▼ Avoid such activities until you have learned how sildenafil affects you because the drug can cause dizziness and altered vision.

 Alcohol
▼ No special problems.

POSSIBLE ADVERSE EFFECTS

Most *adverse effects* of sildenafil are common. However, if priapism (a persistent, painful erection) occurs, you should discontinue the drug and consult your doctor. Sildenafil has been reported to cause muscle aches when taken more frequently than recommended. It is not certain that this effect is due to the drug.

Symptom/effect	Frequency		Discuss with doctor		Stop taking drug now	Call doctor now
	Common	Rare	Only if severe	In all cases		
Headache	●		■			
Flushing	●		■			
Dizziness	●		■			
Indigestion	●		■			
Nasal congestion	●		■			
Blurred vision	●		■			
Altered colour vision	●		■			
Persistent erection		●		■	▲	∎

PROLONGED USE

No problems expected.

INTERACTIONS

Nitrates The effects of these drugs are greatly increased by sildenafil, and they are therefore not prescribed with it.

Cimetidine, erythromycin, and ketoconazole (oral) These drugs increase the blood levels and *toxicity* of sildenafil.

Antihypertensive drugs Sildenafil may enhance the blood-pressure lowering effect of these drugs.

Other drugs for impotence Safety not established. Not recommended.

SIMVASTATIN

Brand name Zocor
Used in the following combined preparations None

GENERAL INFORMATION

Simvastatin is a lipid-lowering drug that was introduced in 1989. It blocks the action of an *enzyme* that is needed for cholesterol to be manufactured in the liver, and as a result the blood levels of cholesterol are lowered. The drug is prescribed for people with hypercholesterolaemia (high levels of cholesterol in the blood) who have not responded to other forms of therapy, such as a special diet, and who are at risk of developing heart disease. At present it is used only for patients with a high cholesterol level that is not caused by another disease; these high levels are often hereditary.

Side effects are usually mild and often wear off with time. In the body, simvastatin is found mainly in the liver, and it may raise the levels of various liver enzymes. This effect does not usually indicate serious liver damage.

INFORMATION FOR USERS

Your drug prescription is tailored for you. Do not alter dosage without checking with your doctor.

How taken

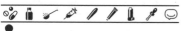

Tablets.

Frequency and timing of doses
Once daily at night.

Adult dosage range
10–40mg daily.

Onset of effect
Within 2 weeks; full beneficial effects may not be felt for 4–6 weeks.

Duration of action
Up to 24 hours.

Diet advice
A low-fat diet is usually recommended.

Storage
Keep in a closed container in a cool, dry place out of the reach of children. Protect from light.

Missed dose
Take as soon as you remember. If your next dose is due within 8 hours, do not take the missed dose, but take the next dose on schedule.

Stopping the drug
Do not stop taking the drug without consulting your doctor. Stopping the drug may lead to worsening of the underlying condition.

Exceeding the dose
An occasional unintentional extra dose is unlikely to cause problems. Large overdoses may cause liver problems. Notify your doctor.

SPECIAL PRECAUTIONS

Be sure to tell your doctor if:
▼ You have liver or kidney problems.
▼ You have eye or vision problems.
▼ You have muscle weakness.
▼ You have a thyroid disorder.
▼ You have had problems with alcohol abuse.
▼ You have porphyria.
▼ You have angina.
▼ You have high blood pressure.
▼ You are taking other medications.

Pregnancy
▼ Not usually prescribed. Safety in pregnancy not established. Discuss with your doctor.

Breast-feeding
▼ Safety not established. Discuss with your doctor.

Infants and children
▼ Not recommended.

Over 60
▼ No special problems.

Driving and hazardous work
▼ No special problems.

Alcohol
▼ Avoid excessive amounts. Alcohol may increase the risk of developing liver problems with this drug.

POSSIBLE ADVERSE EFFECTS

Adverse effects are usually mild and do not last long. The most common are those affecting the gastrointestinal system. Simvastatin may very rarely cause muscle problems, and any muscle pain or weakness should be reported to your doctor at once.

Symptom/effect	Frequency		Discuss with doctor		Stop taking drug now	Call doctor now
	Common	Rare	Only if severe	In all cases		
Abdominal pain	●		■			
Constipation/diarrhoea	●		■			
Nausea/flatulence	●		■			
Headache	●		■			
Rash	●			■	▲	
Muscle pain/weakness	●			■		■

INTERACTIONS

Anticoagulants Simvastatin may increase the effect of anticoagulants. The dose may need to be adjusted, and prothrombin time should be monitored regularly.

Cyclosporin and other immunosuppressant drugs Simvastatin and these drugs are not usually prescribed together because of the risk of muscle *toxicity*.

Other lipid-lowering drugs The use of other lipid-lowering drugs with simvastatin may increase the risk of muscle toxicity.

Itraconazole, ketoconazole, erythromycin Simultaneous administration of these drugs with simvastatin may increase the risk of muscle toxicity.

PROLONGED USE

Prolonged treatment can adversely affect liver function.

Monitoring Regular blood tests to assess liver function and muscle strength are recommended.

SODIUM BICARBONATE

Used in the following combined preparations Alka-Seltzer, Bismag, Bisodol, Carbalax, Dioralyte, Gastrocote, Gaviscon, Mictral, Roter, and many others

GENERAL INFORMATION

Sodium bicarbonate is available without prescription alone or in multi-ingredient preparations for the relief of occasional episodes of indigestion and heartburn. It may also relieve discomfort caused by peptic ulcers. However, it is now seldom recommended by doctors since other drugs are safer and more effective.

Because it also reduces the acidity of the urine, relieving painful urination, it is sometimes recommended for cystitis.

Given by injection, it is effective in reducing the acidity of the blood and body tissues in metabolic acidosis, a potentially fatal condition that may occur in life-threatening illnesses or following cardiac arrest. It should be avoided by people with heart failure and a history of kidney disease. Ear drops containing sodium bicarbonate are sometimes used for the removal of ear wax.

QUICK REFERENCE

Drug group Antacid (p.108)

Overdose danger rating Medium

Dependence rating Low

Prescription needed No

Available as generic Yes

INFORMATION FOR USERS

Follow instructions on the label. Call your doctor if symptoms worsen.

How taken

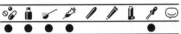

Tablets, capsules, liquid, powder (dissolved in water), injection, ear drops.

Frequency and timing of doses
Indigestion As required (by mouth).

Adult dosage range
Dependent on the condition being treated. As an antacid: 1–5g per dose.

Onset of effect
Within 15 minutes as an antacid.

Duration of action
30–60 minutes as an antacid.

Diet advice
None.

Storage
Keep in a closed container in a cool, dry place out of the reach of children.

Missed dose
No cause for concern.

Stopping the drug
When taken for indigestion, it can be safely stopped. When taken for other disorders, consult your doctor.

Exceeding the dose
An occasional unintentional extra dose is unlikely to cause problems. Large overdoses may cause unusual weakness, dizziness, or headache. Notify your doctor.

POSSIBLE ADVERSE EFFECTS

Belching and stomach pain may arise from the carbon dioxide produced as sodium bicarbonate neutralizes stomach acid, and can be caused by a single dose. The other effects result from the long-term regular use of sodium bicarbonate.

Symptom/effect	Frequency		Discuss with doctor		Stop taking drug now	Call doctor now
	Common	Rare	Only if severe	In all cases		
Belching	●		■			
Abdominal pain		●	■			
Swollen feet/ankles		●		■	▲	
Muscle cramps		●		■	▲	
Tiredness/weakness		●		■	▲	■
Nausea/vomiting		●		■	▲	
Shortness of breath		●		■		

INTERACTIONS

General note Sodium bicarbonate interferes with the absorption or excretion of a wide range of drugs taken by mouth. Consult your doctor if you are taking oral anticoagulants, tetracycline antibiotics, phenothiazine antipsychotics, oral iron preparations, or lithium, and wish to take more than an occasional dose of sodium bicarbonate.

Diuretics The beneficial effects of these drugs may be reduced by use of sodium bicarbonate.

Corticosteroids Large doses of sodium bicarbonate may hasten potassium loss, and increase fluid retention and high blood pressure.

SPECIAL PRECAUTIONS

Be sure to consult your doctor or pharmacist before taking this drug if:
▼ You have long-term liver or kidney problems.
▼ You have heart problems.
▼ You have high blood pressure.
▼ You have severe abdominal pain or vomiting.
▼ You are on a low-sodium diet.
▼ You are taking other medications.

 Pregnancy
▼ No evidence of risk, but it is not likely to help morning sickness, and can encourage fluid retention.

Breast-feeding
▼ No evidence of risk.

 Infants and children
▼ Not recommended under 6 years except on the advice of a doctor. Reduced dose necessary.

 Over 60
▼ Reduced dose may be necessary.

 Driving and hazardous work
▼ Do not take if you are flying. The gas produced expands and may increase stomach distension and belching.

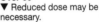 **Alcohol**
▼ Avoid. Alcohol irritates the stomach and may counter the beneficial effects of this drug.

PROLONGED USE

Severe weakness, fatigue, irritability, and muscle cramps may occur when this drug is taken regularly for extended periods. It should not be used daily for longer than 2 weeks without consulting your doctor.

Monitoring Blood and urine tests may be performed during prolonged use.

SODIUM CROMOGLICATE

Brand names Cromogem, Intal, Nalcrom, Opticrom, Rynacrom
Used in the following combined preparations Aerocrom, Intal Compound, Rynacrom Compound

GENERAL INFORMATION

Sodium cromoglicate, introduced in the 1970s, is used primarily to prevent asthma and allergic conditions.

When taken by inhaler as a powder (Spinhaler) or spray, it is commonly used to reduce the frequency and severity of asthma attacks, and is also effective in helping to prevent attacks induced by exercise or cold air. The drug has a slow onset of action, and it may take up to six weeks to produce its full anti-asthmatic effect. It is not effective for the relief of an asthma attack, and aside from its use in asthma prevention, it is also given as eye drops to prevent allergic conjunctivitis. Taken as a nasal spray, the drug is used to prevent allergic rhinitis (hay fever). It is also given, in the form of capsules, for food allergy.

Side effects are mild. Coughing and wheezing occurring on inhalation of the drug may be prevented by using a *sympathomimetic bronchodilator* (p.92) first. Hoarseness and throat irritation can be avoided by rinsing the mouth with water after inhalation.

INFORMATION FOR USERS

Follow instructions on the label. Call your doctor if symptoms worsen.

How taken

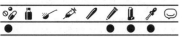

Capsules, eye ointment, inhaler (various types), eye and nose drops, nasal spray.

Frequency and timing of doses
Capsules 4 x daily before meals, swallowed whole or dissolved in water.
Inhaler, nasal preparations 4–6 x daily.
Eye preparations 4 x daily (drops); 2–3 x daily (eye ointment).

Dosage range
800mg daily (capsules); as directed (inhaler); apply to each nostril as directed (nasal preparations); 1–2 drops in each eye per dose (eye drops).

Onset of effect
Varies with dosage, form, and condition treated. Eye conditions and allergic rhinitis may respond after a few days' treatment with drops, while asthma and chronic allergic rhinitis may take take 2–6 weeks to show improvement.

Duration of action
4–6 hours. Some effect persists for several days after treatment is stopped.

Diet advice
Capsules: you may be advised to avoid certain foods. Follow your doctor's advice.

Storage
Keep in a closed container in a cool, dry place out of the reach of children. Protect from light.

Missed dose
Take as soon as you remember. If your next dose is due within 2 hours, take a single dose now and skip the next.

Stopping the drug
Do not stop the drug without consulting your doctor; symptoms may recur.

Exceeding the dose
An occasional unintentional extra dose is unlikely to be a cause for concern. But if you notice any unusual symptoms, or if a large overdose has been taken, notify your doctor.

SPECIAL PRECAUTIONS

Be sure to consult your doctor or pharmacist before taking this drug if:
▼ You are taking other medications.

Pregnancy
▼ No evidence of risk.

Breast-feeding
▼ No evidence of risk.

Infants and children
▼ Reduced dose necessary.

Over 60
▼ No special problems.

Driving and hazardous work
▼ No known problems.

Alcohol
▼ No known problems.

POSSIBLE ADVERSE EFFECTS

Coughing and hoarseness are common with inhalation of sodium cromoglicate. Nasal spray may cause sneezing. These symptoms usually diminish with continued use.

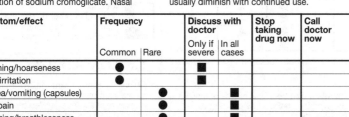

Symptom/effect	Frequency		Discuss with doctor		Stop taking drug now	Call doctor now
	Common	Rare	Only if severe	In all cases		
Coughing/hoarseness	●		■			
Local irritation	●		■			
Nausea/vomiting (capsules)		●		■		
Joint pain		●		■		
Wheezing/breathlessness		●		■		
Rash (capsules)		●		■	▲	

INTERACTIONS

None.

PROLONGED USE

No problems expected.

SODIUM VALPROATE

Brand names Convulex (valproic acid), Epilim, Orlept
Used in the following combined preparations None

GENERAL INFORMATION

Sodium valproate is an anticonvulsant drug that is often used for the treatment of a range of different types of epilepsy. The action of sodium valproate is similar to that of other anticonvulsants, reducing electrical discharges in the brain so that the excessive build-up of discharges that can lead to epileptic fits is prevented.

Beneficial in long-term treatment, this drug does not have a sedative effect. This makes it particularly suitable for children who suffer either from atonic epilepsy (the sudden relaxing of the muscles throughout the body) or from absence seizures (during which the person appears to be daydreaming).

INFORMATION FOR USERS

Your drug prescription is tailored for you. Do not alter dosage without checking with your doctor.

How taken

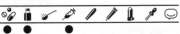

Tablets, capsules, liquid, injection.

Frequency and timing of doses
1–2 x daily.

Dosage range
600mg–2.5g daily, adjusted as necessary.

Onset of effect
Within 60 minutes.

Duration of action
12 hours or more.

Diet advice
None.

Storage
Keep in a tightly closed container in a cool, dry place out of the reach of children. Protect from light.

Missed dose
Take as soon as you remember. If your next dose is due within 2 hours, take a single dose now and skip the next.

Stopping the drug
Do not stop the drug without consulting your doctor; symptoms may recur.

Exceeding the dose
An occasional unintentional extra dose is unlikely to cause problems. Large overdoses may lead to coma. Notify your doctor.

SPECIAL PRECAUTIONS

Be sure to tell your doctor if:
▼ You have long-term liver or kidney problems.
▼ You are taking other medications.

 Pregnancy
▼ Not usually prescribed. May cause abnormalities in the unborn baby. Discuss with your doctor.

 Breast-feeding
▼ The drug passes into the breast milk, but at normal doses adverse effects on the baby are unlikely. Discuss with your doctor.

 Infants and children
▼ Reduced dose necessary.

 Over 60
▼ Reduced dose may be necessary.

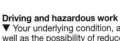 **Driving and hazardous work**
▼ Your underlying condition, as well as the possibility of reduced alertness while taking sodium valproate, may make such activities inadvisable. Discuss with your doctor.

Alcohol
▼ Avoid. Alcohol may increase the sedative effects of this drug.

POSSIBLE ADVERSE EFFECTS

Adverse effects of sodium valproate are uncommon and the most serious ones are rare. They include liver failure, and platelet and bleeding abnormalities. Menstrual periods may become irregular or cease.

Symptom/effect	Frequency		Discuss with doctor		Stop taking drug now	Call doctor now
	Common	Rare	Only if severe	In all cases		
Temporary loss of hair		●	■			
Weight gain		●	■			
Nausea/indigestion		●		■		
Rash		●		■		▮
Drowsiness		●		■		▮
Jaundice		●		■		▮
Vomiting		●		■		▮

INTERACTIONS

Other anticonvulsant drugs These drugs may reduce blood levels of sodium valproate.

Aspirin This drug may increase the effects of sodium valproate

Antidepressants and antipsychotics These drugs may reduce the effectiveness of sodium valproate.

Cholestyramine This drug may reduce the absorption of oral sodium valproate.

Antimalarial drugs Chloroquine and mefloquine reduce the effectiveness of sodium valproate.

Cimetidine This drug may increase the effects of valproate.

Zidovudine When zidovudine and sodium valproate are taken together, the blood levels of zidovudine may increase, leading to increased adverse effects.

PROLONGED USE

Use of this drug may cause liver damage, which is more likely in the first 6 months of use.

Monitoring Periodic checks on blood levels of the drug are usually required. Blood tests of liver function and blood composition may also be carried out.

SOTALOL

Brand names Beta-Cardone, Sotacor
Used in the following combined preparations None

GENERAL INFORMATION

Sotalol is a non-cardioselective beta blocker used in the prevention and treatment of ventricular and supra-ventricular arrhythmias (see p.100). It has an additional anti-arrhythmic action to other beta blockers.

Sotalol is no longer prescribed for the other conditions that beta blockers are prescribed for. This is due to a serious *side effect* called 'torsades de pointes', a kind of ventricular arrhythmia that is serious enough to produce symptoms and, rarely, death. For this reason, anyone taking sotalol will be carefully monitored.

INFORMATION FOR USERS

Your drug prescription is tailored for you. Do not alter dosage without checking with your doctor.

How taken

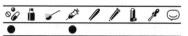

Tablets, injection.

Frequency and timing of doses
2 x daily (tablets); 6-hourly intervals when necessary (injections).

Adult dosage range
80mg daily initially, increased at 2–3-day intervals to 160–320mg daily. Higher doses of 480–640mg under specialist supervision.

Onset of effect
30–60 minutes.

Duration of action
12 hours.

Diet advice
None.

Storage
Keep in a closed container in a cool, dry place out of the reach of children. Protect from light.

Missed dose
Take as soon as you remember. If your next dose is due within 3 hours, take a single dose now and skip the next.

Stopping the drug
Do not stop the drug without consulting your doctor, who will supervise a gradual reduction in dosage. Sudden withdrawal may lead to worsening of your condition.

Exceeding the dose
An occasional unintentional extra dose is unlikely to be a cause for concern. Large overdoses may cause low blood pressure, slow heart rate, heart block, bronchospasm, and heart arrhythmias. Notify your doctor immediately.

SPECIAL PRECAUTIONS

Be sure to tell your doctor if:
▼ You have liver or kidney problems.
▼ You have a breathing disorder such as asthma, bronchitis, or emphysema.
▼ You have heart failure.
▼ You have diabetes.
▼ You have poor circulation in the legs.
▼ You are taking other medications.

Pregnancy
▼ Not usually prescribed. May affect the unborn baby. Discuss with your doctor.

Breast-feeding
▼ The drug passes into the breast milk and may affect the baby. Discuss with your doctor.

Infants and children
▼ Not prescribed.

Over 60
▼ Reduced dose may be necessary.

Driving and hazardous work
▼ Do not undertake such activities until you have learned how sotalol affects you because the drug can cause dizziness and fatigue.

Alcohol
▼ No special problems.

POSSIBLE ADVERSE EFFECTS

A very fast heart rate with palpitations could be a symptom of torsades de pointes; if you experience this you should notify your doctor immediately.

Symptom/effect	Frequency		Discuss with doctor		Stop taking drug now	Call doctor now
	Common	Rare	Only if severe	In all cases		
Lethargy/fatigue/dizziness	●		■			
Cold hands/feet	●		■			
Nightmares/vivid dreams		●		■		
Rash/dry eyes		●		■		
Wheezing/breathlessness		●		■		▮
Palpitations/fainting		●		■		▮

INTERACTIONS

Phenothiazines, antidepressants, terfenadine, vincamine, fenoxedil, and erythromycin (IV) These drugs increase the risk of torsades de pointes with sotalol.

Verapamil and diltiazem Combining these drugs with sotalol will have very adverse effects on heart function.

Anti-arrhythmics such as amiodarone, disopyramide, quinidine, lidocaine, procainamide Taking any of these drugs with sotalol may slow the heart rate and affect heart function.

Calcium channel blockers These may cause low blood pressure, slow heartbeats and heart failure if taken with sotalol.

Potassium-sparing diuretics, amphotericin, corticosteroids, and some laxatives These drugs may lower blood potassium levels, increasing the risk of torsades de pointes.

Sympathomimetics such as adrenaline, noradrenaline and dobutamine There is a risk of severe high blood pressure if these drugs are taken with sotalol.

PROLONGED USE

Sotalol may be taken indefinitely for prevention of ventricular arrhythmias.

Monitoring Periodic blood tests are usually performed to monitor levels of potassium and magnesium. The heartbeat is usually monitored for signs of development of torsades de pointes.

STREPTOKINASE

Brand names Kabikinase, Streptase
Used in the following combined preparation Varidase

GENERAL INFORMATION

Streptokinase, an *enzyme* produced by the streptococcus bacteria, is used in hospitals to dissolve the fibrin (see p.105) of blood clots, especially those in the arteries of the heart and lungs. It is also used on the clots formed in shunts during kidney dialysis.

A fast-acting drug, streptokinase is most effective in dissolving any newly formed clots, and it is often released at the site of the clot via a catheter inserted into an artery. Administered in the early stages of a heart attack to dissolve a clot in the coronary arteries (thrombosis), it can reduce the amount of damage to heart muscle. Because excessive bleeding is a common *side effect*, treatment is closely supervised.

Streptokinase is also used to treat wounds and ulcers in combination with another enzyme called streptodornase. For this use, powder is applied locally.

Streptokinase is a protein, and can cause allergic reactions. To reduce this risk, antihistamines may be given at the start of treatment.

QUICK REFERENCE

Drug group Thrombolytic drug (p.105).

Overdose danger rating Medium

Dependence rating Low

Prescription needed Yes

Available as generic No

INFORMATION FOR USERS

The drug is only given under medical supervision and is not for self-administration.

How taken

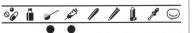

Powder, injection.

Frequency and timing of doses
By a single injection or continuously over a period of 24–72 hours.
Powder 1–2 x daily.

Dosage range
Dosage is determined individually by the patient's condition and response.

Onset of effect
As soon as streptokinase reaches the blood clot, it begins to dissolve within minutes. Most of the clot will be dissolved within a few hours.

Duration of action
Effect disappears within a few minutes of stopping the drug.

Diet advice
None.

Storage
Not applicable. This drug is not normally kept in the home.

Missed dose
Not applicable. This drug is given only in hospital under close medical supervision.

Stopping the drug
The drug is usually given for up to 3 days.

Exceeding the dose
Overdosage is unlikely since treatment is carefully monitored.

SPECIAL PRECAUTIONS

Streptokinase is only prescribed under close medical supervision, usually only in life-threatening circumstances.

Pregnancy
▼ Not usually prescribed. If used during the first 18 weeks of pregnancy there is a risk that the placenta may separate from the wall of the uterus.

Breast-feeding
▼ No evidence of risk.

Infants and children
▼ Reduced dose necessary.

Over 60
▼ Increased likelihood of bleeding into the brain.

Driving and hazardous work
▼ Not applicable.

Alcohol
▼ Not applicable.

POSSIBLE ADVERSE EFFECTS

Streptokinase is given under strict supervision and all adverse effects are closely monitored so that any of the symptoms below can be quickly dealt with.

Symptom/effect	Frequency		Discuss with doctor		Stop taking drug now	Call doctor now
	Common	Rare	Only if severe	In all cases		
Excessive bleeding	●			■		
Nausea/vomiting	●			■		
Rash/itching		●		■	▲	▮
Fever		●		■		
Wheezing		●		■		
Abnormal heart rhythms		●		■		
Collapse		●		■		

PROLONGED USE

Streptokinase is never used long term.

Further instructions Once you have had a dose, you will be given a card which you must keep with you at all times, and present to any doctor in case further treatment is required. A second course of treatment with streptokinase would not normally be given within 6 months of the first.

INTERACTIONS

Anticoagulant drugs There is an increased risk of bleeding when these are taken at the same time as streptokinase.

Antiplatelet drugs There is an increased risk of bleeding if these drugs are given with streptokinase.

SUCRALFATE

Brand name Antepsin
Used in the following combined preparations None

GENERAL INFORMATION

Sucralfate, a drug partly derived from aluminium, is prescribed to treat gastric and duodenal ulcers. The drug does not neutralize stomach acid, but it forms a protective barrier over the ulcer that protects it from attack by digestive juices, giving it time to heal.

If it is necessary during treatment to take antacids to relieve pain, they should be taken at least half an hour before or after taking sucralfate.

Apart from constipation, sucralfate does not have many common *adverse effects*. However, the safety of the drug for long-term use has not yet been confirmed. Therefore, courses of more than 12 weeks are not recommended.

QUICK REFERENCE

Drug group Ulcer-healing drug (p.109).

Overdose danger rating Low

Dependence rating Low

Prescription needed Yes

Available as generic No

INFORMATION FOR USERS

Your drug prescription is tailored for you. Do not alter dosage without checking with your doctor.

How taken

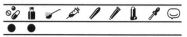

Tablets, liquid.

Frequency and timing of doses
2–4 x daily, 1 hour before each meal and at bedtime, at least 2 hours after food. The tablets may be dispersed in a little water before swallowing. Occasionally, up to 6 x daily.

Dosage range
4–8g daily.

Onset of effect
Some improvement may be noted after one or two doses, but it takes a few weeks for an ulcer to heal.

Duration of action
Up to 5 hours.

Diet advice
Your doctor will advise if supplements are needed.

Storage
Keep in a closed container in a cool, dry place out of the reach of children.

Missed dose
Do not make up the dose you missed. Take your next dose on your original schedule.

Stopping the drug
Do not stop the drug without consulting your doctor; symptoms may recur.

Exceeding the dose
An occasional unintentional extra dose is unlikely to be a cause for concern. But if you notice any unusual symptoms, or if a large overdose has been taken, notify your doctor.

SPECIAL PRECAUTIONS

Be sure to tell your doctor if:
▼ You have a long-term kidney problem.
▼ You are taking other medications.

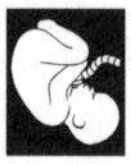

Pregnancy
▼ Safety in pregnancy not established. Discuss with your doctor.

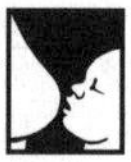

Breast-feeding
▼ No evidence of risk.

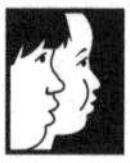

Infants and children
▼ Not usually prescribed.

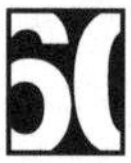

Over 60
▼ No special problems.

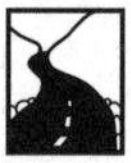

Driving and hazardous work
▼ Usually no problems, but sucralfate may cause dizziness in some people.

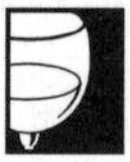

Alcohol
▼ Avoid. Alcohol may counteract the beneficial effect of this drug.

POSSIBLE ADVERSE EFFECTS

Most people do not experience any adverse effects while they are taking sucralfate. The most common is constipation, which will diminish as your body adjusts to the drug.

Symptom/effect	Frequency		Discuss with doctor		Stop taking drug now	Call doctor now
	Common	Rare	Only if severe	In all cases		
Indigestion	●		■			
Constipation	●		■			
Diarrhoea		●	■			
Dry mouth		●	■			
Nausea		●		■		
Rash/itching		●		■		
Dizziness/vertigo		●		■		
Insomnia		●		■		

PROLONGED USE

Not usually prescribed for periods longer than 12 weeks at a time. Prolonged use may lead to deficiencies of vitamins A, D, E, and K.

INTERACTIONS

Antacids and other indigestion remedies These reduce the effectiveness of sucralfate and should be taken more than 30 minutes before or after sucralfate.

Phenytoin The effect of this drug may be reduced if taken with sucralfate.

Warfarin The effects of warfarin may be reduced.

Tetracyclines, ciprofloxacin, norfloxacin, and ofloxacin Sucralfate may reduce the effect of these antibiotics.

Digoxin The effects of digoxin may be reduced.

Thyroxine The effects of thyroxine may be reduced.

SULFASALAZINE

Brand name Salazopyrin
Used in the following combined preparations None

GENERAL INFORMATION

Sulfasalazine, chemically related to the sulphonamide antibacterial drugs, is used to treat two inflammatory disorders affecting the bowel. One is ulcerative colitis (which mainly affects the large intestine); the other is Crohn's disease (which usually affects the small intestine). In recent years, sulfasalazine has also been found effective in the treatment of rheumatoid arthritis.

Adverse effects such as nausea, loss of appetite, and general discomfort are more likely when higher doses are taken. *Side effects* caused by stomach irritation may be avoided by changing to a specially coated tablet form of the drug. Allergic reactions such as fever and skin rash may be avoided or minimized by low initial doses of the drug, followed by gradual increases. Maintenance of adequate fluid intake is important while taking this drug. In rare cases among men, temporary sterility may occur.

QUICK REFERENCE

Drug group Drug for inflammatory bowel disease (p.112) and antirheumatic drug (p.117)

Overdose danger rating Low

Dependence rating Low

Prescription needed Yes

Available as a generic Yes

INFORMATION FOR USERS

Your drug prescription is tailored for you. Do not alter dosage without checking with your doctor.

How taken

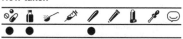

Tablets, liquid, suppositories, enema.

Frequency and timing of doses
4 x daily after meals with a glass of water (tablets); 2 x daily (suppositories); once daily, usually at bedtime (enema).

Adult dosage range
4–8g daily (Crohn's disease/ulcerative colitis); 500mg–3g daily (rheumatoid arthritis).

Onset of effect
Adverse effects may occur within a few days, but full beneficial effects may take 1–3 weeks, depending on the severity of the condition.

Duration of action
Up to 24 hours.

Diet advice
It is important to drink plenty of liquids (at least 1.5 litres a day) during treatment. Sulfasalazine may reduce the absorption of folic acid from the intestine, leading to a deficiency of this vitamin. Eat plenty of green vegetables.

Storage
Keep in a closed container in a cool, dry place out of the reach of children.

Missed dose
Take as soon as you remember. If your next dose is due within 2 hours, take a single dose now and skip the next.

Stopping the drug
Do not stop the drug without consulting your doctor; symptoms may recur.

Exceeding the dose
An occasional unintentional extra dose is unlikely to be a cause for concern. But if you notice any unusual symptoms, or if a large overdose has been taken, notify your doctor.

SPECIAL PRECAUTIONS

Be sure to tell your doctor if:
▼ You have long-term liver or kidney problems.
▼ You have glucose-6-phosphate dehydrogenase (G6PD) deficiency.
▼ You have a blood disorder.
▼ You suffer from porphyria.
▼ You are allergic to sulphonamides or salicylates.
▼ You wear soft contact lenses.
▼ You are taking other medications.

Pregnancy
▼ No evidence of risk to developing fetus. Folic acid supplements may be required. Discuss with your doctor.

Breast-feeding
▼ The drug passes into the breast milk and may affect the baby. Discuss with your doctor.

Infants and children
▼ Not recommended under 2 years. Reduced dose necessary for older children, according to body weight.

Over 60
▼ No special problems.

Driving and hazardous work
▼ No special problems.

Alcohol
▼ No known problems.

POSSIBLE ADVERSE EFFECTS

Adverse effects are common with high doses, but may disappear with a reduction in the dose. Symptoms such as nausea and vomiting may be helped by taking the drug with food. Orange or yellow discoloration of the urine is no cause for alarm.

Symptom/effect	Frequency		Discuss with doctor		Stop taking drug now	Call doctor now
	Common	Rare	Only if severe	In all cases		
Nausea/vomiting	●		■			
Malaise/loss of appetite	●		■			
Headache	●				■	
Joint pain	●				■	
Ringing in the ears		●	■			
Fever/rash		●			■	▮
Bleeding/bruising		●			■	▮

INTERACTIONS

General note 1 Sulfasalazine may increase the effects of a variety of drugs, including oral anticoagulants, oral antidiabetics, anticonvulsants, and methotrexate.

General note 2 Sulfasalazine reduces the absorption and effect of some drugs, including digoxin, folic acid, and iron.

PROLONGED USE

Blood disorders may occur with prolonged use of this drug. Maintenance dosage is usually continued indefinitely.

Monitoring Periodic tests of blood composition and liver function are usually required.

SUMATRIPTAN

Brand name Imigran
Used in the following combined preparations None

GENERAL INFORMATION

Sumatriptan is a highly effective drug for migraine, usually given when people fail to respond to analgesics (such as aspirin and paracetamol). The drug is of considerable value in the treatment of acute migraine attacks, whether or not they are preceded by an aura, but is not meant to be taken regularly to prevent attacks. Sumatriptan is also used for the acute treatment of cluster headache (a form of migraine headache). It should be taken as soon as possible after the onset of the attack, although, unlike other drugs used in migraine, it will still be of benefit at whatever stage of the attack it is taken.

Sumatriptan relieves the symptoms of migraine by preventing the dilation of blood vessels in the brain, which causes the attack.

INFORMATION FOR USERS

Your drug prescription is tailored for you. Do not alter dosage without checking with your doctor.

How taken

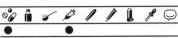

Tablets, injection, nasal spray.

Frequency and timing of doses
Should be taken as soon as possible after the onset of an attack. However, it is equally effective at whatever stage it is taken. DO NOT take a second dose for the same attack. The tablets should be swallowed whole with water.

Adult dosage range
Tablets 50–100mg per attack, up to maximum of 300mg in 24 hours if another attack occurs.
Injection 6mg per attack, up to maximum of 12mg (two injections) in 24 hours if another attack occurs.
Nasal spray 20mg per attack, up to maximum of 40mg (2 puffs) in 24 hours if another attack occurs.

Onset of effect
30 minutes (tablets);10–15 minutes (injection).

Duration of action
Tablets The maximum effect occurs after 2–4 hours.
Injection The maximum effect occurs after 1½–2 hours.

Diet advice
None unless otherwise advised.

Storage
Keep in a closed container in a cool, dry place out of the reach of children. Protect from light.

Missed dose
Not applicable, as it is taken only to treat a migraine attack.

Stopping the drug
Taken only to treat a migraine attack.

Exceeding the dose
An occasional unintentional extra tablet or injection is unlikely to cause problems. But if you notice any unusual symptoms, or if a large overdose has been taken, notify your doctor.

SPECIAL PRECAUTIONS

Be sure to tell your doctor if:
▼ You have liver or kidney problems.
▼ You have heart problems.
▼ You have high blood pressure.
▼ You have had a heart attack.
▼ You have angina.
▼ You are allergic to some medicines.
▼ You are taking other medications.

 Pregnancy
▼ Safety in pregnancy not established. Discuss with your doctor.

 Breast-feeding
▼ Safety not established. Discuss with your doctor.

 Infants and children
▼ Not recommended.

 Over 60
▼ Not recommended for patients over 65 years.

 Driving and hazardous work
▼ Avoid such activities until you have learned how sumatriptan affects you because the drug can cause drowsiness.

 Alcohol
▼ No special problems, but some drinks may provoke migraine in some people (see p.85).

Surgery and general anaesthetics
▼ Notify your doctor or dentist if you have used sumatriptan within 48 hours prior to surgery.

POSSIBLE ADVERSE EFFECTS

Many of the adverse effects will disappear after about 1 hour as your body becomes adjusted to the medicine. If the symptoms persist or are severe, contact your doctor.

Symptom/effect	Frequency		Discuss with doctor		Stop taking drug now	Call doctor now
	Common	Rare	Only if severe	In all cases		
Pain at injection site	●		■			
Feeling of tingling/heat	●		■			
Flushing	●		■			
Feeling of heaviness/weakness	●		■			
Dizziness		●	■			
Fatigue/drowsiness		●	■			
Palpitations/chest pain		●		■	▲	■

INTERACTIONS

Antidepressants Monoamine oxidase inhibitors (MAOIs) and some other antidepressants, such as fluvoxamine, fluoxetine, paroxetine, and sertraline, increase the risk of adverse effects with sumatriptan.

Lithium Patients taking lithium should not take sumatriptan due to the high risk of adverse effects.

Ergotamine must be taken at least 6 hours after sumatriptan, and sumatriptan must be taken at least 24 hours after ergotamine.

PROLONGED USE

Sumatriptan should not be used continuously to prevent migraine but only to treat migraine attacks.

TAMOXIFEN

Brand names Emblon, Fentamox, Nolvadex, Oestrifen, Tamofen
Used in the following combined preparations None

GENERAL INFORMATION

Tamoxifen is an anti-oestrogen drug (oestrogen is a naturally occurring female sex hormone, see p.147). It is used for two conditions: infertility and breast cancer. When given as treatment of certain types of infertility, the drug is taken only on certain days of the menstrual cycle. Used as an anticancer drug for breast cancer, it works against oestrogens. By latching on to cells that recognize these hormones, it can slow the growth of the tumour and even shrink it. It can also be used to prevent the recurrence of a breast cancer that has been surgically removed.

As its effect is specific, tamoxifen has fewer *adverse effects* than most other drugs used for breast cancer. However, it may cause eye damage if high doses are taken for long periods.

QUICK REFERENCE

Drug group Anticancer drug (p.154)
Overdose danger rating Low
Dependence rating Low
Prescription needed Yes
Available as generic Yes

INFORMATION FOR USERS

Your drug prescription is tailored for you. Do not alter dosage without checking with your doctor.

How taken

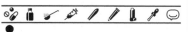

Tablets.

Frequency and timing of doses
1–2 x daily.

Adult dosage range
20mg daily (breast cancer).
20–80mg daily (infertility).

Onset of effect
Side effects may be felt within days, but beneficial effects may take 4–10 weeks.

Duration of action
Effects may be felt for several weeks after stopping the drug.

Diet advice
None.

Storage
Keep in a closed container in a cool, dry place out of the reach of children. Protect from light.

Missed dose
Take as soon as you remember. If your next dose is due within 2 hours, take a single dose now and skip the next.

Stopping the drug
Do not stop the drug without consulting your doctor; stopping the drug may lead to worsening of your underlying condition.

Exceeding the dose
An occasional unintentional extra dose is unlikely to be a cause for concern. But if you notice any unusual symptoms, or if a large overdose has been taken, notify your doctor.

SPECIAL PRECAUTIONS

Be sure to tell your doctor if:
▼ You have cataracts or poor eyesight.
▼ You suffer from porphyria.
▼ You are taking other medications.

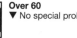

Pregnancy
▼ Not usually prescribed. May have effects on the developing baby. Discuss with your doctor.

Breast-feeding
▼ Not usually prescribed. Discuss with your doctor.

Infants and children
▼ Not prescribed.

Over 60
▼ No special problems.

Driving and hazardous work
▼ Do not drive until you have learned how tamoxifen affects you because the drug can cause dizziness and blurred vision.

Alcohol
▼ No known problems.

POSSIBLE ADVERSE EFFECTS

These are rarely serious and do not usually require treatment to be stopped. Nausea, vomiting, and hot flushes are the most common reactions. There is a small risk of endometrial cancer (cancer of the uterine lining) developing, so you should notify your doctor of any symptoms such as irregular vaginal bleeding as soon as possible.

Symptom/effect	Frequency		Discuss with doctor		Stop taking drug now	Call doctor now
	Common	Rare	Only if severe	In all cases		
Nausea/vomiting	●		■			
Hot flushes	●		■			
Irregular vaginal bleeding	●			■		■
Irregular vaginal discharge	●			■		■
Swollen feet/ankles		●	■			
Bone and tumour pain		●		■		
Rash/itching		●		■		
Blurred vision/headache		●		■		

INTERACTIONS

Anticoagulants People treated with anticoagulants such as warfarin usually need a lower dose of the anticoagulant.

PROLONGED USE

There is a risk of damage to the eye with long-term, high-dose treatment.

There is a small increased risk of endometrial cancer with long-term treatment but this is far outweighed by the benefits of treatment.

Monitoring Eyesight may be tested periodically.

TAMSULOSIN

Brand name Flomax MR
Used in the following combined preparations None

GENERAL INFORMATION

Tamsulosin is a selective alpha-blocker drug used to treat urinary retention due to benign prostatic hypertrophy, or BPH (enlarged prostate gland). The drug, as it passes through the prostate, relaxes the muscle in the wall of the urethra, thereby increasing urine flow.

To exclude other conditions with similar symptoms, your doctor will arrange for you to have a physical examination and a special blood test, which may be repeated at intervals during treatment.

Like other alpha-blockers, tamsulosin may lower blood pressure rapidly after the first dose. For this reason, the first dose should be taken at home so that, if dizziness or weakness occur, you can lie down until they have disappeared.

The drug is not used to treat hypertension (high blood pressure) because the dose used for BPH is low.

QUICK REFERENCE

Drug group Drug for urinary disorders (p166)

Overdose danger rating Medium

Dependence rating Low

Prescription needed Yes

Available as generic No

INFORMATION FOR USERS

Your drug prescription is tailored for you. Do not alter dosage without checking with your doctor.

How taken

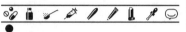

SR-capsules.

Frequency and timing of doses
Once daily after breakfast.

Adult dosage range
400mcg.

Onset of effect
1–2 hours.

Duration of action
24 hours.

Diet advice
None.

Storage
Keep in a closed container in a cool, dry place out of the reach of children.

Missed dose
Taken as soon as you remember. If your next dose is due within 4 hours, take a single dose now and skip the next.

Stopping the drug
Do not stop taking the drug without consulting your doctor; stopping suddenly may lead to a rise in blood pressure.

Exceeding the dose
An occasional unintentional extra dose is unlikely to cause problems. Large overdoses may produce sedation, dizziness, low blood pressure and rapid pulse. Notify your doctor immediately.

SPECIAL PRECAUTIONS

Be sure to tell your doctor if:
▼ You have had low blood pressure.
▼ You have liver or kidney problems.
▼ You have heart failure.
▼ You have a history of depression.
▼ You are taking an MAOI drug.
▼ You are taking drugs for high blood pressure.
▼ You are taking other medications.

Pregnancy
▼ Not prescribed.

Breast-feeding
▼ Not prescribed.

Infants and children
▼ Not prescribed.

Over 60
▼ No special problems.

Driving and hazardous work
▼ Avoid such activities until you have learned how tamsulosin because the drug can cause drowsiness and dizziness.

Alcohol
▼ Avoid until you know how tamsulosin affects you because alcohol can further lower blood pressure.

POSSIBLE ADVERSE EFFECTS

Dizziness seems to be the most common adverse effect, but this usually improves after the first few doses.

Symptom/effect	Frequency		Discuss with doctor		Stop taking drug now	Call doctor now
	Common	Rare	Only if severe	In all cases		
Dizziness/weakness/fainting	●		■			
Ejaculatory problems	●		■			
Headache	●		■			
Drowsiness	●		■			
Palpitations	●		■			
Nausea/vomiting		●	■			
Diarrhoea/constipation		●	■			
Rash/itching		●		■		

INTERACTIONS

Antidepressants, beta-blockers, calcium channel blockers, diuretics, and thymoxamine These drugs are likely to increase the blood-pressure lowering effect of tamsulosin.

PROLONGED USE

No special problems.

TEMAZEPAM

Brand names None
Used in the following combined preparations None

GENERAL INFORMATION

Temazepam belongs to a group of drugs known as the benzodiazepines. The actions and *adverse effects* of this group of drugs are described more fully under Anti-anxiety drugs (p.83).

Temazepam is used in the short-term treatment of insomnia. Because it is a short-acting drug compared with some other benzodiazepines, it is less likely to cause drowsiness and/or lightheadedness the following day.

For this reason, the drug is not usually effective in preventing early wakening, but hangover is less common than with other benzodiazepines.

Like other benzodiazepine drugs, temazepam can be habit-forming if taken regularly over a long period. Its effects also grow weaker with time. For these reasons, treatment with temazepam is usually only continued for a few days at a time.

QUICK REFERENCE

Drug group Benzodiazepine sleeping drug (p.82)

Overdose danger rating Medium

Dependence rating High

Prescription needed Yes

Available as generic Yes

INFORMATION FOR USERS

Your drug prescription is tailored for you. Do not alter dosage without checking with your doctor.

How taken

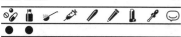

Tablets, liquid.

Frequency and timing of doses
Once daily, 30 minutes before bedtime.

Adult dosage range
10–60mg.

Onset of effect
15–40 minutes, or longer.

Duration of action
6–8 hours.

Diet advice
None.

Storage
Keep in a closed container in a cool, dry place out of the reach of children. Protect from light.

Missed dose
If you fall asleep without having taken a dose and wake some hours later, do not take the missed dose. If necessary, return to your normal dose schedule the following night.

Stopping the drug
If you have been taking the drug continuously for less than 2 weeks, it can be safely stopped as soon as you no longer need it. If you have been taking the drug for longer, consult your doctor, who may supervise a gradual reduction in dosage. Stopping abruptly may lead to *withdrawal symptoms* (see p.82).

Exceeding the dose
An occasional unintentional extra dose is unlikely to be a cause for concern. Large overdoses may cause unusual drowsiness. Notify your doctor.

SPECIAL PRECAUTIONS

Be sure to tell your doctor if:
▼ You have severe respiratory disease.
▼ You suffer from porphyria.
▼ You suffer from depression.
▼ You have liver or kidney problems.
▼ You have myasthenia gravis.
▼ You have had problems with alcohol or drug abuse.
▼ You are taking other medications.

Pregnancy
▼ Safety in pregnancy not established. Discuss with your doctor.

Breast-feeding
▼ The drug passes into the breast milk, but at normal doses adverse effects on the baby are unlikely. Discuss with your doctor.

Infants and children
▼ Not recommended.

Over 60
▼ Reduced dose may be necessary. Increased likelihood of adverse effects.

Driving and hazardous work
▼ Avoid such activities until you have learned how temazepam affects you because the drug can cause reduced alertness and slowed reactions.

Alcohol
▼ Avoid. Alcohol may increase the sedative effect of this drug.

POSSIBLE ADVERSE EFFECTS

The principal adverse effects of this drug are related to its sedative and tranquillizing properties. These effects normally diminish after the first few days of treatment.

Symptom/effect	Frequency		Discuss with doctor		Stop taking drug now	Call doctor now
	Common	Rare	Only if severe	In all cases		
Daytime drowsiness	●		■			
Dizziness/unsteadiness		●		■		
Headache		●		■		
Vivid dreams/nightmares		●		■		
Forgetfulness/confusion		●		■		■

INTERACTIONS

Sedatives All drugs that have a sedative effect on the central nervous system are likely to increase the sedative properties of temazepam. Such drugs include other anti-anxiety and sleeping drugs, *opioid* analgesics, antidepressants, antihistamines, and antipsychotics.

PROLONGED USE

Regular use of this drug over several weeks can lead to a reduction in its effect as the body adapts. It may also be habit-forming when taken for extended periods. Temazepam should not normally be used for longer than 1–2 weeks.

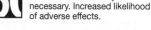

TERBINAFINE

Brand name Lamisil
Used in the following combined preparations None

GENERAL INFORMATION

Terbinafine is an antifungal drug used to treat fungal infections of the skin and nails, particularly tinea (ringworm). It is also used as a cream for candida (yeast) infections.

Terbinafine has largely replaced older drugs such as griseofulvin because it is more easily absorbed and is therefore more effective.

Tinea infections are treated in two to six weeks, but treatment of nail infections may take up to 6 months.

Rare *adverse effects* of terbinafine include *jaundice* and a severe skin rash, both of which should be reported to your doctor without delay.

QUICK REFERENCE

Drug group Antifungal drug (p.138)
Overdose danger rating Low
Dependence rating Low
Prescription needed Yes
Available as generic No

INFORMATION FOR USERS

Your drug prescription is tailored for you. Do not alter dosage without checking with your doctor.

How taken

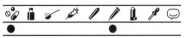

Tablets, cream.

Frequency and timing of doses
Once daily (tablets); 1–2 x daily (cream).

Adult dosage range
Tinea infections 250mg (tablets).
Candida infections As directed (cream).

Onset of effect
1 hour.

Duration of action
24 hours.

Diet advice
None.

Storage
Keep in a closed container in a cool, dry place out of the reach of children. Protect from light.

Missed dose
Take as soon as you remember. If your next dose is due within 4 hours, take a single dose now and skip the next.

Stopping the drug
Take the full course. Even if you feel better, the original infection may still be present and may recur if treatment is stopped too soon.

Exceeding the dose
An occasional unintentional extra dose is unlikely to be a cause for concern. But if you notice any unusual symptoms, or if a large overdose has been taken, notify your doctor.

SPECIAL PRECAUTIONS

Be sure to tell your doctor if:
▼ You have liver or kidney problems.
▼ You are taking other medications.

Pregnancy
▼ Safety in pregnancy not established. Discuss with your doctor.

Breast-feeding
▼ The drug passes into the breast milk and may affect the baby adversely. Discuss with your doctor.

Infants and children
▼ Safety not established. Discuss with your doctor.

Over 60
▼ No special problems.

Driving and hazardous work
▼ No known problems.

Alcohol
▼ No known problems.

POSSIBLE ADVERSE EFFECTS

Side effects of terbinafine are generally mild and transient.

Symptom/effect	Frequency		Discuss with doctor		Stop taking drug now	Call doctor now
	Common	Rare	Only if severe	In all cases		
Nausea/indigestion/bloating	●		■			
Mild abdominal pain/diarrhoea	●		■			
Headache	●		■			
Taste disturbance/loss		●	■			
Dizziness		●	■			
"Pins and needles"		●	■			
Muscle or joint pain		●		■		
Severe skin rash		●		■	▲	▌
Jaundice		●		■	▲	▌

PROLONGED USE

No special problems.

INTERACTIONS

Oral contraceptives "Breakthrough" bleeding may occur when these are taken with terbinafine.

Rifampicin This drug may reduce the blood level and effect of terbinafine.

Cimetidine This drug may increase the blood level of terbinafine.

TERBUTALINE

Brand names Bricanyl, Monovent
Used in the following combined preparations None

GENERAL INFORMATION

Terbutaline is a *sympathomimetic bronchodilator* that dilates the small airways in the lungs. The drug is used in the treatment and prevention of the bronchospasm occurring with asthma, chronic bronchitis, and emphysema. It may be given orally or by inhaler when rapid relief of breathlessness is required.

Muscle tremor, especially of the hands, is common with terbutaline and usually disappears on reduction of the dose or with continued use as the body adapts to the drug. In common with the other sympathomimetic drugs, it may produce nervousness and restlessness.

QUICK REFERENCE

Drug group Bronchodilator (p.92)
Overdose danger rating Low
Dependence rating Low
Prescription needed Yes
Available as generic No

INFORMATION FOR USERS

Your drug prescription is tailored for you. Do not alter dosage without checking with your doctor.

How taken

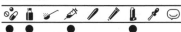

Tablets, liquid, injection, inhaler.

Frequency and timing of doses
3 x daily (tablets); as necessary (inhaler).

Dosage range
Adults 7.5–15mg daily (tablets); up to 2mg daily (inhaler).
Children Reduced dose according to age and weight.

Onset of effect
Within a few minutes (inhaler); within 1–2 hours (tablets).

Duration of action
4–8 hours (tablets).

Diet advice
None.

Storage
Keep in a closed container in a cool, dry place out of the reach of children. Protect from light. Do not puncture or burn aerosol containers.

Missed dose
Do not take the missed dose. Take your next dose as usual.

Stopping the drug
Do not stop the drug without consulting your doctor; symptoms may recur.

Exceeding the dose
An occasional unintentional extra dose is unlikely to be a cause for concern. But if you notice any unusual symptoms, or if a large overdose has been taken, notify your doctor.

SPECIAL PRECAUTIONS

Be sure to tell your doctor if:
▼ You have heart problems.
▼ You have high blood pressure.
▼ You have diabetes.
▼ You have an overactive thyroid.
▼ You are taking other medications.

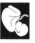

Pregnancy
▼ Safety in early pregnancy not established, although it is used in late pregnancy to prevent premature labour. Discuss with your doctor.

Breast-feeding
▼ The drug passes into the breast milk and may affect the baby adversely. Discuss with your doctor.

Infants and children
▼ Reduced dose necessary.

Over 60
▼ Increased likelihood of adverse effects. Reduced dose may therefore be necessary.

Driving and hazardous work
▼ Avoid such activities until you have learned how terbutaline affects you because the drug can cause tremor of the hands.

Alcohol
▼ No special problems.

POSSIBLE ADVERSE EFFECTS

Possible *adverse effects* include tremor, nervousness, restlessness, and nausea. These may be reduced by adjustment of dosage.

Palpitations and headache, resulting from stimulation of the heart and narrowing of the blood vessels, are rare.

Symptom/effect	Frequency		Discuss with doctor		Stop taking drug now	Call doctor now
	Common	Rare	Only if severe	In all cases		
Nausea/vomiting	●		■			
Tremor	●		■			
Restlessness/anxiety	●		■			
Headache		●	■			
Palpitations		●			■	
Muscle cramps		●			■	

INTERACTIONS

Other sympathomimetics may add to the effects of terbutaline and vice versa, so increasing the risk of adverse effects.

Monoamine oxidase inhibitors (MAOIs) Terbutaline may interact with these drugs to cause a dangerous rise in blood pressure.

Beta blockers may reduce the beneficial effects of terbutaline.

PROLONGED USE

Prolonged use may result in tolerance to the effects of terbutaline. However, failure to respond to the drug may be a result of worsening asthma, requiring prompt medical attention.

TERFENADINE

Brand names Histafen, Seldane, Terfinax, Triludan
Used in the following combined preparations None

GENERAL INFORMATION

Terfenadine is a long-acting antihistamine. Its main use is in the treatment of allergic rhinitis, particularly hay fever, where it reduces sneezing and irritation of the eyes and nose. Allergic skin conditions, such as urticaria (hives), may also be helped by terfenadine.

Unlike the older antihistamines, terfenadine has little sedative effect and is therefore particularly suitable for situations where people need to avoid drowsiness, for example, at work.

Very rarely, terfenadine produces dangerous changes in heart rhythm, especially if taken with other medicines or grapefruit juice. If palpitations develop or you feel faint, seek medical help without delay. Ask your doctor or pharmacist before taking terfenadine with other medications.

QUICK REFERENCE

Drug group Antihistamine (p.124)
Overdose danger rating Medium
Dependence rating Low
Prescription needed Yes
Available as generic Yes

INFORMATION FOR USERS

Your drug prescription is tailored for you. Do not alter dosage without checking with your doctor.

How taken

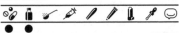

Tablets, liquid.

Frequency and timing of doses
1–2 x daily.

Adult dosage range
60–120mg daily.

Onset of effect
1–3 hours. Some effects may not be felt for 1–2 days.

Duration of action
Up to 12 hours.

Diet advice
Do not take terfenadine with grapefruit juice.

Storage
Keep in a closed container in a cool, dry place out of the reach of children.

Missed dose
No cause for concern, but take as soon as you remember. If your next dose is due within 5 hours, take a single dose now and skip the next.

Stopping the drug
Can be safely stopped as soon as you no longer need it.

Exceeding the dose
An occasional unintentional extra dose is unlikely to cause problems. Large overdoses may cause nausea or drowsiness and have *adverse effects* on the heart. Notify your doctor.

SPECIAL PRECAUTIONS

Be sure to tell your doctor if:
▼ You have a long-term liver problem.
▼ You have any heart problems.
▼ You have had epileptic fits.
▼ You suffer from porphyria.
▼ You have glaucoma.
▼ You are taking other medications.

 Pregnancy
▼ Safety in pregnancy not established. Discuss with your doctor.

 Breast-feeding
▼ No evidence of risk.

 Infants and children
▼ Not recommended for children under 3 years old. Reduced dose necessary in older children.

 Over 60
▼ Increased risk of adverse effects on heart. Reduced dose may be required.

 Driving and hazardous work
▼ Problems are unlikely. However, avoid such activities until you have learned how terfenadine affects you because the drug can cause drowsiness in some people.

Alcohol
▼ Avoid excessive amounts.

POSSIBLE ADVERSE EFFECTS

Indigestion and abdominal pain occur in some cases with terfenadine; other side effects are very unusual. Terfenadine can have adverse effects on the heart; if you have palpitations and/or feel faint while taking the drug, seek medical help without delay.

Symptom/effect	Frequency		Discuss with doctor		Stop taking drug now	Call doctor now
	Common	Rare	Only if severe	In all cases		
Indigestion		●	■			
Headache		●	■			
Drowsiness		●	■			
Dizziness		●		■	▲	▮
Fainting/palpitations		●		■	▲	▮

INTERACTIONS

General note Terfenadine interacts with a wide range of drugs, and with grapefruit juice, to increase the risk of abnormal heart rhythms. Such drugs include antiarrhythmics, anticholinergics, antidepressants, some antibiotics (e.g., erythromycin and clarithromycin), antivirals (e.g., several anti-HIV drugs), antifungals (e.g., ketoconazole and itraconazole), anti-malarials (e.g., halofantrine and quinine), and diuretics (e.g., sotalol and pentamidine isethionate).

Grapefruit juice This may block the breakdown of terfenadine, increasing its effects.

PROLONGED USE

No problems expected. However, use in children should be limited to periods of 1 week unless otherwise directed by a doctor.

Antihistamines should be discontinued approximately 48 hours before allergy skin testing.

TESTOSTERONE

Brand names Andropatch, Primoteston Depot, Restandol, Sustanon, Virormone
Used in the following combined preparations None

GENERAL INFORMATION

Testosterone is a male sex hormone produced by the testes and, in small quantities, by the ovaries in women. The hormone encourages bone and muscle growth in both men and women and stimulates sexual development in men.

The drug is used to initiate puberty in male adolescents if it has been delayed because of a deficiency of the natural hormone. It may help to increase fertility in men suffering from either pituitary or testicular disorders. Rarely, testosterone is used to treat breast cancer.

Testosterone can interfere with growth or cause over-rapid sexual development in adolescents. High doses may cause deepening of the voice, excessive hair growth, or hair loss in women.

QUICK REFERENCE

Drug group Male sex hormone (p.146)

Overdose danger rating Low

Dependence rating Low

Prescription needed Yes

Available as generic Yes

INFORMATION FOR USERS

Your drug prescription is tailored for you. Do not alter dosage without checking with your doctor.

How taken

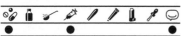

Capsules, injection, patch, implanted pellets.

Frequency and timing of doses
2 x daily (capsules); once every 3 weeks to 2 x weekly (injection) depending on condition being treated; every 6 months (implant); once daily (patch).

Dosage range
Varies with method of administration and the condition being treated.

Onset of effect
2–3 days.

Duration of action
1–2 days (capsules and patch); 1–3 weeks (injection); approximately 6 months (implant).

Diet advice
None.

Storage
Keep in a closed container in a cool, dry place out of the reach of children. Protect from light.

Missed dose
No cause for concern, but take as soon as you remember. If your next dose (by mouth) is due within 3 hours, take a single dose now and skip the next.

Stopping the drug
Do not stop taking the drug without consulting your doctor.

Exceeding the dose
An occasional unintentional extra dose is unlikely to be a cause for concern. But if you notice unusual symptoms, or if a large overdose was taken, notify your doctor.

SPECIAL PRECAUTIONS

Be sure to tell your doctor if:
▼ You have long-term liver or kidney problems.
▼ You have heart problems.
▼ You have prostate trouble.
▼ You have high blood pressure.
▼ You have epilepsy or migraine headaches.
▼ You have diabetes.
▼ You are taking other medications.

Pregnancy
▼ Not prescribed.

Breast-feeding
▼ Not prescribed.

Infants and children
▼ Not prescribed for infants and young children. Reduced dose necessary in adolescents.

Over 60
▼ Rarely required. Increased risk of prostate problems in elderly men. Reduced dose may therefore be necessary.

Driving and hazardous work
▼ No special problems.

Alcohol
▼ No special problems.

POSSIBLE ADVERSE EFFECTS

Most of the more serious *adverse effects* are likely to occur only with long-term treatment with testosterone, and may be helped by a reduction in dosage.

Symptom/effect	Frequency		Discuss with doctor		Stop taking drug now	Call doctor now
	Common	Rare	Only if severe	In all cases		
Jaundice		●		■	▲	
Water retention		●	■			
Men only						
Difficulty in passing urine		●		■		
Abnormal erection	●			■		
Women only						
Unusual hair growth		●	■			
Voice changes		●		■		
Enlarged clitoris		●		■		

PROLONGED USE

Prolonged use of this drug may lead to reduced growth in adolescents.

Monitoring Regular checks of the effects of testosterone treatment are required.

INTERACTIONS

Anticoagulant drugs Testosterone may increase the effect of these drugs. Dosage of anticoagulant drugs may need to be adjusted accordingly.

Antidiabetic agents As testosterone may lower the blood sugar, dosage of antidiabetic drugs and insulin may need to be reduced.

TETRACYCLINE

Brand names Achromycin, Economycin, Tetrachel, Topicycline
Used in the following combined preparations Detaclo, Mysteclin

GENERAL INFORMATION

Tetracyclines were a very widely used group of antibiotics. However, the development of strains of bacteria resistant to these drugs has reduced their effectiveness in many types of infection. Tetracycline is still used for chest infections caused by chlamydia (for example, psittacosis) and myco-plasma microorganisms. It is also used in non-specific urethritis and a number of rarer conditions, such as Q fever, Rocky Mountain spotted fever, cholera, and brucellosis.

Acne improves following long-term treatment with tetracycline drugs either taken by mouth or applied to the skin as a solution.

Common *side effects* of this drug are nausea, vomiting, and diarrhoea. Rashes may also occur. Tetracycline may discolour developing teeth if it is taken by children or by the mother during pregnancy. It is not prescribed for people with poor kidney function as it can cause further deterioration.

INFORMATION FOR USERS

Your drug prescription is tailored for you. Do not alter your dosage without checking with your doctor.

How taken

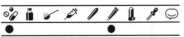

Tablets, capsules, ointment, eye/ear ointment.

Frequency and timing of doses
By mouth 4 x daily, at least 1 hour before or 2 hours after meals. Long-term treatment of acne may require only a single dose daily. *Skin preparations* 1–3 times daily as directed.

Adult dosage range
Infections 1–2g daily.
Acne 250mg–1g daily.

Onset of effect
4–12 hours. Improvement in acne may not be noticed for up to 4 weeks.

Duration of action
Up to 6 hours.

Diet advice
Milk products should be avoided for 1 hour before and 2 hours after taking the drug, since they may impair its absorption.

Storage
Keep in a closed container in a cool, dry place out of the reach of children.

Missed dose
Take as soon as you remember. If your next dose is due within 2 hours, take a single dose now and skip the next.

Stopping the drug
Take the full course. Even if you feel better, the original infection may still be present and may recur if treatment is stopped too soon.

Exceeding the dose
An occasional unintentional extra dose is unlikely to be a cause for concern. But if you notice any unusual symptoms, or if a large overdose has been taken, notify your doctor.

SPECIAL PRECAUTIONS

Be sure to tell your doctor if:
▼ You have long-term liver or kidney problems.
▼ You have previously suffered an allergic reaction to a tetracycline antibiotic.
▼ You are taking other medications.

Pregnancy
▼ Not usually prescribed. May cause discoloured teeth and damage bones of the developing fetus. Discuss with your doctor.

Breast-feeding
▼ The drug passes into the breast milk and may damage developing bones and discolour the baby's teeth. Discuss with your doctor.

Infants and children
▼ Not recommended under 12 years. Reduced dose necessary in older children. May discolour developing teeth.

Over 60
▼ No special problems.

Driving and hazardous work
▼ No known problems.

Alcohol
▼ No known problems.

Taking your tablets
▼ To prevent irritation to the oesophagus, each dose of the drug should be taken with a full glass of water while standing.

POSSIBLE ADVERSE EFFECTS

Adverse effects from skin preparations are rare. When tetracycline is given by mouth, however, it may cause nausea, vomiting, or diarrhoea.

Symptom/effect	Frequency		Discuss with doctor		Stop taking drug now	Call doctor now
	Common	Rare	Only if severe	In all cases		
Nausea/vomiting	●		■			
Diarrhoea	●		■			
Light-sensitive rash		●		■	▲	
Rash/itching		●		■	▲	
Headache/visual disturbance		●		■		

INTERACTIONS

Iron may reduce the effectiveness of tetracycline.

Oral anticoagulants Tetracycline may increase the action of these drugs.

Retinoids may increase the adverse effects of tetracycline.

Oral contraceptives Tetracycline may reduce the effectiveness of oral contraceptives.

Antacids and milk These interfere with the absorption of tetracycline and may reduce its effectiveness. Doses should be separated by 1–2 hours.

PROLONGED USE

No problems expected.

THEOPHYLLINE/AMINOPHYLLINE

Brand names [theophylline] Lasma, Nuelin, Theo-Dur, Uniphyllin; [aminophylline] Amnivent, Phyllocontin
Used in the following combined preparations [theophylline] Do-Do Tablets, Franol, Fanolyn

GENERAL INFORMATION

Theophylline (and aminophylline, which breaks down to theophylline in the body) is used to treat bronchospasm (constriction of the air passages) in patients suffering from asthma, bronchitis, and emphysema.

It is usually taken continuously as a preventative measure, but it is also used to treat acute attacks.

Slow-release formulations of the drugs produce beneficial effects lasting for up to 12 hours. These preparations may be prescribed twice daily, but they are also useful as a single dose taken at night to prevent night-time asthma and early morning wheezing.

Treatment with theophylline must be monitored because the effective dose is very close to the *toxic* dose. Some *adverse effects*, such as indigestion, nausea, headache, and agitation, can be controlled by regulating the dosage and checking blood levels of the drug.

INFORMATION FOR USERS

Your drug prescription is tailored for you. Do not alter dosage without checking with your doctor.

How taken

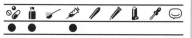

Tablets, SR-tablets, SR-capsules, liquid, injection.

Frequency and timing of doses
3–4 x daily (tablets, liquid); every 12 or 24 hours (SR-tablets/SR-capsules). The drug should be taken at the same time each day in relation to meals.

Dosage range
Adults 375–1,000mg daily, depending on which product is used.

Onset of effect
Within 30 minutes (by mouth); within 90 minutes (SR-tablets/SR-capsules).

Duration of action
Up to 8 hours (by mouth); 12–24 hours (SR-tablets/SR-capsules).

Diet advice
None.

Storage
Keep in a closed container in a cool, dry place out of the reach of children.

Missed dose
Take as soon as you remember. If your next dose is due within 2 hours, take half the dose now (short-acting preparations) or forget about the missed dose and take your next dose now (SR-preparations). Return to your normal dose schedule thereafter.

Stopping the drug
Do not stop taking the drug without consulting your doctor; stopping the drug may lead to worsening of the underlying condition.

OVERDOSE ACTION

 Seek immediate medical advice in all cases. Take emergency action if chest pains, confusion, or loss of consciousness occur.

See Drug poisoning emergency guide (p.494).

SPECIAL PRECAUTIONS

Be sure to consult your doctor or pharmacist before taking this drug if:
▼ You have a long-term liver problem.
▼ You have angina or irregular heart beat.
▼ You have epilepsy.
▼ You have stomach ulcers.
▼ You smoke.
▼ You are taking other medications.

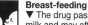 **Pregnancy**
▼ Safety in pregnancy not established. Discuss with your doctor.

 Breast-feeding
▼ The drug passes into the breast milk and may affect the baby. Discuss with your doctor.

 Infants and children
▼ Reduced dose necessary according to age and weight.

 Over 60
▼ Reduced dose may be necessary.

 Driving and hazardous work
▼ No known problems

 Alcohol
▼ Avoid excess as this may alter levels of the drug and may increase gastrointestinal symptoms.

PROLONGED USE

No problems expected.

Monitoring Periodic checks on blood levels of this drug are usually required.

POSSIBLE ADVERSE EFFECTS

Most adverse effects of this drug are related to dosage. These include effects related to the drug's action on the central nervous system, such as agitation and insomnia.

Symptom/effect	Frequency		Discuss with doctor		Stop taking drug now	Call doctor now
	Common	Rare	Only if severe	In all cases		
Agitation		●		■		
Headache	●			■		
Nausea/vomiting	●		■			
Diarrhoea		●	■			
Insomnia		●	■			
Palpitations		●		■	▲	■

INTERACTIONS

General note Many drugs increase the effect of theophylline (e.g., erythromycin and cimetidine); others reduce its effect (e.g., carbamazepine, phenytoin, and rifampicin). Discuss with your doctor.

THIORIDAZINE

Brand names Melleril, Rideril
Used in the following combined preparations None

GENERAL INFORMATION

Thioridazine, one of the phenothiazine antipsychotic group of drugs, was first used in 1959.

This important tranquillizer is widely prescribed to treat a variety of psychiatric conditions. The drug's tranquillizing effect suppresses abnormal behaviour and reduces aggression. Thioridazine is used in the treatment of schizophrenia, mania, dementia, and other disorders where confused or abnormal behaviour may occur. It also helps to relieve the anxiety and depression associated with serious mental disorders. Thioridazine has a similar action to chlorpromazine, but it is less sedating and does not produce movement disorders to the same extent. Consequently, thioridazine is particularly suitable for use in treating the elderly.

The main drawback to the use of this drug is that when given in high doses it can cause eye problems. If large doses are required for long periods, another antipsychotic drug is usually substituted.

INFORMATION FOR USERS

Your drug prescription is tailored for you. Do not alter your dosage without checking with your doctor.

How taken

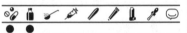

Tablets, liquid.

Frequency and timing of doses
2–4 x daily.

Adult dosage range
30–800mg daily.

Onset of effect
2–3 hours.

Duration of action
4–10 hours. Some effects may last as long as 36 hours.

Diet advice
None.

Storage
Keep in a closed container in a cool, dry place out of the reach of children.

Missed dose
Take as soon as you remember. If your next dose is due within 3 hours, take a single dose now and skip the next.

Stopping the drug
Do not stop the drug without consulting your doctor; symptoms may recur.

Exceeding the dose
An occasional unintentional extra dose is unlikely to cause problems. Large overdoses may cause unusual drowsiness, muscle rigidity, fainting, and agitation. Notify your doctor.

SPECIAL PRECAUTIONS

Be sure to tell your doctor if:
▼ You have liver or kidney problems.
▼ You have heart or circulation problems.
▼ You have had epileptic fits.
▼ You have glaucoma.
▼ You have a heart condition.
▼ You have Parkinson's disease.
▼ You have myasthenia gravis.
▼ You have difficulty in passing urine.
▼ You have porphyria.
▼ You are taking other medications.

Pregnancy
▼ Safety in pregnancy not established. Discuss with your doctor.

Breast-feeding
▼ The drug passes into the breast milk and may affect the baby. Discuss with your doctor.

Infants and children
▼ Not usually prescribed. Reduced dose necessary.

Over 60
▼ Increased likelihood of adverse effects. Reduced dose may therefore be necessary.

Driving and hazardous work
▼ Avoid such activities until you have learned how thioridazine affects you because it may cause drowsiness and blurred vision.

Alcohol
▼ Avoid. Alcohol may increase the sedative effects of this drug.

POSSIBLE ADVERSE EFFECTS

Thioridazine has a strong *anticholinergic* effect that can cause a variety of minor symptoms (see p.79). These often become less marked with time. The most significant adverse effect is a variety of eye problems, such as blurred vision. Adverse effects can be controlled by medically supervised adjustment of dosage, or a change of drug.

Symptom/effect	Frequency		Discuss with doctor		Stop taking drug now	Call doctor now
	Common	Rare	Only if severe	In all cases		
Drowsiness	●		■			
Dry mouth	●		■			
Stuffy nose	●			■		
Blurred vision		●		■		
Muscle stiffness/tremor		●		■		
Unsteadiness		●		■		
Dizziness/fainting		●		■		▲

INTERACTIONS

Sedatives All drugs that have a sedative effect are likely to increase the sedative properties of thioridazine.

Drugs used for parkinsonism Thioridazine may counter the beneficial effect of these drugs.

Anticholinergic drugs The side effects of drugs with anticholinergic properties may be increased by thioridazine.

Antihistamines The risk of terfenadine producing abnormal heart rhythms is increased by thioridazine.

PROLONGED USE

Use of this drug for more than a few months may lead to eye problems and abnormal movements of the face and limbs known as *tardive dyskinesia*. Occasionally, *jaundice* may occur.

Monitoring Eye examinations should be carried out at intervals if the drug is taken long term.

THYROXINE

Brand name Eltroxin
Used in the following combined preparations None

GENERAL INFORMATION

Thyroxine is the major hormone produced by the thyroid gland. A deficiency of the natural hormone causes hypothyroidism and may sometimes lead to myxoedema, a condition characterized by slowing of body functions and facial puffiness. A synthetic preparation is used to replace the natural hormone when it is deficient.

Certain types of goitre (an enlarged thyroid gland) are helped by thyroxine, and it may be prescribed to prevent the development of goitre during treatment with antithyroid drugs. Thyroxine is also prescribed for some forms of thyroid cancer.

Adults who have a severe thyroid deficiency are sensitive to thyroid hormones, so treatment is introduced gradually, and increased slowly, to prevent *adverse effects*. Particular care is required in patients with heart problems such as angina.

QUICK REFERENCE

Drug group Thyroid hormone (p.144)

Overdose danger rating Medium

Dependence rating Low

Prescription needed Yes

Available as generic Yes

INFORMATION FOR USERS

Your drug prescription is tailored for you. Do not alter dosage without checking with your doctor.

How taken

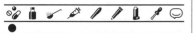

Tablets.

Frequency and timing of doses
Once daily.

Dosage range
Adults Doses of 50–100mcg daily, increased at 3–4-week intervals as required. The maximum dose is 200mcg daily.

Onset of effect
Within 48 hours. Full beneficial effects may not be felt for several weeks.

Duration of action
1–3 weeks.

Diet advice
None.

Storage
Keep in a closed container in a cool, dry place out of the reach of children. Protect from light.

Missed dose
Take as soon as you remember. If your next dose is due within 8 hours, take a single dose now and skip the next.

Stopping the drug
Do not stop the drug without consulting your doctor; symptoms may recur.

Exceeding the dose
An occasional unintentional extra dose is unlikely to cause problems. Large overdoses may cause palpitations during the next few days. Notify your doctor.

SPECIAL PRECAUTIONS

Be sure to tell your doctor if:
▼ You have high blood pressure.
▼ You have heart problems.
▼ You have diabetes.
▼ You are taking other medications.

Pregnancy
▼ No evidence of risk.

Breast-feeding
▼ The drug passes into the breast milk, but at normal doses adverse effects on the baby are unlikely. Discuss with your doctor.

Infants and children
▼ Dosage depends on age and weight.

Over 60
▼ Reduced dose usually necessary.

Driving and hazardous work
▼ No known problems.

Alcohol
▼ No known problems.

POSSIBLE ADVERSE EFFECTS

Adverse effects are rare with thyroxine and are usually the result of overdosage causing thyroid overactivity. These effects diminish as the dose is lowered. Too low a dose of thyroxine may cause signs of thyroid underactivity.

Symptom/effect	Frequency		Discuss with doctor		Stop taking drug now	Call doctor now
	Common	Rare	Only if severe	In all cases		
Anxiety/agitation		●		■		
Diarrhoea		●		■		
Weight loss		●		■		
Sweating/flushing		●		■		
Muscle cramps		●		■		
Palpitations/chest pain		●		■		■

INTERACTIONS

Oral anticoagulants Thyroxine may increase the effect of these drugs.

Cholestyramine This drug may reduce the absorption of thyroxine.

Sucralfate The absorption of thyroxine may be reduced by sucralfate.

Antidiabetic agents The doses of these drugs may need increasing once thyroxine treatment is started.

PROLONGED USE

No special problems.

Monitoring Periodic tests of thyroid function are usually required.

TIBOLONE

Brand name Livial
Used in the following combined preparations None

GENERAL INFORMATION

Tibolone is used for treating symptoms of natural or surgical menopause, such as sweating, depressed mood, and decreased sex drive, and is particularly effective in controlling hot flushes. The drug is taken continuously and, unlike most of the other available hormone replacement therapies, the treatment does not require a cyclical course of progestogen to be taken as well. This is because the drug has both oestrogenic and progestogenic activity.

Tibolone has a low incidence of *side effects* and does not cause *withdrawal* bleeding in post-menopausal women. However, this drug is not used long term for preventing osteoporosis after the menopause.

INFORMATION FOR USERS

Your drug prescription is tailored for you. Do not alter dosage without checking with your doctor.

How taken

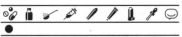

Tablets.

Frequency and timing of doses
Daily, preferably at the same time each day. Swallow the tablets whole – do not chew.

Adult dosage range
2.5mg daily.

Onset of effect
You may notice improvement of symptoms within a few weeks but the best results are obtained when the drug is taken for at least 3 months.

Duration of action
A few days.

Diet advice
None.

Storage
Keep in a closed container in a cool, dry place out of the reach of children. Protect from light.

Missed dose
Take as soon as you remember.

Stopping the drug
Do not stop the drug without consulting your doctor; symptoms may recur.

Exceeding the dose
An occasional unintentional extra dose is unlikely to be a cause for concern. If several tablets are taken together, they may cause a stomach upset. Notify your doctor.

SPECIAL PRECAUTIONS

Be sure to tell your doctor if:
▼ You have long-term liver or kidney problems.
▼ You suffer from epilepsy or migraine.
▼ You have diabetes.
▼ You have a tumour.
▼ You have a history of cardiovascular or cerebrovascular disease.
▼ You have a high cholesterol level.
▼ You have vaginal bleeding.
▼ You have had a period in the last 12 months.
▼ You are taking other medications.

 Pregnancy
▼ Not prescribed.

 Breast-feeding
▼ Not prescribed.

 Infants and children
▼ Not prescribed.

 Over 60
▼ No special problems.

 Driving and hazardous work
▼ No problems expected.

 Alcohol
▼ No known problems.

POSSIBLE ADVERSE EFFECTS

Tibolone is well tolerated and the incidence of adverse effects is low. Vaginal bleeding is more likely if it is less than one year since the menopause. For this reason, the drug is not recommended if less than 12 months have passed since your last period.

Symptom/effect	Frequency		Discuss with doctor		Stop taking drug now	Call doctor now
	Common	Rare	Only if severe	In all cases		
Weight increase	●		■			
Ankle swelling	●		■			
Dizziness	●		■			
Acne	●			■		
Vaginal bleeding	●			■		
Headache	●		■			
Stomach upset	●		■			
Facial hair growth	●		■			
Jaundice		●		■	▲	∎

INTERACTIONS

Some anticonvulsants Phenytoin, phenobarbitone, primidone, and carbamazepine can accelerate the metabolism of tibolone and so decrease blood levels of the drug and its effectiveness.

Rifampicin This can accelerate the metabolism of tibolone and so decrease blood levels of the drug and its effectiveness.

PROLONGED USE

Monitoring Periodic examination by your doctor is advised.

TIMOLOL

Brand names Betim, Blocadren, Glau-opt, Timoptol
Used in the following combined preparations Moducren, Prestim

GENERAL INFORMATION

Timolol is a beta blocker prescribed to treat hypertension (high blood pressure) and angina (pain due to narrowing of the coronary arteries). It may be given after a heart attack to prevent further damage to the heart muscle. When used to treat hypertension, it may also be given with a diuretic. Timolol is commonly administered as eye drops to people with certain types of glaucoma, and is occasionally given to prevent migraine.

Timolol can cause breathing difficulties, especially in people who have asthma, chronic bronchitis, or emphysema. This problem is more likely in people taking the drug in tablet form, although it can also occur in individuals using timolol eye drops. As with other beta blockers, timolol may mask the body's response to low blood sugar and, for that reason, is prescribed with caution to diabetics.

INFORMATION FOR USERS

Your drug prescription is tailored for you. Do not alter dosage without checking with your doctor.

How taken

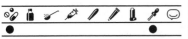

Tablets, eye drops.

Frequency and timing of doses
1–3 x daily.

Adult dosage range
By mouth 10–60mg daily (hypertension); 10–45mg daily (angina); 10–20mg daily (after a heart attack); 10–20mg daily (migraine prevention).

Onset of effect
Within 30 minutes (by mouth).

Duration of action
Up to 24 hours.

Diet advice
None.

Storage
Keep in a closed container in a cool, dry place out of the reach of children.

Missed dose
Take as soon as you remember. If your next dose is due within 3 hours, take a single dose now and skip the next.

Stopping the drug
Do not stop the drug without consulting your doctor; stopping the drug may lead to worsening of the underlying condition.

OVERDOSE ACTION

Seek immediate medical advice in all cases of overdose by mouth. Take emergency action if breathing difficulties, palpitations, or loss of consciousness occur.

See Drug poisoning emergency guide (p.494).

POSSIBLE ADVERSE EFFECTS

Timolol taken by mouth can occasionally provoke or worsen heart problems and asthma. Fainting may be a sign that the drug has slowed the heartbeat excessively. Eye drops cause these problems only rarely; headache or blurred vision is more likely.

Symptom/effect	Frequency		Discuss with doctor		Stop taking drug now	Call doctor now
	Common	Rare	Only if severe	In all cases		
Lethargy/fatigue/headache	●			■		
Blurred vision (eye drops)	●			■		
Eye irritation (eye drops)		●		■		
Cold hands/feet		●		■		
Dizziness/fainting		●			■	
Nightmares/vivid dreams		●			■	
Wheezing/breathlessness		●			■	▲	■

SPECIAL PRECAUTIONS

Be sure to tell your doctor if:
▼ You have a lung disorder such as asthma, bronchitis, or emphysema.
▼ You have diabetes.
▼ You have myasthenia gravis.
▼ You have poor circulation.
▼ You have allergies.
▼ You are taking other medications.

Pregnancy
▼ Safety in pregnancy not established. Discuss with your doctor.

Breast-feeding
▼ The drug passes into the breast milk, but at normal doses *adverse effects* on the baby are unlikely. Discuss with your doctor.

Infants and children
▼ Not usually prescribed.

Over 60
▼ Reduced dose may be necessary.

Driving and hazardous work
▼ Avoid such activities until you have learned how timolol affects you because the tablets may cause drowsiness and the eye drops may cause blurred vision.

Alcohol
▼ May enhance lowering of blood pressure; avoid excessive amounts.

Surgery and general anaesthetics
▼ Timolol by mouth may need to be stopped before you have a general anaesthetic. Discuss with your doctor or dentist before any surgery.

INTERACTIONS

Sympathomimetics Present in many cough and cold remedies, these drugs can cause a dangerous rise in blood pressure when taken with timolol.

Salbutamol, salmeterol, and other beta agonists The effects of these drugs may be reduced by timolol.

PROLONGED USE

No problems expected.

TOLBUTAMIDE

Brand name None
Used in the following combined preparations None

GENERAL INFORMATION

Tolbutamide is an antidiabetic agent that lowers blood sugar by stimulating insulin secretion from the pancreas. Taken by mouth, it is used to treat adult (maturity-onset or Type 2) diabetes in which active insulin-secreting cells are still present. Where these are lacking, as in juvenile diabetes, the drug is ineffective.

Tolbutamide does not act in isolation, but is administered in conjunction with a special diabetic diet that limits the patient's carbohydrate intake.

Shorter-acting than many other oral antidiabetic drugs, tolbutamide may help in the initial control of diabetes. It may also be given to people with impaired kidney function because it is less likely to build up in the body and cause excessive lowering of blood sugar. As with other oral antidiabetic drugs, tolbutamide may need to be replaced with insulin during serious illnesses, injury, or surgery, when diabetic control is lost.

QUICK REFERENCE

Drug group Antidiabetic drug (p.142)

Overdose danger rating High

Dependence rating Low

Prescription needed Yes

Available as generic Yes

INFORMATION FOR USERS

Your drug prescription is tailored for you. Do not alter dosage without checking with your doctor.

How taken

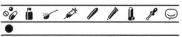

Tablets.

Frequency and timing of doses
Taken with meals either once daily in the morning, or 2 x daily in the morning and evening.

Adult dosage range
500mg–2g daily.

Onset of effect
Within 1 hour.

Duration of action
6–10 hours.

Diet advice
A low-fat, low-carbohydrate diet must be maintained for the drug to be fully effective. Follow the advice of your doctor.

Storage
Keep in a closed container in a cool, dry place out of the reach of children. Protect from light.

Missed dose
Take as soon as you remember. If your next dose is due within 2 hours, take a single dose now and skip the next.

Stopping the drug
Do not stop the drug without consulting your doctor; stopping the drug may lead to worsening of the underlying condition.

OVERDOSE ACTION

Seek immediate medical advice in all cases. If faintness, confusion, or headache occur, eat something sugary. Take emergency action if fits or loss of consciousness occur.

See Drug poisoning emergency guide (p.494).

SPECIAL PRECAUTIONS

Be sure to tell your doctor if:
▼ You have long-term liver or kidney problems.
▼ You are allergic to sulphonamides.
▼ You have thyroid problems.
▼ You are taking other medications.

Pregnancy
▼ Not usually prescribed. May cause birth defects if taken in the first 3 months of pregnancy. Discuss with your doctor.

Breast-feeding
▼ The drug passes into the breast milk and may affect the baby. Discuss with your doctor.

Infants and children
▼ Not prescribed.

Over 60
▼ Increased risk of low blood sugar. Reduced dose is therefore usually necessary.

Driving and hazardous work
▼ Usually no problem. Avoid these activities if you have warning signs of low blood sugar.

Alcohol
▼ Keep consumption low. Alcohol may upset diabetic control.

Surgery and general anaesthetics
▼ Notify your doctor that you are diabetic before any surgery; insulin treatment may need to be substituted.

PROLONGED USE

No problems expected.

Monitoring Regular monitoring of urine and/or blood sugar is required.

POSSIBLE ADVERSE EFFECTS

Serious *adverse effects* are rare with this drug. Symptoms such as dizziness, sweating, weakness, and confusion may indicate low blood sugar levels.

Symptom/effect	Frequency		Discuss with doctor		Stop taking drug now	Call doctor now
	Common	Rare	Only if severe	In all cases		
Dizziness/confusion	●			■		
Weakness/sweating	●			■		
Headache		●	■			
Nausea/vomiting		●		■		
Jaundice		●		■	▲	▮
Rash/itching		●		■	▲	▮

INTERACTIONS

General note A variety of drugs may oppose the effect of tolbutamide and so may raise blood sugar levels. Such drugs include corticosteroids, oestrogens, diuretics, and rifampicin. Other drugs increase the risk of low blood sugar. These include warfarin, sulphonamides, beta blockers, chloramphenicol, clofibrate, aspirin and other non-steroidal anti-inflammatory drugs (NSAIDs), and monoamine oxidase inhibitors (MAOIs).

TOLTERODINE

Brand name Detrusitol
Used in the following combined preparations None

GENERAL INFORMATION

Tolterodine is an *anticholinergic* and antispasmodic drug that is similar to atropine (p.203). It is used to treat urinary frequency and incontinence in adults. Tolterodine works by reducing contraction of the bladder, allowing it to expand and hold more. It also stops spasms and delays the desire to empty the bladder.

Tolterodine's usefulness is limited to some extent by its *side effects*, and dosage needs to be reduced in the elderly. Children are more susceptible than adults to the drug's anticholinergic effects. Tolterodine can also trigger glaucoma.

INFORMATION FOR USERS

Your drug prescription is tailored for you. Do not alter dosage without checking with your doctor.

How taken

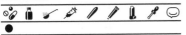

Tablets.

Frequency and timing of doses
2 x daily.

Dosage range
4mg daily, reduced to 2mg daily, if necessary, to minimize side effects.

Onset of effect
1 hour.

Duration of action
12 hours.

Diet advice
None.

Storage
Keep in a closed container in a cool, dry place out of the reach of children.

Missed dose
Take as soon as you remember. If your next dose is due within 2 hours, take a single dose now and skip the next.

Stopping the drug
Do not stop taking the drug without consulting your doctor; symptoms may recur.

Exceeding the dose
An occasional unintentional extra dose is unlikely to cause problems. Large overdoses may cause visual disturbances, urinary difficulties, hallucinations, convulsions, and breathing difficulties. Notify your doctor.

SPECIAL PRECAUTIONS

Be sure to tell your doctor if:
▼ You have liver or kidney problems.
▼ You have thyroid problems.
▼ You have heart problems.
▼ You have porphyria.
▼ You have hiatus hernia.
▼ You have ulcerative colitis.
▼ You have glaucoma.
▼ You have myasthenia gravis.
▼ You are taking other medications.

Pregnancy
▼ Safety in pregnancy not established. May harm the unborn baby. Discuss with your doctor.

Breast-feeding
▼ Safety not established. Discuss with your doctor.

Infants and children
▼ Not recommended. Safety not established.

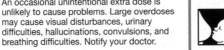

Over 60
▼ Reduced dose may be necessary.

Driving and hazardous work
▼ Avoid. Tolterodine may cause drowsiness, disorientation, and blurred vision.

Alcohol
▼ Avoid. Alcohol increases the drug's sedative effects.

POSSIBLE ADVERSE EFFECTS

The most common side effects, such as dry mouth, digestive upset, and dry eyes, are the result of the drug's anticholinergic action.

Symptom/effect	Frequency		Discuss with doctor		Stop taking drug now	Call doctor now
	Common	Rare	Only if severe	In all cases		
Dry mouth/digestive upset	●		■			
Constipation/abdominal pain	●		■			
Headache	●		■			
Dry eyes/blurred vision	●		■			
Drowsiness/nervousness	●		■			
Chest pain		●			■	
Confusion		●			■	
Urinary difficulties		●			■	

INTERACTIONS

General note All drugs that have an anticholinergic effect will have increased side effects when taken with tolterodine.

Cisapride, domperidone and metoclopramide The effects of these drugs may be decreased by tolterodine.

Erythromycin, clarithromycin, itraconazole, ketoconazole, and miconazole These drugs may increase blood levels of tolterodine.

PROLONGED USE

No special problems. Effectiveness of the drug, and continuing clinical need for it, are usually reviewed after 6 months.

Monitoring Periodic eye tests for glaucoma may be performed.

TRAMADOL

Brand names Tramake, Zamadol, Zydol
Used in the following combined preparations None

GENERAL INFORMATION

Tramadol is a synthetic *opioid* analgesic chemically similar to natural opioids. It is used to prevent or treat moderate pain and severe pain of, for example, a heart attack, injury, surgery, or cancer.

The painkilling effect of tramadol wears off after about 4 hours, but the drug can be given in a slow-release (long-acting) form, which gives relief for up to 12 hours.

Tramadol can be habit-forming, and dependence may occur. But most people who take it for a short time do not become dependent and are able to stop taking it without difficulty. The drug is said to be less likely than the older opioids to cause breathing problems and constipation. Its *side effects* include hallucinations and confusion.

INFORMATION FOR USERS

Your drug prescription is tailored for you. Do not alter dosage without checking with your doctor.

How taken

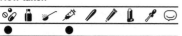

Tablets, SR-tablets, capsules, SR-capsules, injection, sachets.

Frequency and timing of doses
Up to 6 x daily.

Adult dosage range
Up to 400mg daily (by mouth); 600mg daily (injection).

Onset of effect
30–60 minutes (by mouth); 15–30 minutes (injection).

Duration of action
4 hours.

Diet advice
None.

Storage
Keep in a closed container in a cool, dry place out of the reach of children.

Missed dose
Take as soon as you remember, and return to your normal schedule as soon as possible.

Stopping the drug
If the reason for taking tramadol no longer exists, you may stop taking the drug and notify your doctor. If you have been taking it for a long time, you may experience withdrawal effects.

OVERDOSE ACTION

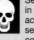 Seek immediate medical advice in all cases. Take emergency action if breathing difficulties, severe drowsiness, or loss of consciousness occur.

See Drug poisoning emergency guide (p.494).

SPECIAL PRECAUTIONS

Be sure to tell your doctor if:
▼ You have had a head injury.
▼ You have liver or kidney problems.
▼ You have heart or circulatory problems.
▼ You have a lung disorder such as asthma or bronchitis.
▼ You have thyroid disease.
▼ You have a history of epileptic fits.
▼ You are taking other medications.

 Pregnancy
▼ Safety not established. Discuss with your doctor.

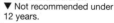 **Breast-feeding**
▼ The drug passes into the breast milk and may make the baby drowsy. Discuss with your doctor.

 Infants and children
▼ Not recommended under 12 years.

 Over 60
▼ Reduced dose may be necessary.

 Driving and hazardous work
▼ Avoid. Tramadol can cause drowsiness.

Alcohol
▼ Avoid. Alcohol increases the sedative effects of tramadol.

POSSIBLE ADVERSE EFFECTS

Adverse effects such as drowsiness seem more common than with some other opioids.

Symptom/effect	Frequency		Discuss with doctor		Stop taking drug now	Call doctor now
	Common	Rare	Only if severe	In all cases		
Nausea/vomiting	●		■			
Dry mouth	●		■			
Tiredness	●		■			
Drowsiness	●		■			
Dizziness/headache		●	■			
Confusion/hallucinations		●		■		
Convulsions		●		■	▲	▮
Wheezing/breathlessness		●		■	▲	▮

PROLONGED USE

Dependence may occur if tramadol is taken for long periods.

INTERACTIONS

Antidepressants Some antidepressants may increase the risk of convulsions if taken with tramadol.

Carbamazepine This drug may reduce blood levels and effects of tramadol.

Sedatives All drugs that have a sedative effect are likely to increase the sedative effects of tramadol. Such drugs include antidepressants, antipsychotics, antihistamines, and sleeping drugs.

TRAZODONE

Brand name Molipaxin
Used in the following combined preparations None

GENERAL INFORMATION

Trazodone is one of many drugs used to treat depression. It helps to elevate the patient's mood and restore interest in everyday activities. Because the drug has a strong sedative effect, it is particularly useful when the depression is accompanied by anxiety, insomnia, or both. Consequently, when taken at night trazodone helps to reduce the need for sleeping drugs.

The drug is less likely to cause *side effects* than tricyclic antidepressants. Trazodone is also safer for people with heart problems, and is therefore commonly used to treat depression in elderly patients.

QUICK REFERENCE

Drug group Antidepressant (p.84)
Overdose danger rating Medium
Dependence rating Low
Prescription needed Yes
Available as generic No

INFORMATION FOR USERS

Your drug prescription is tailored for you. Do not alter dosage without checking with your doctor.

How taken

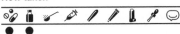

Tablets, capsules, liquid.

Frequency and timing of doses
1–3 x daily with food.

Adult dosage range
150mg daily (starting dose), increased to 200–300mg, occasionally up to 600mg, daily (maintenance dose).

Onset of effect
Some benefits and adverse effects may appear within a few days of starting treatment, but full antidepressant effect may not be felt for 2–4 weeks.

Duration of action
Adverse effects may last up to 24 hours after stopping the drug. Following cessation of prolonged treatment, the antidepressant effect may persist for up to 6 weeks.

Diet advice
None.

Storage
Keep in a closed container in a cool, dry place out of the reach of children. Protect from light.

Missed dose
Take as soon as you remember. If your next dose is due within 3 hours, take a single dose now and skip the next.

Stopping the drug
Do not stop the drug without consulting your doctor; symptoms may recur.

Exceeding the dose
An occasional unintentional extra dose is unlikely to cause problems. Large doses may cause unusual drowsiness. Notify your doctor.

SPECIAL PRECAUTIONS

Be sure to tell your doctor if:
▼ You have had epileptic fits.
▼ You have long-term liver or kidney problems.
▼ You have heart disease or are recovering from a recent heart attack.
▼ You are taking other medications.

Pregnancy
▼ Safety in pregnancy not established. Discuss with your doctor.

Breast-feeding
▼ The drug passes into the breast milk, but at normal doses adverse effects on the baby are unlikely. Discuss with your doctor.

Infants and children
▼ Not recommended.

Over 60
▼ Increased likelihood of adverse effects. Reduced dose may therefore be necessary.

Driving and hazardous work
▼ Avoid such activities until you have learned how trazodone affects you because the drug can cause drowsiness.

Alcohol
▼ Avoid. Alcohol may increase the sedative effects of this drug.

POSSIBLE ADVERSE EFFECTS

Trazodone has fewer common adverse effects than some of the other antidepressants, mainly because it has a much weaker *anticholinergic* action.

Symptom/effect	Frequency		Discuss with doctor		Stop taking drug now	Call doctor now
	Common	Rare	Only if severe	In all cases		
Drowsiness	●			■		
Constipation/diarrhoea		●		■		
Dry mouth		●		■		
Dizziness/fainting		●		■		
Headache		●		■		
Rash		●		■	▲	
Painful/prolonged erection		●		■	▲	■

INTERACTIONS

Sedatives All drugs that have a sedative effect on the central nervous system are likely to increase the sedative properties of trazodone. Such drugs include sleeping drugs, antipsychotic drugs, antihistamines, and *opioid* analgesics.

Anticonvulsants Trazodone may reduce the effects of these drugs.

Monoamine oxidase inhibitors (MAOIs) Trazodone may cause serious adverse effects if given with these antidepressants.

PROLONGED USE

No problems expected.

TRIAMTERENE

Brand name Dytac
Used in the following combined preparations Dyazide (co-triamterzide), Dytide, Frusene, Kalspare, Triam-Co, TriamaxCo

GENERAL INFORMATION

Triamterene belongs to the class of drugs known as potassium-sparing diuretics. In combination with thiazide or loop diuretics, this drug is given for the treatment of hypertension and oedema (fluid retention). Triamterene, either on its own or, more commonly, with a thiazide diuretic, may be used to treat oedema as a complication of heart failure, nephrotic syndrome, or cirrhosis of the liver.

Triamterene is quick to act; its effect on urine flow is apparent within two hours. For this reason, you should avoid taking the drug after about 4 pm. As with other potassium-sparing diuretics, unusually high levels of potassium may build up in the blood if the kidneys are functioning abnormally. Therefore, triamterene is prescribed with caution to people with kidney failure.

QUICK REFERENCE

Drug group Potassium-sparing diuretic (p.99)

Overdose danger rating Low

Dependence rating Low

Prescription needed Yes

Available as generic No

INFORMATION FOR USERS

Your drug prescription is tailored for you. Do not alter dosage without checking with your doctor.

How taken

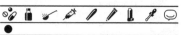

Tablets.

Frequency and timing of doses
1–2 x daily after meals or on alternate days.

Adult dosage range
50–250mg daily.

Onset of effect
Within 2 hours.

Duration of action
9–12 hours.

Diet advice
Avoid foods that are high in potassium, such as dried fruit and salt substitutes.

Storage
Keep in a closed container in a cool, dry place out of the reach of children.

Missed dose
Take as soon as you remember. However, if it is late in the day, do not take the missed dose, or you may need to get up at night to pass urine. Take the next scheduled dose as usual.

Stopping the drug
Do not stop the drug without consulting your doctor; symptoms may recur.

Exceeding the dose
An occasional unintentional extra dose is unlikely to be a cause for concern. But if you notice any unusual symptoms, or if a large overdose has been taken, notify your doctor.

SPECIAL PRECAUTIONS

Be sure to tell your doctor if:
▼ You have long-term liver or kidney problems.
▼ You have had kidney stones.
▼ You have gout.
▼ You are taking other medications.

Pregnancy
▼ Not usually prescribed. May cause a reduction in the blood supply to the developing fetus. Discuss with your doctor.

Breast-feeding
▼ The drug passes into breast milk and may affect the baby. It could also reduce your milk supply. Discuss with your doctor.

Infants and children
▼ Not usually prescribed. Reduced dose necessary.

Over 60
▼ Increased likelihood of adverse effects. Reduced dose may therefore be necessary.

Driving and hazardous work
▼ No special problems.

Alcohol
▼ No known problems.

POSSIBLE ADVERSE EFFECTS

Triamterene has few adverse effects; the main problem is the possibility of potassium being retained by the body, causing muscle weakness and numbness. Triamterene may colour your urine blue but this is not a cause for concern.

Symptom/effect	Frequency		Discuss with doctor		Stop taking drug now	Call doctor now
	Common	Rare	Only if severe	In all cases		
Digestive disturbance		●	■			
Headache		●	■			
Muscle weakness		●		■		
Rash		●		■		
Dry mouth		●	■			

INTERACTIONS

Lithium Triamterene may increase the blood levels of lithium, leading to an increased risk of lithium *toxicity*.

Non-steroidal anti-inflammatory drugs (NSAIDs) may increase the risk of raised blood levels of potassium.

ACE inhibitors These drugs increase the risk of raised blood levels of potassium with triamterene.

Cyclosporin This drug may increase levels of potassium with triamterene.

PROLONGED USE

Serious problems are unlikely, but levels of salts such as sodium and potassium may occasionally become abnormal during prolonged use.

Monitoring Blood tests may be performed to check on kidney function and levels of body salts.

TRIMETHOPRIM

Brand names Monotrim, Trimogal, Trimopan, Triprimix
Used in the following combined preparations Comixco, Co-trimoxazole, Fectrim, Septrin, and others

GENERAL INFORMATION

Trimethoprim is an antibacterial drug that became popular in the 1970s for prevention and treatment of infections of the urinary and respiratory tracts. The drug has been used for many years in combination with another antibacterial, sulfamethoxazole, in a preparation known as co-trimoxazole (see p.246). Trimethoprim, however, has fewer *adverse effects* than co-trimoxazole and is equally effective in treating many conditions. The drug can also be given by injection to treat severe infections.

Although *side effects* of trimethoprim are not usually troublesome, tests to monitor blood composition are often advised when the drug is taken for prolonged periods.

QUICK REFERENCE

Drug group Antibacterial drug (p.131)

Overdose danger rating Low

Dependence rating Low

Prescription needed Yes

Available as generic Yes

INFORMATION FOR USERS

Your drug prescription is tailored for you. Do not alter dosage without checking with your doctor.

How taken

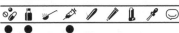

Tablets, liquid, injection.

Frequency and timing of doses
1–2 x daily.

Adult dosage range
300–400mg daily (treatment);
100–200mg daily (prevention).

Onset of effect
1–4 hours.

Duration of action
Up to 24 hours.

Diet advice
None.

Storage
Keep in a closed container in a cool, dry place out of the reach of children. Protect from light.

Missed dose
Take as soon as you remember.

Stopping the drug
Take the full course. Even if you feel better, the original infection may still be present and symptoms may recur if treatment is stopped too soon.

Exceeding the dose
An occasional unintentional extra dose is unlikely to be a cause for concern. But if you notice any unusual symptoms, or if a large overdose has been taken, notify your doctor.

SPECIAL PRECAUTIONS

Be sure to tell your doctor if:
▼ You have long-term liver or kidney problems.
▼ You have a blood disorder.
▼ You have porphyria.
▼ You are taking other medications.

Pregnancy
▼ Safety in pregnancy not established. Discuss with your doctor.

Breast-feeding
▼ The drug passes into the breast milk, but at normal doses adverse effects on the baby are unlikely. Discuss with your doctor.

Infants and children
▼ Reduced dose necessary.

Over 60
▼ Increased likelihood of adverse effects. Reduced dose may be required.

Driving and hazardous work
▼ No known problems.

Alcohol
▼ No known problems.

POSSIBLE ADVERSE EFFECTS

Trimethoprim taken on its own rarely causes side effects. However, additional adverse effects may occur when trimethoprim is taken in combination with sulfamethoxazole.

Symptom/effect	Frequency		Discuss with doctor		Stop taking drug now	Call doctor now
	Common	Rare	Only if severe	In all cases		
Nausea/vomiting		●		■		
Rash/itching		●			■	▲
Sore throat/fever		●			■	▲

INTERACTIONS

Phenytoin Taken with trimethoprim, this drug may increase the risk of folic acid deficiency, resulting in blood abnormalities.

Warfarin Trimethoprim may increase the anticoagulant effect of warfarin.

Cyclosporin Trimethoprim increases the risk of this drug causing kidney damage.

Antimalarials containing pyrimethamine Drugs such as fansidar or maloprim may increase the risk of folic acid deficiency, resulting in blood abnormalities, if they are taken with trimethoprim.

PROLONGED USE

Long-term use of this drug may lead to folate deficiency, which, in turn, may lead to blood abnormalities. Folate supplements may be prescribed.

Monitoring Periodic blood tests to monitor blood composition are usually advised.

VENLAFAXINE

Brand name Efexor
Used in the following combined preparations None

GENERAL INFORMATION

Venlafaxine is a new antidepressant with a chemical structure unlike any other available antidepressant. It combines the therapeutic properties of both the tricyclic antidepressants and selective serotonin reuptake inhibitors (SSRIs), without *anticholinergic adverse effects*.

As with other antidepressants, this drug acts to elevate mood, increase physical activity, and restore interest in everyday activities.

Nausea, dizziness, drowsiness or insomnia, and restlessness are common adverse effects. Weight loss may occur due to decreased appetite. The drug can cause an elevation of blood pressure, which should be monitored during the course of treatment.

INFORMATION FOR USERS

Your drug prescription is tailored for you. Do not alter dosage without checking with your doctor.

How taken

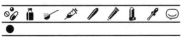

Tablets.

Frequency and timing of doses
2–3 x daily (tablets); once daily (SR-tablets). The tablets should be taken with food.

Dosage range
75–150mg daily for outpatients; up to 375mg daily in severely depressed patients.

Onset of effect
Can appear within days, although full antidepressant effect may not be felt for 2–4 weeks, or longer.

Duration of action
About 8–12 hours; 24 hours for SR-tablets. Following prolonged treatment, antidepressant effects may persist for up to 6 weeks.

Diet advice
None.

Storage
Keep in the original container in a cool, dry place out of the reach of children.

Missed dose
Do not make up for a missed dose. Just take your next regularly scheduled dose.

Stopping the drug
Do not stop the drug without consulting your doctor, who may supervise a gradual reduction in dosage.

OVERDOSE ACTION

 Seek immediate medical advice in all cases. Take emergency action if fits, slow or irregular pulse, or loss of consciousness occur.

See Drug poisoning emergency guide (p.494).

SPECIAL PRECAUTIONS

Be sure to tell your doctor if:
▼ You have had an adverse reaction to any other antidepressants.
▼ You have long-term liver or kidney problems.
▼ You have a heart problem or elevated blood pressure.
▼ You have had epileptic fits.
▼ You have had problems with alcohol or drug misuse/abuse.
▼ You are taking other medications.

 Pregnancy
▼ Safety in pregnancy not established. Discuss with your doctor.

 Breast-feeding
▼ Not recommended. Discuss with your doctor.

 Infants and children
▼ Not recommended under 18 years.

 Over 60
▼ Increased likelihood of adverse effects. Reduced dose may therefore be necessary.

Driving and hazardous work
▼ Avoid such activities until you have learned how venlafaxine affects you because the drug can cause dizziness, drowsiness, and blurred vision.

 Alcohol
▼ Avoid. Alcohol may increase the sedative effects of this drug.

PROLONGED USE

No problems expected.

Monitoring Blood pressure should be measured periodically.

POSSIBLE ADVERSE EFFECTS

The most common adverse effects are weakness, nausea, restlessness, and drowsiness. Some of these effects may wear off within a few days. Restlessness may include anxiety, nervousness, tremor, abnormal dreams, agitation, and confusion.

Symptom/effect	Frequency		Discuss with doctor		Stop taking drug now	Call doctor now
	Common	Rare	Only if severe	In all cases		
Nausea	●			■		
Restlessness/insomnia	●			■		
Weakness/blurred vision	●			■		
Drowsiness/dizziness	●			■		
Decreased appetite		●	■			
Sexual dysfunction		●	■		▲	
Rash/itching		●	■		▲	■

INTERACTIONS

Sedatives All drugs with a sedative effect are likely to increase the sedative effects of venlafaxine.

Antihypertensive drugs Treatment with venlafaxine may reduce the effectiveness of these drugs.

Monoamine oxidase inhibitors (MAOIs) Venlafaxine may interact with these drugs to produce a dangerous rise in blood pressure. Therefore, at least 14 days should elapse between stopping MAOIs and starting venlafaxine.

VERAPAMIL

Brand names Berkatens, Cordilox, Ethimil, Securon-SR, Univer, Verapress
Used in the following combined preparations None

GENERAL INFORMATION

Verapamil belongs to a group of drugs known as calcium channel blockers, which interfere with the conduction of signals in the muscles of the heart and blood vessels. It is used in the treatment of hypertension, abnormal heart rhythms, and angina. It reduces the frequency of angina attacks but does not work quickly enough to help relieve pain while an attack is in progress. Verapamil increases the ability to tolerate physical exertion, and unlike some drugs it does not affect breathing so it can be used safely by asthmatics.

Because of its effects on the heart, verapamil is also prescribed for certain types of abnormal heart rhythm. For such disorders it can be administered by injection as well as in tablet form.

Verapamil is not generally prescribed for people with low blood pressure, slow heart beat, or heart failure, because it may worsen these conditions. The drug may also cause constipation.

INFORMATION FOR USERS

Your drug prescription is tailored for you. Do not alter dosage without checking with your doctor.

How taken

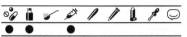

Tablets, SR-tablets, SR-capsules liquid, injection.

Frequency and timing of doses
2–3 x daily (tablets, liquid); 1–2 x daily (SR-tablets).

Adult dosage range
120–480mg daily.

Onset of effect
1–2 hours (tablets); 2–3 minutes (injection).

Duration of action
6–8 hours. During prolonged treatment some beneficial effects may last for up to 12 hours. SR-tablets act for 12–24 hours.

Diet advice
Avoid grapefruit juice which may increase blood levels of verapamil.

Storage
Keep in a closed container in a cool, dry place out of the reach of children.

Missed dose
Take as soon as you remember. If your next dose is due within 3 hours (tablets, liquid) or 8 hours (SR-tablets, SR-capsules), take a single dose now and skip the next.

Stopping the drug
Do not stop the drug without consulting your doctor; symptoms may recur.

Exceeding the dose
An occasional unintentional extra dose is unlikely to be a cause for concern. Large overdoses may cause dizziness. Notify your doctor.

POSSIBLE ADVERSE EFFECTS

Verapamil has fewer *adverse effects* than other calcium channel blockers, but it can still cause a variety of minor symptoms, such as nausea, constipation, and headache.

Symptom/effect	Frequency		Discuss with doctor		Stop taking drug now	Call doctor now
	Common	Rare	Only if severe	In all cases		
Constipation	●			■		
Headache	●			■		
Nausea/vomiting	●			■		
Ankle swelling	●			■		
Flushing		●		■		
Dizziness		●			■	
Rash		●			■	■

INTERACTIONS

Beta blockers When verapamil is taken with these drugs, there is a slight risk of abnormal heart beat and heart failure.

Carbamazepine The effects of this drug may be enhanced by verapamil.

Cyclosporin The blood levels of this drug may be increased by verapamil and its dose may need to be reduced.

Antihypertensive drugs Blood pressure may be further lowered when these drugs are taken with verapamil.

Digoxin The effects of this drug may be increased if it is taken with verapamil. The dosage of digoxin may need to be reduced.

SPECIAL PRECAUTIONS

Be sure to tell your doctor if:
▼ You have a long-term liver problem.
▼ You have porphyria.
▼ You are taking other medications.

Pregnancy
▼ Not usually prescribed. May inhibit labour if taken during later stages of pregnancy. Discuss with your doctor.

Breast-feeding
▼ The drug passes into the breast milk, but at normal doses adverse effects on the baby are unlikely. Discuss with your doctor.

Infants and children
▼ Reduced dose necessary.

Over 60
▼ No special problems.

Driving and hazardous work
▼ Avoid such activities until you have learned how verapamil affects you because the drug can cause dizziness.

Alcohol
▼ Avoid. Alcohol may further reduce blood pressure, causing dizziness or other symptoms.

Surgery and general anaesthetics
▼ Verapamil may need to be stopped before surgery. Consult your doctor or dentist.

PROLONGED USE

No problems expected.

WARFARIN

Brand name Marevan
Used in the following combined preparations None

GENERAL INFORMATION

Warfarin is an anticoagulant used to prevent blood clots, mainly in areas where blood flow is slowest, particularly in the leg and pelvic veins. Such clots can break off and travel through the bloodstream to the lungs, where they lodge and cause pulmonary embolism. The drug is also used to reduce the risk of clots forming in the heart in people with atrial fibrillation, or after insertion of artificial heart valves. These clots may travel to the brain and cause a stroke.

A widely used oral anticoagulant drug, warfarin requires regular monitoring to ensure proper maintenance dosage. As its full beneficial effects are not felt for two to three days, a faster-acting drug such as heparin is often used to complement the effects of warfarin at the start of treatment.

The most serious *adverse effect*, as with all anticoagulants, is the risk of excessive bleeding, which is usually the result of excessive dosage.

QUICK REFERENCE

Drug group Anticoagulant drug (p.104)

Overdose danger rating High

Dependence rating Low

Prescription needed Yes

Available as generic Yes

INFORMATION FOR USERS

Your drug prescription is tailored for you. Do not alter dosage without checking with your doctor.

How taken

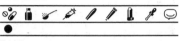

Tablets.

Frequency and timing of doses
Once daily, taken at the same time each day.

Dosage range
10–15mg daily according to age and weight (starting dose); 3–9mg daily, as determined by blood tests (maintenance dose).

Onset of effect
Within 24–48 hours, with full effect after several days.

Duration of action
2–3 days.

Diet advice
None.

Storage
Keep in a closed container in a cool, dry place out of the reach of children. Protect from light.

Missed dose
Take as soon as you remember. Take the following dose on your original schedule.

Stopping the drug
Do not stop taking the drug without consulting your doctor; stopping the drug may lead to worsening of the underlying condition.

OVERDOSE ACTION

Seek immediate medical advice in all cases. Take emergency action if severe bleeding or loss of consciousness occur.

See Drug poisoning emergency guide (p.494).

SPECIAL PRECAUTIONS

Be sure to tell your doctor if:
▼ You have long-term liver or kidney problems.
▼ You have high blood pressure.
▼ You have peptic ulcers.
▼ You bleed easily.
▼ You are taking other medications.

Pregnancy
▼ Not usually prescribed. If given in early pregnancy, the drug can cause malformations in the unborn child. Taken near the time of delivery, it may cause the mother to bleed excessively. Discuss with your doctor.

Breast-feeding
▼ The drug passes into the breast milk, but at normal doses adverse effects on the baby are unlikely. Discuss with your doctor.

Infants and children
▼ Reduced dose necessary.

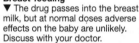

Over 60
▼ No special problems.

Driving and hazardous work
▼ Use caution. Even minor bumps can cause bad bruises and excessive bleeding.

Alcohol
▼ Avoid excessive amounts. Alcohol may increase the effects of this drug.

Surgery and general anaesthetics
▼ Warfarin may need to be stopped before surgery. Discuss with your doctor or dentist.

POSSIBLE ADVERSE EFFECTS

Bleeding is the most common adverse effect with warfarin. Any bruising, dark stools, dark urine, or bleeding should be reported to your doctor at once.

Symptom/effect	Frequency		Discuss with doctor		Stop taking drug now	Call doctor now
	Common	Rare	Only if severe	In all cases		
Fever		●		■	▲	∎
Nausea/vomiting		●		■	▲	∎
Abdominal pain/diarrhoea		●		■		
Rash		●		■		
Hair loss		●		■		
Bleeding/bruising	●			■	▲	∎

INTERACTIONS

General note A wide variety of drugs, such as aspirin, barbiturates, oral contraceptives, cimetidine, diuretics, certain laxatives, certain antidepressants, and certain antibiotics interact with warfarin, either by increasing or decreasing the anticlotting effect. Consult your pharmacist before using over-the-counter medicines.

PROLONGED USE

No special problems.

Monitoring Regular blood tests are performed during treatment.

ZALCITABINE

Brand name Hivid
Used in the following combined preparations None

GENERAL INFORMATION

Zalcitabine is a nucleoside reverse transcriptase inhibitor – an antiviral drug used in the treatment of HIV (human immunodeficiency virus) which causes AIDS (acquired immunodeficiency syndrome). The drug interferes with reverse transcriptase, an *enzyme* used by the virus to produce genetic material.

Treatment for HIV is now usually begun with triple therapy, which consists of two nucleoside transcriptase inhibitors and a third drug from another class, such as ritonavir, a protease inhibitor.

If the treatment is started before the immune system becomes too badly damaged, this combination can be very effective in slowing down the progress of the infection.

INFORMATION FOR USERS

Your drug prescription is tailored for you. Do not alter dosage without checking with your doctor.

How taken

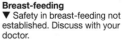

Tablets.

Frequency and timing of doses
3 x daily.

Adult dosage range
2,250mcg daily.

Onset of effect
Within a few hours. Full beneficial effect may not be felt for several weeks or months.

Duration of action
Approximately 8 hours.

Diet advice
None.

Storage
Keep in a closed container in a cool, dry place out of the reach of children.

Missed dose
Take as soon as you remember. If your next dose is due within 3 hours, take a single dose now and skip the next.

Stopping the drug
Do not stop taking the drug without consulting your doctor; stopping the drug may lead to worsening of the underlying condition.

Exceeding the dose
An occasional unintentional extra dose is unlikely to cause problems. But if you notice any unusual symptoms or if a large overdose has been taken, notify your doctor.

POSSIBLE ADVERSE EFFECTS

Most *adverse effects* are minor, but some, such as damage to the nerves, pancreas, or liver, are more serious. Therefore, treatment must be closely monitored.

Symptom/effect	Frequency		Discuss with doctor		Stop taking drug now	Call doctor now
	Common	Rare	Only if severe	In all cases		
Diarrhoea/constipation	●		■			
Loss of appetite	●		■			
Nausea/vomiting	●			■		
Pallor/fatigue	●			■		
Muscle/joint pain		●		■		
Sore throat/fever		●		■		
Mouth ulcers		●		■		
Numbness/unusual sensation		●		■		

INTERACTIONS

General note A wide range of other drugs may increase the risk of harmful effects with zalcitabine. These include drugs that damage the nerves or pancreas or affect blood production. Do not take any other medications without consulting your doctor or pharmacist.

SPECIAL PRECAUTIONS

Be sure to tell your doctor if:
▼ You have long-term liver or kidney problems.
▼ You have a history of blood disorders.
▼ You have heart problems.
▼ You have had pancreatitis.
▼ You are taking other medications.

 Pregnancy
▼ Safety in pregnancy not established. Discuss with your doctor.

 Breast-feeding
▼ Safety in breast-feeding not established. Discuss with your doctor.

 Infants and children
▼ Not recommended.

 Over 60
▼ Not recommended.

 Driving and hazardous work
▼ No known problems.

 Alcohol
▼ Keep consumption low. Excessive consumption increases the risk of liver damage.

PROLONGED USE

There is an increased risk of nerve, liver, and pancreatic damage and blood abnormalities with prolonged treatment.

Monitoring Regular blood tests are performed to check blood cell production and liver and pancreatic function.

ZANAMIVIR

Brand name Relenza
Used in the following combined preparations None

GENERAL INFORMATION

Zanamivir is a new type of antiviral drug used to treat Influenza (flu), a virus that infects and multiplies in the lungs. The drug works by attacking the virus, preventing it from multiplying and spreading in the lungs.

Flu causes fever, chills, headache, aches and pains. Other symptoms include sore throat, cough, and nasal symptoms. Taken by inhaler, zanamivir helps to clear these symptoms and may shorten the duration of the illness. There is no benefit, however, if you do not have a fever. Therefore, treatment should begin as soon as possible, and certainly within 48 hours of the onset of symptoms.

Symptoms usually subside in two to seven days, unless complications such as a chest infection occur. The elderly and those with long-term illnesses, such as chronic lung and heart disease, are at most risk of complications.

Zanamivir is also being investigated for flu prevention. The drug should be used with caution by asthmatic patients because it may provoke wheezing requiring urgent use of a *bronchodilator*.

INFORMATION FOR USERS

Your drug prescription is tailored for you. Do not alter dosage without checking with your doctor.

How taken

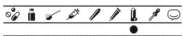
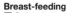

Inhaler.

Frequency and timing of doses
2 x daily. Inhale the contents of the blisters one at a time.

Adult dosage range
20mg (4 x 5mg blisters) daily for 5 days.

Onset of effect
Within 7 days.

Duration of action
Up to 12 hours.

Diet advice
None.

Storage
Keep in a cool, dry place out of the reach of children.

Missed dose
Take as soon as you remember. If your next dose is due within 2 hours, take a single dose now and skip the next.

Stopping the drug
Do not stop taking the drug without consulting your doctor; symptoms may recur.

Exceeding the dose
An occasional unintentional dose is unlikely to cause problems. However, if you notice any unusual symptoms, or if a large overdose has been taken, notify your doctor.

SPECIAL PRECAUTIONS

Be sure to tell your doctor if:
▼ You have ever had an allergic reaction to zanamivir or lactose monohydrate.
▼ You have a long-term illness.
▼ You have a lung disease such as asthma.
▼ You have poor immunity to infections.
▼ You suffer from asthma.
▼ You are taking other medications.

Pregnancy
▼ Safety in pregnancy not established. Discuss with your doctor.

Breast-feeding
▼ Safety in breast-feeding not established. Discuss with your doctor.

Infants and children
▼ Not recommended.

Over 60
▼ No special problems.

Driving and hazardous work
▼ No known problems.

Alcohol
▼ No known problems.

POSSIBLE ADVERSE EFFECTS

Adverse effects are uncommon. Such effects that occur are similar to signs and symptoms of flu and may therefore sometimes be caused by the influenza virus rather than zanamivir.

Symptom/effect	Frequency		Discuss with doctor		Stop taking drug now	Call doctor now
	Common	Rare	Only if severe	In all cases		
Headache		●	■			
Sore throat		●	■			
Cough		●	■			
Nasal symptoms		●	■			
Wheezing/breathlessness		●		■	▲	

INTERACTIONS

Inhaled drugs (e.g., salbutamol and beclometasone) These should be inhaled just before zanamivir is administered.

PROLONGED USE

This drug should only be used for 5 days and is not prescribed for long-term use.

ZIDOVUDINE

Brand name Retrovir
Used in the following combined preparation Combivir

GENERAL INFORMATION

Zidovudine, formerly known as azidothymidine, or AZT, is an antiviral drug used in the treatment of HIV (human immunodeficiency virus) which causes AIDS (acquired immunodeficiency syndrome). It is a nucleoside reverse transcriptase inhibitor which interferes with an *enzyme* used by the virus to produce genetic material.

Treatment for HIV is now usually begun with triple therapy, which consists of two nucleoside transcriptase inhibitors and a third drug from another class, such as ritonavir, a protease inhibitor.

When treatment is started before the immune system is too badly damaged, this combination is very effective in slowing the progress of HIV infection.

INFORMATION FOR USERS

Your drug prescription is tailored for you. Do not alter dosage without checking with your doctor.

How taken

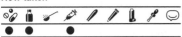

Tablets, capsules, liquid, injection.

Frequency and timing of doses
2–5 times daily.

Adult dosage range
0.5–1g daily.

Onset of effect
Within 48 hours.

Duration of action
About 4 hours.

Diet advice
None.

Storage
Keep in a tightly closed container in a cool, dry place out of the the reach of children. Protect from light.

Missed dose
Take as soon as you remember. If your next dose is due within 2 hours, take a single dose now and skip the next.

Stopping the drug
Do not stop taking the drug without consulting your doctor; symptoms may recur.

Exceeding the dose
An occasional unintentional extra dose is unlikely to cause problems. Serious *adverse effects* from large overdoses are unusual, but notify your doctor.

POSSIBLE ADVERSE EFFECTS

The most common adverse effect of this drug is anaemia. Symptoms include pallor, fatigue, and shortness of breath. Sore throat and fever are less frequent effects, and result from a decreased number of white blood cells. All of these problems are the result of reduced blood cell production in the bone marrow.

Symptom/effect	Frequency		Discuss with doctor		Stop taking drug now	Call doctor now
	Common	Rare	Only if severe	In all cases		
Nausea/vomiting/headache	●		■			
Loss of appetite	●		■			
Pallor/fatigue	●			■		
Numbness/unusual sensation		●		■		■
Insomnia		●		■		
Aching muscles		●		■		
Sore throat/fever		●		■		

INTERACTIONS

General note A wide range of drugs may increase the risk of harmful effects with zidovudine. These include drugs that act on the kidneys or affect blood production. Do not take other medications without consulting your doctor or pharmacist.

Probenecid Blood levels of zidovudine are increased by probenecid, increasing the risk of *toxic* effects.

SPECIAL PRECAUTIONS

Be sure to tell your doctor if:
▼ You have long-term liver or kidney problems.
▼ You have had a previous allergic reaction to zidovudine.
▼ You have a history of blood disorders.
▼ You are taking other medications.

 Pregnancy
▼ Safety in pregnancy not fully established. Discuss with your doctor. Zidovudine may be used during pregnancy to prevent transmission of HIV from mother to baby.

 Breast-feeding
▼ The drug passes into the breast milk and may affect the baby. Discuss with your doctor.

 Infants and children
▼ Reduced dose necessary.

 Over 60
▼ Increased likelihood of adverse effects. Reduced dose may therefore be necessary.

 Driving and hazardous work
▼ No special problems.

 Alcohol
▼ No known problems.

PROLONGED USE

There is an increased risk of serious blood disorders with prolonged use of zidovudine.

Monitoring Regular blood checks are required during treatment.

ZOPICLONE

Brand names Zileze, Zimovane
Used in the following combined preparations None

GENERAL INFORMATION

Zopiclone is a hypnotic (sleeping drug) used for the short-term treatment of insomnia. Sleep problems can take the form of difficulty in falling asleep, frequent night-time awakenings, and/or early morning awakenings. Hypnotic drugs are given only when non-drug measures – for example, avoidance of caffeine – have proved ineffective.

Unlike benzodiazepines, zopiclone possesses no anti-anxiety properties. Therefore, it may be suited for instances of insomnia that are not accompanied by anxiety – for example, international travel or change in shift work routine.
Hypnotics are intended for occasional use only. *Dependence* can develop after as little as one week of continuous use.

QUICK REFERENCE

Drug group Sleeping drug (p.82)
Overdose danger rating Medium
Dependence rating Medium
Prescription needed Yes
Available as generic Yes

INFORMATION FOR USERS

Your drug prescription is tailored for you. Do not alter dosage without checking with your doctor.

How taken

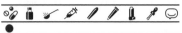

Tablets.

Frequency and timing of doses
Once daily at bedtime when required.

Dosage range
3.75–7.5mg.

Onset of effect
Within 30 minutes.

Duration of action
4–6 hours.

Diet advice
None.

Storage
Keep in a closed container in a cool, dry place out of the reach of children. Protect from light.

Missed dose
If you fall asleep without having taken a dose and wake some hours later, do not take the missed dose.

Stopping the drug
If you have been taking the drug continuously for less than 1 week, it can be safely stopped as soon as you feel you no longer need it. However, if you have been taking the drug for longer, consult your doctor.

Exceeding the dose
An occasional, unintentional extra dose is unlikely to cause problems. Large overdoses may cause prolonged sleep, drowsiness, lethargy, and poor muscle coordination and reflexes. Notify your doctor immediately.

SPECIAL PRECAUTIONS

Be sure to tell your doctor if:
▼ You have or have had any problems with alcohol or drug misuse/abuse.
▼ You have myasthenia gravis.
▼ You have had epileptic fits.
▼ You have liver or kidney problems.
▼ You are taking other medications.

Pregnancy
▼ Not recommended.

Breast-feeding
▼ Not recommended.

Infants and children
▼ Not recommended.

Over 60
▼ Increased likelihood of adverse effects. Reduced dose may therefore be necessary.

Driving and hazardous work
▼ Avoid such activities until you have learned how zopiclone affects you because the drug can cause drowsiness, reduced alertness, and slowed reactions.

Alcohol
▼ Avoid. Alcohol increases the sedative effects of this drug.

POSSIBLE ADVERSE EFFECTS

The most common *adverse effects* of zopiclone are daytime drowsiness, which normally diminishes after the first few days of treatment, and a bitter taste in the mouth. Persistent morning drowsiness or impaired coordination are signs of excessive dose.

Symptom/effect	Frequency		Discuss with doctor		Stop taking drug now	Call doctor now
	Common	Rare	Only if severe	In all cases		
Bitter taste	●		■			
Daytime drowsiness/headache	●		■			
Dizziness/weakness		●	■			
Nausea/vomiting/diarrhoea		●	■			
Amnesia/confusion		●		■	▲	
Rash		●		■	▲	■

INTERACTIONS

Sedatives All drugs, including alcohol, that have a sedative effect on the central nervous system are likely to increase the sedative effects of zopiclone. Such drugs include other sleeping and anti-anxiety drugs, antihistamines, antidepressants, *opioid* analgesics, and antipsychotics.

PROLONGED USE

Intended for occasional use only. Continuous use of zopiclone – or any other sleeping drug – for as little as one week may cause *dependence*.

A–Z OF VITAMINS AND MINERALS

This section gives detailed information on 24 of the major vitamins and minerals that are required by the body for good health – chemicals that are essential, but which the body cannot make by itself. These include the main vitamins – A, C, D, E, K, H (biotin), and the B vitamins – together with eleven essential minerals.

The section on vitamins in Part 3 (p.149) gives in general terms the main sources of the major vitamins and minerals and their roles in the body, while the following profiles discuss each vitamin and mineral in detail.

The following pages may be particularly useful as a guide for those who think their diet lacks sufficient amounts of a certain vitamin or mineral, and for those with disorders of the digestive tract or liver, who may need larger amounts of certain vitamins. The table on p.150 gives the good dietary sources of each one.

The vitamin and mineral profiles

The profiles are arranged in alphabetical order and give information under standard headings. These include the different names by which each chemical is known; whether it is available over the counter or by prescription only; its role in body maintenance; specific foods in which it can be found; the recommended daily amounts; how to detect a deficiency; how and when to supplement your diet; and the risks that are associated with excessive intake of a particular vitamin or mineral.

Normal daily vitamin and mineral requirements are usually based on the Reference Nutrient Intake (RNI), which is the amount of the nutrient thought to be enough for about 97 per cent of people. The dosages for treating deficiency are usually considerably higher, but need to be determined by your doctor.

HOW TO UNDERSTAND THE PROFILES

Each vitamin and mineral profile contains information arranged under standard headings to enable you to find the information you need.

Availability
Tells you whether the vitamin or mineral is available over the counter or only by prescription.

Other names — Lists the chemical and non-chemical names by which the vitamin or mineral is also known.

Dietary and other natural sources — Tells you how the vitamin or mineral is obtained naturally.

When supplements are helpful — Suggests when your doctor may recommend that you take supplements.

Dosage range for treating deficiency — Gives a usual recommended dosage of vitamin or mineral supplements.

Actions on the body — Explains the role played by each vitamin or mineral in maintaining healthy body function.

Normal daily requirement — Gives you a guide to the reference nutrient intake (RNI) of each vitamin or mineral.

Symptoms of deficiency — Describes the common signs of deficiency.

Symptoms and risks of excessive intake — Explains the risks that may accompany excessive intake of each vitamin or mineral and warning signs to look out for.

PANTOTHENIC ACID

Other names Calcium pantothenate, panthenol, pantothenol, vitamin B₅.

Availability
Pantothenic acid, calcium pantothenate, and panthenol are available without prescription in a variety of multivitamin and mineral preparations.

Actions on the body
Pantothenic acid plays a vital role in the activities of many enzymes. It is essential for the production of energy from sugars and fats, for the manufacture of fats, corticosteroids, and sex hormones, for the utilization of other vitamins, for the proper function of the nervous system and the adrenal glands, and for normal growth and development.

Dietary and other natural sources
Pantothenic acid is present in almost all vegetables, cereals, and animal foods. Liver, kidney, heart, fish, and egg yolks are good dietary sources. Brewer's yeast, wheat germ, and royal jelly (the substance on which queen bees feed) are also rich in the vitamin.

Normal daily requirement
No reference nutrient intake (RNI) for pantothenic acid has ever been established, but adult requirements are met by a 3–7mg intake daily.

When supplements are helpful
Most diets provide adequate amounts of pantothenic acid. Any deficiency is likely to occur in malnutrition together with other B vitamin deficiency diseases such as pellagra (see niacin), beriberi (see thiamine), or with alcoholism, and will be treated with B complex supplements. There is no firm evidence that large doses help, as some believe, in the prevention of greying hair, nerve disorders in diabetes, or psychiatric illness.

Symptoms of deficiency
Pantothenic acid deficiency is unlikely to occur unless a person is suffering from malnutrition. However, deficiency produced under experimental conditions can cause malaise, abdominal discomfort, and burning feet.

Dosage range for treating deficiency
Usually 5–20mg per day.

Symptoms and risks of excessive intake
In tests, doses of 1,000mg or more of pantothenic acid have not caused toxic effects. The risk of toxicity is considered to be very low, since pantothenic acid is a water-soluble vitamin that does not accumulate in the tissues. Any excess is eliminated rapidly in the urine. However, very high intakes of 10–20g can cause diarrhoea.

POTASSIUM

Other names Potassium acetate, potassium chloride, potassium citrate, potassium gluconate

Availability
Salts of potassium in small doses are available in a number of multivitamin and mineral supplements. They are available at higher doses in prescription-only drugs given as dietary supplements and in some diuretics given to offset the loss of potassium in the urine (for example, Burinex-K). Potassium salts are also widely available in sodium-free salt (used as a salt substitute).

Actions on the body
Potassium works together with sodium in the control of the body's water balance, conduction of nerve impulses, contraction of muscle, and maintenance of a normal heart rhythm. Potassium is essential for maintenance of normal blood sugar.

Dietary and other natural sources
The best dietary sources of potassium are leafy green vegetables, tomatoes, oranges, potatoes, and bananas. Lean meat, pulses, chocolate, coffee, and milk are also rich in the mineral. Many methods of food processing may lower the potassium levels found in fresh food.

Normal daily requirement
The reference nutrient intakes (RNI) for potassium are: 0.8g (birth–3 months); 0.85g (4–6 months); 0.7g (7–12 months); 0.8g (1–3 years); 1.1g (4–6 years); 2g (7–10 years); 3.1g (11–14 years); 3.5g (15 years and over). There are no extra requirements in pregnancy or breast-feeding.

When supplements are helpful
Most diets contain adequate amounts of potassium, and supplements are rarely required in normal circumstances. However, people who drink large amounts of alcohol or eat lots of salty foods may become marginally deficient. People with a condition called diabetic ketoacidosis or with certain types of kidney disease may be deficient in potassium, but the most common cause is prolonged treatment with diuretics. Long-term use of corticosteroids may also deplete the body's potassium. Prolonged vomiting and diarrhoea also cause potassium deficiency, so people who abuse laxatives may be affected. Supplements are usually advised only when symptoms suggest deficiency, or for people at particular risk.

Dosage range for treating deficiency
Depends on the preparation, the individual, and the cause and severity of deficiency. In general, daily doses equivalent to 2–4g of potassium chloride are given to prevent deficiency (for example, in people treated with diuretics that deplete potassium). Doses equivalent to 3.0–7.2g of potassium chloride daily are used to treat deficiency.

Symptoms of deficiency
Early symptoms of potassium deficiency may include muscle weakness, fatigue, dizziness, and mental confusion. Impairment of nerve and muscle function may progress to cause disturbances of the heart rhythm and paralysis of the skeletal muscles and those of the bowel, which leads to constipation.

Symptoms and risks of excessive intake
Blood potassium levels are normally regulated by the kidneys, and any excess is rapidly eliminated in the urine. Massive doses cause serious disturbances of the heart rhythm and muscular paralysis. In people with impaired kidney function, excess potassium may build up and the risk of potassium poisoning is increased. People on haemodialysis treatment need to take a carefully controlled low-potassium diet.

443

BIOTIN

Other names Coenzyme R, vitamin H

Availability
Biotin is available without a prescription, alone and in a wide variety of multivitamin and mineral preparations.

Actions on the body
Biotin plays a vital role in the activities of several *enzymes*. It is essential for the breakdown of carbohydrates and fatty acids in the diet for conversion into energy, for the manufacture of fats, and for excretion of the products of protein breakdown.

Dietary and other natural sources
Traces of biotin are present in a wide variety of foods. Dietary sources rich in this vitamin include liver, nuts, peas, beans, egg yolks, cauliflower, and mushrooms. A large proportion of the biotin we require is manufactured by bacteria in the intestine.

Normal daily requirement
A reference nutrient intake (RNI) has not been established, but a daily dietary intake of 10–200mcg is safe.

When supplements are helpful
Adequate amounts of biotin are provided in most diets and by the bacteria living in the intestine, so supplements are rarely needed. However, deficiency can occur with prolonged, excessive consumption of raw egg whites (as in eggnogs), because these contain a protein – avidin – that prevents absorption of the vitamin in the intestine. The risk of deficiency is also increased during long-term treatment with antibiotics or sulphonamide antibacterial drugs, which may destroy the biotin-producing bacteria in the intestine. However, additional biotin is not usually necessary with a balanced diet.

Symptoms of deficiency
Deficiency symptoms include weakness, tiredness, poor appetite, hair loss, and depression. Severe deficiency may cause eczema of the face and body, and inflammation of the tongue.

Dosage range for treating deficiency
Depends on the individual and on the nature and severity of the disorder. Dietary deficiency can be treated with doses of 150–300mcg of biotin daily. Deficiency of biotin resulting from a genetic defect that limits use of the vitamin by body cells can be treated with very large doses of 5mg given once or twice daily.

Symptoms and risks of excessive intake
None known.

CALCIUM

Other names Calcium carbonate, calcium chloride, calcium citrate, calcium glubionate, calcium gluceptate, calcium gluconate, calcium lactate, calcium phosphate

Availability
Oral forms are available without a prescription. Injectable forms of calcium are available only under medical supervision.

Actions on the body
The most abundant mineral in the body, calcium makes up more than 90 per cent of the hard matter in bones and teeth. It is essential for the formation and maintenance of strong bones and healthy teeth, as well as blood clotting, transmission of nerve impulses, and muscle contraction.

Dietary and other natural sources
The main dietary sources of calcium are milk and dairy products, sardines, dark green leafy vegetables, beans, peas, and nuts. Calcium may also be obtained by drinking water in hard water areas.

Normal daily requirement
The reference nutrient intakes (RNI) for calcium are: 525mg (birth–1 year); 350mg (1–3 years); 450mg (4–6 years); 550mg (7–10 years); 1,000mg (males aged 11–18 years); 800mg (females aged 11–18 years); and 700mg (19 years and older). Daily requirements of calcium do not increase markedly during pregnancy, but rise by 550mg during breast-feeding.

When supplements are helpful
Unless a sufficient amount of dairy products is consumed (a pint of milk contains approximately 600mg) the diet may not contain enough calcium, and supplements may be needed. Breast-feeding women are especially vulnerable to calcium deficiency because breast-feeding demands large amounts of calcium, which may be extracted from the skeleton if intake is not adequate. Osteoporosis (fragile bones) has been linked to dietary calcium deficiency in some cases, but may not be helped by supplements in all women. Hormone replacement therapy or other treatment may also be necessary (see Drugs for bone disorders, p.122).

Symptoms of deficiency
Deficiency symptoms do not develop because, when dietary intake is inadequate, the body obtains the calcium it needs from the skeleton. Long-term deficiency of calcium may lead to increased fragility of the bones. Osteoporosis also results in increased risk of fractures, particularly of the vertebrae, hip, and wrist. Severe deficiency, resulting in low levels of calcium in the blood, causes abnormal stimulation of the nervous system, resulting in cramp-like spasms in the hands, feet, and face. Vitamin D deficiency is the main cause of the bone-softening diseases rickets and osteomalacia.

Dosage range for treating deficiency
Vitamin D is needed for treatment of rickets and osteo-malacia (p.122), but oral supplements of up to 800mg daily may be advised for children with rickets, and 1,000mg or more daily may be given for osteoporosis and osteomalacia. Severe deficiency is treated in hospital by intravenous injection of calcium.

Symptoms and risks of excessive intake
Excessive intake of calcium may reduce the amount of iron and zinc absorbed and may also cause constipation and nausea. There is an increased risk of palpitations and, for susceptible people, of calcium deposits in the kidneys leading to kidney stones and kidney damage. These symptoms do not usually develop unless calcium is taken with large amounts of vitamin D.

CHROMIUM

Other names Chromium trichloride, chromium picolinate

Availability
Chromium supplements are available without prescription.

Actions on the body
Chromium plays a vital role in the activities of several *enzymes*. It is involved in the breakdown of sugar for conversion into energy and in the manufacture of certain fats. The mineral works together with insulin and is thus essential to the body's ability to use sugar. Chromium may also be involved in the manufacture of proteins in the body.

Dietary and other natural sources
Traces of chromium are present in a wide variety of foods. Meat, dairy products, and wholemeal cereals are good sources of this mineral.

Normal daily requirement
Only minute quantities of chromium are required. A reference nutrient intake (RNI) has not been determined, but a safe intake for adults is about 25mcg.

When supplements are helpful
Most people who eat a healthy diet containing plenty of fresh or unprocessed foods receive adequate amounts of chromium. The use of chromium in diabetes is under investigation, but diabetics and those with diabetes-like symptoms may benefit from additional chromium. Supplements may also be helpful if symptoms suggest chromium deficiency.

Symptoms of deficiency
Chromium deficiency is very rare in Britain. A diet of too many processed foods may contribute to chromium deficiency. Inadequate intake of chromium over a prolonged period may impair the body's ability to use sugar, leading to high blood sugar levels. However, in most cases, there are no symptoms. In some people, there may be diabetes-like symptoms such as tiredness, mental confusion, and numbness or tingling of the hands and feet. Deficiency may worsen pre-existing diabetes and may depress growth in children. It has also been suggested that chromium deficiency may contribute to the development of atherosclerosis (narrowing of the arteries).

Dosage range for treating deficiency
Severe chromium deficiency may be treated with daily doses of up to 10mcg.

Symptoms and risks of excessive intake
Chromium is poisonous in excess. Levels that produce symptoms are usually obtained from occupational exposure or industrial waste in drinking water or the atmosphere, not from excessive dietary intake. Symptoms include inflammation of the skin and, if inhaled, damage to the nasal passages. People who are repeatedly exposed to chromium fumes have a higher-than-average risk of developing lung cancer. High levels may reduce reduce kidney function.

COPPER

Other names Copper chloride, copper chloride dihydrate, copper gluconate, copper sulphate

Availability
Copper supplements are available in oral forms without a prescription. Copper chloride is an injectable form and is available only on prescription. Copper chloride dihydrate is part of a multiple-ingredient preparation for hospital use.

Actions on the body
Copper is an essential constituent of several proteins and *enzymes*. It plays an important role in the development of red blood cells, helps to form the dark pigment that colours hair and skin, and helps the body to use vitamin C. It is essential for the formation of collagen and elastin – proteins found in ligaments, blood vessel walls, and the lungs – and for the proper formation and maintenance of strong bones. It is also required for central nervous system activity.

Dietary and other natural sources
Most unprocessed foods contain copper. Liver, shellfish, nuts, mushrooms, wholemeal cereals, and dried pulses are particularly rich sources. Soft water may dissolve copper from pipes.

Normal daily requirement
The reference nutrient intakes (RNI) for copper are: 0.2mg (birth–3 months); 0.3mg (4 months–1 year); 0.4mg (1–3 years); 0.6mg (4–6 years); 0.7mg (7–10 years); 0.8mg (11–14 years); 1.0mg (15–18 years); and 1.2mg (19 years and over). Daily requirements do not change during pregnancy, but rise by 0.3mg when breast-feeding.

When supplements are helpful
A diet that regularly includes a selection of the foods mentioned above provides sufficient copper. Supplements are rarely necessary. However, doctors may advise additional copper for malnourished infants and children.

Symptoms of deficiency
Copper deficiency is very rare. The major change is *anaemia* due to failure of production of red blood cells, the main symptoms of which are pallor, fatigue, shortness of breath, and palpitations. In severe cases, abnormal bone changes may occur. An inherited copper deficiency disorder called Menke's syndrome (kinky hair disease) results in brain degeneration, retarded growth, sparse and brittle hair, and weak bones.

Dosage range for treating deficiency
This depends on the individual and on the nature and severity of the disorder.

Symptoms and risks of excessive intake
As little as 250mg of copper sulphate taken by mouth in a single dose can produce toxic effects. Symptoms of poisoning include nausea, vomiting, abdominal pain, diarrhoea, and general aches and pains. Large overdoses of copper may cause destruction of red blood cells (haemolytic anaemia), and liver and kidney damage. In Wilson's disease, an inherited disorder, the patient cannot excrete copper and suffers from long-term copper poisoning and gradually develops liver and brain damage. The disease is treated with *chelating agents* such as penicillamine. Acute copper poisoning may occur in people who regularly drink homemade alcohol distilled through copper tubing.

FLUORIDE

Other names Calcium fluoride, sodium fluoride, sodium monofluorophosphate, stannous fluoride

Availability
Sodium fluoride may be added to drinking water and is available over the counter in single- or multiple-ingredient preparations. Mouth rinses and toothpastes containing sodium fluoride, sodium monofluorophosphate, or stannous fluoride are available over the counter. Calcium fluoride is a naturally occurring form of the mineral.

Actions on the body
Fluoride helps to prevent tooth decay and contributes to the strength of bones. It is thought to work on the teeth by strengthening the mineral composition of the tooth enamel, making it more resistant to attack by acid in the mouth. Fluoride is most effective when taken during the formation of teeth in childhood, since it is then incorporated into the tooth itself. It may also strengthen developing bones.

Dietary and other natural sources
Fluoride has been added to drinking water in many areas, and water is therefore a prime source of this mineral (fluoride levels in water vary from area to area, and untreated water also contains a small amount of fluoride). Foods and beverages grown or prepared in areas with fluoride-treated water may also contribute fluoride. Tea and sea fish are also rich in fluoride.

Normal daily requirement
No reference nutrient intake (RNI) has been established, but an intake of approximately 0.15mg is a safe level for infants (under 3 months), and about 0.5mg up to 2 years.

When supplements are helpful
Most diets typically provide 0.9–2.6mg of fluoride per day, depending on whether or not the water supply contains fluoride. Drinking water containing fluoride at 1 part per million (ppm) provides an additional 1.4–1.8mg per day for adults and 0.4–0.8mg per day for young children. If the level is inadequate, children may be given fluoride drops or tablets. The use of fluoride supplements for the prevention and treatment of osteoporosis (fragile bones) is currently under investigation.

Symptoms of deficiency
Fluoride deficiency increases the risk of tooth decay, especially in children.

Dosage range for treating deficiency
Dietary supplements may be given to children when the concentration of fluoride in the water supply is less than 0.7ppm. When fluoride is present at less than 0.3ppm, the recommended daily dose is: 0.25 micrograms (mcg) (6 months–3 years); 0.5mcg (3–6 years); and 1mcg (over 6 years). When the concentration is 0.3–0.7ppm, supplements are not recommended in infants under 3 years, and the recommended daily dose in older children is 0.25mcg (3–6 years) and 0.5mg (over 6 years).

Symptoms and risks of excessive intake
In large quantities, fluoride may cause slow poisoning, known as fluorosis. Prolonged intake of water containing more than 2ppm fluoride may lead to mottled or brown discoloration of the enamel in developing teeth. Very high levels (over 8ppm) may also lead to bone disorders and calcification of ligaments and tendons. Suggestions of a link between fluoridation of the water supply and cancer are without foundation. A child who has taken a number of fluoride tablets may vomit and lose consciousness. Give milk if the child is conscious, and seek immediate medical help (see p.496).

FOLIC ACID

Other names Folacin, vitamin B_9, B_{11}, sodium folate, folates

Availability
Folic acid is available without prescription, alone and in a variety of multivitamin and mineral preparations. Strengths of 500mcg and over are available only on prescription.

Actions on the body
Folic acid is essential for the activities of several *enzymes*. It is required for the manufacture of nucleic acids – the genetic material of cells – and thus for the processes of growth and reproduction. It is vital for the formation of red blood cells by the bone marrow and the development and proper function of the central nervous system.

Dietary and other natural sources
The best sources are leafy green vegetables, yeast extract, and liver. Root vegetables, oranges, nuts, dried pulses, and egg yolks are also rich sources.

Normal daily requirement
The reference nutrient intakes (RNI) for folic acid, as folate, in micrograms (mcg) are: 50mcg (birth–1 year); 70mcg (1–3 years); 100mcg (4–6 years); 150mcg (7–10 years); 200mcg (11 years and over); 400mcg per day to prevent first occurrence of neural tube defects, then 5mg per day to prevent recurrence (pregnancy and breast-feeding).

When supplements are helpful
A varied diet containing fresh fruit and vegetables usually provides adequate amounts. However, minor deficiency is fairly common, and can be corrected by the addition of one uncooked fruit or vegetable or a glass of fruit juice daily. Supplements are now routinely recommended for women planning a pregnancy and during the first 12 weeks of pregnancy for the prevention of neural tube defects such as spina bifida. Supplements may also be needed in premature or low-birth-weight infants and those fed on goat's milk (breast and cow's milk contain adequate amounts of the vitamin). Doctors may recommend additional folic acid for people on haemodialysis, those who have certain blood disorders, psoriasis, certain conditions in which absorption of nutrients from the intestine is impaired, severe alcoholism, or liver disease. Supplements may be helpful if you are a heavy drinker or if you are taking certain drugs that deplete folic acid. Such drugs include anticonvulsants, antimalarial drugs, oestrogen-containing contraceptives, certain analgesics, corticosteroids, and sulphonamide antibacterial drugs.

Symptoms of deficiency
Folic acid deficiency leads to abnormally low numbers of red blood cells (*anaemia*). The main symptoms include fatigue, loss of appetite, nausea, diarrhoea, and hair loss. Mouth sores are common and the tongue is often sore. Deficiency may also cause poor growth in infants and children.

Dosage range for treating deficiency
Symptoms of anaemia are usually treated with 15mg of folic acid daily, together with vitamin B_{12}. A lower maintenance dose may be substituted after symptoms have subsided.

Symptoms and risks of excessive intake
Excessive folic acid is not toxic. However, it may worsen the symptoms of a coexisting vitamin B_{12} deficiency and should never be taken to treat anaemia without a full medical investigation of the cause of the anaemia.

IODINE

Other names Potassium iodide, potassium iodate, sodium iodide

Availability
Iodine supplements are available without prescription as kelp tablets and in several multivitamin and mineral preparations. Iodine skin preparations are also available without a prescription for antiseptic use. A small amount of iodine is routinely added to most table salts in order to prevent iodine deficiency from occurring. Treatments for thyroid suppression are available only on prescription.

Actions on the body
Iodine is essential for the formation of thyroid hormone, which regulates the body's energy production, promotes growth and development, and helps burn excess fat.

Dietary and other natural sources
Seafood is the best source of iodine, but bread and dairy products such as milk are the main sources of this mineral in most diets. Iodized table salt is also a good source. Iodine may also be inhaled from the atmosphere in coastal regions.

Normal daily requirement
The reference nutrient intakes (RNI) for iodine in micrograms (mcg) are: 50mcg (birth–3 months); 60mcg (4–12 months); 70mcg (1–3 years); 100mcg (4–6 years); 110 mcg (7–10 years); 130mcg (11–14 years); and 140mcg (15 years and over). Requirements increase very slightly during breast-feeding; one vitamin tablet with calcium and iodine daily is recommended for nursing mothers.

When supplements are helpful
Most diets contain adequate amounts of iodine and use of iodized table salt can usually make up for any deficiency. Supplements are rarely necessary except on medical advice. However, excessive intake of raw cabbage or nuts reduces uptake of iodine into the thyroid gland and it may lead to deficiency if iodine intake is otherwise low. Kelp supplements may be helpful.

Adults exposed to radiation from radioactive iodine released into the environment may be given 100mg of iodine as a single dose (as potassium iodate 170mg); a lower dose is given to children according to age.

Iodine is used to treat people with thyrotoxicosis before surgery on the thyroid gland.

Symptoms of deficiency
Deficiency may result in a goitre (enlargement of the thyroid gland) and hypothyroidism (deficiency of thyroid hormone). Symptoms of hypothyroidism include tiredness, physical and mental slowness, weight gain, facial puffiness, and constipation. Babies born to iodine-deficient mothers are lethargic and difficult to feed. Left untreated, many show poor growth and mental retardation.

Dosage range for treating deficiency
Iodine deficiency may be treated with doses of 150mcg of iodine daily, and then followed up by ensuring that iodized table salt is used.

Symptoms and risks of excessive intake
The amount of iodine that occurs naturally in food is non-toxic, but prolonged use of large amounts (6mg or more daily) may suppress the activity of the thyroid gland. Large overdoses of iodine compounds may cause abdominal pain, vomiting, bloody diarrhoea, and swelling of the thyroid and salivary glands.

IRON

Other names Ferrous fumarate, ferrous gluconate, ferrous sulphate, iron dextran, iron-polysaccharide complex

Availability
Ferrous sulphate, ferrous fumarate, ferrous gluconate, and iron-polysaccharide complex are all available without prescription, alone and in multivitamin and mineral preparations. Iron dextran, an injectable form, is available only on prescription.

Actions on the body
Iron has an important role in the formation of red blood cells (which contain two-thirds of the body's iron) and is a vital component of the oxygen-carrying pigment haemoglobin. It is involved in the formation of myoglobin, a pigment that stores oxygen in muscles for use during exercise. It is also an essential component of several *enzymes*, and is involved in the uptake of oxygen by the cells and the conversion of blood sugar to energy.

Dietary and other natural sources
Liver is the best dietary source of iron. Meat (especially organ offal), eggs, chicken, fish, leafy green vegetables, dried fruit, enriched or wholemeal cereals, breads and pastas, nuts, and dried pulses are also rich sources. Iron is better absorbed from meat, eggs, chicken, and fish than from vegetables. Foods containing vitamin C enhance iron absorption.

Normal daily requirement
The reference nutrient intakes (RNI) for iron are: 1.7mg (birth–3 months); 4.3mg (4–6 months); 7.8mg (7–12 months); 6.9mg (1–3 years); 6.1mg (4–6 years); 8.7mg (7–10 years); 11.3mg (males aged 11–18 years); 14.8mg (females aged 11–50 years); and 8.7mg (males aged 19 and over, and females aged 51 and over). Requirements may be increased during pregnancy and for 2 to 3 months after childbirth.

When supplements are helpful
Most average diets supply adequate amounts of iron. However, larger amounts are necessary during pregnancy. Supplements may be given throughout pregnancy and for 2 to 3 months after childbirth to maintain and replenish adequate iron stores in the mother. Premature babies may be prescribed supplements from a few weeks after birth to prevent deficiency. Supplements may be helpful in young vegetarians, women with heavy menstrual periods, and people with chronic blood loss due to disease (for example, peptic ulcer).

Symptoms of deficiency
Iron deficiency causes *anaemia*. Symptoms of anaemia include pallor, fatigue, shortness of breath, and palpitations. Apathy, irritability, and lowered resistance to infection may also occur. Iron deficiency may also affect intellectual performance and behaviour.

Dosage range for treating deficiency
Depends on the individual and the nature and severity of the condition. In adults, iron-deficiency anaemia is usually treated with 100–200mg of iron (usually as ferrous sulphate or gluconate) daily. In children, the dose is reduced according to age and weight. Iron supplements of 30–60mg daily may be given during pregnancy.

Symptoms and risks of excessive intake
An overdose of iron tablets is extremely dangerous. Pain in the abdomen, nausea, and vomiting may be followed by abdominal bloating, dehydration, and dangerously lowered blood pressure. Immediate medical attention must be sought (see p.496).

Excessive long-term intake, especially when it is taken with large amounts of vitamin C, may in susceptible individuals cause iron to accumulate in organs, causing congestive heart failure, cirrhosis of the liver, and diabetes mellitus. This condition is known as haemochromatosis.

MAGNESIUM

Other names Magnesium gluconate, magnesium hydroxide, magnesium oxide, magnesium sulphate

Availability
Magnesium is available without prescription in a variety of multivitamin and mineral preparations. Magnesium is also an ingredient of numerous over-the-counter antacid and laxative preparations, but it is not absorbed well from these sources.

Actions on the body
About 60 per cent of the body's magnesium is found in bones and teeth. Magnesium is essential for the formation of healthy bones and teeth, the transmission of nerve impulses, and the contraction of muscles. It activates several *enzymes*, and is important in the conversion of carbohydrates, fats, and proteins into energy.

Dietary and other natural sources
The best dietary sources of magnesium are leafy green vegetables. Nuts, wholemeal cereals, soya beans, cheese, and seafood are also rich in magnesium. Drinking water in hard water areas is also a source of this mineral.

Normal daily requirement
The reference nutrient intakes (RNI) for magnesium are: 55mg (birth–3 months); 60mg (4–6 months); 75mg (7–9 months); 80mg (10–12 months); 85mg (1–3 years); 120mg (4–6 years); 200mg (7–10 years); 280mg (11–14 years); 300mg (males aged 15 and over, and females aged 15–18 years); and 270mg (females aged 19 and over). Daily requirements do not increase during pregnancy but rise by 50mg during breast-feeding.

When supplements are helpful
A varied diet provides adequate amounts of magnesium, particularly in hard water areas. Supplements are usually necessary only on medical advice for deficiency of magnesium associated with certain conditions in which absorption from the intestine is impaired, which occurs in repeated vomiting or diarrhoea, advanced kidney disease, severe alcoholism, or prolonged treatment with certain diuretic drugs. Magnesium is used to treat eclampsia, cardiac arrhythmias, and myocardial infarction.

Oestrogens and oestrogen-containing oral contraceptives may reduce blood magnesium levels, but women who are on adequate diets do not need supplements.

Symptoms of deficiency
The symptoms of magnesium deficiency include anxiety, restlessness, tremors, confusion, palpitations, irritability, depression, and disorientation. Severe magnesium deficiency causes marked overstimulation of the nervous system, and results in fits and cramp-like spasms of the hands and feet. Inadequate intake may be a factor in the development of coronary heart disease, and may also lead to calcium deposits in the kidneys, resulting in kidney stones.

Dosage range for treating deficiency
This depends on the individual and on the nature and severity of the disorder. Severe deficiency is usually treated in hospital by injection of magnesium sulphate.

Symptoms and risks of excessive intake
Magnesium toxicity (hypermagnesaemia) is rare, but can occur in people with impaired kidney function after prolonged intake of the large amounts that are found in antacid or laxative preparations. Symptoms include nausea, vomiting, dizziness (due to a drop in blood pressure), and muscle weakness. Very large increases in magnesium in the blood may cause fatal respiratory failure or heart arrest.

NIACIN

Other names Niacinamide, nicotinamide, nicotinic acid, nicotinyl alcohol tartrate, vitamin B_3

Availability
Niacin is available without prescription in a wide variety of single-ingredient and multivitamin and mineral preparations. However, high doses of nicotinic acid are available only on prescription.

Actions on the body
Niacin plays a vital role in the activities of many *enzymes* and is important in producing energy from blood sugar, and in the manufacture of fats. Niacin is essential for the proper working of the nervous system, for a healthy skin and digestive system, and for the manufacture of steroid hormones.

Dietary and other natural sources
Liver, lean meat, poultry, fish, wholemeal cereals, nuts, and dried pulses are the best dietary sources of niacin.

Normal daily requirement
The reference nutrient intakes (RNI) for niacin are: 3mg (birth–3 months); 4mg (7–9 months); 5mg (10–12 months); 8mg (1–3 years); 11mg (4–6 years); 12mg (males aged 7–10 years and females aged 7–14 years); 15mg (males aged 11–14 years); 18mg (males aged 15–18 years); 14mg (females aged 15–18 years); 17mg (males aged 19–50 years); 13mg (females aged 19–50 years); 16mg (males aged 51 and over); and 12mg (females aged 51 and over). Daily requirements do not increase during pregnancy, but rise by 2mg during breast-feeding.

When supplements are helpful
Most British diets provide adequate amounts of niacin, and dietary deficiency is rare. Supplements are required for niacin deficiency associated with bowel disorders in which absorption from the intestine is impaired, and for people with liver disease or severe alcoholism. They may also be required for elderly people on poor diets. Large doses of niacin (up to 6g daily) are sometimes used in the treatment of hyperlipidaemia (raised blood fat levels). There is no convincing medical evidence that niacin helps psychiatric disorders (except those associated with pellagra).

Symptoms of deficiency
Severe niacin deficiency causes pellagra (literally, rough skin). Symptoms include sore, red, cracked skin in areas exposed to sun, friction, or pressure, inflammation of the mouth and tongue, abdominal pain and distension, nausea, diarrhoea, and mental disturbances such as depression, anxiety, and dementia.

Dosage range for treating deficiency
For severe pellagra, adults are usually treated with 100–500mg nicotinamide daily by mouth, and children are usually given 100–300mg daily. For less severe deficiency, doses of 25–50mg are given.

Symptoms and risks of excessive intake
At doses of over 50mg, niacin (nicotinic acid) may cause transient itching, flushing, tingling, or headache. Niacinamide in the form that occurs naturally in the body (nicotinamide), is free of these effects. Large doses of niacin may cause nausea and may aggravate a peptic ulcer. Side effects may be reduced by taking the drug on a full stomach. At doses of over 2g daily (which have been used to treat hyperlipidaemia), there is a risk of gout, liver damage, and high blood sugar levels, leading to extreme thirst.

PANTOTHENIC ACID

Other names Calcium pantothenate, panthenol, pantothenol, vitamin B_5

Availability
Pantothenic acid, calcium pantothenate, and panthenol are available without prescription in a variety of multivitamin and mineral preparations.

Actions on the body
Pantothenic acid plays a vital role in the activities of many *enzymes*. It is essential for the production of energy from sugars and fats, for the manufacture of fats, corticosteroids, and sex hormones, for the utilization of other vitamins, for the proper function of the nervous system and the adrenal glands, and for normal growth and development.

Dietary and other natural sources
Pantothenic acid is present in almost all vegetables, cereals, and animal foods. Liver, kidney, heart, fish, and egg yolks are good dietary sources. Brewer's yeast, wheat germ, and royal jelly (the substance on which queen bees feed) are also rich in the vitamin.

Normal daily requirement
No reference nutrient intake (RNI) for pantothenic acid has ever been established, but adult requirements are met by a 3–7mg intake daily.

When supplements are helpful
Most diets provide adequate amounts of pantothenic acid. Any deficiency is likely to occur in malnutrition together with other B vitamin deficiency diseases such as pellagra (see niacin), beriberi (see thiamine), or with alcoholism, and will be treated with B complex supplements. There is no firm evidence that large doses help, as some believe, in the prevention of greying hair, nerve disorders in diabetes, or psychiatric illness.

Symptoms of deficiency
Pantothenic acid deficiency is unlikely to occur unless a person is suffering from malnutrition. However, deficiency produced under experimental conditions can cause malaise, abdominal discomfort, and burning feet.

Dosage range for treating deficiency
Usually 5–20mg per day.

Symptoms and risks of excessive intake
In tests, doses of 1,000mg or more of pantothenic acid have not caused toxic effects. The risk of toxicity is considered to be very low, since pantothenic acid is a water-soluble vitamin that does not accumulate in the tissues. Any excess is eliminated rapidly in the urine. However, very high intakes of 10–20g can cause diarrhoea.

POTASSIUM

Other names Potassium acetate, potassium chloride, potassium citrate, potassium gluconate

Availability
Salts of potassium in small doses are available in a number of multivitamin and mineral supplements. They are available at higher doses in prescription-only drugs given as dietary supplements and in some diuretics given to offset the loss of potassium in the urine (for example, Burinex-K). Potassium salts are also widely available in sodium-free salt (used as a salt substitute).

Actions on the body
Potassium works together with sodium in the control of the body's water balance, conduction of nerve impulses, contraction of muscle, and maintenance of a normal heart rhythm. Potassium is essential for maintenance of normal blood sugar.

Dietary and other natural sources
The best dietary sources of potassium are leafy green vegetables, tomatoes, oranges, potatoes, and bananas. Lean meat, pulses, chocolate, coffee, and milk are also rich in the mineral. Many methods of food processing may lower the potassium levels found in fresh food.

Normal daily requirement
The reference nutrient intakes (RNI) for potassium are: 0.8g (birth–3 months); 0.85g (4–6 months); 0.7g (7–12 months); 0.8g (1–3 years); 1.1g (4–6 years); 2g (7–10 years); 3.1g (11–14 years); 3.5g (15 years and over). There are no extra requirements in pregnancy or breast-feeding.

When supplements are helpful
Most diets contain adequate amounts of potassium, and supplements are rarely required in normal circumstances. However, people who drink large amounts of alcohol or eat lots of salty foods may become marginally deficient. People with a condition called diabetic ketoacidosis or with certain types of kidney disease may be deficient in potassium, but the most common cause is prolonged treatment with diuretics. Long-term use of corticosteroids may also deplete the body's potassium. Prolonged vomiting and diarrhoea also cause potassium deficiency, so people who abuse laxatives may be affected. Supplements are usually advised only when symptoms suggest deficiency, or for people at particular risk.

Symptoms of deficiency
Early symptoms of potassium deficiency may include muscle weakness, fatigue, dizziness, and mental confusion. Impairment of nerve and muscle function may progress to cause disturbances of the heart rhythm and paralysis of the skeletal muscles and those of the bowel, which leads to constipation.

Dosage range for treating deficiency
Depends on the preparation, the individual, and the cause and severity of deficiency. In general, daily doses equivalent to 2–4g of potassium chloride are given to prevent deficiency (for example, in people treated with diuretics that deplete potassium). Doses equivalent to 3.0–7.2g of potassium chloride daily are used to treat deficiency.

Symptoms and risks of excessive intake
Blood potassium levels are normally regulated by the kidneys, and any excess is rapidly eliminated in the urine. Massive doses cause serious disturbances of the heart rhythm and muscular paralysis. In people with impaired kidney function, excess potassium may build up and the risk of potassium poisoning is increased. People on haemodialysis treatment need to take a carefully controlled low-potassium diet.

PYRIDOXINE

Other names Pyridoxine hydrochloride, vitamin B_6

Availability
Pyridoxine and pyridoxine hydrochloride are available without prescription in a variety of single-ingredient and multivitamin and mineral preparations.

Actions on the body
Pyridoxine plays a vital role in the activities of many enzymes. This B vitamin is essential for the release of carbohydrates stored in the liver and muscles for energy; for the breakdown and use of proteins, carbohydrates, and fats from food; and for the manufacture of niacin (vitamin B_3). It is needed for the production of red blood cells and antibodies, for healthy skin. It is also important for normal function of the central nervous system.

Dietary and other natural sources
Liver, chicken, fish, wholemeal cereals, wheat germ, and eggs are rich in this vitamin. Bananas, avocados, and potatoes are also good sources.

Normal daily requirement
The reference nutrient intakes (RNI) for pyridoxine are: 0.2mg (birth–6 months); 0.3mg (7–9 months); 0.4mg (10 months– 1 year); 0.7mg (1–3 years); 0.9mg (4–6 years); 1mg (males aged 7–10 years and females aged 7–14 years); 1.2mg (males aged 11–14 years); 1.5mg (males aged 15–18 years); 1.2mg (females aged 15 and over); and 1.4mg (males aged 19 and over). There are no extra requirements in pregnancy or breast-feeding.

When supplements are helpful
Most balanced diets contain adequate amounts of pyridoxine, and it is also manufactured in small amounts by bacteria that live in the intestine. However, breast-fed infants and elderly people may require additional pyridoxine. Supplements may be given on medical advice together with other B vitamins to people with certain conditions in which absorption from the intestine is impaired. They may also be used to treat a form of anaemia (sideroblastic) and certain rare genetic disorders termed pyridoxine dependency conditions. Supplements may also be recommended to prevent or treat deficiency caused by alcoholism, oral contraceptives, and treatment with drugs such as isoniazid, penicillamine, and hydralazine.

Symptoms of deficiency
Pyridoxine deficiency is rare unless it is due to drug treatment Deficiency may cause weakness, nervousness, irritability, depression, skin disorders, inflammation of the mouth and tongue, and cracked lips. In adults, it may cause *anaemia* (abnormally low levels of red blood cells). Convulsions may occur in infants.

Dosage range for treating deficiency
Depends on the individual and the nature and severity of the disorder. In general, deficiency is treated with 20–50mg up to 3 times per day for three weeks followed by 1.5–2.5mg daily in a multivitamin preparation for as long as necessary. Deficiency resulting from genetic defects that prevent use of the vitamin is treated with doses of 10–100mg daily in infants and 10–250mg daily in adults and children. Daily doses of 50–100mg (given with other B vitamins from day 10 of a menstrual cycle) to day 3 of the following cycle may help relieve premenstrual syndrome.

Symptoms and risks of excessive intake
Daily doses of over 500mg taken over a prolonged period may severely damage the nervous system, resulting in unsteadiness, numbness, and clumsiness of the hands.

RIBOFLAVIN

Other names Vitamin B_2, vitamin G

Availability
Riboflavin is available without a prescription, alone and in a wide variety of multivitamin and mineral preparations.

Actions on the body
Riboflavin plays a vital role in the activities of several *enzymes*. It is involved in the breakdown and utilization of carbohydrates, fats, and proteins and in the production of energy in cells using oxygen. It is needed for utilization of other B vitamins and for production of steroid hormones (by the adrenal glands).

Dietary and other natural sources
Riboflavin is found in most foods. Good dietary sources are liver, milk, cheese, eggs, leafy green vegetables, wholemeal cereals, and pulses. Brewer's yeast is also a rich source of the vitamin.

Normal daily requirement
The reference nutrient intakes (RNI) for riboflavin are: 0.4mg (birth–1 year); 0.6mg (1–3 years); 0.8mg (4–6 years); 1mg (7–10 years); 1.2mg (males aged 11–14 years); 1.1mg (females aged 11 and over); and 1.3mg (males aged 15 and over). Daily requirements rise by 0.3mg in pregnancy and by 0.5mg when breast-feeding.

When supplements are helpful
A balanced diet generally provides adequate amounts of riboflavin. Supplements may be beneficial in people on very low-calorie diets and elderly people on poor diets. Riboflavin requirements may also be increased by prolonged use of phenothiazine antipsychotics, tricyclic antidepressants, and oestrogen-containing oral contraceptives. Supplements are required for riboflavin deficiency associated with chronic diarrhoeal illnesses in which absorption of nutrients from the intestine is impaired. Riboflavin deficiency is also common among alcoholics. As with other B vitamins, the need for riboflavin is increased by injury, surgery, severe illness, and psychological stress. In all cases, treatment with supplements works best in a complete B-complex formulation.

Symptoms of deficiency
Prolonged deficiency may lead to chapped lips, cracks, and sores in the corners of the mouth, a red, sore tongue, and skin problems in the genital area. The eyes may itch, burn, and become unusually sensitive to light.

Dosage range for treating deficiency
Usually treated with 1–2mg daily in combination with other B vitamins.

Symptoms and risks of excessive intake
Excessive intake does not appear to have harmful effects.

SELENIUM

Other names Selenious acid, selenium sulphide, selenium yeast, selenomethionine, sodium selenite

Availability
Selenium is available without a prescription as 200mcg tablets and in a multivitamin and mineral preparation. Selenium sulphide is the active ingredient of several antidandruff shampoos.

Actions on the body
Selenium is an trace element that is an essential part of an enzyme system that protects cells against damage by oxygen radicals (it is an *antioxidant* like vitamins A, C, and E).

Dietary and other natural sources
Meat, fish, wholemeal cereals, and dairy products are good dietary sources. The amount of selenium found in vegetables depends on the content of the mineral in the soil where they were grown. Selenium is found in foodstuffs combined in amino acids.

Normal daily requirement
The reference nutrient intakes (RNI) for selenium are: 10mcg (birth–3 months); 13mcg (4–6 months); 10mcg (7–12 months); 15mcg (1–3 years); 20mcg (4–6 years); 30mcg (7–10 years); 45mcg (11–14 years); 70mcg (males aged 15–18 years); 60mcg (females aged 15 and over); and 75mcg (males aged 19 and over). There is no extra requirement during pregnancy, but 15mcg extra daily are required when breast-feeding.

When supplements are helpful
Most normal diets provide adequate amounts of selenium, and supplements are, therefore, rarely necessary. At present, there is no conclusive medical evidence to support some claims that selenium may provide protection against cancer or that it prolongs life. A daily intake of more than 150mcg is not recommended, except on the advice of a doctor.

Symptoms of deficiency
Long-term lack of selenium may result in loss of stamina and degeneration of tissues, leading to premature ageing. Severe deficiency may cause muscle pain and tenderness, and can eventually lead to a fatal form of heart disease in children in areas where selenium levels in the diet are very low – for example in one remote part of China.

Dosage range for treating deficiency
Depends on the individual and on the nature and severity of the disorder. Severe selenium deficiency may be treated with doses of up to 200mcg daily.

Symptoms and risks of excessive intake
Excessive intake may cause hair and nail loss, tooth decay and loss, fatigue, nausea, vomiting, and garlic breath. Total daily intake should not exceed 400mcg; large overdoses may be fatal.

SODIUM

Other names Sodium bicarbonate (baking soda), sodium chloride (table salt), sodium lactate, sodium phosphate

Availability
Sodium is widely available in the form of common table salt (sodium chloride). Sodium bicarbonate is used in many over-the-counter antacids. Sodium lactate is a prescription-only drug used in intravenous infusion fluid. Sodium phosphate is a laxative available only on prescription.

Actions on the body
Sodium works with potassium in control of the water balance in the body, conduction of nerve impulses, contraction of muscles, and maintenance of a normal heart rhythm.

Dietary and other natural sources
Sodium is present in almost all foods as a natural ingredient, or as an extra ingredient added during processing. The main sources are table salt, processed foods, cheese, breads and cereals, and smoked, pickled, or cured meats and fish. High concentrations are found in pickles and snack foods, including potato crisps and olives. Sodium is also present in water that has been treated with water softeners. Manufactured foods may also contain sodium compounds such as monosodium glutamate.

Normal daily requirement
The daily reference nutrient intakes (RNI) for sodium are: 0.21g (birth–3 months); 0.28g (4–6 months); 0.32g (7–9 months); 0.35g (10–12 months); 0.5g (1–3 years); 0.7g (4–6 years); 1.2g (7–10 years); and 1.6g (11 years and over). Most British diets contain far more sodium than this: the average consumption of sodium is 3–7g daily. One teaspoon of table salt contains about 2g of sodium.

When supplements are helpful
The need for supplementation is rare in temperate climates, even with "low-salt" diets. In tropical climates, however, sodium supplements may help to prevent cramps and possibly heatstroke occurring as a result of sodium lost through excessive perspiration during heavy work. Sodium supplements may be given on medical advice to replace salt loss due to prolonged diarrhoea and vomiting, particularly in infants. They may also be given to prevent or treat deficiency due to certain kidney disorders, cystic fibrosis, adrenal gland insufficiency, use of diuretics, or severe bleeding (as intravenous infusion).

Symptoms of deficiency
Sodium deficiency caused by dietary insufficiency is rare. It is usually a result of conditions that increase loss of sodium from the body, such as diarrhoea, vomiting, and excessive perspiration. Early symptoms include lethargy, muscle cramps, and dizziness. In severe cases, there may be a marked drop in blood pressure leading to confusion, fainting, and palpitations.

Dosage range for treating deficiency
Depends on the individual and on the nature and severity of symptoms. In extreme cases, intravenous sodium chloride may be required.

Symptoms and risks of excessive intake
Excessive sodium intake is thought to contribute to the development of high blood pressure, which may increase the risk of heart disease, stroke, and kidney damage. Other adverse effects include abnormal fluid retention, which leads to swelling of the legs and face. Large overdoses, even of table salt, may cause fits or coma and could be fatal. Table salt should never be used as an *emetic*.

THIAMINE

Other names Thiamin, thiamine hydrochloride, thiamine mononitrate, vitamin B$_1$

Availability
Thiamine is available without prescription in single-ingredient and a variety of multivitamin and mineral preparations.It is also available on prescription only as an injection.

Actions on the body
Thiamine plays a vital role in the activities of many *enzymes*. It is essential for the breakdown and utilization of fats, alcohol, and carbohydrates. It is important for a healthy nervous system, healthy muscles, and normal heart function.

Dietary and other natural sources
Thiamine is present in all unrefined food. Good dietary sources include wholemeal or enriched cereals and breads, brown rice, pasta, liver, kidneys, meat, fish, beans, nuts, eggs, and most vegetables. Wheat germ and bran are excellent sources.

Normal daily requirement
The reference nutrient intakes (RNI) for thiamine are: 0.2mg (birth–9 months); 0.3mg (10–12 months); 0.5mg (1–3 years); 0.7mg (males aged 4–10 years and females aged 4–14 years); 0.9mg (males aged 11–14 years); 1.1mg (males aged 15–18 years); 0.8mg (females aged 15 and over); 1mg (males aged 19–50 years); and 0.9mg (males aged 51 and over). Daily requirements rise by 0.1mg in the last three months of pregnancy and by 0.2mg when breast-feeding.

When supplements are helpful
A balanced diet generally provides adequate amounts of thiamine. However, supplements may be helpful in elderly people on poor diets or those with high energy requirements caused, for example, by overactivity of the thyroid or heavy manual work. As with other B vitamins, requirements of thiamine are increased during severe illness, surgery, serious injury, and prolonged psychological stress. Additional thiamine is usually necessary on medical advice for deficiency associated with conditions in which absorption of nutrients from the intestine is impaired, and for prolonged liver disease or severe alcoholism.

Symptoms of deficiency
Deficiency may cause fatigue, irritability, loss of appetite, and disturbed sleep, confusion, loss of memory, depression, abdominal pain, constipation, and beriberi, a disorder that affects the nerves, brain, and heart. Symptoms of beriberi include tingling or burning sensations in the legs, cramps and tenderness in the calf muscles, incoordination, palpitations, fits, and heart failure. In chronic alcoholics and in malnutrition, thiamine deficiency may lead to a characteristic deterioration of central nervous system function known as Wernicke Korsakoff's syndrome. The syndrome results in paralysis of the eye muscles, severe memory loss, and dementia, for which urgent treatment is needed.

Dosage range for treating deficiency
Depends on the nature and severity of the disorder but, in general, for mild chronic deficiency 10–25mg by mouth should be taken daily. Injections of the vitamin are sometimes given when deficiency is very severe or when symptoms have appeared suddenly.

Symptoms and risks of excessive intake
The risk of adverse effects is very low because any excess is rapidly eliminated in the urine. However, prolonged use of large doses of thiamine may deplete other B vitamins and should therefore be taken in a vitamin B complex formulation. There is a risk of allergic reactions with thiamine injections.

VITAMIN A

Other names Beta-carotene, carotenoids, retinoic acid, retinoids, retinol, retinol palmitate

Availability
Retinol, retinol palmitate, and beta-carotene are available without prescription in various single-ingredient and multi-vitamin and mineral preparations. Retinoids are used in prescription-only treatments for acne and psoriasis.

Actions on the body
Vitamin A is essential for normal growth and strong bones and teeth in children. It is necessary for normal vision and healthy cell structure. It helps to keep skin healthy and protect the linings of the mouth, nose, throat, lungs, and digestive and urinary tracts against infection. Vitamin A is also necessary for fertility in both sexes. Beta-carotene is an important anti-oxidant (i.e., it protects the body from cell damage).

Dietary and other natural sources
Liver (the richest source), fish liver oils, eggs, dairy products, orange and yellow vegetables and fruits (carrots, tomatoes, apricots, and peaches), and leafy green vegetables are good dietary sources. Vitamin A is also added to margarine.

Normal daily requirement
The reference nutrient intakes (RNI) for vitamin A are: 350mcg (up to 1 year); 400mcg (1–3 years); 500mcg (4–10 years); 600mcg (males aged 11–14 years, females aged 11 and over); 700mcg (males aged 15 and over, and pregnant women); 950mcg (breast-feeding).

When supplements are helpful
Most diets provide adequate amounts of vitamin A. Diets very low in fat or protein can lead to deficiency. Supplements are often given to young children in developing countries. They may also be needed by people with cystic fibrosis, obstruction of the bile ducts, overactivity of the thyroid gland, and certain intestinal disorders, and by people on long-term treatment with certain lipid-lowering drugs (e.g., cholestyramine), which reduce absorption of the vitamin from the intestine. They are recommended with other vitamins for pregnant women, children under 5 years, and nursing mothers.

Symptoms of deficiency
Night blindness (difficulty in seeing in dim light) is the earliest symptom of deficiency; others include dry, rough skin, loss of appetite, and diarrhoea. Resistance to infection is decreased. Eyes may become dry and inflamed. Severe deficiency may lead to corneal ulcers.

Dosage range for treating deficiency
Deficiency is treated by intramuscular injection of 100,000 units monthly.

Symptoms and risks of excessive intake
Prolonged excessive intake (7.5–15mg daily) in adults can cause loss of appetite, diarrhoea, dry or itchy skin, and hair loss. Fatigue and irregular menstruation are common. Headache, weakness, and vomiting may result from increased pressure of the fluid surrounding the brain. In extreme cases, bone pain and enlargement of the liver and spleen may occur. High doses of beta-carotene may turn the skin orange but are not dangerous. Excessive intake in pregnancy may lead to birth defects (see box, below).

VITAMIN A AND PREGNANCY

Very large doses of vitamin A in the early weeks of pregnancy can, rarely, cause defects in the baby, leading to damage of the central nervous system, face, eyes, ears, or palate. Pregnant women and those considering pregnancy should keep to the prescribed dose and not take extra vitamin A or eat liver products such as pâté (one serving of liver may contain 4–12 times the dose recommended for pregnancy). No other dietary restrictions are considered necessary.

VITAMIN B12

Other names Cobalamin, cobalamins, cyanocobalamin, hydroxocobalamin

Availability
Vitamin B_{12} is available without prescription in a wide variety of preparations. Hydroxocobalamin is given only by injection under medical supervision.

Actions on the body
Vitamin B_{12} plays a vital role in the activities of several *enzymes*. It is essential for the manufacture of the genetic material of cells and thus for growth and development. The formation of red blood cells by the bone marrow is particularly dependent on this vitamin. It is also involved in the utilization of folic acid and carbohydrates in the diet, and is necessary for maintaining a healthy nervous system.

Dietary and other natural sources
Liver is the best dietary source of vitamin B_{12}. Almost all animal products, as well as seaweed, are also rich in the vitamin, but vegetables are not.

Normal daily requirement
Only minute quantities of vitamin B_{12} are required. Reference nutrient intakes (RNI) are: 0.3mcg (birth–6 months); 0.4mcg (7–12 months); 0.5mcg (1–3 years); 0.8mcg (4–6 years); 1mcg (7–10 years); 1.2mcg (11–14 years); 1.5mcg (15 years and over); 2mcg (breast-feeding). Requirements of vitamin B_{12} are unchanged in pregnancy.

When supplements are helpful
A balanced diet usually provides more than adequate amounts of this vitamin, and deficiency is generally due to impaired absorption from the intestine rather than low dietary intake. However, a strict vegetarian or vegan diet lacking in eggs or dairy products is likely to be deficient in vitamin B_{12}, and supplements are usually needed. The most common cause of deficiency is pernicious *anaemia*, in which absorption of the vitamin is impaired due to inability of the stomach to secrete a special substance – known as intrinsic factor – that normally combines with the vitamin so that it can be taken up in the intestine. Supplements are also prescribed on medical advice in certain bowel disorders, such as coeliac disease and various other causes of malabsorption, after surgery to the stomach or intestine, and in fish tapeworm infestation.

Symptoms of deficiency
Vitamin B_{12} deficiency usually develops over months or years – the liver can store up to 6 years' supply. Deficiency leads to anaemia. The mouth and tongue often become sore. The brain and spinal cord may also be affected, leading to numbness and tingling of the limbs, memory loss, and depression.

Dosage range for treating deficiency
Depends on the individual and on the type and severity of deficiency. Pernicious anaemia (due to impaired absorption of vitamin B_{12}) is treated in adults with 0.25mg–1mg (250–1,000mcg) on alternate days for 1–2 weeks, then 0.25mg per week until blood counts are normal, then 1mg every 2–3 months. Higher monthly doses of up to 1,000mcg of B_{12}, together with folic acid, may be given if the deficiency is severe. Children are treated with a total of 30–50mcg daily. Dietary deficiency is usually treated with oral supplements of 50–150mcg or more daily (35–50mcg twice daily in infants). Deficiency that results from a genetic defect preventing use of the vitamin is treated with 250mcg every three weeks throughout life.

Symptoms and risks of excessive intake
Harmful effects from high doses of vitamin B_{12} are rare. Allergic reactions may in rare cases occur with preparations given by injection.

VITAMIN C

Other names Ascorbic acid, calcium ascorbate, sodium ascorbate

Availability
Vitamin C is available without prescription in a wide variety of single-ingredient and multivitamin and mineral preparations. Sodium ascorbate is given only by injection under specialized medical supervision.

Actions on the body
Vitamin C plays an essential role in the activities of several *enzymes*. It is vital for the growth and maintenance of healthy bones, teeth, gums, ligaments, and blood vessels, and is an important component of all body organs. Vitamin C is also recognized as an important antioxidant (i.e., it protects the body against cell damage and may prevent fat deposits from building up in the blood vessels) and is important for the manufacture of certain *neurotransmitters* and adrenal hormones. It is required for the utilization of folic acid and absorption of iron. This vitamin is also necessary for normal immune responses to infection and for wound healing.

Dietary and other natural sources
Vitamin C is found in most fresh fruits and vegetables. Citrus fruits, tomatoes, potatoes, and leafy green vegetables are good dietary sources. This vitamin is easily destroyed by cooking; some fresh, uncooked fruit and vegetables should be eaten daily. Adding a daily source of vitamin C, such as a glass of orange juice, is also recommended.

Normal daily requirement
The reference nutrient intakes (RNI) for vitamin C are: 25mg (birth–1 year); 30mg (1–10 years); 35mg (11–14 years); 40mg (15 years and over); 50mg (pregnancy); and 70mg (breast-feeding).

When supplements are helpful
A healthy diet generally contains sufficient quantities of vitamin C. However, it is used up more rapidly after a serious injury, major surgery, burns, and in extremes of temperature. Supplements may be necessary to prevent or treat deficiency in the elderly and chronically sick, for smokers, and in severe alcoholism. They are recommended with other vitamins for pregnant women, children under 5 years, and nursing mothers. Women taking oestrogen-containing contraceptives may also require supplements. Although many people take larger doses (1g daily) for the prevention or treatment of colds, there is no convincing evidence that vitamin C in large doses prevents them, although it may reduce the severity of symptoms.

Symptoms of deficiency
Mild deficiency may cause weakness and aches and pains. Severe deficiency results in scurvy, the symptoms of which include inflamed, bleeding gums, nosebleeds, excessive bruising, and internal bleeding. In adults, teeth become loose. In children, there is abnormal bone and tooth development. Wounds fail to heal and become infected. Deficiency of vitamin C often leads to *anaemia* (abnormally low levels of red blood cells), the symptoms of which are pallor, fatigue, shortness of breath, and palpitations. Untreated scurvy may cause fits, coma, and death.

Dosage range for treating deficiency
For scurvy, at least 250mg of vitamin C is given daily for several weeks.

Symptoms and risks of excessive intake
The risk of harmful effects is low, since excess vitamin C is excreted in the urine. However, doses of over 3g daily may cause diarrhoea, nausea, and stomach cramps. Kidney stones may occasionally develop.

VITAMIN D

Other names Alfacalcidol, calcifediol, calciferol, calcitriol, cholecalciferol, ergocalciferol, vitamin D_2, vitamin D_3

Availability
Vitamin D is available without prescription in a variety of multivitamin and mineral preparations. Injections are given only under medical supervision.

Actions on the body
Vitamin D (together with parathyroid hormone) helps regulate the balance of calcium and phosphate in the body. It aids in the absorption of calcium from the intestinal tract, and is essential for strong bones and teeth.

Dietary and other natural sources
Margarine (to which vitamin D is added by law), oily fish (sardines, herring, salmon, and tuna), liver, dairy products, and egg yolks are usually good sources of this vitamin. It is also formed by the action of ultraviolet rays in sunlight on chemicals naturally present in the skin. Sunlight is one main source of vitamin D for most people.

Normal daily requirement
The reference nutrient intakes (RNI) for vitamin D are: 8.5mcg (birth–6 months); 7mcg (7 months–3 years); 10mcg (over 65 years, and women who are pregnant or breast-feeding). Most people outside these groups do not require dietary supplements of vitamin D. 1mcg of vitamin D equals 40 international units (IU).

When supplements are helpful
Vitamin D requirements are small and are usually adequately met by dietary sources and normal exposure to sunlight. However, a poor diet and inadequate sunlight may lead to deficiency; dark-skinned people (particularly those living in smoggy urban areas) and night-shift workers are more at risk. In areas of moderate sunshine, supplements may be given to infants. Premature infants, strict vegetarians, vegans, and the elderly may benefit from supplements of this vitamin. Supplements are usually necessary on medical advice to prevent and treat vitamin D deficiency-related bone disorders, and for conditions in which absorption from the intestine is impaired, deficiency due to liver disease, certain kidney disorders, prolonged use of certain drugs, and genetic defects. They are also used in the treatment of hypoparathyroidism. Supplements are recommended with other vitamins for pregnant women, children under 5 years, and nursing mothers, and with calcium to prevent or treat osteoporosis.

Symptoms of deficiency
Long-term deficiency leads to low blood levels of calcium and phosphate, which results in softening of the bones. In children, this causes abnormal bone development (rickets), and in adults, osteomalacia, causing backache, muscle weakness, bone pain, and fractures.

Dosage range for treating deficiency
In general, rickets caused by dietary deficiency is treated initially with 1,500–6,000 IU of vitamin D daily, depending on the age of the child, followed by a maintenance dose of 400 IU. Osteomalacia caused by deficiency of vitamin D is treated initially with 3,000–40,000 IU daily, followed by a daily maintenance dose of 400 IU. Deficiency caused by impaired intestinal absorption is treated with doses of 10,000–40,000 IU daily (adults) and 10,000–25,000 IU daily (children).

Symptoms and risks of excessive intake
Doses of over 400 IU of vitamin D daily are not beneficial in most people and may increase the risk of adverse effects. Prolonged excessive use disrupts the balance of calcium and phosphate in the body and may lead to abnormal calcium deposits in the soft tissues, blood vessel walls, and kidneys and retarded growth in children. Excess calcium may lead to symptoms such as weakness, unusual thirst, increased urination, gastrointestinal disturbances, and depression.

VITAMIN E

Other names Alpha tocopherol, Alpha tocopheryl acetate, tocopherol, tocopherols

Availability
Vitamin E is available without prescription in many single-ingredient and multivitamin and mineral preparations. It is also included in skin creams. Alpha tocopherol is the most powerful form.

Actions on the body
Vitamin E, a potent anti-oxidant, is vital for healthy cell structure, for slowing the effects of the ageing process on cells, and for maintaining the activities of certain *enzymes*. Vitamin E protects the lungs and other tissues from damage caused by pollutants, and protects red blood cells against destruction by poisons in the bloodstream. It also helps to maintain healthy red blood cells, and is involved in the production of energy in the heart and muscles. There is some evidence that vitamin E may protect against coronary heart disease and cancer, but further research is required.

Dietary and other natural sources
Some vegetable oils are good sources. Other sources rich in this vitamin include leafy green vegetables, wholemeal cereals, and wheat germ.

Normal daily requirement
Vitamin E is measured in milligrams of alpha-tocopherol equivalents (mg alpha-TE). Approximately 3–15mg daily are recommended. However, no UK recommendations have been made as vitamin E requirement depends on intake of poly-unsaturated fatty acid, which varies widely. Recommended daily allowances (RDA) in the USA are: 3mg alpha-TE (birth–6 months); 4mg alpha-TE (7–12 months); 6mg alpha-TE (1–3 years); 7mg alpha-TE (4–10 years); 10mg alpha-TE (males aged 11 and over); 8mg alpha-TE (females aged 11 and over); 10mg alpha-TE (pregnancy); 12mg alpha-TE (first 6 months of breast-feeding); and 11mg alpha-TE (second 6 months of breast-feeding).

When supplements are helpful
A normal diet supplies adequate amounts of vitamin E, and supplements are rarely necessary. However, people who consume large amounts of polyunsaturated fats in vegetable oils, especially if used in cooking at high temperatures, may need supplements. Supplements of vitamin E are also recommended for premature infants and people with impaired intestinal absorption, liver disease in children, or cystic fibrosis.

Symptoms of deficiency
Vitamin E deficiency leads to destruction of red blood cells (haemolysis) and eventually *anaemia* (abnormally low levels of red blood cells), symptoms of which may include pallor, fatigue, shortness of breath, and palpitations. In infants, deficiency may cause irritability and fluid retention.

Dosage range for treating deficiency
Doses are generally four to five times the RDA in adults and children, for the relevant sex and age group.

Symptoms and risks of excessive intake
Harmful effects are rare, but there is a risk of diarrhoea and abdominal pain with doses of than 1g per day. Prolonged use of over 250mg daily may lead to nausea, abdominal pain, vomiting, and diarrhoea. Large doses may also reduce the amounts of vitamin A, D, and K absorbed from the intestines; they can also increase the tendency to bleed in patients taking oral anticoagulants.

VITAMIN K

Other names Menadione, phytomenadione, vitamin K_1, vitamin K_2, vitamin K_3

Availability
Vitamin K is available without prescription as a dietary supplement in several multivitamin and mineral preparations. Injectable and oral preparations of vitamin K alone are used to treat bleeding disorders are available only on prescription.

Actions on the body
Vitamin K is necessary for the formation in the liver of several substances that promote the formation of blood clots (blood clotting factors), including prothrombin (clotting factor II).

Dietary and other natural sources
The best dietary sources of vitamin K are leafy green vegetables and root vegetables, fruits, seeds, cow's milk, and yoghurt. Alfalfa is also an excellent source. In adults and children, the intestinal bacteria manufacture a large part of the vitamin K that is required.

Normal daily requirement
The safe reference nutrient intake (RNI) for vitamin K in newborn infants is 10mcg. No RNI has been set for other age groups; however, in the USA, the recommended daily allowances (RDA) are: 10mcg (6–12 months); 15mcg (1–3 years); 20mcg (4–6 years); 30mcg (7–10 years); 45mcg (11–14 years); 65mcg (males aged 15–18); 55 mcg (females aged 15–18); 70mcg (males aged 19–24); 60mcg (females aged 19–24); 80mcg (males aged 25 and over); and 65mcg (females aged 25 and over). There are no extra requirements in pregnancy or breast-feeding.

When supplements are helpful
Vitamin K requirements are generally met adequately by dietary intake and by manufacture of the vitamin by bacteria that live in the intestine. Supplements are given routinely to newborn babies, since they lack intestinal bacteria capable of producing the vitamin and are therefore more at risk of deficiency than adults are. In adults and children, additional vitamin K is usually necessary only on medical advice for deficiency associated with prolonged use of antibiotics or sulphonamide antibacterials that destroy bacteria in the intestine, or when absorption of nutrients from the intestine is impaired. These conditions include liver disease, obstruction of the bile duct, and intestinal disorders causing chronic diarrhoea. Vitamin K may also be given to reduce blood loss during labour or after surgery in people who have been taking oral anticoagulants. Vitamin K also reverses the effect of an overdose of oral anticoagulants.

Symptoms of deficiency
Vitamin K deficiency leads to low levels of prothrombin (hypoprothrombinaemia) and other clotting factors, resulting in delayed blood clotting and a tendency to bleed. This may cause easy bruising, oozing from wounds, nosebleeds, and bleeding from the gums, intestine, urinary tract, and, rarely, in the brain.

Dosage range for treating deficiency
Depends on the individual and on the nature and severity of the disorder.

Symptoms and risks of excessive intake
Excess dietary intake of vitamin K has no known harmful effects. Synthetic vitamin K (menadione) may cause rupture of red blood cells (haemolysis) in people who have glucose-6-phosphate dehydrogenase (G6PD) deficiency. This may lead to reddish brown urine, *jaundice*, and, in extreme cases, *anaemia*. Adverse effects are extremely rare with vitamin K preparations taken by mouth.

ZINC

Other names Zinc acetate, zinc chloride, zinc gluconate, zinc oxide, zinc sulphate

Availability
Zinc supplements are available without prescription in single-ingredient and multivitamin and mineral preparations. Zinc chloride is used in ocular solutions and mouthwashes and as an injectable preparation given only under medical supervision during intravenous feeding. Zinc is also one ingredient included in a variety of topical formulations used for the treatment of minor skin irritations, dandruff, acne, haemorrhoids, and fungal infections.

Actions on the body
Zinc plays a vital role in the activities of over 100 *enzymes*. It is essential for the manufacture of proteins and nucleic acids (the genetic material of cells), and is involved in the function of the hormone insulin in the utilization of carbohydrates. It is necessary for normal functioning of the immune system, a normal rate of growth, development of the reproductive organs, normal function of sperm, and healing of wounds and burns.

Dietary and other natural sources
Zinc is present in small amounts in a wide variety of foods. The mineral is better absorbed from animal sources than from plant sources. Protein-rich foods such as lean meat and seafood are the best sources of the mineral. Wholemeal breads and cereals, as well as dried pulses, are also good dietary sources.

Normal daily requirement
The reference nutrient intakes (RNI) for zinc are: 4mg (birth–6 months); 5mg (7 months–3 years); 6.5mg (4–6 years); 7mg (7–10 years); 9mg (11–14 years); 9.5mg (males aged 15 and over); and 7mg (females aged 15 and over). There is no extra requirement during pregnancy, but the RNI is 13mg in the first 4 months of breast-feeding and 9.5mg thereafter.

When supplements are helpful
A balanced diet containing natural, unprocessed foods usually provides adequate amounts of zinc. Dietary deficiency is rare in Britain, and is likely only in people who are generally malnourished, such as debilitated elderly people on poor diets. Supplements are usually recommended on medical advice for those with reduced absorption of the mineral due to certain intestinal disorders, such as cystic fibrosis; for those with increased zinc requirements due to sickle cell disease or major burns; and for those with liver damage occurring, for example, as a result of excessive alcohol intake. There is evidence that zinc supplements may shorten the duration of the common cold.

Symptoms of deficiency
Deficiency may cause loss of appetite and impair the sense of taste. In children, it may also lead to poor growth and, in severe cases, to delayed sexual development and short stature. Severe, prolonged lack of zinc may result in a rare skin disorder involving hair loss, rash, inflamed areas of skin with pustules, and inflammation around the mouth, tongue, eyelids, and around the fingernails.

Dosage range for treating deficiency
Depends on the individual and on the cause and severity of the deficiency. In general, 30–50mg daily is sufficient, usually in the form of zinc sulphate.

Symptoms and risks of excessive intake
Large overdoses of zinc salts in powder form are corrosive to tissues and may cause burns in the mouth and throat. Prolonged use of high doses may interfere with the absorption of copper, leading to deficiency, and may cause nausea, vomiting, headache, fever, malaise, and abdominal pain.

DRUGS OF ABUSE

The purpose of these pages is to clarify the medical facts concerning certain drugs (or classes of drugs) that are commonly abused in the UK. Their physical and mental effects, sometimes combined with a dangerous habit-forming potential, have led to their use outside a medical context. Some of the drugs listed in this section are illegal, while others have legitimate medical uses – such as anti-anxiety and sleeping drugs – and are also discussed in other parts of the book. Alcohol, nicotine, and solvents, although not medical drugs, are all substances that have drug-like effects and high abuse potential. These substances are not illegal, but the sale of alcohol and tobacco products to young people is regulated by law, and the sale of solvents by voluntary agreement.

The individual profiles are designed to instruct and inform the reader, enabling him or her to understand how these drugs affect the body, to become more aware of the hazards of drug abuse, and to be able to recognize signs of drug abuse in other people.

Since a large proportion of drug abusers are young people, the following pages may serve as a useful source of reference for parents and teachers who are concerned that young people in their charge may be taking drugs.

The drugs of abuse profiles

The profiles are arranged in alphabetical order under their medical names, with street names, drug categories, and cross-references to other parts of the book where appropriate. Each profile contains information on that drug under standard headings. Topics covered include the various ways it is taken, its habit-forming potential, its legitimate medical uses, its legal status, its effects and risks, the signs of abuse, and interactions with other drugs.

HOW TO UNDERSTAND THE PROFILES

Each drug of abuse profile contains standard headings under which you will find information covering important aspects of the drug.

Drug category
Categorizes the drug according to its principal effects on the body, with cross-references to other parts of the book where relevant.

Other common names
Lists the usual, alternative, and street names of each drug.

How taken
Tells you the various forms in which each substance is taken.

Short-term effects
Explains the immediate mental and physical effects of the drug.

Signs of abuse
Describes the outward effects of taking the drug, both short- and long-term, that concerned observers may notice.

Practical points
Gives tips on how to avoid abuse of the drug and suggests ways to stop or reduce intake.

Habit-forming potential
Explains to what extent the drug is likely to produce physical or psychological *dependence.*

Legitimate uses
Describes the accepted medical uses of the substance, if any.

Long-term effects and risks
Explains the serious long-term effects on health and the risks involved with regular use of the drug.

Interactions
Describes interactions that may occur with other drugs.

BENZODIAZEPINES

Other common names Tranquillizers, temmies
Drug category Central nervous system depressants (see Sleeping drugs, p.82, and Anti-anxiety drugs, p.83)

Habit-forming potential
The addictive potential of benzodiazepines is much lower than that of some other central nervous system depressants such as barbiturates. However, regular long-term use of these drugs can lead to physical and psychological dependence on their sedative effects.

How taken
By mouth as tablets or capsules, or by injection. Temazepam is the most widely abused benzodiazepine.

Legitimate uses
Benzodiazepines are commonly prescribed mainly for short-term treatment of anxiety and stress, as well as for relief of sleeplessness. They are also used in anaesthesia, both as premedication and for induction of general anaesthesia. Other medical uses include the management of alcohol withdrawal, control of epileptic fits, and relief of muscle spasms. Most benzodiazepines are classified under Class C and Schedule IV of the Misuse of Drugs legislation, although temazepam is under Schedule III.

Short-term effects
Benzodiazepines can reduce mental activity. In moderate doses, they may also cause unsteadiness, reduce alertness, and slow the body's reactions, thus impairing driving ability as well as increasing the risk of accidents. Benzodiazepines may also cause amnesia (loss of memory regarding events that occurred while the person was under the influence of the drug). Any benzodiazepine in a high-enough dose induces sleep. Very large overdoses may cause depression of the breathing mechanism and death can occur.

Long-term effects and risks
Benzodiazepines tend to lose their sedative effect with long-term use. This may lead the user to increase the dose progressively, a manifestation of tolerance and physical dependence. Older people may become apathetic or confused when taking these drugs. On stopping the drug, the chronic user may develop *withdrawal* symptoms that may include anxiety, panic attacks, palpitations, shaking, insomnia, headaches, dizziness, aches and pains, nausea, loss of appetite, and clumsiness. Symptoms can last for days or weeks. Babies born to women who use benzodiazepines regularly may suffer withdrawal symptoms during the first week of life.

Signs of abuse
Abuse can occur by injection in young people. Another type of abuser is a middle-aged or elderly person who may have been taking these drugs by prescription for months or years. He or she is usually unaware of the problem, and may freely admit to taking "nerve" or sleeping pills in normal or large quantities. Problems usually occur only if people attempt to cut down or stop taking the drugs without medical advice.

Interactions
Benzodiazepines increase the risk of sedation with any drug that has a sedative effect on the central nervous system. These include other anti-anxiety and sleeping drugs, alcohol, opioid analgesics, antipsychotics, tricyclic antidepressants, and antihistamines.

Practical points
Benzodiazepines should normally be used for courses of two weeks' duration or less. If these drugs have been taken for longer than two weeks, it is usually best to reduce the dose gradually, to minimize the risk of withdrawal symptoms. If you have been taking benzodiazepines for many months or years, it is best to consult your doctor to work out a dose reduction programme. If possible, it will help to tell your family and friends and enlist their support.

CANNABIS

Other common names Marijuana, grass, pot, dope, reefers, weed, hash, ganja, skunk, skunkweed
Drug category Central nervous system depressant, hallucinogen, anti-emetic

Habit-forming potential
There is evidence that regular users of cannabis can become physically and psychologically dependent on its effects.

How taken
Usually smoked, either like tobacco or through a "bong" pipe. May be eaten, often in cakes or biscuits, or brewed like tea and drunk.

Legitimate uses
Preparations of the leaves and resin of the cannabis plant (marijuana) have been in use for over 2,000 years. Introduced into Western medicine in the mid-19th century, cannabis was formerly taken for a wide variety of complaints, including anxiety, insomnia, rheumatic disorders, migraine, painful menstruation, strychnine poisoning, and opioid withdrawal. Today, cannabis derivatives – for example, nabilone – can be prescribed with certain restrictions for the relief of nausea and vomiting caused by treatment with anticancer drugs. Cannabis itself is listed under Class B and Schedule I of the Misuse of Drugs legislation.

Short-term effects
These partly depend on the effects expected by the user as well as on the amount and strength of the preparation used. Some types of cannabis available today (such as skunk) are more potent than that of a few years ago. In small doses, the drug promotes a feeling of relaxation and well-being, enhances auditory and visual perception, and increases talkativeness. Appetite is usually increased. However, in some individuals the drug may have little or no effect.
Under the influence of the drug, short-term memory may be impaired and driving ability and coordination are disrupted. Confusion, emotional distress, and loss of the sense of time can result. Hallucinations may occur in rare cases. The effects last for one to three hours after smoking cannabis and for up to 12 hours or longer after it is eaten, but reaction times remain slowed for 24 hours after a single use of the drug. Death from overdose is unknown.

Long-term effects and risks
Cannabis smoking, like tobacco smoking, increases the risk of bronchitis and lung cancer. Regular users may become apathetic and lethargic, and neglect their work or studies and personal appearance. In susceptible people, heavy use may trigger a temporary psychiatric disturbance. Cannabis is thought by some doctors to increase the likelihood of experimentation with other drugs.
Since cannabis may lower blood pressure and increase the heart rate, people with heart disorders may be at risk from adverse effects of this drug. Regular use of cannabis may reduce fertility in both men and women and, if used during pregnancy, may contribute to premature birth.

Signs of abuse
The cannabis user may appear unusually talkative or drunk under the influence of the drug. Appetite is increased. The user may become defensive or aggressive when challenged about use of the drug.
Cannabis smoke has a distinct herbal smell that may linger in the hair and clothes of those who use it. Burns may occur on clothing as a result of pieces of lighted cannabis falling from the cigarette.

Interactions
Cannabis may increase the risk of sedation with any drugs that have a sedative effect on the central nervous system. These include anti-anxiety drugs, sleeping drugs, general anaesthetics, opioid analgesics, antipsychotics, tricyclic antidepressants, antihistamines, and alcohol.

453

ALCOHOL

Other common names Booze, drink (includes beer, wine, and spirits); also known as ethyl alcohol or ethanol
Drug category Central nervous system depressant; sedative

Habit-forming potential
Because individual responses vary so widely, it is difficult to measure the habit-forming potential of alcohol. But there is certainly a disease called alcoholism, characterized by a person's inability to control intake. Regular drinking and heavy drinking do not cause alcoholism so much as indicate that it may be present. Alcoholism involves psychological and physical *dependence,* evidenced by large daily consumption, heavy weekend drinking, or periodic binges.

How taken
By mouth, usually in the form of wines, beers, and a wide range of spirits and liqueurs.

Legitimate uses
There are no legal restrictions on the consumption of alcohol, but the sale of alcoholic beverages is restricted to those over the age of 18. The manufacture and sale of alcoholic drinks is closely regulated, both because it is a source of government revenue and to prevent the production of alcoholic drinks containing methanol (methyl alcohol), which is toxic and can cause blindness.

Medically, surgical spirit (strongly concentrated alcohol that contains methanol) is widely used as an *antiseptic* before injections to minimize the risk of infection. It is also used to harden the skin and thus prevent pressure sores in bedridden people and foot sores in hikers or runners. It can be extremely harmful if ingested regularly.

Short-term effects
Alcohol acts as a central nervous system depressant, thus reducing anxiety, tension, and inhibitions. In moderate quantities, it creates a feeling of relaxation and confidence and increases sociability and talkativeness, but does not improve mental performance. Moderate amounts also dilate small blood vessels, especially in the skin, leading to flushing and a feeling of warmth. Increasing amounts progressively impair concentration and judgment and the body's reactions are increasingly slowed. Accidents, particularly driving accidents, are more likely. As blood alcohol levels rise, violent or aggressive behaviour is possible. Speech is slurred, and the person becomes unsteady, staggers, and may experience double vision and loss of balance. Nausea and vomiting are frequent; incontinence may occur. Loss of consciousness may follow if blood alcohol levels continue to rise, and there is a risk of death occurring as a result of inhalation of vomit or cessation of breathing.

Long-term effects and risks
Heavy drinkers risk developing liver diseases, for example, alcoholic hepatitis, liver cancer, cirrhosis, or fatty liver (excess fat deposits that may lead to cirrhosis). High blood pressure and strokes may also result from heavy drinking. Inflammation of the stomach (gastritis) and peptic ulcers are more common in alcoholics, who also have a higher than average risk of developing dementia (irreversible mental deterioration).

Long-term heavy drinking is generally associated with physical dependence. An alcoholic may appear to be sober, even after heavy drinking, because of built-up tolerance. But a reverse tolerance effect is frequently seen in long-term alcoholics, where relatively little alcohol can rapidly produce a state of intoxication. As well as health problems, alcohol dependence is associated with a range of personal and social problems. Alcoholics may suffer from anxiety and depression, and since they often eat poorly, they are at risk of various nutritional deficiency diseases, particularly deficiency of thiamine (see p.436).

Drinking during pregnancy can cause fetal abnormalities and poor physical and mental development in infants; even taking moderate amounts of alcohol can lead to miscarriage, low birth weight, and mental retardation.

Signs of abuse
Alcohol consumption may be getting out of control if any or all of the following signs are noted: changes in drinking pattern (for example, early morning drinking or a switch from beer to spirits); changes in drinking habits (such as drinking alone or having a drink before an appointment or interview); neglect of personal appearance; personality changes; poor eating habits; furtive behaviour; and increasingly frequent or prolonged bouts of intoxication with memory lapses ("blackouts") about events that occurred during drinking episodes. Physical symptoms may include nausea, vomiting, or shaking in the morning, abdominal pain, cramps, redness and enlarged blood vessels in the face, weakness in the legs and hands, unsteadiness, poor memory, and incontinence. The sudden discontinuation of heavy drinking, if not treated, can lead to delirium tremens (severe shaking, confusion, hallucinations, and occasionally fatal convulsions) beginning after one to four days of abstinence and lasting for up to three days. *Withdrawal symptoms* can be controlled by drugs such as chlormethiazole, atenolol, or benzodiazepines, such as diazepam, given short term under medical supervision.

Interactions
Alcohol interacts with a wide variety of drugs. In particular, it increases the risk of sedation with any drug that has a *sedative* effect on the central nervous system. These include anti-anxiety drugs, sleeping drugs, *general anaesthetics*, *opioid* analgesics, antipsychotics, tricyclic antidepressants, antihistamines, and certain antihypertensive drugs (clonidine and methyldopa). Taking alcohol with other depressant drugs of abuse, particularly opioids, barbiturates, or solvents, can lead to coma and may be fatal.

Taken with aspirin and similar analgesics, alcohol increases the risk of bleeding from the stomach, particularly in people who have had stomach ulcers.

People taking disulfiram (Antabuse), a drug used to help people stay in an alcohol-free state, will experience highly unpleasant reactions if they then take even a small amount of alcohol. The results include flushing of the face, throbbing headache, palpitations, nausea, and vomiting.

Excessive alcohol may slow down the breakdown of some oral antidiabetic drugs and oral anticoagulants, and thereby increase their effects.

Taken with monoamine oxidase inhibitors (MAOIs), some alcoholic drinks, particularly in the form of red wine, may cause a dangerous rise in blood pressure.

Practical points
If you drink, know what your limits are. They vary from person to person, and your capacity depends a good deal on your body weight, age, experience, and mental and emotional state. However, you can use a "rule of thumb" guide to judge the body's ability to break down alcohol. Generally, the body can break down only about one unit of alcohol (i.e., one measure of spirits, one glass of wine, or one-half pint of beer) per hour. If you drink faster than this, your blood alcohol is likely to rise above the "legal limit" for driving. Even lower levels of alcohol than this can affect judgment and reaction times, so the safest advice is not to drink at all if you plan to drive. Men should not drink a total of more than 20 units per week, and women should not exceed 15 units per week. If you are a woman and are pregnant, or you are trying to conceive, the safest course is abstinence.

If you find that you are having trouble controlling your drinking, seek help and advice from your doctor or from an organization, such as Alcoholics Anonymous, dedicated to helping people with this problem. Even if you do not have a control problem, do not drink heavily because alcohol can have harmful effects on many parts of your body, including your liver and brain.

AMPHETAMINE

Other common names Speed, uppers, bennies, whizz, blues
Drug category Central nervous system stimulant (see p.88)

Habit-forming potential
Regular use of amphetamine or methamphetamine rapidly leads to the development of *tolerance*, so that higher and higher doses are required to achieve the same effect. Users become psychologically dependent on the drug's effects. Toxic effects can occur at relatively low doses.

How taken
Usually swallowed as tablets or powder. Sometimes sniffed or mixed with water and injected.

Legitimate uses
During the 1950s and 1960s, amphetamine was widely given as an appetite suppressant. This use of the drug has largely been abandoned because of the risk of *dependence* and abuse. Amphetamine was also used to maintain wakefulness by drivers and pilots. It is still prescribed for attention deficit disorder (hyperactivity) and narcolepsy (see also Nervous system stimulants, p.88). Amphetamine is classified under Class B and Schedule II of the Misuse of Drugs legislation.

Short-term effects
In small doses, amphetamine increases mental alertness and physical energy. Breathing and heart rate speed up, the pupils dilate, appetite decreases, and dryness of the mouth is common. As these effects wear off, depression and fatigue may follow. At high doses, amphetamine may cause tremor, sweating, anxiety, headache, palpitations, and chest pain. Large doses may cause delusions, confusion, hallucinations, delirium, collapse, aggressive behaviour, convulsions, coma, and death.

Long-term effects and risks
Regular use frequently leads to muscle damage, weight loss, and constipation. People who use amphetamine regularly may also become emotionally unstable. Severe depression and suicide are associated with withdrawal. Heavy long-term use reduces resistance to infection and also carries a risk of damage to the heart and blood vessels, leading to strokes and heart failure.

Use of amphetamine in early pregnancy may increase the risk of birth defects, especially in the heart. Taken throughout pregnancy, amphetamine leads to premature birth and low birth weight.

Signs of abuse
The amphetamine user may appear unusually energetic, cheerful, and excessively talkative while under the influence of the drug. Restlessness, agitation, and a lack of interest in food are typical symptoms; personality changes, psychotic reactions, and paranoid delusions may also occur. Regular users may exhibit unusual sleeping patterns, staying awake for two or three nights at a stretch, then sleeping for up to 48 hours afterwards. Mood swings are common.

Interactions
Amphetamine interacts with a variety of drugs. It causes an increase in blood pressure, thus opposing the effect of antihypertensive drug treatments. Taken with monoamine oxidase inhibitors (MAOIs), it may lead to a dangerous rise in blood pressure. It also increases the risk of abnormal heart rhythms with digitalis drugs, levodopa, and certain anaesthetics that are given by inhalation. Amphetamine counteracts the *sedative* effects of drugs that depress the central nervous system.

BARBITURATES

Other common names Barbs, downers
Drug category Central nervous system depressant (see also Sleeping drugs, p.82), sedative

Habit-forming potential
Long-term, regular use of barbiturates can be habit-forming. Both physical and psychological *dependence* may occur.

How taken
By mouth in the form of capsules or tablets. Occasionally mixed with water and injected.

Legitimate uses
In the past, barbiturates were widely prescribed as sleeping drugs. Since the 1960s, however, they have been increasingly replaced by benzodiazepines, which may also be addictive but are less likely to cause death from overdose.

The widest uses of barbiturates today are in *anaesthesia* (thiopentone) and for epilepsy (phenobarbitone).

Most barbiturates are listed under Class B and Schedule III of the Misuse of Drugs Legislation.

Short-term effects
The short-term effects are similar to those of alcohol. A low dose produces relaxation, while larger amounts make the user more intoxicated and drowsy. Coordination is impaired and slurred speech, clumsiness, and confusion may occur. Increasingly large doses may produce loss of consciousness, coma, and death caused by depression of the person's breathing mechanism.

Long-term effects and risks
The greatest risk of long-term barbiturate use is physical dependence. In an addicted person, sudden withdrawal of the drug precipitates a withdrawal syndrome that varies in severity, depending partly on the type of barbiturate, its dose, and the duration of use, but primarily on the availability and administration of supportive treatment, including appropriate medication. Symptoms may include irritability, disturbed sleep, nightmares, nausea, vomiting, weakness, tremors, and extreme anxiety. Abrupt withdrawal after several months of use may cause convulsions, delirium, fever, and coma lasting for up to one week. Long-term, heavy use of barbiturates increases the risk of accidental overdose. The risk of chest infections is also increased because the cough reflex is suppressed by long-term, heavy use of these drugs.

Use of barbiturates during pregnancy may cause fetal abnormalities and, used regularly in the last three months, may lead to *withdrawal symptoms* in the newborn baby.

Signs of abuse
Long-term heavy use of barbiturates may cause prolonged bouts of intoxication with memory lapses ("blackouts"), neglect of personal appearance and responsibilities, personality changes, and episodes of severe depression.

Interactions
Barbiturates interact with a wide variety of drugs and increase the risk of sedation with any drug that has a *sedative* effect on the central nervous system. These include anti-anxiety drugs, *opioid* analgesics, antipsychotics, antihistamines, and tricyclic antidepressants. High doses taken with alcohol can lead to a fatal coma.

Barbiturates also increase the activity of certain enzymes in the liver, leading to an increase in the breakdown of certain drugs, thus reducing their effects. Tricyclic antidepressants, phenytoin, griseofulvin, and corticosteroids are affected in this way. However, the toxicity of a paracetamol overdose is likely to be greater in people taking barbiturates.

BENZODIAZEPINES

Other common names Tranquillizers, temmies
Drug category Central nervous system depressants (see Sleeping drugs, p.82, and Anti-anxiety drugs, p.83)

Habit-forming potential
The addictive potential of benzodiazepines is much lower than that of some other central nervous system depressants such as barbiturates. However, regular long-term use of these drugs can lead to physical and psychological *dependence* on their *sedative* effects.

How taken
By mouth as tablets or capsules, or by injection. Temazepam is the most widely abused benzodiazepine.

Legitimate uses
Benzodiazepines are commonly prescribed mainly for short-term treatment of anxiety and stress, as well as for relief of sleeplessness. They are also used in *anaesthesia*, both as *premedication* and for induction of general anaesthesia. Other medical uses include the management of alcohol withdrawal, control of epileptic fits, and relief of muscle spasms. Most benzodiazepines are classified under Class C and Schedule IV of the Misuse of Drugs legislation, although temazepam is under Schedule III.

Short-term effects
Benzodiazepines can reduce mental activity. In moderate doses, they may also cause unsteadiness, reduce alertness, and slow the body's reactions, thus impairing driving ability as well as increasing the risk of accidents. Benzodiazepines may also cause amnesia (loss of memory regarding events that occurred while the person was under the influence of the drug). Any benzodiazepine in a high-enough dose induces sleep. Very large overdoses may cause depression of the breathing mechanism and death can occur.

Long-term effects and risks
Benzodiazepines tend to lose their sedative effect with long-term use. This may lead the user to increase the dose progressively, a manifestation of tolerance and physical dependence. Older people may become apathetic or confused when taking these drugs. On stopping the drug, the chronic user may develop *withdrawal symptoms* that may include anxiety, panic attacks, palpitations, shaking, insomnia, headaches, dizziness, aches and pains, nausea, loss of appetite, and clumsiness. Symptoms can last for days or weeks. Babies born to women who use benzodiazepines regularly may suffer withdrawal symptoms during the first week of life.

Signs of abuse
Abuse can occur by injection in young people. Another type of abuser is a middle-aged or elderly person who may have been taking these drugs by prescription for months or years. He or she is usually unaware of the problem, and may freely admit to taking "nerve" or sleeping pills in normal or large quantities. Problems usually occur only if people attempt to cut down or stop taking the drugs without medical advice.

Interactions
Benzodiazepines increase the risk of sedation with any drug that has a sedative effect on the central nervous system. These include other anti-anxiety and sleeping drugs, alcohol, *opioid* analgesics, antipsychotics, tricyclic antidepressants, and antihistamines.

Practical points
Benzodiazepines should normally be used for courses of two weeks' duration or less. If these drugs have been taken for longer than two weeks, it is usually best to reduce the dose gradually to minimize the risk of withdrawal symptoms. If you have been taking benzodiazepines for many months or years, it is best to consult your doctor to work out a dose reduction programme. If possible, it will help to tell your family and friends and enlist their support.

CANNABIS

Other common names Marijuana, grass, pot, dope, reefers, weed, hash, ganja, skunk, skunkweed
Drug category Central nervous system depressant, hallucinogen, anti-emetic

Habit-forming potential
There is evidence that regular users of cannabis can become physically and psychologically *dependent* on its effects.

How taken
Usually smoked, either like tobacco or through a "bong" pipe. May be eaten, often in cakes or biscuits, or brewed like tea and drunk.

Legitimate uses
Preparations of the leaves and resin of the cannabis plant have been in use for over 2,000 years. Introduced into Western medicine in the mid-19th century, cannabis was formerly taken for a wide variety of complaints, including anxiety, insomnia, rheumatic disorders, migraine, painful menstruation, strychnine poisoning, and *opioid* withdrawal. Today, cannabis derivatives – for example, nabilone – can be prescribed with certain restrictions for the relief of nausea and vomiting caused by treatment with anticancer drugs. Cannabis itself is listed under Class B and Schedule I of the Misuse of Drugs legislation.

Short-term effects
These partly depend on the effects expected by the user as well as on the amount and strength of the preparation used. Some types of cannabis available today (such as skunk) are more potent than that of a few years ago. In small doses, the drug promotes a feeling of relaxation and well-being, enhances auditory and visual perception, and increases talkativeness. Appetite is usually increased. However, in some individuals the drug may have little or no effect.

Under the influence of the drug, short-term memory may be impaired and driving ability and coordination are disrupted. Confusion, emotional distress, and loss of the sense of time can result. Hallucinations may occur in rare cases. The effects last for one to three hours after smoking cannabis and for up to 12 hours or longer after it is eaten, but reaction times remain slowed for 24 hours after a single use of the drug. Death from overdose is unknown.

Long-term effects and risks
Cannabis smoking, like tobacco smoking, increases the risk of bronchitis and lung cancer. Regular users may become apathetic and lethargic, and neglect their work or studies and personal appearance. In susceptible people, heavy use may trigger a temporary psychiatric disturbance. Cannabis is thought by some doctors to increase the likelihood of experimentation with other drugs.

Since cannabis may lower blood pressure and increase the heart rate, people with heart disorders may be at risk from adverse effects of this drug. Regular use of cannabis may reduce fertility in both men and women and, if used during pregnancy, may contribute to premature birth.

Signs of abuse
The cannabis user may appear unusually talkative or drunk under the influence of the drug. Appetite is increased. The user may become defensive or aggressive when challenged about use of the drug.

Cannabis smoke has a distinct herbal smell that may linger in the hair and clothes of those who use it. Burns may occur on clothing as a result of pieces of lighted cannabis falling from the cigarette.

Interactions
Cannabis may increase the risk of sedation with any drugs that have a *sedative* effect on the central nervous system. These include anti-anxiety drugs, sleeping drugs, *general anaesthetics*, opioid analgesics, antipsychotics, tricyclic antidepressants, antihistamines, and alcohol.

COCAINE

Other common names Coke, crack, nose candy, snow
Drug category Central nervous system stimulant and local anaesthetic (p.80)

Habit-forming potential
Taken regularly, cocaine is habit-forming. Users may become psychologically dependent on its physical and psychological effects, and may step up their intake to maintain or increase these effects or to prevent the feelings of severe fatigue and depression that may occur after the drug is stopped. The risk of *dependence* is especially pronounced with the form of cocaine known as "freebase" or "crack" (see below).

How taken
Smoked, sniffed "snorted", or occasionally injected.

Legitimate uses
Cocaine was formerly widely used as a *local anaesthetic*. It is still sometimes given for *topical* anaesthesia in the eye, mouth, and throat prior to minor surgery or other procedures. However, because of its *side effects* and potential for abuse, cocaine has now been replaced in most cases by safer local anaesthetic drugs. Cocaine is classified under Class A and Schedule II of the Misuse of Drugs legislation.

Short-term effects
Cocaine is a central nervous system stimulant. In moderate doses it overcomes fatigue and produces feelings of well-being and elation. Appetite is reduced. Physical effects include an increase in heart rate and blood pressure, dilation of the pupils, tremor, and increased sweating. Large doses can lead to agitation, anxiety, paranoia, and hallucinations. Paranoia may cause violent behaviour. Very large doses of cocaine may cause convulsions and death due to heart attacks or heart failure.

Long-term effects and risks
Heavy, regular use of cocaine can cause restlessness, anxiety, hyperexcitability, nausea, insomnia, and weight loss. Continued use may cause increasing paranoia and psychosis. Repeated sniffing also damages the membranes lining the nose and may eventually lead to the destruction of the septum (the structure separating the nostrils).

Regular cocaine use leads to increased atheroma (fatty deposits in the arteries) and consequent risk of heart attacks.

Signs of abuse
The cocaine user may appear unusually energetic and exuberant under the influence of the drug and show little interest in food. Heavy, regular use may lead to disturbed eating and sleeping patterns. Agitation, mood swings, aggressive behaviour, and suspiciousness of other people may also be signs of a heavy user.

Interactions
Cocaine can increase blood pressure, thus opposing the effect of antihypertensive drugs. Taken with monoamine oxidase inhibitors (MAOIs), it can cause a dangerous rise in blood pressure. It also increases the risk of adverse effects on the heart when taken with certain general anaesthetics.

CRACK

This potent form of cocaine is taken in the form of crystals that are smoked. Highly addictive, crack appears to have more intense effects than other forms of cocaine and it is associated with an increased risk of abnormal heart rhythms, high blood pressure, heart attacks, stroke, and death. Other consequences of crack abuse include coughing of black phlegm, wheezing, irreversible lung damage, hoarseness, and parched lips, tongue, and throat from inhaling the hot fumes. Mental deterioration, personality changes, social withdrawal, paranoia or violent behaviour, and suicide attempts may occur.

ECSTASY

Other common names E, MDMA, XTC. Other slang names vary from place to place.
Drug category Central nervous system stimulant

Habit-forming potential
As with other amphetamines, regular use leads to tolerance, so that higher doses are required to achieve the same effect. Users may become psychologically dependent on the effects of the drug and the lifestyle that surrounds its use.

How taken
By mouth in tablet or capsule form.

Legitimate uses
Although there have been claims that ecstasy may have a place in psychotherapy, it currently has no legitimate medical use. The drug is classified under Class A and Schedule I in the Misuse of Drugs legislation.

Short-term effects
Ecstasy is most commonly used as a dance drug at "raves" or parties to increase the emotional effects of dancing to fast music and to enable users to dance for many hours. Adverse effects are more commonly due to "recreational" doses rather than to an overdose. Ecstasy stimulates the central nervous system, leading to increased wakefulness and energy and suppression of thirst, tiredness, and sleep. It can produce tight clenching of the jaw muscles (sometimes leading to involuntary tooth grinding) and stiffness in other muscles. The drug also increases the heart rate and raises the blood pressure. Various complications may occur, in particular, heatstroke due to prolonged dancing without replacing fluids lost by sweating. Heatstroke can lead to muscle breakdown, kidney failure, problems with the blood clotting mechanism, convulsions, and death. In some cases there may be low sodium levels and brain swelling due to excessive intake of fluid in the absence of sufficient exertion to sweat it off. These patients may experience vomiting, headaches, and drowsiness. Liver damage and stroke have also occurred.

Long-term effects and risks
Little is known about the long-term effects. Some cases of psychiatric illness have been reported, such as schizophrenia and depression, in addition to sleep disturbances, dental problems, and a craving for chocolate. Because ecstasy causes damage to certain types of nerve cell in animals, it may possibly lead to mental illnesses. There may be an increased likelihood of developing depression even years after stopping the drug.

Signs of abuse
The ecstasy user may experience weight loss, tooth damage as a result of jaw-clenching, and anxiety.

Interactions
Ecstasy interacts with a variety of drugs. If it is taken with monoamine oxidase inhibitors (MAOIs), ecstasy may lead to a dangerous rise in blood pressure. It also increases the risk of abnormal heart rhythms with digitalis drugs, levodopa, and certain anaesthetics given by inhalation. Ecstasy tends to counteract the *sedative* effects of drugs that depress the central nervous system, and its effect on the mind is reduced by these drugs.

GHB

Other common names Liquid X, GBH, Liquid E, gamma hydroxybutyrate
Drug category Central nervous system depressant

Habit-forming potential
GHB is not known to be addictive.

How taken
By mouth. Often sold as a liquid in bottles, but it may be presented in a capsule or as a powder that is commonly dissolved in water to produce a clear, colourless liquid.

Legitimate uses
GHB is a naturally occurring chemical produced in the body in small amounts. Originally developed as an anaesthetic, it has been used in the treatment of narcolepsy, insomnia, and alcohol and *opioid* withdrawal, but currently has no recognized medical use. It is controlled under the Medicines Act, and unauthorized manufacture and distribution could be classed as an offence. However, since GHB is not controlled under the Misuse of Drugs legislation, possession is not illegal and the drug can be imported for personal use.

Short-term effects
GHB is a central nervous system depressant. Its effects are somewhat similar to alcohol, with talkativeness, cheerfulness, and euphoria occurring soon after taking an average dose. Most people become drowsy but recover within 8 hours of ingestion. Some users may experience confusion, headache, or gastrointestinal symptoms such as vomiting or stomach pain. Excessive doses may cause unconsciousness, but this typically lasts only 1–2 hours.

Long-term effects and risks
Users may suffer a "hung-over" state for 2–3 days, and insomnia and dizziness may linger for up to 2 weeks. Longer-term effects of the drug have not been well studied.

Signs of abuse
As the drug is taken in liquid form it is difficult to estimate the correct dose, and the response to a low dose varies widely. Many abusers simply "guzzle" it until they reach an adequate high. This is often achieved only shortly before becoming unconscious, so sudden unconsciousness on the dance floor, for example, may be caused by GHB intoxication. Abnormally long-lasting hangovers and dizziness may be signs of abuse.

Interactions
The effects will be increased by other central nervous system depressants – for example, alcohol, benzodiazepines, and antipsychotics. GHB may also add to the effects of opioid analgesic drugs and muscle relaxants. It is sometimes mixed with amphetamines to prolong the "high" for several hours.

KETAMINE

Other common names Kit-Kat, Special K, Super K
Drug category General anaesthetic with analgesic properties (see p.80)

Habit-forming potential
Low.

How taken
Usually swallowed as the liquid pharmaceutical preparation or as tablets/capsules, produced mainly by heating the liquid anaesthetic to evaporate the water, leaving ketamine crystals. Sometimes smoked or sniffed as a powder.

Legitimate uses
A *general anaesthetic* with analgesic properties, used both in human and veterinary medicine. It is related to phencyclidine.

Short-term effects
The effects may depend on mood and environment, but have a rapid onset. Ketamine stimulates the cardiovascular system, producing a racing heart. There are a number of psychological effects that may occur, including a feeling of paralysis in which the user cannot move or speak but is still fully conscious and can see and hear. Actions or words may be repeated persistently, or the user may have an "out of body" experience. Users may be unconcerned whether they live or die. Due to the analgesic effects, the user is unlikely to feel pain. Severe reactions, usually due to overdose, may include convulsions, depression of the breathing mechanism, or heart failure.

Long-term effects and risks
The long-term use of ketamine may interfere with memory, learning, and attention span. Users may also experience flashbacks.

Signs of abuse
Strange behaviour may suggest the psychological effects of ketamine. Painful injuries (such as cigarette burns) appear to go unnoticed.

Interactions
Barbiturates lengthen the duration of action that results from ketamine use, and in combination there is a risk of respiratory depression. Use of ketamine together with theophylline or aminophylline may increase the likelihood of convulsions. Alcoholics tend to be resistant to ketamine, although the psychological effects may be exaggerated during the recovery period.

KHAT

Other common names Cat, chaat, mriaa, quat
Drug category Central nervous system stimulant

Habit-forming potential
Dependence on khat is exclusively psychological.

How taken
Khat is composed of the leaves and small twigs of a plant (*Catha edulis*) that grows on high ground in many tropical countries. A large amount of the leaves or stems are chewed, and the plant material is kept in the cheek while the juice is swallowed. Occasionally it is brewed and drunk as tea.

Legitimate uses
The drug is widely used as a social stimulant in many Middle East and African countries, and is often taken at celebrations and gatherings. It has also been used as a traditional remedy to treat depression, fatigue, obesity, and gastric ulcers. However, the authorities in these countries are increasingly concerned about its adverse effects on health.

Short-term effects
Khat produces euphoria, increased alertness, talkativeness, and hyperactivity. Gastrointestinal *side effects* are common, as well as a mild rise in the blood pressure, pulse, respiratory rate, and temperature. Insomnia, poor concentration, and malaise are also common side effects. Aggressive verbal outbursts and hallucinations may occur as a result of khat use, but severe psychosis is rare. Mental depression and sedation may follow withdrawal after heavy or regular use.

Long-term effects and risks
Constipation is a very common side effect and stomach ulcers are quite common in regular users of khat. Men may experience impotence and reduced sex drive. Khat use may contribute to the risk of high blood pressure in young adults. Chronic use during pregnancy may lead to low birth weight, and the drug is excreted in breast milk.

Signs of abuse
The drug causes a brown staining of the teeth. Weight loss may occur as a result of appetite suppression.

Interactions
It may interact with amphetamine or phenylpropanolamine to cause a fast heart rate and high blood pressure.

LSD

Other common names Lysergide, diethylamide, lysergic acid, acid, haze, microdots
Drug category Hallucinogen

Habit-forming potential
Although it is not physically addictive, LSD may cause psychological *dependence*. After several days of regular use, a person develops a tolerance to its actions. A waiting period must pass before resumption of the drug will produce the original effects.

How taken
By mouth, as tiny coloured tablets (known as "microdots"), or absorbed onto small squares of paper, gelatin sheets, or sugar cubes.

Legitimate uses
None. Early interest of the medical profession in LSD focused on its possible use in psychotherapy, but additional studies suggested that it could lead to psychosis in susceptible people. LSD is listed under Class A and Schedule I of the Misuse of Drugs legislation.

Short-term effects
The effects of usual doses of LSD last for about 4–12 hours, beginning almost immediately after taking the drug. Initial effects include restlessness, dizziness, a feeling of coldness with shivering, and an uncontrollable desire to laugh. The subsequent effects include distortions in vision and, in some cases, in the perception of sound. Introspection is often increased and mystical, pseudoreligious experiences may occur. Loss of emotional control, unpleasant or terrifying hallucinations, and overwhelming feelings of anxiety, despair, or panic may occur, particularly if the user is suffering from underlying anxiety or depression. Suicide may be attempted. Driving and other hazardous tasks are extremely dangerous. Some people under the influence of this drug have fallen off high buildings, mistakenly believing they could fly.

Long-term effects and risks
The effects of long-term LSD use include an increase in the risk of mental disturbances, including severe depression. In those with existing psychological difficulties, it may lead to lasting mental problems (e.g., permanent psychosis). In addition, for months or even years after last taking the drug, some frequent users experience brief but vivid recurrences of LSD's effects ("flashbacks"), which cause anxiety and disorientation. There is no evidence of lasting physical ill-effects from LSD use.

Signs of abuse
A person under the influence of LSD may be behaving strangely but rarely shows any other outward signs of intoxication. Occasionally, a user who is drugged with LSD may seem overexcited, or appear withdrawn or confused.

Interactions
Chlorpromazine reduces the effects of LSD, so it can be used to treat a person who is acutely disturbed. Interactions with other drugs acting on the brain, such as alcohol, may increase the likelihood of unpredictable or violent behaviour. Lysergide abusers who are given SSRI antidepressants (e.g., fluoxetine, paroxetine, or sertaline) may experience onset or worsening of flashbacks.

MESCALINE

Other common names Peyote, cactus buttons, big chief
Drug category Hallucinogen

Habit-forming potential
Mescaline has a low habit-forming potential; it does not cause physical *dependence* and does not usually lead to psychological dependence. After several days of taking mescaline, the user develops a tolerance for further doses of the drug, thus discouraging regular daily use.

How taken
By mouth as capsules, or in the form of peyote cactus buttons, eaten fresh or dried, drunk as tea, or ground up and smoked with cannabis.

Legitimate uses
The peyote cactus has been used by Native Mexicans for over 2,000 years, both in religious rituals and as a herbal remedy for various ailments ranging from wounds and bronchitis to failing vision. Mescaline is classified under Schedule I of the Misuse of Drugs legislation.

Short-term effects
Mescaline alters visual and auditory perception, although true hallucinations are rare. Appetite is reduced under the influence of this drug. There is also a risk of unpleasant mental effects, particularly in people who are anxious or depressed.

Peyote may have additional effects caused by several other active substances (in addition to mescaline) in the plant. Strychnine-like chemicals may cause nausea, vomiting, and, occasionally, tremors and sweating, which usually precede the perceptual effects of mescaline by up to 2 hours.

Long-term effects and risks
The long-term effects of mescaline have not been well studied. It may increase the risk of mental disturbances, particularly in people with existing psychological problems. Studies have shown that, after taking mescaline, most of the drug concentrates in the liver rather than in the brain, and it may therefore have special risks for people with impaired liver function.

Signs of abuse
Mescaline or peyote abuse may not have obvious signs. Users might sometimes appear withdrawn, disoriented, or confused.

Interactions
The combination of alcohol and peyote, although common, is recognized to be dangerous. There is a risk of temporary derangement, leading to disorientation, panic, and violent behaviour. Vomiting is likely to occur.

NICOTINE

Other common names Found in tobacco products
Drug category Central nervous system stimulant (see also p.351)

Habit-forming potential
The nicotine in tobacco is largely responsible for tobacco *addiction* in over one-third of the population who are cigarette smokers. Most are also probably psychologically *dependent* on the process of smoking. Most people who start go on to smoke regularly, and most become physically dependent on nicotine. Stopping can produce temporary *withdrawal symptoms* that include nausea, headache, diarrhoea, hunger, drowsiness, fatigue, insomnia, irritability, depression, inability to concentrate, and craving for cigarettes.

How taken
Usually smoked in the form of cigarettes, cigars, and pipe tobacco. Sometimes sniffed (tobacco snuff) or chewed (chewing tobacco).

Legitimate uses
There are no legal restrictions on tobacco use. Its sale, however, is restricted to those over the age of 16. Nicotine chewing gum or slow-release patches may be prescribed on a temporary basis along with behaviour modification therapy to help people who want to give up smoking. Nicotine is also used commercially as an insecticide (it is a very potent poison).

Short-term effects
Nicotine stimulates the sympathetic nervous system (see p.79). In regular tobacco users, it increases concentration, relieves tension and fatigue, and counters boredom and monotony. These effects are short-lived, thus encouraging frequent use. Physical effects include narrowing of blood vessels, increase in heart rate and blood pressure, and reduction in urine output. First-time users often feel dizzy and nauseated, and may vomit.

Long-term effects and risks
Nicotine taken regularly may cause a rise in fatty acids in the bloodstream. This effect, combined with the effects of the drug on heart rhythm and blood vessel size, may increase the risk of diseases of the heart and circulation, including angina, high blood pressure, peripheral vascular disease, stroke, and coronary thrombosis. In addition, its stimulatory effects may lead to excess production of stomach acid, and thereby increase the risk of peptic ulcers.

Other well-known risks of tobacco smoking, such as chronic lung diseases, adverse effects on pregnancy, and cancers of the lung, mouth, and throat, may be due to other harmful ingredients in tobacco smoke. It is now believed that the cancer-causing chemical in tobacco smoke is benzo (a) pyrene diol epoxide.

Signs of abuse
Regular smokers often have yellow, tobacco-stained fingers and teeth and bad breath. The smell of tobacco may linger on hair and clothes. A smoker's cough or shortness of breath are early signs of lung damage or heart disease.

Interactions
Cigarette smoking reduces the blood levels of a variety of drugs and reduces their effects. Such drugs include the benzodiazepines, tricyclic antidepressants, theophylline, propranolol, heparin, and caffeine. Diabetics may require larger doses of insulin. The health risks involved in taking oral contraceptives are increased by smoking.

Practical points
▼ Don't start smoking; nicotine is highly addictive.
▼ If you smoke already, give up now even if you have not yet suffered *adverse effects*.
▼ Ask your doctor for advice and support.
▼ Inquire about self-help groups in your neighbourhood for people trying to give up smoking.

NITRITES

Other common names Amyl nitrite, butyl nitrite, poppers, snappers
Drug category Vasodilators (see also p.98)

Habit-forming potential
Nitrites do not seem to cause physical *dependence*; major *withdrawal symptoms* have never been reported. However, users may become psychologically dependent on the stimulant effect of these drugs.

How taken
By inhalation, usually from small bottles with screw or plug tops or from small glass ampules that are broken.

Legitimate uses
Amyl nitrite was originally introduced as a treatment for angina but has now largely been replaced by safer, longer-acting drugs. It is still used as an *antidote* for cyanide poisoning. Butyl and isobutyl nitrites are not used medically.

Short-term effects
Nitrites increase the flow of blood by relaxing blood vessel walls. They give the user a rapid "high", felt as a strong rush of energy. Less pleasant effects include an increase in heart rate, intense flushing, dizziness, fainting, pounding headache, nausea, and coughing. High doses may cause fainting, and regular use may produce a blue discoloration of the skin due to alteration of haemoglobin in the red blood cells.

Long-term effects and risks
Nitrites are very quick-acting drugs. Their effects start within 30 seconds of inhalation and last for about 5 minutes. Regular users may become *tolerant* to these drugs, thus requiring higher doses to achieve the desired effects. Lasting physical damage, including cardiac problems, can result from chronic use of these drugs, and deaths have occurred.

The risk of *toxic* effects is increased in those with low blood pressure. Nitrites may also precipitate the onset of glaucoma in susceptible people, by increasing pressure inside the eye.

Signs of abuse
Nitrites have a pungent, fruity odour. They evaporate quickly; the contents of a small bottle left uncapped in a room usually disappear within 2 hours. Unless someone is actually taking the drug or is suffering from an overdose, the only sign of abuse is a bluish skin discoloration.

Interactions
The blood pressure-lowering effects of these drugs may be increased by alcohol, beta blockers, calcium channel blockers, and tricyclic antidepressants, thus increasing the risk of dizziness and fainting.

OPIOIDS (HEROIN)

Other common names Horse, junk, smack, scag, H, diamorphine, morphine, opium
Drug category Central nervous system depressant

Habit-forming potential
Opioid analgesics include not only those drugs derived from the opium poppy (opium and morphine) but also synthetic drugs whose medical actions are similar to those of morphine (pethidine, methadone, and dextropropoxyphene). Frequent use of these drugs leads to *tolerance*, and all have a potential for *dependence*. Among them, heroin is the most potent, widely abused, and dangerous. It is also associated with criminal behaviour.

After only a few weeks of use, *withdrawal symptoms* may occur when the drug is stopped; fear of such withdrawal effects may be a strong inducement to go on using the drug. In heavy users, the drug habit is often coupled with a lifestyle that revolves around its use.

How taken
A white or speckled brown powder, heroin is smoked, sniffed, or injected. Other opioids may be taken by mouth.

Legitimate uses
Heroin is widely used both in Britain and Belgium for the treatment of acute severe pain, such as the pain following a heart attack. It is not used medically in other countries. Other opioids, such as morphine and methadone, are used as analgesics. Most opioids are listed under Class A and Schedule II of the Misuse of Drugs legislation. Mild opioids such as codeine are also sometimes included in cough suppressant and antidiarrhoeal medications and are listed under Schedule V.

Short-term effects
Strong opioids induce a feeling of contentment and well-being. Pain is dulled and the activity of the nervous system is depressed; breathing and heart rate are slowed and the cough reflex is inhibited. First-time users often feel nauseated and vomit. With higher doses, there is increasing drowsiness, sometimes leading to coma and, in rare cases, death from respiratory arrest.

Long-term effects and risks
The long-term regular use of opioids leads to constipation, reduced sexual drive, disruption of menstrual periods, and poor eating habits. Poor nutrition and personal neglect may lead to general ill health.

Street drugs are often mixed ("cut") with other substances, such as caffeine, quinine, talcum powder, and flour, that can damage blood vessels and clog the lungs. There is also a risk of abscesses at the injection site. Dangerous infections, such as hepatitis, syphilis, and human immunodeficiency virus (HIV), may be transmitted via unclean or shared needles.

After several weeks of regular use, sudden withdrawal of opioids produces a flu-like withdrawal syndrome beginning 6–24 hours after the last dose. Symptoms may include runny nose and eyes, hot and cold sweats, sleeplessness, aches, tremor, anxiety, nausea, vomiting, diarrhoea, muscle spasms, and abdominal cramps. These effects are at their worst 48–72 hours after withdrawal and fade after 7–10 days.

Signs of abuse
An opioid abuser may exhibit such signs as apathy, neglect of personal appearance and hygiene, loss of appetite and weight, loss of interest in former hobbies and social activities, personality changes, and furtive behaviour. Users resort to crime to continue financing their habit. Signs of intoxication include pinpoint pupils and a drowsy or drunken appearance.

Interactions
Opioids dangerously increase the risk of sedation with any drug that has a sedative effect on the central nervous system, including barbiturates and alcohol.

PHENCYCLIDINE

Other common names PCP, angel dust, crystal, ozone
Drug category General anaesthetic (see p.80), hallucinogen

Habit-forming potential
There is little evidence that phencyclidine causes physical *dependence*. Some users become psychologically dependent on this drug and *tolerant* to its effects.

How taken
May be sniffed, used in smoking mixtures (in the form of angel dust), eaten (as tablets), or, in rare cases, injected.

Legitimate uses
Although it was once used as an anaesthetic, it no longer has any medical use. Its only legal use now is in veterinary medicine. It is classified under Class A and Schedule II of the Misuse of Drugs legislation. Phencyclidine's effects on behaviour (see below) make it one of the most dangerous of all drugs of abuse. Fortunately, it is rarely abused in Europe.

Short-term effects
Phencyclidine taken in small amounts generally produces a "high", but sometimes leads to anxiety or depression. Coordination of speech and movement deteriorates, and thinking and concentration are impaired. Hallucinations and violent behaviour may occur. Other possible effects include increases in blood pressure and heart rate, dilation of the pupils, dryness of the mouth, tremor, numbness, and greatly reduced sensitivity to pain, which may make it difficult to restrain a person who has become violent under the influence of the drug. Shivering, vomiting, muscle weakness, and rigidity may also occur. Higher doses lead to coma or stupor. The recovery period is often prolonged, with alternate periods of sleep and waking, usually followed by memory blackout of the whole episode.

Long-term effects and risks
Repeated phencyclidine use may lead to paranoia, auditory hallucinations, violent behaviour, anxiety, severe depression, and schizophrenia. While depressed, the user may attempt suicide by overdosing on the drug. Heavy users may also develop brain damage, which may cause memory blackouts, disorientation, visual disturbances, and speech difficulties.

Deaths due to prolonged convulsions, cardiac or respiratory arrest, and ruptured blood vessels in the brain have been reported. After high doses or prolonged coma, there is also a risk of mental derangement, which may be permanent.

Signs of abuse
The phencyclidine user may appear drunk while under the influence of the drug. Hostile or violent behaviour and mood swings with bouts of depression may be more common with heavy use.

Interactions
Using phencyclidine may inhibit the effects of *anticholinergic* drugs, as well as beta blockers and antihypertensive drugs.

SOLVENTS

Other common names Inhalants, glue
Drug category Central nervous system depressant

Habit-forming potential
There is a low risk of physical *dependence* with solvent abuse, but regular users may become psychologically dependent. Young people with family and personality problems are at particular risk of becoming habitual users of solvents.

How taken
By breathing in the fumes, usually from a plastic bag placed over the nose and/or mouth or from a cloth or handkerchief soaked in the solvent.

Legitimate uses
Solvents are used in a wide variety of industrial, domestic, and cosmetic products. They function as aerosol propellants for spray paints, hair lacquer, lighter fuel, and deodorants. They are used in adhesives, paints, paint stripper, lacquers, petrol, and cleaning fluids. Most products containing solvents may not be sold to people under the age of 18.

Short-term effects
The short-term effects of solvents include lightheadedness, dizziness, confusion, and progressive drowsiness; loss of coordination occurs with increasing doses. Accidents of all types are more likely. Heart rhythm might be disturbed, sometimes fatally. Large doses can lead to disorientation, hallucinations, and loss of consciousness. Nausea, vomiting, and headaches may also occur. There are over 100 deaths every year in Britain from solvent abuse.

Long-term effects and risks
One of the greatest risks of solvent abuse is accidental death or injury while intoxicated. Some products, especially aerosol gases, butane gas, and cleaning fluids, may seriously disrupt heart rhythm or cause heart failure and sometimes death. Aerosols and butane gas can also cause suffocation by sudden cooling of the airways and these are particularly dangerous if squirted into the mouth. Butane gas has been known to ignite in the mouth. Aerosol products, such as deodorant and paint, may suffocate the user by coating the lungs. People have suffocated while sniffing solvents from plastic bags placed over their heads. There is also a risk of death from inhalation of vomit and depression of the breathing mechanism.

Long-term misuse of solvent-based cleaning fluids can cause permanent liver or kidney damage, while long-term exposure to benzene (found in plastic cements, lacquers, paint remover, petrol, and cleaning fluid) may lead to blood and liver disorders. Hexane-based adhesives may cause nerve damage leading to numbness and tremor. Repeated sniffing of leaded petrol may cause lead poisoning.

Regular daily use of solvents can lead to pallor, fatigue, and forgetfulness. Heavy use may affect the student's school performance and lead to weight loss, depression, and general deterioration of health.

Signs of abuse
Most abusers are adolescents between the ages of 10 and 17, although the average age, 14–15, for this type of drug abuse is thought to be falling.

Obvious signs of solvent abuse include a chemical smell on the breath and traces of glue or solvents on the body or clothes. Other signs include furtive behaviour, uncharacteristic moodiness, unusual soreness or redness around the mouth, nose, or eyes, and a persistent cough.

Interactions
Sniffing solvents increases the risk of sedation with any drug that has a *sedative* effect on the central nervous system. Such drugs include anti-anxiety and sleeping drugs, *opioids*, tricyclic antidepressants, antipsychotics, and alcohol.

ALTERNATIVE MEDICINE

Alternative, or complementary, medicine has become increasingly popular in recent years. A growing number of people consult alternative practitioners as well as, or instead of, their own doctors, and the use of alternative remedies has become considerably more widespread. Doctors are also more likely to refer some patients to alternative practitioners or to recommend the use of alternative treatments. However, there is little evidence of how alternative medicines work or of the safety and effectiveness of many of these remedies. Although the number of studies being carried out on alternative medicines is increasing, little research has been done into the incidence and severity of adverse effects caused by the different alternative remedies.

Although many medicines are derived from plant matter, the use of plants and other natural substances to aid healing can be found in different cultures all around the world. Modern alternative remedies are based on these traditional therapies. Most alternative practitioners believe that an illness is caused by an imbalance within the body, and that to treat the illness this balance must be restored. Many treat the whole body rather than just particular symptoms.

Buying alternative medicines
Many alternative medicines are available over the counter from chemists, health shops, and supermarkets. Only buy products from a reputable manufacturer who will usually provide information leaflets and instructions for use with their products. Other medicines can only be dispensed by practitioners who are suitably trained and registered. Some are also medically qualified.

Using alternative medicines
You may be able to treat yourself for minor, short-lived conditions, such as a cold, but professional advice should be sought for more serious or persistent complaints. Always follow the instructions given when taking alternative medicines, and never exceed the recommended dose. Certain herbs and preparations contain ingredients that can be harmful if not used with care.

Some alternative medicines can interact with other drugs or affect pre-existing disorders in an adverse way. You should tell your practitioner about any drugs you are taking and any pre-existing illnesses. You should also inform your doctor or pharmacist about any alternative remedies you are taking before you start taking conventional drugs. Do not stop or reduce conventional treatment without asking your doctor's advice.

HOMEOPATHY

The aim of homeopathy is to stimulate the body's powers of self-healing. Treatment is based on the concept of "like cures like" and uses the principle that the body's immune system can be stimulated to overcome illness if a patient is given dilute doses of a substance that, at full strength, would produce symptoms of the illness. For example, minute doses of pollen are used to treat hayfever and allergic asthma.

Homeopathy has had royal patronage for many years and is the only form of alternative medicine that was included in the National Health Service when it started in 1948. Doctors who practise homeopathy can prescribe homeopathic remedies using NHS prescriptions.

Creating homeopathic remedies
There are at least 2000 homeopathic remedies. They are made from extracts of plants, animals, or minerals. These extracts are infused in alcohol and water to make a tincture. This is then diluted repeatedly, a process that is known as potentiation. Homeopathic practitioners believe that the more dilute the remedy, the stronger the effect. A few drops of the tincture are usually added to sugar tablets, creams, or other substances.

How homeopathy works
One theory of how homeopathy works is that an electromagnetic imprint of the substance remains after dilution, even though no molecules of the original substance are present. This imprint is believed to stimulate a response in the body. Some practitioners believe that the imprint acts on the flow of energy in the body rather than on physical processes.

Some studies indicate homeopathy is successful in relieving symptoms. In particular, trials have produced positive results in favour of homeopathic treatment compared with a placebo (see p.15), and homeopathy has been shown to be especially effective in relieving the symptoms of hayfever. However, these findings have not always been repeated and the basic principles underlying homeopathy are still generally regarded with scepticism.

Common homeopathic remedies
Examples of common homeopathic remedies include arnica for bruises and soft tissue injuries, aconite for coughs and colds, and nux vomica for indigestion (see right).

Using homeopathic remedies
Homeopathic remedies are available as sugar tablets, powders, tinctures, oils, creams, and ointments. Oral remedies should be taken at least 30 minutes before or after eating, drinking, smoking, or using toothpaste and should never be touched with the hands. Tablets should be sucked or chewed. Tinctures are usually diluted and taken internally or applied externally. Oils, creams, and ointments are applied externally.

Many homeopathic medicines are taken every few hours at the start of treatment. The interval between successive doses is then increased as symptoms improve. Some conditions may require many months of treatment.

Homeopathic remedies have a good safety record and do not interact with conventional medicines. Due to the dilute nature of the remedies, they are very unlikely to cause side effects. Symptoms may, however, briefly worsen after treatment begins.

COMMON HOMEOPATHIC REMEDIES

Coughs, colds, and 'flu Aconite Bryonia Gelsemium	**Bruises, sprains, and minor injuries** Arnica Hypericum Ruta.grav.
Hayfever Allium Arsen. alb. Euphrasia Nat. mur.	**Menopause** Calcarea Graphites Sepia Sulphur
Indigestion Acid. phos. Bryonia Carbo veg. Nux vom.	**Insomnia and exhaustion** Arnica Arsen. alb. Coffea Nux vom.
Irritable bowel syndrome Argent. nit. Arsen. alb. Cantharis Nux vom.	**Stress** Ignatia Nux vom. Sepia
Headaches and migraine Aconite Belladonna Hypericum Nat. mur.	**Depression** Lycopodium Nat. mur. Pulsatilla Sulphur
Eczema and dermatitis Graphites Nat. mur.	**Anxiety** Argent. nit. Arsen. alb. Gelsemium Phos.

WESTERN HERBAL MEDICINE

Western herbal medicines are extracted from the leaves, flowers, roots, seeds, berries, fruits, or bark of whole plants. They differ from modern drugs derived from herbs in that they use parts of the whole plant instead of isolating a single active ingredient. Many herbalists believe that the therapeutic effect of the whole plant is greater and safer than that of its isolated constituents. Several herbs may be combined in one remedy, and products should indicate which part of the plant has been used. The World Health Organization acknowledges that Western herbal medicine plays an important role in healthcare.

How Western herbal medicine works

The use of specific herbs is based on their recognized actions on the body. Although research into the use of herbal medicines is limited, evidence supports the claims made for the effectiveness of several herbal medicines. These include echinacea, which appears to stimulate the immune system; garlic, which lowers the level of cholesterol and other fats in the blood; and St John's wort (hypericum perforatum), which seems to be very effective in treating depression.

Common Western herbal remedies

Examples of common herbal remedies include meadowsweet and marshmallow for digestive disorders, devil's claw and celery seed for arthritis, and camomile for its relaxant effects (see top right).

Using Western herbal remedies

Herbal remedies are available in a range of forms including infusions or teas, decoctions, tinctures, tablets, creams, lotions, ointments, and oils. Treatment is individually prescribed by a herbal practitioner, although you can treat yourself for simple, short-lived illnesses.

Remedies are most often taken three times a day. They should only be taken for short periods as the effects of long-term use are not known. Side effects are not common, although allergic reactions may occur. In general, herbal remedies should be avoided during pregnancy or breast-feeding, and they should not be taken by young children or by elderly people without professional advice.

Some interactions between herbal medicines and conventional drugs have been reported; other potential interactions can be predicted from the known effects of a plant. For example, liquorice, which is used to treat coughs and heal peptic ulcers, can raise blood pressure and interfere with antihypertensive medication. Other plant remedies that could interfere with drugs affecting the heart and circulation include blue cohosh, broom, and ginger.

COMMON WESTERN HERBAL REMEDIES

Minor injuries and bruises
Comfrey
Marigold
St John's wort

Coughs and colds
Echinacea
Garlic
Ginger

Nausea and vomiting
Chamomile
Fennel
Ginger
Peppermint

Headaches and migraine
Chamomile
Feverfew
Lavender

Acne
Echinacea
Dandelion root
Nettle

Premenstrual syndrome
Agnus castus
Cramp bark
Dandelion
Marigold

Chronic fatigue
Astralgus
Echinacea
Ginseng
Goldenseal
Yellow dock root

Stress
Chamomile
Ginseng
Hops
Motherwort
Passion flower
Valerian
Vervain

CHINESE HERBAL MEDICINE

Chinese herbal medicine is part of the ancient system of healing known as Traditional Chinese Medicine (TCM). Medicines are derived from hundreds of different plant species. Parts used may include the flowers, leaves, fruits, stalks, seeds, or bark. Chinese herbal medicine is different from Western medicine in that it regards symptoms as being due to disharmony in the body and tries to treat the underlying cause in order to restore balance. Western medicine tends to concentrate on specific symptoms. In China, TCM is taught at university level and practised in all hospitals.

How Chinese herbal medicine works

TCM is based around the concepts of *ying* and *yang*, two complementary but opposing forces. If these forces are disturbed, disease occurs. Different symptoms indicate excess *ying* or *yang*. Another belief is that of the five elements – fire, earth, metal, water, and wood. Each internal organ is associated with one of these elements.

Herbal remedies are used to restore balance between all these forces within the body. Herbs are classified under one of the five elements and according to their *ying* and *yang* qualities.

Although some studies have shown an improvement in symptoms following the use of Chinese herbal medicines, the concepts underlying traditional Chinese medicine cannot be explained by Western science and many Western doctors are still sceptical.

Common Chinese herbal remedies

Herbal remedies are commonly used to treat eczema and another skin conditions, as well as migraine, fatigue, and digestive disorders. Some people with AIDS claim that Chinese herbal remedies improve their overall well-being (see below).

Using Chinese herbal remedies

Herbs are generally prescribed by the practitioner as a formula containing several different ingredients, usually up to 15 in combination. Each herb performs a particular function and is used for a specific purpose. The herbs are usually boiled in water to make a decoction or tea but may also be available as tablets, pills, powders, pastes, ointments, creams, and lotions. Medicine is usually taken daily at the start of treatment. The prescription may then be altered and the dose reduced according to the response.

A large range of Chinese herbal medicines for minor conditions can be bought over the counter from health shops, chemists, Chinese herbalists, or Chinese medicine centres. More complex remedies and formulas are prescribed by a practitioner.

Although side effects are uncommon, some Chinese medicinal plants can have toxic effects. In particular, some remedies have been associated with liver damage. Additionally, recent analysis of a small sample of Chinese herbal cream showed that a significant proportion contained potent corticosteroids, which can be harmful if used inappropriately.

COMMON CHINESE HERBAL REMEDIES

Coughs and colds
Astragalus root
Balloon flower
Fritillary
Plantain

Eczema
Chinese gentian
Chinese wormwood
Peony root
Rehmannia

Irritable bowel syndrome
Chinese angelica
Chinese rhubarb
Dandelion
Magnolia bark
Poria

Arthritis
Aconite
Chinese angelica
Cinnamon
Ginger
Liquorice

Headaches and migraine
Cassia
Chrysanthemum

Menopause
Chinese angelica
Ginseng
Peony
Rehmannia
Thorowax root

Insomnia
Fleeceflower
Poria
Wild jujube

AIDS
Chinese bitter melon
Ginseng
Lentinan
Red sage
White peony

DRUGS IN SPORT

The use of drugs to improve athletic performance has been universally condemned by the sporting authorities. The deliberate use of certain drugs gives the athlete an unfair advantage and may also endanger health. On 1 January 2000 the whole of the International Olympic Movement adopted a common Olympic Movement Antidoping Code. If traces of a prohibited substance are found by means of a urine test, the athlete is banned from the competition and risks lifelong exclusion from the sport. Not only strong, prescribed medications affect athletic performance; everyday items such as cigarettes, alcohol, tea, and coffee can also have an effect. Drugs of any kind should be taken by athletes only under strict medical supervision and must be declared in writing to the relevant medical authority before the competition.

Many drugs affect the performance of athletes who are taking them. Some are medications that have been prescribed by doctors to treat specific medical conditions but are abused by athletes who want to benefit from the body-building and general performance-improving effects of these drugs. Others are everyday non-prescribed substances, such as caffeine and nicotine, which have a relatively minor effect on performance. However, even these substances can cause drug levels in the athlete's body to rise to unacceptable levels if they are taken in excess.

Detecting drugs
Drugs can be detected in the urine and other body fluids. Increasingly sensitive tests are constantly being devised to check for prohibited substances. These tests are performed frequently in most sports, both during competitions and in training.

Prohibited substances
The International Olympic Committee completely prohibits five classes of drugs and these are listed as: stimulants, *opioid analgesics*, diuretics, anabolic agents (steroids and beta-agonists), and peptide hormones and analogues. Many other drugs are banned in most sports – for example, alcohol, cannabis, *local anaesthetics*, corticosteroids, and beta blockers. In addition to these drugs, substances and methods that alter the validity of tests are illegal.

Legitimate medications
Certain prescribed drugs are allowed to be taken legitimately by athletes for certain medical disorders, such as asthma or epilepsy. Prescribed medicines must be declared in writing to the appropriate medical authority before any competition. Other prescribed drugs – for example, antibiotics – may not make any noticeable difference to athletic performance, but the underlying disorder for which the drugs are being taken may make strenuous exercise inadvisable. The athlete should also be careful when using certain over-the-counter preparations, as many contain low doses of prohibited substances.

TYPES OF DRUGS AND PRACTICES

Antibiotics
These drugs may occasionally impair ability by causing nausea or diarrhoea.

Antihistamines
Preparations containing chlorphenamine or diphenhydramine may cause drowsiness, dizziness, or blurred vision.

Anti-inflammatory drugs
Using anti-inflammatory drugs to relieve pain in muscles, tendons, or ligaments can be dangerous; masking pain may result in aggravation of an injury.

Asthma drugs
An asthma drug should not contain isoprenaline, ephedrine, or phenylephrine, which are prohibited stimulants. However, inhalers containing salbutamol, steroids, terbutaline, or salmeterol may be used.

Blood doping
This illegal practice involves removing blood from an athlete during training and replacing it shortly before a competition. After the blood is removed, the volume and number of red blood cells in the remaining blood is naturally replenished. When stored blood is reinfused, the haemoglobin content of the blood is increased, enhancing the blood's ability to deliver oxygen to muscles. A similar effect is achieved by epoetin (erythropoietin), which stimulates extra blood production.

Caffeine
Although caffeine is listed as a prohibited stimulant, disqualification results only if large quantities (more than 12 mg/litre) are detected in the urine sample.

Cocaine
This illegal and highly addictive stimulant is prohibited in sport. Dangerous side effects include heart arrhythmias, negative personality changes, and damage to the nasal lining after regular inhalation. A high dose can trigger convulsions or psychosis and may cause death.

Cough and cold remedies
Avoid preparations that contain codeine, ephedrine, pseudoephedrine, phenylpropanolamine, or phenylephrine for 12 hours before a competition. Drugs used legally include antibiotics and antihistamines, steam inhalations, dextromethorphan, guaiphenesin, and pholcodine.

Diarrhoea remedies
Any preparation containing opioids, such as morphine, must be avoided. However, diphenoxylate, loperamide, or electrolytes may be used.

Dieting drugs
Most diet drugs contain a prohibited stimulant or diuretic.

Hay fever remedies
Many remedies contain the prohibited stimulants ephedrine, pseudoephedrine, phenylephrine, or phenylpropanolamine. However, nasal sprays that contain steroids or xylometazoline and sodium cromoglycate can be used legally. See also Antihistamines.

Liniment
Used as a counter irritant on the pain receptors in the skin, it is important that application of liniment does not mask pain to the point where further damage to an injury may result after exertion.

Nicotine
Available from tobacco products as well as from nicotine gum and transdermal patches, this drug reduces the flow of blood through the muscles. Carbon monoxide from smoking decreases the available oxygen carried round the body, reducing the capacity for exercise.

Painkillers
Strong painkillers such as pethidine and morphine, known as opioid analgesics, are prohibited in sport. Weaker painkillers, – for example, paracetamol, ibuprofen, aspirin, and local anaesthetics in spray, ointment, or cream form – are permitted, but their use can mask pain, resulting in the aggravation of an injury.

Sleeping drugs
Many sports authorities ban sedatives, so a sleeping drug should not be taken less than 24 hours before a competition.

MEDICINES AND TRAVEL

Low cost air transport has resulted in enormous growth in international travel for both business and pleasure in recent years. This expansion has been paralleled by a more adventurous approach to leisure destinations. Few areas of the world are not on someone's itinerary and travellers are more likely than ever before to visit destinations with health hazards they have not encountered before and with poorly developed health services. Although few travellers run into serious medical problems, it is worth paying a little attention to the health aspects of travel when planning a trip. This should help to prevent problems later on and to ensure that any that do arise will not be serious. Risks can be minimized by seeking information about the country you are visiting, checking out facilities before you travel, and being prepared for both minor and major medical emergencies.

BEFORE YOU GO

If you take medicines regularly
Pack sufficient supplies to last for the duration of the trip. Some drugs may not be available at your destination or may require a local prescription. If any of your medicines are schedule II or III controlled drugs (see p.13), check with your doctor or pharmacist because there may be stopped by Customs in some countries. It might be helpful for your doctor to give you a letter with details of the drugs you have been prescribed to show to Customs abroad, as well as to British Customs on your return. If you are worried about taking a prescription medicine into another country, you could ask the relevant embassy whether there might be a problem.

... and even if you don't
Take a few everyday medicines with you, including:
- a motion sickness remedy
- simple painkillers
- an antidiarrhoeal and rehydration salts for traveller's diarrhoea
- a laxative for constipation caused by changes in diet or routine
- an antiseptic cream for small injuries
- a bite/sting relief spray or cream for insect bites
- a high-protection factor (SPF 25+) sunscreen lotion
- an insect repellent

If you are going to a high risk area for malaria, start taking antimalarial drugs (p.137) a week or two before going to ensure that any intolerable side effects become apparent before departure.

If you are going outside the usual tourist routes, backpacking, or living among the local people, you might need to carry an emergency sterile syringe and needle kit. If you are intending to stay away for a long time, see your dentist for a check-up before you leave.

Vaccinations
Vaccinations are not normally necessary when travelling to Western Europe, North America, Australia, or New Zealand (although you should make sure that your tetanus and poliomyelitis boosters are up to date). However, consult your doctor if you are visiting other destinations. If you are taking children with you, check that they have had the full set of routine childhood vaccinations as well as any vaccinations that are necessary for the areas you will be travelling in.

If you are visiting an area where there is yellow fever, an International Certificate of Vaccination will be needed. You may also need this certificate in the future. Many countries that you might want to visit require an International Certificate of Vaccination if you have already been to a country where yellow fever is present.

You are at risk of other infectious diseases in many parts of the world and appropriate vaccinations are a wise precaution. For example, there is a zone across northern India, Nepal, Bhutan, Pakistan, continuing in a wide band across Africa from the Sahara down to Kenya, that is called the "Meningitis Belt". Meningococcal vaccine A and C should be given to anyone who intends to visit this zone. Visitors who are going to Saudi Arabia at certain times of the year may also be required to have had the meningitis group A and C vaccine.

You may need extra vaccinations if you are planning to stay for a long time or backpacking. For example, hepatitis A vaccine would be sensible for anyone travelling to a developing country, but a long-stay traveller should consider having hepatitis B vaccine and BCG (tuberculosis) as well. Anyone travelling into remote areas is recommended to have rabies vaccination.

All immunization should be completed well before departure as the vaccinations do not give instant protection (BCG needs 3 months), and some need more than one dose to be effective, for example typhoid.

The Department of Health (see Further sources, p.468) publishes a booklet called "Health Advice for Travellers Anywhere in the World". This booklet gives information on requirements for vaccination and is available from some travel agents and post offices.

Outbreaks of disease
Some infectious diseases are endemic (constantly or generally present). For example, dengue fever is found throughout the tropics; only the severity of the illness varies. Other diseases appear as definite outbreaks or epidemics; influenza is an example. While we are accustomed to think of influenza as a winter illness, it may occur at any time, especially in the tropics. If you or family members are likely to be at special risk and did not get the latest influenza booster, it would be worth checking whether there is an outbreak of influenza (or any other serious infectious disease) in the area you are planning to visit.

You could ask your doctor or travel insurance company about the risk of disease in the country you are visiting. If you have access to the Internet, the best source of information on serious outbreaks of disease is the website of the Centers for Disease Control and Prevention (see Further sources, p.468).

Insurance
Being taken ill when you are abroad can be expensive. This is especially so outside the European Union (where healthcare is available to all EU citizens, so remember to take your form E.111). Even in the European Union, repatriation by air ambulance in the event of serious illness or accident is rarely included in state healthcare. You should always take out travel insurance, which can be inexpensive, before you leave. If you have a regular annual policy, check that it is kept up to date and is valid for the entire travel period and for any activities that you may be undertaking (such as skiing or watersports).

WHILE YOU ARE TRAVELLING

Travel sickness
If you are prone to travel sickness, take a travel sickness medicine about half an hour before you start your journey. Ask your doctor or pharmacist for advice on which drug to choose. Do not drink alcohol if you are taking travel sickness drugs because alcohol can interact with the drugs and may make you excessively sleepy.

Dehydration and other cabin problems
The dry atmosphere inside the cabin of a passenger plane makes it very easy to become dehydrated, especially if you

over-indulge in alcoholic drinks. Drink plenty of non-alcoholic fluids and limit alcoholic drinks, and you will feel fresher when you reach your destination.

Sitting still in a cramped seat during a long-haul flight may lead to thrombosis (a blood clot) in the leg veins; try to get up and walk around the cabin now and again; you could also practise ankle- and knee-flexing exercises to try to help your circulation.

Taking medicines

International travel in which time zones are crossed and airline meals are served at apparently random intervals may make it difficult to decide when to take regular medicines. Fortunately, precise timing is not critical with most medicines; take them at the correct intervals (e.g. every 8 hours for a drug normally taken 3 times a day) regardless of the clock time, then adjust to the original schedule upon arrival at your destination.

The timing of some drugs is much more crucial. For example, progestogen-only oral contraceptives (p.161), must be taken at intervals of almost exactly 24 hours to remain effective; a delay of more than 3 hours will interfere with contraceptive protection. Timing is less critical with the combined (oestrogen and progestogen) oral contraceptives.

People with insulin-dependent diabetes also face problems when travelling as their insulin dosage regimen is governed by the clock and by the timing of their meals (p.142). Such individuals should always consult their doctor or diabetic nurse before travelling long distances.

Jet lag

Rapid travel across time zones can cause physical and psychological stress. Business travellers should try to avoid major decisions during the first day after arrival, and all travellers should give themselves a quiet adjustment period of at least a day to settle in to the new day/night timing. Those on regular medication should seek advice from their doctor about dosage adjustment before travelling.

Although some people feel they are helped by taking melatonin, there are at present no licensed drugs that are effective to prevent or correct jet lag. Short-acting sleeping tablets may help you to overcome unwanted wakefulness due to time zone shifts before travelling, during flights, or on arrival.

TRAVEL IMMUNIZATION

The immunizations that you will need before travelling depend on the area of the world you intend to visit, although some diseases can be contracted almost anywhere. Wherever you are planning to go, make sure that you have been immunized against tetanus and polio and have had booster doses if necessary. Advice on other necessary immunizations may change from time to time. Before you travel, it is advisable to ask your doctor, pharmacist, or travel clinic about vaccination for specific areas of the world as they should have the most up-to-date information.

Disease	Number of doses	When effective	Period of protection	Who should be immunized
Diphtheria	1 injection	Immediately	10 years	People travelling to the countries of the former USSR and expatriates living in developing countries.
Hepatitis A	1 injection (gamma globulin)	Immediately	3–6 months	People travelling to the Mediterranean or developing countries on a single occasion.
	2 injections (active vaccine)	2–4 weeks after 1st dose	10 years	Frequent travellers to the Mediterranean or developing countries.
Hepatitis B	3 injections over 6 months, at least 4 weeks apart	Immediately after 2nd dose	3–5 years	People travelling to countries in which hepatitis B is prevalent; those who might need medical or dental treatment while travelling in a developing country; and people likely to have unprotected sex.
Japanese B encephalitis	2–3 injections 1–2 weeks apart	10–14 days after last dose	About 2 years	People staying for an extended period in rural areas of the Indian subcontinent, China, Southeast Asia, and the Far East.
Meningitis A and C	1 injection	After 15 days	3–5 years	People travelling to Saudi Arabia and remote areas of sub-Saharan Africa, Nepal, and Brazil; immunization certificate needed if travelling to Mecca.
Rabies	3 injections. 1 week between 1st and 2nd doses, 3 weeks between 2nd and 3rd doses	Immediately after 3rd dose	2–3 years	People travelling to areas where rabies is endemic and who are at high risk (veterinary surgeons, people working with animals, and those travelling into remote country).
Typhoid	1 or 2 injections or 3 oral doses	10 days after last dose or injection	3 years	People travelling to areas with poor sanitation.
Yellow fever	1 injection	After 10 days	10 years	People travelling to parts of South America and Africa.

ON ARRIVAL

Insect bites

Many microbial and viral diseases are spread by insect bites; taking steps to prevent these bites can help minimize risks. Ticks, sand flies, simulium flies, tsetse flies, and mosquitoes are among the insect carriers of disease. Although usually thought of as tropical problems, ticks, sand flies, and mosquitoes may spread some of the diseases mentioned here as far from the tropics as North America and the Mediterranean basin.

Viral diseases borne by insects include dengue fever, yellow fever, Japanese encephalitis, phlebotomus fever (sand fly fever), Colorado tick fever, and many others. Insects also transmit protozoal parasitical diseases, for example: malaria, filariasis, leishmaniasis, Lyme disease, river blindness, and trypanosomiasis (African sleeping sickness).

To reduce the chance of being bitten wear long sleeved shirts and trousers, apply insect repellent regularly, and sleep under an insecticide-impregnated mosquito bed net or in screened accommodation sprayed with an insecticide just before bedtime and protected by an insecticide vaporizer.

Malaria prevention

Travellers to malaria-affected areas should protect themselves by taking antimalarial tablets regularly (p.137) and taking steps to prevent mosquito bites (see above).

Traveller's diarrhoea

This unpleasant, although usually short-lived, condition affects up to 50 per cent of all travellers to the developing world and is usually the result of different local bacteria. The condition is largely avoidable by drinking only mineral water and other bottled beverages or sterilized water and avoiding ice in drinks, uncooked and unpeeled fruit and vegetables, salads, and meat that is not freshly and thoroughly cooked. Be cautious about shellfish, even if it seems to have been cooked. Avoid buying cooked food from street traders. When brushing teeth, rinse with bottled water, not tap water. People who are careful about water often overlook this.

If you do get traveller's diarrhoea, it normally disappears quickly without medicines, and so your primary concern should be on preventing the dehydration that may accompany it, especially in young children, by using rehydration salts. Commercial packs of oral rehydration salts are available from pharmacies in the UK.

Although antidiarrhoeal drugs are of no value in reducing the overall duration of traveller's diarrhoea, they might be useful for people who wish to reduce the frequency of bowel movements. Loperamide (p.326) and co-phenotrope are often used for this purpose. Remember that severe diarrhoea can reduce both the absorption and the effectiveness of medicines that are taken by mouth.

Typhoid and cholera are two serious diseases and are spread by contaminated food and drink that may start like traveller's diarrhoea. No effective vaccine is available for cholera. If you are going to a country where typhoid is endemic, you should be vaccinated against it before you travel, but you must still observe all precautions. Do not hesitate to call local medical help if diarrhoea seems to be getting out of control.

Eating raw, salted, dried, or pickled fish may lead to liver fluke or tapeworm infestations, particularly in the Far East.

Sun

In the UK, more than 40,000 people develop skin cancer each year, and this figure is increasing by 8 per cent annually. Sun-induced skin damage can be avoided by following a few simple precautions. Travellers, especially those with fair skins, should avoid exposure to the hottest sun (from 11 am to 3 pm), apply a high-protection factor (25+) sunscreen protecting against both UVA and UVB to exposed skin, and use a wide-brimmed hat and clothing for additional sun protection. There is no such thing as a healthy tan.

A traveller who is unaccustomed to hot climates may experience heat exhaustion and even sunstroke, causing weakness, dizziness, nausea, muscle cramps, and eventually unconsciousness. Rarely, severe sunstroke may be fatal. Drinking plenty of non-alcoholic fluids, limiting exposure to the sun, especially during the hottest part of the day, and avoiding physical exertion until you are acclimatized to the hotter climate can usually prevent this condition developing.

Bites and stings

Seek expert advice if stung or bitten by any unfamiliar wildlife or by any mammal, and try to avoid such incidents by following local advice on where it is safe to walk or swim. Tropical and subtropical rivers and lakes may contain parasitic flukes such as bilharzia that will infest visitors who drink, bathe, or swim in them. Walking outdoors with bare feet is a bad idea in many parts of the world; hookworms and threadworms in the soil are able to penetrate the skin and enter the body, passing through tissues, the bloodstream, and the lungs before parasitizing the intestines to suck blood. If out hiking, always wear good walking shoes or boots and long trousers with the bottoms tucked into your socks. Keep to paths and avoid walking in long grass.

ON RETURN

If you have any unusual symptoms such as persistent diarrhoea or fever after you have travelled, tell a doctor exactly where you went. If you were taking antimalarials while you were away, continue to take them for 4 weeks after your return.

INTERACTIONS OF TRAVEL DRUGS

Two or more drugs taken at the same time may interact and so, if you are taking regular medication, it is advisable to consider what the potential interaction might be when it is combined with some common drugs that may be taken while you are travelling. For more details on the interactions of particular drugs consult your doctor or pharmacist.

Travel (motion) sickness drugs
• **Hyoscine** Nitrates (taken sublingually) may have a reduced effect because of dry mouth, which is a side effect of hyoscine. Alcohol and sedative drugs will increase the sedative effect of hyoscine.
• **Antihistamines** These drugs may negate the effect of anti-arrhythmics and increase the effect of sedatives.

Painkillers
• **Paracetamol** The effect of anticoagulant drugs may be increased if taken with paracetamol. The anti-diarrhoea drug colestyramine reduces absorption of paracetamol.
• **Aspirin and other NSAIDs** When taken with other NSAIDs, the effect is increased; there is an increased risk of bleeding if taken with anticoagulants. Aspirin and NSAIDs increase the toxicity of methotrexate. When taken with ACE inhibitors, these drugs may reduce their antihypertensive effects. The effects of lithium may be increased when combined with aspirin and other NSAIDs.

Antidiarrhoeal drugs
Alcohol increases the sedative effects of opioid analgesics when they are taken as antidiarrhoeals. Antidiarrhoeal drugs may increase the adverse effects of MAOIs and the overall effects of anti-epileptic drugs. There is a greater risk of toxicity when antiviral (HIV) drugs are taken with antidiarrhoeal drugs.

Drugs for malaria prevention
• **Chloroquine and mefloquine** The effect of amiodarone and quinidine may be decreased with chloroquine, and mefloquine may antagonize anti-epileptic drugs. Chloroquine and mefloquine may increase digoxin levels and toxicity.
• **Proguanil** This may increase the effects of warfarin.
• **"Maloprim"** This may lead to folic acid deficiency when taken with trimethoprim or co-trimoxazole.

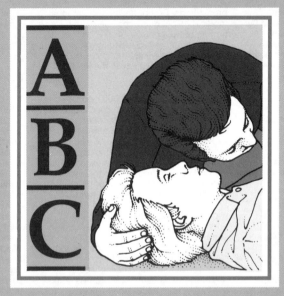

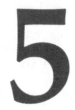

5

GLOSSARY
AND INDEX

FURTHER INFORMATION
GLOSSARY
GENERAL INDEX
DRUG POISONING EMERGENCY GUIDE

FURTHER INFORMATION

It is important to have as much information as possible about any medicines that you, or someone that you are caring for, are taking. All medicines, whether prescribed or bought over-the-counter should come with a patient information leaflet. Always read these leaflets. If you are still in doubt about anything to do with a medicine, you should ask your doctor or pharmacist.

Organizations should be able to provide general information on medicines. Some of these societies are listed below. Further information is usually also available from your local hospital, as well as social services and local libraries. If you have access to the Internet you will also be able to find hundreds of websites that offer information.

Although much of the available advice on medicines and drugs is useful and reliable, some information may sometimes be misleading, oversimplified, or even wrong. Always be careful of following advice that does not appear to be from a qualified source, and discuss the matter with your doctor or pharmacist if you are unsure.

GENERAL INFORMATION

BBC Online Health and Fitness
Online: www.bbc.co.uk/health

British Medical Association
BMA House
Tavistock Square
London WC1H 9JP
Tel: (020) 7387 4499
E-mail: smanley@bma.org.uk
Online: www.bma.org.uk

Child Health (US)
Online: kidshealth.org/

Department of Health
Richmond House
79 Whitehall
London SW1A 2NS
Tel: (020) 7210 4850
Online: www.doh.gov.uk

Food and Drug Administration (US)
5600 Fishers Lane
Rockville
MD 20857
USA
Tel: 001 800 463 6332
E-mail: webmail@oc.fda.gov
Online: www.fda.gov

HealthAnswers (US)
Online: www.healthanswers.com

Health Education Authority
Trevelyan House
30 Great Peter Street
London SW1P 2HW
Tel: (020) 7222 5300
Online: www.hea.org.uk

Medicines Control Agency
Market Towers
1 Nine Elms Lane
London SW8 5NQ
Tel: (020) 7273 0000
E-mail: info@mca.gov.uk
Online: www.open.gov.uk/mca

National Pharmaceutical Association
Mallinson House
38–42 St Peter's Street
St Albans
Herts AL1 3NP
Tel: (01727) 832161
Fax: (01727) 840858
E-mail: npa@npa.co.uk
Online: npa.co.uk

NHS Direct Online
Online: www.nhsdirect.nhs.uk

Patient UK
E-mail: info@patient.co.uk
Online: www.patient.org.uk

Pharm Web
School of Pharmacy and
   Pharmaceutical Services
University of Manchester
Manchester M13 9PL
Tel/Fax: (0161) 275 2333
Online: www.pharmweb.net

Royal College of General Practitioners
14 Princes Gate
Hyde Park
London SW7 1PU
Tel: (020) 7581 3232
E-mail: info@rcgp.org.uk
Online: www.rcgp.org.uk

Royal Pharmaceutical Society of Great Britain
1 Lambeth High Street
London SE1 7JN
Tel: (020) 7735 9141
Fax: (020) 7735 7629
E-mail: enquiries@rpsgb.org.uk
Online: www.rpsgb.org.uk

World Health Organization
Avenue Appia 20
1211 Geneva 27
Switzerland
Tel: 0041 22 791 2111
E-mail: info@who.ch
Online: www.who.int

DRUG DEPENDENCE

Addiction Recovery Foundation
122A Wilton Road
London SW1V 1JZ
Tel: (020) 7233 5333
E-mail: acw@easynet.co.uk
Online: easyweb.easynet.co.uk/~acw

Alcoholics Anonymous
PO Box 1
Stonebow House
York Y01 7NJ
Tel: (01904) 644 026
Online: www.alcoholics-anonymous.org.uk

The Centre for Recovery
1 North Parade
Aberystwyth
Ceredigion
SY23 2JH
Tel/Fax: (01970) 626470
E-mail: office@recovery.org.uk
Online: www.recovery.org.uk

European Association for the Treatment of Addiction
PO Box 1381
Rugby
Warwickshire CV21 1ZF
Tel: (01788) 536389
Fax: (01788) 550152
E-mail: secretariat@eata.org.uk
Online: www.box-1.freeserve.co.uk

Institute for the Study of Drug Dependence
Waterbridge House
32–36 Loman Street
London SE1 0EE
Tel: (020) 7928 1211
Fax: (020) 7928 1771
E-mail: services@isdd.co.uk
Online: www.isdd.co.uk

Narcotics Anonymous
Helpline: (020) 7730 0009
Online: www.na.org

DRUG REACTIONS

British Allergy Foundation
30 Bellegrove Road
Welling
Kent DA16 3PY
Helpline: (0189) 516500
Tel: (020) 8303 8525
Online: www.allergyfoundation.com

Medic Alert Foundation
1 Bridge Wharf
156 Caledonian Road
London N1 9UU
Tel: (020) 7833 3034
Online: www.medicalert.co.uk

SPECIFIC CONDITIONS

Arthritis Research Campaign
Copeman House
St Mary's Court
St Mary's Gate
Chesterfield
Derbyshire S41 7TD
Tel: (01246) 558033
E-mail: info@arc.org.uk
Online: www.arc.org.uk

British Brain and Spine Foundation
7 Winchester House
Kennington Park
Cranmer Road
London SW9 6EJ
Helpline: (0800) 328 5758
Tel: (020) 7793 5900
E-mail: info@bbsf.org.uk
Online: www.bbsf.org.uk

British Heart Foundation
14 Fitzhardinge Street
London W1H 4DH
Heartline: (0990) 200656
Tel: (020) 7935 0185
Online: www.bhf.org.uk

British Lung Foundation
78 Hatton Garden
London EC1N 8LD
Tel: (020) 7831 5831
E-mail: blf_user@gpiag-asthma.org
Online: www.lunguk.org

British Red Cross Society
9 Grosvenor Crescent
London SW1X 7EJ
Tel: (020) 7235 5454
Online: www.redcross.org.uk

Cancer Research Campaign
10 Cambridge Terrace
London NW1 4JL
Tel: (020) 7224 1333
E-mail: crcinformation@crc.org.uk
Online: www.crc.org.uk

The Digestive Disorders Foundation
3 St Andrews Place
London NW1 4LB
Tel: (020) 7486 0341
E-mail: ddf@digestivedisorders.org.uk
Online: www.digestivedisorders.org.uk

The Mental Health Foundation
UK Office
20/21 Cornwall Terrace
London NW1 4QL
Tel: (020) 7535 7400
E-mail: mhf@mentalhealth.org.uk
Online: www.mentalhealth.org.uk

Pain Relief Foundation
Rice Lane
Liverpool L9 1AE
Tel: (0151) 523 1486
Online: www.liv.ac.uk/pri

Royal National Institute for Deaf People
PO Box 16464
London EC1Y 8TT
Helpline: 0870 605 0123
Textphone: 0870 603 3007
E-mail: helpline@rnid.org.uk
Online: www.rnid.org.uk

Royal National Institute for the Blind
224 Great Portland Street
London W1N 6AA
Helpline: 0845 766 9999
Tel: (020) 7388 1266
Textphone: 0800 515152
Online: www.rnib.org.uk

ALTERNATIVE MEDICINE

British Herbal Medicine Association
PO Box 304
Bournemouth
Dorset BH7 6JZ
Tel: (01202) 433691
Online: www.ex.ac.uk/phytonet/bhma.html

The Institute of Chinese Medicine
44/46 Chandos Place
London WC2N 4HS
Tel: (020) 7836 5220
E-mail: icm@drtmli.netkonect.co.uk

The UK Homeopathic Medical Association
6 Livingstone Road
Gravesend
Kent DA12 5DZ
Tel: (01474) 560336
E-mail: info@the-hmg.org
Online: www.the-hma.org

DRUGS IN SPORT

British Olympic Association
1 Wandsworth Plain
London SW18 1EH
Tel: (020) 8871 2677
Online: www.olympics.org.uk

UK Sport
Walkden House
10 Melton Street
London NW1 2EB
Tel: (020) 7380 8000
Fax: (020) 7380 8005
E-mail: info@uksport.gov.uk
Online: www.uksport.gov.uk

MEDICINES AND TRAVEL

British Airways Travel Clinics
Tel: (01276) 685040
Online: www.british-airways.com/
travelqa/fyi/health/health.shtml

Centers for Disease Control and Prevention (US)
1600 Clifton Road NE
Atlanta
GA 30333
USA
Tel: 001 404 639 3534
E-mail: netinfo@cdc.org
Online: www.cdc.gov/travel

Department of Health: Health Advice for Travellers
Online: www.doh.gov.uk/hat

Foreign and Commonwealth Office Travel Advice Unit
1 Palace Street
London SW1E 5HE
Tel: (020) 7238 4503/4504
Fax: (020) 7238 4545
Online: www.fco.gov.uk/travel

London School of Hygiene and Tropical Medicine
Keppel Street
London WC1E 7HT
Tel: (020) 7636 8636
Fax: (020) 7436 5389
Online: www.lshtm.ac.uk

MASTA (Medical Advisory Services for Travellers Abroad)
Tel: (020) 7631 4408
Online: www.masta.org

Tropical Medical Bureau
5 Northumberland Avenue
Dun Laoghaire
Co. Dublin
Ireland
Tel: 003 531 280 4996
Online: www.tmb.ie

GLOSSARY

The following pages contain definitions of drug-related terms whose technical meanings are not explained in detail elsewhere in the book, or for which an easily located precise explanation may be helpful. These are words that may not be familiar to the general reader, or that have a slightly different meaning in a medical context from that in ordinary use. Some of the terms included refer to particular drug actions or effects; others describe methods of drug administration. A few medical conditions that may occur as a result of drug use are also defined. All words printed in *italics* in the main text are included as entries in this glossary.

The glossary is arranged in alphabetical order. To avoid repetition, where relevant, entries include cross-references to further information on that topic located in other sections of the book, or to another glossary term.

A

Activator
See *Agonist*.

Addiction
A term referring to compulsive use of a drug that can cover anything from intense, habitual cravings for caffeine (the drug in coffee and tea) to physical and psychological dependence on drugs such as nicotine (in tobacco) and *opioids*. See also *Dependence* and Drug dependence (p.23).

Adjuvant
A drug or chemical that enhances the therapeutic effect of another drug. An example is aluminium, which is added to certain vaccines to enhance the immune response, thereby increasing the protection that is given by the vaccine.

Adrenergic
See *Sympathomimetic*.

Adverse effect
Like side effect and adverse reaction, this is a term that refers to unwanted effects of a drug. When drugs are taken, they are distributed throughout the body and their actions are unlikely to be restricted to just the intended organ or tissue. Other parts of the body contain *receptors* like those at which the drug is aimed. The drug molecule may fit other, different, receptors well enough to affect them too. Most unwanted effects are dose-related, increasing as the dose is increased. Other unwanted adverse effects appear not to be dose-related, such as an *idiosyncrasy* or an *allergic reaction*. See also Adverse effects (p.15).

Adverse reaction
See *Adverse effect*.

Agonist
A term meaning to have a stimulating effect. An agonist drug (often called an activator) is one that binds to a *receptor* and triggers or increases a particular activity in that cell.

Allergic reaction
An allergic reaction or allergy is one that appears not on first exposure to a drug but on a subsequent occasion. The causes and symptoms are similar to a reaction caused by other allergens. See also Allergy (p.123) and *Anaphylaxis*.

Amoebicide
A drug that kills amoebae (single-celled microorganisms). See also Antiprotozoal drugs (p.136).

Anaemia
A condition in which the concentration of haemoglobin, the oxygen-carrying pigment of the blood, is below normal. Many different disorders may cause anaemia, and it may sometimes occur as a result of drug treatment. Severe anaemia may cause pallor, fatigue, and, occasionally, breathing difficulty.

Anaesthetic, general
A drug or drug combination given to produce unconsciousness before and during surgery or potentially painful investigative procedures. General anaesthesia is usually induced initially by injection of a drug such as thiopental, and maintained by inhalation of the fumes of a volatile liquid such as halothane or a gas such as nitrous oxide mixed with oxygen. See also *Premedication*.

Anaesthetic, local
A drug applied topically or injected to numb sensation in a small area. See also Local anaesthetics (p.80).

Analeptic
A drug given in hospital to stimulate breathing. See also Respiratory stimulants (p.88).

Analgesia
Relief of pain, usually by drugs. See also Analgesics (p.80).

Anaphylaxis
A severe reaction to an allergen such as a bee sting or a drug (see Allergy, p.123). Symptoms may include rash, swelling, breathing difficulty, and collapse. See also Anaphylactic shock (p.496).

Antagonist
A term meaning to have an opposing effect. An antagonist drug (often called a blocker) binds to a *receptor* without stimulating cell activity and prevents any other substance from occupying that receptor.

Antibiotic
A substance that kills particular bacteria or fungi. Originally, antibiotics were produced by microorganisms such as moulds, but most are now produced synthetically. See also Antibiotics (p.128), Antifungal drugs (p.138), and Antibacterial drugs (p.131).

Antibody
A protein manufactured by lymphocytes (a type of white blood cell) to neutralize an antigen (foreign protein) in the body. The formation of antibodies against an invading microorganism is part of the body's defence against infection. *Immunization* carried out to increase the body's resistance to a specific disease involves either injection of specific antibodies or administration of a *vaccine* that stimulates antibody production. See also Vaccines and immunization (p.134).

Anticholinergic
A drug that blocks the action of acetylcholine. Acetylcholine, a neurotransmitter secreted by the endings of nerve cells, allows certain nerve impulses to be transmitted, including those that relax some involuntary muscles, tighten others, and affect the release of saliva. Anticholinergic drugs are used to treat urinary incontinence because they relax the bladder's squeezing muscles while tightening those of the sphincter. Anticholinergic drugs also relax the muscles of the intestinal wall, helping to relieve irritable bowel syndrome (p.110). See also Autonomic nervous system (p.79).

Antidote
A substance used to neutralize or counteract the effects of a poison. Very few poisons have a specific antidote.

Antineoplastic
An anticancer drug (p.154).

Antioxidant
A substance that delays deterioration due to free radicals (unstable oxygen atoms). Free radicals are generated by the body's normal processes and are thought to play a role in aging and disease. Vitamins A, C, and E are antioxidants. See also Vitamins (p.149)

Antiperspirant
A substance applied to the skin to reduce excess sweating. Antiperspirants reduce the activity of the sweat glands or block ducts carrying sweat to the skin surface.

Antipyretic
A type of drug that reduces fever. The most commonly used antipyretic drugs are aspirin and paracetamol.

Antiseptic
A chemical that destroys bacteria and sometimes other microorganisms.

Antiseptics may be applied to the skin or other areas to prevent infection. See also Anti-infective skin preparations (p.175).

Antispasmodic
A type of drug that reduces spasm (abnormally strong or inappropriate contraction) of the digestive-tract muscles. The pain caused by intestinal spasm is known as colic. These drugs may be used to relieve irritable bowel syndrome (p.110).

Antitussive
A drug that prevents or relieves a cough. See also Drugs to treat coughs (p.94).

Aperient
A mild laxative. See also Laxatives (p.111).

Astringent
A substance that causes tissue to dry and shrink by reducing its ability to absorb water. Astringents are used in a number of antiperspirants and skin tonics to remove excessive moisture from the skin surface. They are also used in ear drops for inflammation of the outer ear because they promote healing of inflamed tissue.

B

Bactericidal
A term used to describe a drug that kills bacteria. See also Antibiotics (p.128) and Antibacterials (p.131).

Bacteriostatic
A term used to describe a drug that stops the growth or multiplication of bacteria. See also Antibiotics (p.128) and Antibacterials (p.131).

Balm
A soothing or healing preparation applied to the skin.

Bioavailability
The proportion of a dose of a drug that enters the bloodstream and so reaches the body tissues, usually expressed as a percentage of the dose given. Injection of a drug directly into a vein produces 100 per cent bioavailability. Drugs given by mouth generally have a lower bioavailability because some of the drug may not pass through the gut wall, and some may be broken down in the liver before reaching the rest of the body.

Bladder instillation/irrigation
A term used to describe the placement of *sterile* liquids inside the bladder via a catheter. Bladder instillations may be held inside the bladder for a short time to treat the bladder wall; this is in effect a *topical* application. Bladder irrigations are run into the bladder and allowed to run out again in order to wash the bladder walls and urethra.

Blocker
See *Antagonist*.

Body salts
Also known as electrolytes, these are minerals that are present in body fluids such as blood, urine, and sweat, and within cells. These salts play an important role in regulating water balance, acidity of the blood, conduction of nerve impulses, and muscle contraction. The balance between the salts can be upset by such conditions as diarrhoea and vomiting. The balance may also be altered by the action of drugs such as diuretics (p.99).

Brand name
The name chosen by a manufacturer for its version of a product containing a generic drug. For example, Viagra is a brand name for the generic drug sildenafil. See also *Generic name* and How drugs are classified (p.13).

Bronchoconstrictor
A substance that causes the airways in the lungs to narrow. An attack of asthma may be caused by the release of bronchoconstrictor substances such as histamine or certain *prostaglandins*.

Bronchodilator
A type of drug that widens the airways. See also Bronchodilators (p.92).

C

Capsule
See p.19.

Cathartic
A type of drug that stimulates bowel action to produce a soft or liquid bowel movement. See also Laxatives (p.111).

Chelating agent
A chemical used in the treatment of poisoning by metals such as iron, lead, arsenic, and mercury. It combines with the metal to form a less poisonous substance and in some cases increases excretion in the urine. Penicillamine is a commonly used chelating agent.

Chemotherapy
The drug treatment of cancer or infections. *Cytotoxic* drugs (see also p.154) and *antibiotics* (see also p.128) are examples of drugs used in chemotherapy.

Cholinergic
A type of drug, also called *parasympathomimetic*, that acts by stimulating the parasympathetic nervous system. See also Autonomic nervous system (p.79).

Coma
A state of unconsciousness and unresponsiveness to external stimuli such as noise and pain. Coma results from damage to, or disturbance of, part of the brain, for example by trauma or drug overdose.

Contraindication
A factor in a person's current condition, medical history, or genetic make-up that may increase the risks of an *adverse effect* from a drug, to the extent that the drug should not be prescribed (called an absolute contraindication), or should only be prescribed with great caution (called a relative contraindication).

Counter-irritant
Another term for *rubefacient*.

Cycloplegic
The action of paralysing the ciliary muscle in the eye. This muscle alters the shape of the lens when it contracts, enabling the eye to focus on objects. A cycloplegic drug prevents this action, thereby making both examination of, and surgery on, the eye easier. See also Drugs affecting the pupil (p.170).

Cytotoxic
A drug that kills or damages cells. Drugs with this action are most commonly used to treat cancer. Although these drugs are primarily intended to affect abnormal cells, they may also kill or damage healthy ones. See also Anticancer drugs (p.154).

D

Dependence
A term that relates to psychological or physical dependence on a substance, or both. Psychological dependence involves intense mental cravings if a drug is unavailable or withdrawn. Physical dependence causes physical withdrawal symptoms (sweating, shaking, abdominal pain, and convulsions) if the substance is not taken. Dependence also implies loss of control over intake. See also Drug dependence (p.23).

Depot injection
Injection into a muscle of a drug that has been specially formulated to provide for a slow, steady absorption of its active ingredients by the surrounding blood vessels. The drug may be mixed with oil or wax. Alternatively, some drugs may be injected under the skin using an applicator. This is known as an implant injection. The release period can be made to last up to several weeks for both methods. See also Methods of administration (p.17).

Designer drugs
A group of unlicensed substances whose only purpose is to duplicate the effects of certain illegal drugs of abuse or to provide even stronger ones. Designer drugs differ chemically in some minor degree from the original drug, enabling the user and supplier to evade prosecution for dealing in, or possession of, an illegal drug. They are very dangerous because their effects are unpredictable, they are often highly potent, and they may contain impurities.

Double-blind
A test used to determine the effectiveness of a new drug compared to an existing medicine or a *placebo*. Neither the patients nor the doctors administering the drug know who is receiving which substance. Only after the test is completed and the patients' responses are recorded is the identity of those who received the new drug revealed. Double-blind trials are performed for all new drugs. See also Testing and approving new drugs (p.12).

Drip
A non-medical term for *intravenous infusion*.

E

Electrolyte
See *Body salts*.

Elixir
A clear, sweetened liquid, often containing alcohol, which forms the base for many liquid medicines such as those used to treat coughs.

Embrocation
An ointment or liniment rubbed on to the skin to relieve joint pain, muscle cramp, or muscle injury. An embrocation usually contains a *rubefacient*.

Emetic
Any substance that causes a person to vomit. An emetic may work by irritating the lining of the stomach and/or by stimulating the part of the brain that controls vomiting. Emetics such as ipecac (ipecacuanha) may be used in the treatment of drug overdose but are not generally very effective. See also Drug poisoning emergency guide (p.494).

Emollient
A substance having a soothing, softening effect when applied to the skin. An emollient also has a moisturizing effect, preventing loss of water from the skin surface by forming an oily film. See also Bases for skin preparations (p.175).

Emulsion
A combination of two liquids that do not normally mix together but, on the addition of a third substance (known as an emulsifying agent), can be mixed to give a complex liquid consisting of droplets of one liquid suspended in the other. An example of an emulsion is liquid paraffin. The medicine bottle may have to be shaken each time before use to ensure that the two liquids are thoroughly mixed.

Endorphins
A group of substances occurring naturally in the brain. Released in response to pain, they bind to specialized receptors and reduce the perception of pain. *Opioid* analgesics such as morphine work by mimicking the action of endorphins. See also Analgesics (p.80).

Enteric coated
Treatment of a drug to give it a coating so that, after being taken orally, it passes safely and unaltered through the stomach and affects the intestine.

Enzyme
A protein that controls the rate of one or more chemical reactions in the body. There are thousands of enzymes active in the body. Each type of cell produces a specific range of enzymes. Cells in the liver contain enzymes that stimulate the breakdown of nutrients and drugs; cells in the digestive tract release enzymes that help digest food. Some drugs work by altering the activity of enzymes – for example, certain anticancer drugs halt tumour growth by altering enzyme function in cancer cells.

Excitatory
A term that means having a stimulating or enhancing effect. A chemical released from a nerve ending that causes muscle contraction is having an excitatory effect. See also *Inhibitory*.

Expectorant
A type of cough remedy that enhances the production of sputum (phlegm) and is used in the treatment of a productive (sputum-producing) cough. See also Drugs to treat coughs (p.94).

F

Formula, chemical
A way of expressing the constituents of a chemical in the form of symbols and numbers. Every chemical substance has a formula. Water has the formula H_2O, indicating that it is composed of two hydrogen atoms (H_2) and one oxygen atom (O). All drugs have much more complicated formulas than that of water.

Formulary
A list of drugs produced as a guide to prescribers and other health professionals with the intention of aiding choice. Local formularies are frequently found in hospitals and sometimes used by groups of GPs. The British National Formulary is jointly produced by the British Medical Association and the Royal Pharmaceutical Society as a non-promotional guide to what is available and considered worth prescribing for most common conditions.

G

Generic name
The official name for a substance that is therapeutically active. The term generic is distinct from a *brand name*, which is a term chosen by a manufacturer for its version of a product containing a generic drug. For example: diazepam is a generic name;

Valium is a brand name for a product that contains diazepam. See also How drugs are classified (p.13).

GSL (General Sales List) medicines
Over-the-counter medicines considered suitable for sale by any retail outlet because of their safety record. Examples include aspirin and paracetamol. See also Managing your drug treatment (p.25).

H

Half-life
A term used in *pharmacology* for the time taken to reduce the concentration of the drug in the blood by half. Knowledge of the half-life of a drug helps to determine frequency of dosage.

Hallucinogen
A drug that causes hallucinations (unreal perceptions of surroundings and objects). Common hallucinogens include the drugs of abuse LSD and cannabis (p.454). Alcohol taken in large amounts may have an hallucinogenic effect; hallucinations may also occur during withdrawal from alcohol (p.451). Certain prescribed drugs may in rare cases cause hallucinations.

Hormone
A chemical released directly into the bloodstream by a gland or tissue. The body produces numerous hormones, each of which has a specific range of functions – for example, controlling the *metabolism* of cells, growth, sexual development, and the body's response to stress or illness. Hormone-producing glands make up the endocrine system; the kidneys, intestine, and brain also release hormones. See also Hormones and endocrine system (p.140).

I

Idiosyncrasy
Some *adverse effects* appear not to be dose related. Where such an effect happens on the first use of a drug and is unexpected, the phenomenon is called idiosyncrasy, or an idiosyncratic reaction. This happens because people are different genetically; they may lack a particular enzyme or an enzyme may be less active than usual. Because of this difference they may react differently when they take a drug.

Immunization
The process of inducing immunity (resistance to infection) as a preventive measure against the spread of infectious diseases. See also Vaccines and immunization (p.134).

Indication
The term used to describe a disorder, symptom, or condition for which a drug or treatment may be prescribed. For example,

indications for the use of beta blockers include angina and high blood pressure (hypertension).

Infusion pump
A machine for administering a continuous, controlled amount of a drug or other fluid through a needle that is inserted into a vein or under the skin. It consists of a small battery-powered pump that controls the flow of fluid from a syringe into the needle. The pump may be strapped to the patient and pre-programmed to deliver the fluid at a constant rate. See also Methods of administration (p.17).

Inhaler
A device for administering a drug in powder or vapour form. Inhalers are used principally in the treatment of respiratory disorders such as asthma and chronic bronchitis. The kinds of drugs that are often administered by this method include corticosteroids and bronchodilators. See also Methods of administration (p.17) and Inhalers (p.92).

Inhibitory
A term meaning to have a blocking effect on cell activity, e.g., a chemical that prevents muscle contraction has an inhibitory effect. See also *Antagonist* and *Excitatory*.

Inoculation
A method of administering biological substances, such as microorganisms, to produce immunity to disease by scratching the *vaccine* into the skin. See also Vaccines and immunization (p.134).

Interaction
See p.16.

Intramuscular injection
Injection of a drug into a muscle, usually located in the upper arm or buttock. The drug is absorbed into the bloodstream from the muscle. See also Methods of administration (p.17).

Intravenous infusion
Prolonged, slow injection of fluid (often a drug solution) into a vein. The fluid flows at a controlled rate from a bag or bottle through a fine tube inserted into an opening in a vein. An intravenous infusion may also be administered via an *infusion pump*.

Intravenous injection
Direct injection of a drug into a vein, putting the drug immediately into the circulation. Because it has a rapid effect, intravenous injection is useful in an emergency. See also Methods of administration (p.17).

JL

Jaundice
A condition in which the skin and whites of the eyes take on a yellow coloration. It can be caused by an accumulation in the blood of the yellow-brown bile pigment bilirubin. Jaundice is a sign of many disorders of the liver. A drug may cause jaundice as an *adverse effect* either by damaging the liver or by causing an increase in the breakdown of red blood cells in the circulation. See also Liver and kidney disease, p.22.

Liniment
A liquid medicine for application to the skin with friction, that is, to be rubbed in. See also *Embrocation*.

Lotion
A liquid preparation that may be applied to large areas of skin. See also Bases for skin preparations (p.175).

M

Medication
Any substance prescribed to treat illness. See also *Medicine*.

Medicine
A medication or drug that is taken in order to maintain, improve, or restore health.

Metabolism
The term used to describe all chemical processes in the body that involve either the formation of new substances or the breakdown of substances to release energy or detoxify foreign substances. The metabolism provides the energy that is required to keep the body functioning at rest – that is, to maintain breathing, heart beat, and body temperature and to replace worn tissues. It also provides the energy needed during exertion. This energy is produced by metabolism from the breakdown of foods.

Miotic
A drug that constricts (narrows) the pupil. *Opioid* drugs such as morphine have a miotic effect, and someone who is taking one of these drugs has very small, pinpoint pupils. The pupil is sometimes deliberately narrowed by other miotic drugs, such as pilocarpine, in the treatment of glaucoma. See also Drugs for glaucoma (p.168) and Drugs affecting the pupil (p.170).

Mucolytic
A drug that liquefies mucus secretions (phlegm) in the airways, making them less sticky and easier to cough up. See also Drugs to treat coughs (p.94).

Mydriatic
A drug that dilates (widens) the pupil. *Anticholinergic* drugs, such as atropine, have this effect and they may cause *photophobia* as a consequence. Mydriatic drugs may occasionally provoke the onset of glaucoma. These drugs are also used to facilitate examination of the retina (at the back of the eye). See also Drugs affecting the pupil (p.170).

N

Narcotic
Originating from the Greek word for numbness or stupor and, once applied to drugs derived from the opium poppy, the word narcotic no longer has a precise medical meaning; some American sources use the term to mean any potent abused drug. Narcotic analgesic, a term largely replaced by *opioid* analgesic, is used to refer to opium-derived and synthetic drugs that have pain-relieving properties and other effects similar to those of morphine (see Analgesics, p.80). See also Opioids (p.458).

Nebulizer
A method of administering a drug to the airways and lungs in aerosol form through a facemask. The apparatus includes an electric or hand-operated pump that sends a stream of air or oxygen through a length of tubing into a small canister containing the drug in liquid form. This inflow of gas causes the drug to be dispersed into a fine mist, which is then carried through another tube into the facemask. Inhalation of this drug mist is much easier than inhaling from a pressurized aerosol. See also *Inhaler*.

Neuroleptic
A drug used to treat psychotic illness. See also Antipsychotic drugs (p.85).

Neurotransmitter
A chemical released from a nerve ending after receiving an electrical impulse. A neurotransmitter may carry a message from the nerve to another nerve so that the electrical impulse passes on, or to a muscle to stimulate contraction, or to a gland to stimulate secretion of a particular hormone. Acetylcholine and noradrenaline are examples of neurotransmitters. Many drugs either mimic or block the action of neurotransmitters. See also Brain and nervous system (p.78).

O

Opioid
A group of drugs (also known as *narcotic analgesics*) that are given to relieve pain, treat diarrhoea, and suppress coughs. See also Opioids (p.458).

Orphan drug
A drug that is effective for a rare medical condition, but that may not be marketed by a drug manufacturer because of the small profit potential compared with the high costs of development and production.

OTC
The abbreviation for over-the-counter. Over-the-counter drugs can be bought from a pharmacy without a prescription. See also GSL, *P medicines*, *POM*, and Managing your drug treatment (p.25)

P

Parasympathomimetic
A drug that is prescribed to stimulate the parasympathetic nervous system (see Autonomic nervous system, p.79). These drugs (also called *cholinergics*) are used as *miotics* and to stimulate bladder contraction in urinary retention. See also Drugs used in urinary disorders (p.166).

Parkinsonism
Neurological symptoms, including tremor of the hands, muscle rigidity, and slowness of movement, that resemble Parkinson's disease. Parkinsonism may be caused by prolonged treatment with an antipsychotic drug. See also Drugs for parkinsonism (p.87).

Patch
See *Transdermal patch*.

Pharmacist
A registered health professional (often called a "chemist") concerned with the development, preparation, manufacture, and dispensing of drugs. Pharmacists can advise on the correct use of drugs.

Pharmacodynamics
A word used to describe the effects or actions that a drug produces in the body. For example, bronchodilation and pain relief are some pharmacodynamic effects that may stem from a drug.

Pharmacokinetics
The term used to describe how the body deals with a drug, including how the drug is absorbed into the bloodstream, distributed to different tissues, broken down, and excreted from the body.

Pharmacologist
A scientist concerned with the study of the actions and *pharmacokinetics* of drugs. Pharmacologists form one of the groups responsible for scientific research into new drugs and new uses for existing drugs. Clinical pharmacologists are usually qualified doctors.

Pharmacology
The science of the origin, appearance, chemistry, action, and use of drugs.

Pharmacopoeia
A publication (in book or electronic form) that describes drugs used in medicine. The term pharmacopoeia usually refers to an official publication (such as the British Pharmacopoeia) that sets standards and describes the methods used to identify drugs and determine their purity. These publications are used for reference by the medical profession.

Pharmacy
A term that is used to describe the science and technology involved in the study of drugs. The term is also used to refer to the place where the practice of preparing drugs, making up prescriptions, and dispensing the drugs is carried out.

Photophobia
Dislike of bright light. Certain drugs (notably *mydriatics*) and diseases may induce photophobia.

Photosensitivity
An abnormal reaction of the skin to light, often causing reddening. Photosensitivity may be caused by certain drugs.

Placebo
A "medicine", often in tablet or capsule form, that contains no medically active ingredient. Placebos are frequently used in clinical trials of new drugs (see *Double-blind*). A doctor may sometimes prescribe a placebo because of the emotional or psychological uplift it may give to a patient convinced that his or her condition calls for drug treatment. See also Placebo response (p.15).

P medicines
These are over-the-counter drugs that may only be sold in a *pharmacy*. Most drugs that are not *POMs* are P (pharmacy) medicines. See also Managing your drug treatment (p.25).

Poison
A substance that, in relatively small amounts, disrupts the structure and/or function of cells, causing harmful and sometimes fatal effects. Many drugs are poisonous if taken in overdose.

POM
An abbreviation for Prescription Only Medicine. These drugs cannot be bought without a prescription from a doctor or dentist. See also Prescription drugs (p.26)

Premedication
The term applied to drugs given to patients to prepare them for surgery between one and two hours before an operation. The premedication usually contains an *opioid* analgesic to help relieve pain and anxiety and to reduce the dose of anaesthetic needed to produce unconsciousness (see also *Anaesthetic, general*). In some cases, an *anticholinergic* drug is also included to reduce secretions in the airways.

Prescription
A written instruction from the doctor to the pharmacist, detailing the name of the drug to be dispensed, the dosage, how often it has to be taken, and other instructions as necessary. A prescription is written and signed by a doctor and carries the name and address of the patient for whom the drug is prescribed. The pharmacist keeps a record, often computerized, of all prescriptions dispensed to each patient. See also Managing your drug treatment (p.25).

Prophylactic
A drug, procedure, or piece of equipment used to prevent disease. The process of prevention is called prophylaxis. For example, a course of drugs taken by a traveller to prevent malarial infection is known as malaria prophylaxis.

Proprietary
A term now applied to a drug that is sold over the counter and having its name registered to a private manufacturer, i.e., a proprietor.

Prostaglandin
A fatty (organic) acid that acts in a similar way to a hormone. Prostaglandins occur in many different tissues and have various effects. These include causing inflammation in damaged tissue, lowering blood pressure, and stimulating contractions in labour.

Purgative
A drug that helps eliminate faeces from the body in order to relieve constipation or to empty the bowel/intestine before surgery. See also *Cathartic* and Laxatives (p.111).

Pyrogen
A substance that causes a rise in temperature.

R

Receptor
A specific site on the surface of a cell with a characteristic chemical and physical structure. Natural body chemicals such as *neurotransmitters* bind to cell receptors to initiate a response in the cell. Many drugs also have an effect on cells by binding to a receptor. They may promote cell activity or may block it. See also *Agonist* and *Antagonist*.

Replication
The duplication of genetic material (DNA or RNA) in a cell as part of the process of cell division that enables a tissue to grow or a virus to multiply.

Rubefacient
A preparation, also known as a counter-irritant, that, when applied to an area of skin, causes it to redden by increasing blood flow in vessels in that area. A rubefacient such as methyl salicylate may be included in an *embrocation* or a *liniment*.

S

Sedative
A drug that dampens the activity of the central nervous system. Sleeping drugs (p.82) and anti-anxiety drugs (p.83) have a sedative effect, and many other drugs, including antihistamines (p.124) and antidepressants (p.84), can produce sedation as a side effect.

Side effect
See *Adverse effect*.

Sterile
A term meaning free from living micro-organisms. Drugs that are administered by certain methods, such as injection and *bladder irrigation/instillation*, must be sterile to avoid causing infection. See also *Pyrogen*.

Subcutaneous injection
A method of giving a drug by which the drug is injected just under the skin. The drug is then slowly absorbed over a few hours into the surrounding blood vessels. Insulin is given in this way. See also Methods of administration (p.17).

Sublingual
A term meaning under the tongue. Some drugs are taken sublingually in tablet or spray form. The drug is rapidly absorbed into the bloodstream through the lining of the mouth. Nitrate drugs may be given this way to provide rapid relief of an angina attack. See also Methods of administration (p.17).

Suppository
A bullet-shaped pellet usually containing a drug for insertion into the rectum. See also Methods of administration (p.17).

Sympatholytic
A term that means blocking the effect of the sympathetic nervous system. Sympatholytic drugs work either by reducing the release of the stimulatory *neurotransmitter* norepinephrine (noradrenaline) from nerve endings, or by occupying the *receptors* to which the neurotransmitters epinephrine (adrenaline) and norepinephrine normally bind, thereby preventing their normal actions. Beta blockers are examples of sympatholytic drugs. See also Autonomic nervous system (p.79).

Sympathomimetic
Having the same effect as stimulation of the sympathetic nervous system to cause, for example, an increase in the heart rate and widening of the airways. A drug having a sympathomimetic action may work either by causing the release of the stimulatory *neurotransmitter* noradrenaline from the nerve endings or by mimicking neurotransmitter action (see Autonomic nervous system, p.79). The sympathomimetic drugs include certain bronchodilators (p.92) and decongestants (p.93).

Syrup
A solution of sucrose (sugar) in water. Syrup is used a basis for some liquid medicines because it acts as an *antioxidant*; bacteria, fungi, and moulds do not grow in it; and its sweetness hides the taste of some drugs. Syrups are not suitable for diabetics.

Systemic
Having a generalized effect, causing physical or chemical changes in tissues throughout the body. For a drug to have a systemic effect it must be absorbed into the bloodstream, usually via the digestive tract, by injection, or by rectal suppository.

T

Tablet
See p.19.

Tardive dyskinesia
Abnormal, uncontrolled movements, mainly of the face, tongue, mouth, and neck, that may be caused by prolonged treatment with antipsychotic drugs. This condition is distinct from *parkinsonism*, which may also be caused by such drugs. See also Antipsychotic drugs (p.85).

Tolerance
The need to take a higher dosage of a specific drug to maintain the same physical or mental effect. Tolerance occurs during prolonged treatment with *opioid* analgesics and benzodiazepines. See also Drug tolerance (p.23).

Tonics
A diverse group of remedies prescribed or bought over the counter for relieving vague symptoms such as malaise, lethargy, and loss of appetite, for which no obvious cause can be found. Tonics sometimes contain vitamins and minerals, but there is no scientific evidence that such ingredients have anything other than a *placebo* effect. Nevertheless, many individuals feel better after taking a tonic for a few weeks, and this does no harm.

Topical
The term used to describe the application of a drug directly to the site where it is intended that it should have its effect. Disorders of the skin, eye, outer ear, nasal passages, anus, and vagina are often treated with drugs applied topically.

Toxic reaction
Unpleasant and possibly dangerous symptoms caused by a drug, the result of an overdose. See also The effects of drugs (p.15).

Toxin
A poisonous substance such as a harmful chemical released by bacteria.

Tranquillizer, major
A drug used to treat a psychotic illness such as schizophrenia. See also Antipsychotic drugs (p.85).

Tranquillizer, minor
A sedative drug used to treat anxiety and emotional tension. See also Anti-anxiety drugs (p.83).

Transdermal patch
An adhesive patch that is impregnated with a drug and placed on the skin. The drug is slowly absorbed through the skin into the underlying blood vessels. Drugs administered in this way include nicotine, nitrates, travel sickness remedies, and oestrogens. See also Methods of administration (p.17).

V

Vaccine
A substance administered to induce active immunity against a specific infectious disease. See also Vaccines and immunization, p.134.

Vasoconstrictor
A drug that narrows blood vessels, often prescribed to reduce nasal congestion (see Decongestants, p.93). These drugs are also frequently given with injected local anaesthetics (p.80) (see also *Anaesthetic, local*). Ephedrine is a commonly prescribed vasoconstrictor.

Vasodilator
A drug that widens blood vessels. See also Vasodilators (p.98).

W

Wafer
A thin wafer that is impregnated with a drug and placed on the tongue. The wafer slowly dissolves and the drug is absorbed through the lining of the mouth into the surrounding blood vessels.

Withdrawal symptom
Any symptom caused by abrupt stopping of a drug. These symptoms occur as a result of physical *dependence* on a drug. Drugs that may cause withdrawal symptoms after prolonged use include *opioids*, benzodiazepines, and nicotine. Withdrawal symptoms vary according to each drug, but common examples include sweating, shaking, anxiety, nausea, and abdominal pain. See also Drug dependence (p.23).

THE GENERAL INDEX

This General Index contains references to the information in all sections of the book. It can be used to look up topics such as groups of drugs, diseases, and conditions. References for generic and brand-name drugs are also listed, with references to either the appropriate drug profile or the listing in the Drug Finder (pp.48–75). For brand-name drugs that are pictured in the Colour Identification Guide (pp.34–47), there is also an italicized reference to the page number and grid letter where the photograph will be found. Entries that contain a page reference followed by the letter "g" indicate that the entry is defined in the Glossary on the page specified (pp.470–475).

DRUG POISONING EMERGENCY GUIDE

The information on the following pages is intended to give practical advice for dealing with a known or suspected drug poisoning emergency. Although many of the first-aid techniques described can be used in a number of different types of emergency, these instructions apply specifically to drug overdose or poisoning.

Emergency action is necessary in any of the following circumstances:

● If a person has taken an overdose of any of the high-danger drugs listed in the box on p.496.
● If a person has taken an overdose of a less dangerous drug, but has one or more of the danger symptoms listed (right).
● If a person has taken, or is suspected of having taken, an overdose of an unknown drug.
● If an infant or child has swallowed, or is suspected of having swallowed any medicines or any drug of abuse.

What to do

If you are faced with a drug poisoning emergency, it is important to carry out first aid and arrange immediate medical help in the correct order. The Priority Action Decision Chart (below left) will help you to assess the situation and to determine your priorities. The following information should help you to remain calm in an emergency if you ever need to deal with a case of drug poisoning.

DANGER SYMPTOMS

Take emergency action if the person has one or more of the following symptoms:
● Drowsiness or unconsciousness
● Shallow, irregular, or stopped breathing
● Vomiting
● Fits or convulsions

PRIORITY ACTION DECISION CHART

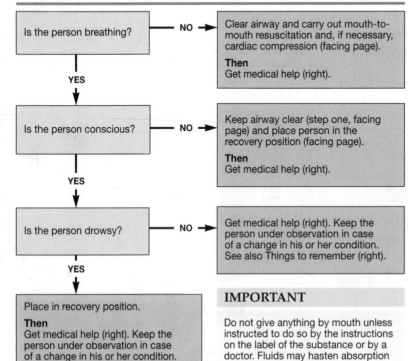

Is the person breathing? — **NO** → Clear airway and carry out mouth-to-mouth resuscitation and, if necessary, cardiac compression (facing page).
Then
Get medical help (right).

YES

Is the person conscious? — **NO** → Keep airway clear (step one, facing page) and place person in the recovery position (facing page).
Then
Get medical help (right).

YES

Is the person drowsy? — **NO** → Get medical help (right). Keep the person under observation in case of a change in his or her condition. See also Things to remember (right).

YES

Place in recovery position.
Then
Get medical help (right). Keep the person under observation in case of a change in his or her condition. See also Things to remember (right).

IMPORTANT

Do not give anything by mouth unless instructed to do so by the instructions on the label of the substance or by a doctor. Fluids may hasten absorption of the drug, increasing the danger.

GETTING MEDICAL HELP

In an emergency, a calm person who is competent in first aid should stay with the victim, while others summon help. However, if you have to deal with a drug poisoning emergency on your own, use first aid (see the Priority Action Decision Chart, left) before getting help.

Calling an ambulance may be the quickest method of transport to hospital. Then call your doctor or a hospital accident and emergency department for advice. If possible, tell them what drug has been taken and how much, and the age of the victim. Follow the doctor's or hospital's instructions precisely.

THINGS TO REMEMBER

Effective treatment of drug poisoning depends on the doctor making a rapid assessment of the type and amount of drug taken. Collecting evidence that will assist the diagnosis will help. After you have carried out first aid, look for empty or opened medicine (or other) containers. Keep any of the drug that is left, together with its container (or syringe), and give these to the nurse or doctor. Save any vomit for analysis by the hospital.

ESSENTIAL FIRST AID

AIRWAY CLEARANCE AND MOUTH-TO-MOUTH RESUSCITATION

When there is no rise and fall of the chest and you can feel no movement of exhaled air, open the airway and immediately start mouth-to-mouth resuscitation.

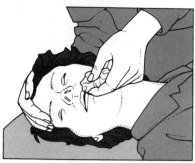

1 Lay the victim on his or her back on a firm surface. Wipe any vomit from around the mouth and clear the mouth of any obvious obstruction that might block the airway.

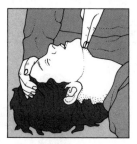

2 To open the airway, place two fingers under the point of the victim's chin and lift his or her jaw. At the same time, place your other hand on the victim's forehead and gently tilt the head well back.

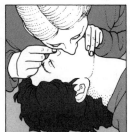

3 Pinch the victim's nostrils closed with the hand that is placed on the forehead. Take a deep breath, seal your mouth over that of the victim, and give a breath twice in quick succession. Check the pulse or for other signs of life (see Checking pulse, below). If signs are present, continue by giving one full breath every 5 seconds.

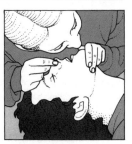

4 After each breath, turn to watch the chest falling while you listen for the sound of air leaving the victim's mouth. Continue until the victim starts to breathe regularly on his or her own, or until medical help arrives.

CARDIAC COMPRESSION

This technique is used in conjunction with mouth-to-mouth resuscitation to continue output of blood from a stopped heart. It does not usually restart a heart that has stopped. It should normally be done only by someone who has received training.

Cardiac compression involves putting repeated, strong pressure on the centre of the chest with the heels of both hands, at a rate of 80 compressions per minute for adult victims (right). After each set of 15 compressions, two breaths should be given using mouth-to-mouth resuscitation

(above). This sequence should be continued until breathing restarts.

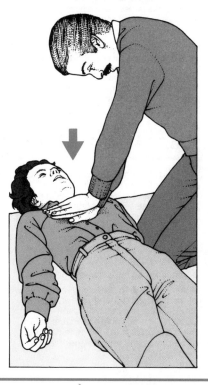

CHECKING PULSE

If the victim does not start breathing after you give two breaths of mouth-to-mouth resuscitation, check the pulse in the neck and check for other signs of life. If there is none present, start cardiac compression if you have been trained in this technique.

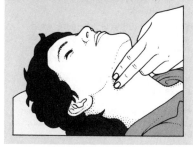

THE RECOVERY POSITION

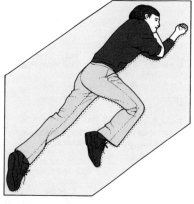

The recovery position is the safest position for an unconscious or drowsy person. It allows the person to breathe easily and will help to prevent choking if vomiting occurs. A drug poisoning victim should be placed in the recovery position if more urgent first aid, such as mouth-to-mouth resuscitation, is not necessary and when shock (p.496) is not suspected. Place the victim on his or her front with one leg bent. Turn the head to the side, tilt it back to keep the airway open, and support it in this position by placing the victim's hand under the cheek. Cover him or her with a blanket for warmth.

DEALING WITH A FIT

Certain types of drug poisoning may provoke fits. These may occur whether the person is conscious or not. The victim usually falls to the ground twitching or making uncontrolled movements of the limbs and body. If you witness a fit, remember the following points:

● Do not try to hold the person down.

● Loosen clothing around neck if possible.

● Do not attempt to put anything into the person's mouth.

● Try to ensure that the person does not suffer injury by keeping him or her away from dangerous objects or furniture.

● Once the fit is over, place the person in the recovery position (p.495).

HIGH-DANGER DRUGS

The following is a list of drugs given a high overdose rating in the drug profiles or included in the drugs of abuse. If you suspect that someone has taken an overdose of any of these drugs, seek immediate medical attention.

Amitriptyline
Aspirin
Atropine

Betahistine

Chloral hydrate
Chloroquine
Chlorpropamide
Clomipramine
Codeine
Colchicine
Co-proxamol

Digoxin
Dothiepin

Epinephrine
  (adrenaline)

Fenfluramine/
  dexfenfluramine

Glibenclamide
Gliclazide

Heparin

Imipramine
Insulin
Isoniazid
Isoprenaline

Lithium

Mefloquine
Metformin
Moclobemide
Morphine

Neostigmine

Orphenadrine

Paracetamol
Pethidine
Phenobarbitone

Phenylpropanol
  amine
Primidone
Procyclidine
Propranolol
Pyridostigmine

Quinine

Theophylline/
  aminophylline
Timolol
Tolbutamide

Venlafaxine

Warfarin

Drugs of abuse
Alcohol
Amphetamine
Barbiturates
Benzodiazepines
Cannabis
  (marijuana)
Cocaine
  (including crack)
Ecstasy
GHB
Ketamine
Khat
LSD
Mescaline
Nicotine
Nitrites
Opioids
  (including heroin)
Phencyclidine
Solvents

DEALING WITH ANAPHYLACTIC SHOCK

Anaphylactic shock can occur as the result of a severe allergic reaction to a drug (such as penicillin). Blood pressure drops dramatically and the airways may become narrowed. The reaction usually occurs within minutes of taking the drug. The main symptoms are:

● Extreme anxiety
● Pallor
● Tightness in the chest
● Breathing difficulty
● Rash
● Facial swelling
● Collapse

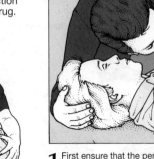

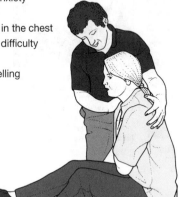

1 First ensure that the person is breathing. If breathing has stopped, immediate mouth-to-mouth resuscitation should be carried out as described on p.495.

2 If the person is conscious but having breathing difficulties, he or she is usually more comfortable sitting up. If the breathing is normal, lay him or her down, face up, with legs raised above the level of the heart to ensure the adequate circulation of the blood.

3 Phone for medical help. While waiting, cover the person with a blanket or other article of clothing. If you have to leave the person, place him or her in the recovery position. Do not attempt to administer anything by mouth.

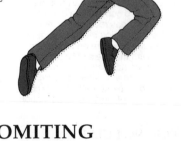

DEALING WITH VOMITING

Vomiting is the body's response to many things, including contaminated food, viral infections, and severe pain. It also occurs as an adverse effect of some drugs and as a result of drug overdose.

Do not attempt to provoke vomiting by pushing fingers down the victim's throat. When vomiting does occur, remember the following:

● Vomiting can be a sign of poisoning.

● Vomiting due to drugs is usually a result of an overdose rather than a side effect. Check in the relevant drug profile whether vomiting is a possible adverse effect of the suspected drug. If vomiting appears to be due to an overdose, get medical help urgently.

● Even if vomiting has stopped, keep the person under observation in case he or she loses consciousness or has a fit.

● If the person is unconscious and is vomiting, place him or her in the recovery position (p.495).

1 Ensure that the victim leans well forward to avoid either choking or inhaling vomit. If the victim appears to be choking, encourage coughing.

2 Keep the vomit for later analysis (see Things to remember, p.494).

3 Give water to rinse the mouth. This water should be spat out; it should not be swallowed.